School of Nursing
& Midwifery

Handbook of

THERAPEUTIC
INTERVENTIONS

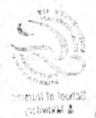

Handbook of

THERAPEUTIC INTERVENTIONS

Springhouse Corporation
Springhouse, Pennsylvania

Staff

Executive Director, Editorial
Stanley Loeb

Publisher
Barbara F. McVan

Editorial Director
Helen Klusek Hamilton

Art Director
John Hubbard

Drug Information Editor
George J. Blake, RPh, MS

Clinical Project Editor
Judith A. Schilling McCann

Clinical Editors
Roseann Barrett, Sherri Izes Becker, Paulette Dorney, Mary C. Gyetvan, Patricia Holmes, Eileen E. Jaskuta, Joan E. Mason, Candace Rehnert, Beverly Ann Tscheschlog, Eileen M. Wenkus

Copy Editors
Christina P. Ponczek, Mary T. Durkin, Kathryn A. Marino, Dorothy E. Oren

Designers
Stephanie Peters (associate art director), Maryanne Buschini (book designer), Janice Nawn, Lesley Weissman-Cook

Illustrators
Jacalyn Facciolo, Jean Gardner, Bob Jackson, Bob Neumann, Judy Newhouse

Typography
David C. Kosten (director), Diane Paluba (manager), Elizabeth Bergman, Joyce Rossi Biletz, Phyllis Marron, Robin Mayer, Valerie Rosenberger

Manufacturing
Deborah C. Meiris (manager), Kate Davis, T. A. Landis

Production Coordination
Margaret A. Rastiello

Editorial Assistants
Maree DeRosa, Beverly Lane, Mary Madden

Indexer
Barbara Hodgson

Library of Congress Cataloging-in-Publication Data
Handbook of therapeutic interventions.
   p.   cm.
  Includes index.
  1. Therapeutics—Handbooks, manuals, etc.
2. Nursing—Handbooks, manuals, etc. I. Springhouse Corporation.
   [DNLM: 1. Therapeutics—handbooks.   WB 39
H23643 1994]
RM104.H36   1994
615.5—dc20
DNLM/DLC   93-18459
ISBN 0-87434-480-8   CIP

Contents

Therapeutic interventions

Selected references and index

Physicians, nurses, pharmacists, and other consultants

Ruth E. Blauer, RN, BSN, CNA
Nurse Coordinator
Vanderbilt University Medical Center
Nashville, Tenn.

Mary Ann Cali-Ascani, RN, MSN, OCN
Nurse Manager, Oncology Unit
Easton (Pa.) Hospital

Jeanette K. Chambers, RN, PhD, CS
Renal Medicine Clinical Nurse Specialist
Riverside Methodist Hospitals
Adjunct Instructor, College of Nursing
Ohio State University
Columbus

Kathleen K. Collins, RN,C, BSN
Medical-Surgical Nurse Educator
Rutland (Vt.) Regional Medical Center

Tammy Croom-Brumfield, RN,C
Quality Assurance Coordinator
Ochsner Hospital
New Orleans

Stephen C. Duck, MD
Associate Professor, Pediatrics
Northwestern University Medical School
Evanston, Ill.

Stanley J. Dudrick, MD
Clinical Professor, Surgery
University of Texas Health Science Center
at Houston
Surgeon-in-Chief
Hermann Hospital
Houston

Sandra D. Durkin, RD, MS
Consulting Dietician
Nutrition Consult Services, Inc.
Washington Crossing, Pa.

Nancy G. Evans, RN, BSN, CGRN
Nurse Manager, Gastroenterology
Department
Daniel Freeman Memorial and Marina
Hospitals
Inglewood, Calif.

Susan Ezzone, RN, MS, OCN
Clinical Nurse Specialist, Bone Marrow
Transplant
The Arthur G. James Cancer Hospital and
Research Institute
Columbus, Ohio

Nancy M. Flynn, RN,C, MSN
Clinical Educator
Bryn Mawr (Pa.) Hospital

Ellie Z. Franges, RN, MSN, CCRN, CNRN
Head Nurse, Central Nervous System Unit
The Allentown (Pa.) Hospital–Lehigh Valley
Hospital Center

Susan P. Gauthier, RN, MSN, PhD
Assistant Professor, Department of Nursing
Temple University
Philadelphia

Shirley A. Grieshaber, RN
Advanced Clinical Nurse
Warren G. Magnuson Clinical Center
National Institutes of Health
Bethesda, Md.

Gunter R. Haase, MD
Neurologist
Pennsylvania Hospital
Philadelphia

Paul M. Kirschenfeld, MD, FACP, FCCP
Medical Director, Intensive Care Units
Program Director, Internal Medicine Resi-
dency Program
Atlantic City (N.J.) Medical Center

Lixing Lao, MD, PhD, RAc
Research Assistant Professor
University of Maryland Pain Center
Baltimore

David B. Messinger, MD
Clinical Cardiology Fellow, Instructor in Medi-
cine
The New York Hospital, Cornell Medical
Center

Margaret E. Miller, RN, MSN
Clinical Service Manager
Department of Otolaryngology
Head and Neck Surgery
Northwestern Medical Faculty Foundation
Chicago

Randie Oberlender, RPh
Pharmacy Coordinator
Pennsylvania Hospital
Philadelphia

Norman E. Peterson, MD
Professor, Department of Surgery
University of Colorado Health Sciences
Center
Associate Director of Surgery
Urology Division Chief
Denver General Hospital

Kathleen Pippel, RN, MAEd, NHA
Staff Nurse
Department of Psychiatry
Medical College Hospitals, Bucks County
Campus
Warminster, Pa.

Mina Ricciardelli, RPh
Drug Information Pharmacist
Pennsylvania Hospital
Philadelphia

Kathleen A. Rorapaugh, RN, BSN
Nurse Manager
Riverside Methodist Hospitals
Columbus, Ohio

Marilyn Sawyer Sommers, RN, PhD, CCRN
Assistant Professor
College of Nursing and Health
University of Cincinnati

Steven J. Schweon, RN, BSN, CCRN
Staff Nurse
Horsham Clinic
Ambler, Pa.

Janice Selekman, RN, DNS
Chairman, Department of Advanced Nursing Science
University of Delaware, College of Nursing
Newark

Denise A. Silvasi, RN, BSN
Research Nurse Coordinator
Coronary Care Unit
The New York Hospital, Cornell Medical
Center

Naomi Walpert, RN, MS, CDE
Clinical Nurse Specialist, Endocrinology
Sinai Hospital
Baltimore

Contributors

Theresa L. Abernathy, RN
Community Health Nurse II
Baltimore City Health Department

Marjorie L. Beck, RN
Nurse Manager
GI Procedure Unit
Abington (Pa.) Memorial Hospital

Sherri Izes Becker, RN, MBA, CCRN
Clinical Consultant
Blue Bell, Pa.

Linda Bellmore, RN, BS, CVNS
Nurse Manager
Cardiac Catheterization Laboratory
Clinical Monitoring Services
St. Joseph's Hospital and Medical Center
Phoenix, Ariz.

Vicki L. Buchda, RN, MS
Director, Special Care Unit
Maryvale Samaritan Medical Center
Phoenix, Ariz.

Margaret Budziszewski, RN, BSN, CCRN, CHT
Clinical Coordinator, Hyperbaric Medicine
St. Luke's Medical Center
Milwaukee

Janice M. Buelow, RN, MS
Clinical Nurse Specialist
Surgical Epilepsy Program
Rush-Presbyterian-St. Luke's Medical
Center
Chicago

Julia K. Burns, RN
Patient Care Coordinator
Atkins, Keane, Rowe, and Rosen
Otolaryngic Associates
Philadelphia

Barbara H. Cabrera, RN, BSN
Nursing Instructor
Phoenix (Ariz.) Children's Hospital

Mary Ann Cali-Ascani, RN, MSN, OCN
Nurse Manager, Oncology Unit
Easton (Pa.) Hospital

Patricia Carroll, RN,C, MS, CEN, RRT
Nursing Consultant
Educational Medical Consultants
Middletown, Conn.
Staff Nurse
Emergency Department
Manchester (Conn.) Memorial Hospital

Carla M. Clark, RN, MS
Nurse Research Clinician
Good Samaritan Regional Medical Center
Phoenix, Ariz.

Debora A. Conrad, RD
Chief Clinical-Nutrition Support Dietitian
The Wood Company at Easton (Pa.)
Hospital

Stephen V. Fabus, CHT
Supervisor, Hyperbaric Medicine
St. Luke's Medical Center
Milwaukee

Nancy M. Flynn, RN,C, MSN
Clinical Educator
Bryn Mawr (Pa.) Hospital

Marybeth L. Gentry, RN
Nurse Manager
Otolaryngology Head and Neck Surgery
Clinic
Greater Baltimore Medical Center
Towson, Md.

Frank Hyland, PT, BS, MS
Director of Physical Therapy
Good Shepherd Rehabilitation Hospital
Allentown, Pa.

Eileen E. Jaskuta, RN, BSN
Nurse Recruiter
Suburban General Hospital
Norristown, Pa.

Selma Kendrick, RN, MS, OCN
Director, Oncology and Hematology
Good Samaritan Regional Medical Center
Phoenix, Ariz.

Robin L. Keyack, RPh, BS
Assistant Director, Pharmacy
Pennsylvania Hospital
Philadelphia

Susan Lyons, RN, ADN
Staff Research Nurse
Proton Beam Therapy Group
Massachusetts General Hospital
Boston

Deirdre P. Mountjoy, RN, MSN
Instructor, Education
Maryvale Samaritan Medical Center
Phoenix, Ariz.

Teresa E. Omert, RN, MS
Clinical Nurse Specialist for Neuroscience
Chicago Neurosurgical Center at Columbus
Hospital

Janet N. Pavel, RN
Chief Nurse, Blood Services
Department of Transfusion Medicine
Bethesda, Md.

Jody Pelusi, RN, MSN, OCN, RT
Clinical Nurse Specialist, Oncology
Maryvale Samaritan Medical Center
Phoenix, Ariz.

Stevelynn J. Pogue, RN, BSN
Assistant Head Nurse
The Methodist Hospital
Houston

Christine A. Quigel, RN
Supervisor, Specialty Services
Focus Health Care Services
Highlands Ranch, Colo.

Rose Ravalli, RN, BSN, CURN
Urology Nurse Clinician
Long Island Jewish Medical Center
New Hyde Park, N.Y.

Pamela Sue Reed, RN, MS
Clinical Nurse Specialist, Medical-Surgical
St. Joseph Mercy Hospital
Pontiac, Mich.

Candace Rehnert, RN, CDE
Certified Diabetic Educator
Abington (Pa.) Hospital

Paula Trahan Rieger, RN, MSN, OCN
Clinical Nurse Specialist
University of Texas M.D. Anderson Cancer
Center
Houston

Mary Faut Rodts, RN, MS, ONC
Assistant Professor
Rush College of Nursing, Rush University
Chicago

Melinda M. Schuster, RN, BSN
Head Nurse, Electrophysiology
Hahnemann University Hospital
Philadelphia

Gwendolyn A. Smith, RN, MBA, MSM
Clinical Coordinator
Nathan Speare Regional Burn Treatment
Center
Crozer-Chester Medical Center
Chester, Pa.

Sharon K. Spreitzer, RN, ADN, CGC, CLS
Nurse Educator
St. Joseph's Hospital and Medical Center
Phoenix, Ariz.

Lori J. Strauss, RN, MSA, CCRN, CNA
Nurse Manager, Coronary Care Unit
Chester County Hospital
West Chester, Pa.

Juanita Taylor, RN, MSN, CRNP
Assistant Professor of Nursing
Lehigh County Community College
Schecksville, Pa.

Elaine G. Warner, RN, MS, CCRN, CS
Regional Clinical Coordinator—Midatlantic
Region
Genentech, Inc.
Yardley, Pa.

Foreword

In today's climate, which demands cost-efficient use of resources, the wise health care professional should be comprehensively informed about the vast array of available therapeutic options. Necessary information about each intervention includes its indications, efficacy, application, potential adverse consequences, and follow-up care. Patients and their families, other medical professionals, and regulatory agencies and other third parties will demand no less.

Although such comprehensive information has been available to those with the time and other resources to seek it in numerous scientific journals and textbooks, a single source has not existed until now. *Handbook of Therapeutic Interventions* provides concise, accurate, and up-to-date entries on virtually all medically useful interventions and treatments commonly used by doctors, nurses, physical therapists, respiratory therapists, and other health care professionals. The options discussed include drug and diet therapies, surgical procedures, complementary and alternative healing techniques, and other therapeutic strategies.

Interventions are presented in alphabetical entries. Each entry begins with a description of the treatment, tells how or why it works, and (if appropriate) compares it with related options. Then the entry provides the following elements:

• *Purpose,* which lists the clinical rationales for using the treatment.

• *Indications,* which identifies the conditions for which the treatment is typically recommended. Within this section, the final paragraph summarizes contraindications for the procedure, drug regimen, or other treatment.

• *Procedure,* which briefly describes the usual method for implementing the treatment. For example, surgical entries include patient preparation and positioning, the anesthesia required, the usual anatomical approach, and any special requirements.

• *Complications,* which describes the associated risks of each treatment, with recommendations for preventing or overcoming them. (In drug treatment entries, this section is called *Adverse reactions* and describes the risks of using each drug.)

• *Care considerations,* which provides detailed recommendations for concomitant patient care needed for safe and effective treatment. As appropriate, this section specifies patient care, routine and special monitoring, and other clinical interventions needed before, during, and after the treatment. For example, the entry on laser surgery includes detailed recommendations for protecting the eyes of the patient, the surgeon, and the assisting staff.

• *Home care instructions,* which provides information for continuing patient care after discharge.

These headings, which mark each section of an entry, can speed the user to the needed information.

The treatments in this volume include surgeries, such as angioplasty; procedures, such as hemodialysis; techniques, such as range-of-motion exercises; devices, such as hearing aids; drugs, such as histamine-2 receptor antagonists; complementary treatments, such as hydrotherapy; and alternative treatments, such as milieu therapy. The information for both new and established therapies has been scrupulously reviewed for accuracy and timeliness by doctors, nurses, and clinical technicians. Data reflect these reviewers' experiences.

To assist the reader further, the editors have added many charts and illustrations that summarize, explain, or demonstrate. In the entry on biotherapy, for example, a detailed chart compares the uses and adverse reactions of the biological response modifiers, a new group of drugs that are becoming widely used. The entry on chest physiotherapy includes illustrations of the positions for postural drainage.

A comprehensive index lists all therapies, including alternative names of surgical procedures; specific generic drugs and drug groups; major signs, symptoms, and syndromes; special equipment; and other significant concepts. It also indicates charts and illustrations.

Handbook of Therapeutic Interventions will prove to be an indispensable resource for health care professionals at all levels of training, experience, and expertise. We believe that it can significantly improve the quality and appropriateness of the care delivered by those who rely on it.

David B. Messinger, MD
Denise A. Silvasi, RN, BSN
The New York Hospital,
Cornell Medical Center

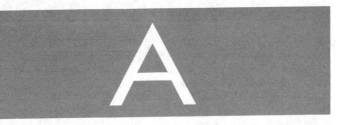

ABDOMINAL THRUST

An abdominal thrust relieves sudden airway obstruction such as occurs when a foreign body lodges in the throat or bronchus or when the patient aspirates blood, mucus, or vomitus. A subdiaphragmatic abdominal thrust applies pressure that elevates the diaphragm and forces sufficient air from the lungs to create a forceful cough, which expels the obstruction. A variation of the abdominal thrust, the chest thrust, is used if the patient is in advanced pregnancy or markedly obese.

Obstruction of an airway by a foreign body most often occurs when the patient is eating. In adults, the most common cause is an accidentally aspirated piece of meat, although various other foods and foreign bodies can cause airway obstruction.

Foreign bodies can cause complete or partial airway obstruction. The abdominal thrust and its variations are contraindicated in a patient with partial airway obstruction who has sufficient air exchange to maintain adequate ventilation and to dislodge the foreign body by effective coughing. The patient with sufficient air exchange can cough forcefully. Partial airway obstruction can progress to poor air exchange and complete obstruction; therefore, if the partial obstruction with good air exchange persists, activate the emergency medical service (EMS) system. The EMS is a coordinated, community-wide system for responding to emergency situations and is usually activated with a phone call.

Recognize progression to poor air exchange and the need for an abdominal thrust when the patient develops a weak, ineffective cough and a high-pitched noise when inhaling and has increased difficulty breathing. In complete airway obstruction, the patient cannot speak, breathe, or cough, and often clutches his neck with his thumbs and fingers, the universal distress signal.

An obstructed airway causes anoxia, which can lead to brain damage and death in minutes without successful intervention. For this reason, it's necessary to call for emergency rescue as soon as airway obstruction is identified. In the hospital, follow established policy for this occurrence. Outside of the hospital, activate the EMS system.

Purpose

• To relieve airway obstruction caused by aspiration of a foreign body.

Indications

The abdominal thrust is indicated for conscious or unconscious adults who have suddenly developed a foreign body airway obstruction. If the victim is in an advanced stage of pregnancy or is markedly obese, a variation of the abdominal thrust, the chest thrust, is indicated to expel the foreign body.

Procedure

The abdominal thrust can be performed by anyone who has been taught the technique. Before performing it, make sure the patient has a completely obstructed airway or a partially obstructed airway with poor air exchange. The patient who has a complete obstruction won't be able to answer when you ask if he's choking; if he has poor air exchange, coughing will be ineffective, and he may not be able to speak easily. If the patient is unconscious and his airway is obstructed, he will not be breathing, and the air that you attempt to blow into the patient's lungs will meet resistance.

When you've established that the patient requires an abdominal thrust, perform forceful inward and upward subdiaphragmatic abdominal thrusts or chest thrusts until the foreign body is dislodged. Once dislodged, the foreign body is usually visible in the patient's mouth and can be removed by the rescuer with a finger sweep if the patient is unable to remove the object himself.

If you come upon an unconscious victim, proceed as you would for adult cardiopulmonary resuscitation (CPR). If the airway is obstructed, you will meet resistance when you attempt to ventilate the patient. Because the tongue is the most common cause of airway obstruction, and you may not have properly opened the airway, reposition the airway and again attempt ventilation. If you still meet resistance, try to clear the obstructed airway by performing five abdominal thrusts (or chest thrusts, if indicated); then perform a blind finger sweep and try to ventilate. Repeat this sequence—thrusts, finger sweep, ventilate—until ventilation succeeds or the obstruction is relieved. For a child or infant, the sequence and procedures are different. (See *Clearing an obstructed airway*.)

Complications

A major complication associated with abdominal or chest thrusts is damage to the underlying organs. Abdominal or chest thrusts can lacerate or rupture such organs as the liver or lungs. Vomiting may also result.

Care considerations
Before the procedure
• Activate the EMS system or, if in the hospital, follow hospital policy for getting help.
• Verify foreign body airway obstruction before performing this maneuver.
During the procedure
• When performing an abdominal thrust on a conscious victim, ensure that each thrust is a separate and distinct movement forceful enough to create an artificial cough that will dislodge the obstruction.
• Keep a firm grip on the conscious victim because he may lose consciousness and need to be lowered to the floor.
• If the victim vomits, turn him on his side, quickly perform a finger sweep, return him to supine position, and repeat the maneuver as necessary.
• Even if efforts to clear the airway don't seem effective, keep trying. As oxygen deprivation increases, smooth and skeletal muscles relax, which makes the maneuver more likely to succeed.
• For a child, perform a finger sweep only if you can see the object.
• For an unconscious infant in whom you have established partial or complete obstruction, perform five back blows and five chest thrusts identical to the chest compressions recommended for infant CPR. Next, look into the mouth, and finger sweep if you see the obstructing object; then try to ventilate. Repeat this sequence until you successfully ventilate or relieve the obstruction.
• For a conscious infant, perform only back blows and chest thrusts.
After the procedure
• If the patient was unconscious, observe him closely. Nausea and regurgitation may develop after the patient regains consciousness and can breathe independently. The patient should also be evaluated for injuries that may have occurred. If the incident happens outside the hospital, the EMS team will

(Text continues on page 7.)

Clearing an obstructed airway

If you determine that the patient's airway is totally obstructed, follow these guidelines.

To perform the procedure on a conscious adult
- Tell the patient you're going to try to dislodge the foreign body.
- Standing behind the patient, wrap your arms around her waist. Make a fist with one hand and place the thumb side against her abdomen, slightly above the umbilicus and well below the xiphoid process. Then grasp your fist with the other hand, and squeeze the patient's abdomen with a quick inward and upward thrust (see below).

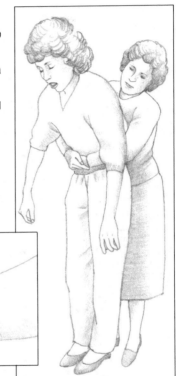

- Repeat this maneuver until the object is dislodged or the patient becomes unconscious. If the patient becomes unconscious, lower her carefully to the floor and continue trying to dislodge the obstruction using the technique for an unconscious patient, beginning with a finger sweep.

To perform the procedure on an unconscious adult
- If you come upon an unconscious patient, ask any witnesses what happened. Begin cardiopulmonary resuscitation (CPR) and attempt to ventilate the patient. If you're unable to ventilate her, reposition her head and try again.
- If you still can't ventilate the patient, kneel astride her thighs.

(continued)

Clearing an obstructed airway *(continued)*

• Place the heel of one hand on top of the other. Then place your hands between her umbilicus and the tip of her xiphoid process at the midline. Push inward and upward with five quick abdominal thrusts.

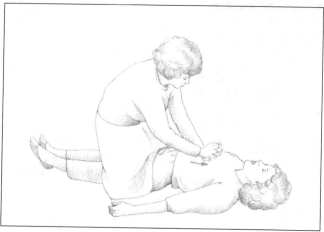

• After delivering the abdominal thrusts, open the patient's airway by grasping the tongue and lower jaw with your thumb and fingers. Lift the jaw to draw the tongue away from the back of the throat and perform a finger sweep (see below).

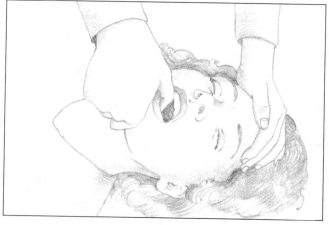

Clearing an obstructed airway *(continued)*

• If you can see the object, remove it by inserting your index finger deep into the throat at the base of her tongue. Using a hooking motion, remove the obstruction. Keep in mind that some clinicians object to a blind finger sweep—using your finger when you can't see the obstruction—because the finger acts as a second obstruction. They believe that, in most cases, the jaw lift described above should be enough to dislodge the obstruction.

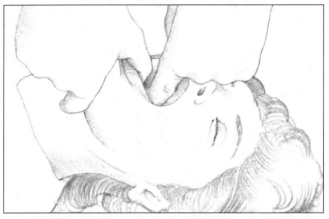

• If the object is not removed, try to ventilate the patient. If you can't, repeat the abdominal thrust maneuver described above in sequence until you clear the airway.
• If you are able to remove the obstruction, determine if the patient is breathing; if not, proceed with CPR.

To perform the procedure on an obese patient or one who is in advanced stages of pregnancy

• If the patient is conscious, stand behind her and place your arms under her armpits and around her chest.
• Place the thumb side of your clenched fist against the middle of the sternum, avoiding the margins of the ribs and the xiphoid process. Grasp your fist with your other hand, and perform a chest thrust with enough force to expel the foreign body (see right). Continue until the patient expels the obstruction or loses consciousness.

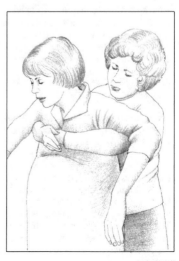

(continued)

Clearing an obstructed airway   *(continued)*

• If the patient loses consciousness, carefully lower her to the floor.
• Kneel close to the patient's side and place the heel of one hand just above the bottom of the patient's sternum. The long axis of the heel of your hand should align with the long axis of the patient's sternum (see below). Place the heel of your other hand on top of that, making sure your fingers don't touch the patient's chest. Deliver each thrust forcefully enough to remove the obstruction.

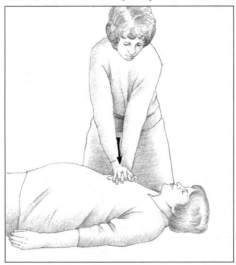

To perform the procedure on a child
• If the child is conscious and can stand, perform abdominal thrusts using the same technique as you would with an adult, but with less force.
• If he's unconscious or lying down, kneel at his feet; if he's a large child, kneel astride his thighs. If he's lying on a treatment table, stand by his side. Deliver abdominal thrusts as you would for an adult patient, but use less force. (Never perform a blind finger sweep on a child because you risk pushing the foreign body farther back into the airway.)

To perform the procedure on an infant
• Whether or not the infant is conscious, place him face down and straddling your arm with his head lower than his trunk. Rest your forearm on your thigh and deliver five back blows with the heel of your hand between the infant's shoulder blades.
• If you haven't removed the obstruction, place your free hand on the infant's back. Supporting his neck, jaw, and chest with your other hand, turn him over onto your thigh, keeping his head lower than his trunk.
• Position your fingers. To do so, imagine a line between the infant's nipples; place the index finger of your free hand on his sternum, just below this imaginary line. Then place your middle and ring fingers next to your index finger and lift the index finger off his chest. Deliver five chest thrusts as you would for chest compression, but at a slower rate. (As with a child, never perform a blind finger sweep.)

transport the patient to the hospital for further evaluation.

• Tell the patient to expect achiness, which often follows this procedure.

• Strongly encourage the patient who was conscious during the procedure to go to an emergency department for careful evaluation.

Home care instructions

• Explain precautions that will help prevent airway obstruction by a foreign body. Tell the patient to cut food into small pieces and to chew it thoroughly before swallowing, not to laugh or talk when chewing or swallowing, and to avoid drinking excessive amounts of alcohol before or during meals.

• Advise parents not to permit their children to walk, run, or play when they have food or anything else in their mouths and to keep small foreign objects away from infants and small children.

• Tell parents the importance of learning how to perform the abdominal thrust correctly and teach them the universal sign of foreign body airway obstruction.

ACUPUNCTURE

Although primarily used to relieve pain, the ancient Chinese technique of acupuncture is also used to treat symptoms such as diarrhea, hiccups, insomnia, and stress reactions. For this procedure, fine needles are inserted at selected points on the body. Acupuncture provides symptomatic relief that varies from permanent and complete to temporary or inadequate. Typically, several treatments are required.

Many Western pain experts who favor acupuncture explain its effectiveness in terms of the gate theory of pain control. They suggest that the needles used in acupuncture stimulate large

sensory nerve fibers that carry pain-inhibiting impulses, thereby blocking impulses from the smaller pain-conducting fibers at the spinal level. Other researchers suggest that acupuncture produces analgesia by triggering the release of opioid-like compounds, such as enkephalins and endorphins.

Purpose

• To relieve pain
• To regulate the autonomic nervous system
• To activate the immune system.

Indications

The World Health Organization has published a list of indications for acupuncture therapy. The list includes acute and chronic gastritis, colitis, and pharyngitis; acute sinusitis; acute bacterial dysentery; acute tonsillitis, conjunctivitis, rhinitis, and acute bronchitis; acquired immunodeficiency syndrome; bronchial asthma (in children and in patients without concomitant disease); cataract (without complications); central retinitis; chronic duodenal ulcer; common cold; constipation or diarrhea; facial paralysis; gastric hyperacidity; gastroptosis; headache; hiccups; intercostal neuralgia; lumbar back pain; Ménière's syndrome; migraine; myopia (in children); neurogenic bladder dysfunction; nocturnal enuresis; pain after tooth extraction; paralysis caused by poliomyelitis or after apoplectic fit; paralytic ileus; periarthritis humeroscapularis; peripheral neuropathy; rheumatoid arthritis; sciatica; spasms of the esophagus and cardia; tennis elbow; toothache; and trigeminal neuralgia.

Acupuncture should be avoided in patients with bleeding disorders or in those with certain psychiatric disorders such as paranoia that may preclude the elective use of any invasive procedure. Acupuncture may also be contraindicated in pregnant women because of the risk of precipitating uterine contractions. Electrical acupuncture should be used with caution in patients with pacemakers.

Procedure

The treatment should be performed only by a doctor trained in acupuncture or by an acupuncturist who, depending on state law, may practice independently or with a doctor.

The patient is typically placed in a reclining position, and the clinician inserts 4 to 20 fine disposable needles under the skin either directly into the painful area or into remote areas. Insertion of the needles may cause sensations of pinpricks, warmth, and stinging or a dull aching throb. (If dizziness occurs, the needles should be removed immediately.) When all the needles are in place, the clinician stimulates them, either electrically or manually. Typically, needles remain in the sites for 15 to 30 minutes before they are removed.

The first treatment may provide only transient relief or none at all, but the pain relief should persist longer with successive treatments.

Complications

Acupuncture causes few complications if performed correctly. Possible complications include hyperemia or hematoma at a needle insertion site; syncope, particularly in nervous, tense, or tired patients; internal organ injury from deep needle insertion over vital organs, such as the lungs; local infection from improper needle insertion or use of nondisposable needles; and soreness at needle insertion sites.

Care considerations
Before therapy
• Ensure that the patient understands the procedure, the risks, and the expected outcome.
• Evaluate the patient's pain level before treatment to establish a baseline.

During therapy
• Tell the patient to inform the clinician of dizziness or increased pain. The therapy can be stopped if the patient desires.
After therapy
• Observe the insertion sites for a hematoma. If one occurs, apply pressure.
• Have the patient sit or stand up slowly to avoid syncope and light-headedness.
• If needles were inserted into the patient's thorax, observe for signs of pneumothorax, such as dyspnea or tachypnea.
• Compare the patient's level of pain with the pretreatment baseline.

Home care instructions

• Teach the patient to identify signs of local infection, such as redness, swelling, and discharge. Infection is unlikely but, if it occurs, the patient should notify the clinician immediately.
• Instruct the patient who has had needles placed in the thorax to immediately report any shortness of breath or painful breathing.
• Instruct the patient to note the duration and effectiveness of pain relief, and to report these observations at the next appointment. Full analgesic effect may require 8 to 16 treatments. However, if analgesia hasn't occurred after a reasonable number of sessions, the clinician may terminate treatment.

ADRENALECTOMY

Adrenalectomy is the surgical resection or removal of one or both adrenal glands. An adrenalectomy may be performed when an adrenal tumor overproduces any of the adrenal hormones. The glucocorticoids, a class of adrenal hormones, are normally produced in response to the stimulation of the adrenal cortex by pituitary secretion of adrenocorticotropic hormone (ACTH). Overproduction of glucocorticoids can be secondary to an overproduction of ACTH by a pituitary adenoma (Cushing's disease) or due to a primary adrenal disorder (an adrenal adenoma), causing Cushing's syndrome. The treatment for Cushing's syndrome is adrenalectomy; the treatment for Cushing's disease is removal of the pituitary adenoma.

Purpose

• To remove adrenal tissue, reducing adrenal hormone hypersecretion
• To resect a malignant tumor.

Indications

Adrenalectomy is the treatment of choice for adrenal hyperfunction caused by adrenal hyperplasia or an adrenal adenoma. The prognosis is good when adrenalectomy is used to treat a benign adrenal adenoma. The prognosis is less favorable for adrenal cancer.

The procedure can also be used to treat a pheochromocytoma (a catecholamine-secreting tumor of the adrenal medulla) in one or both adrenal glands, and it has also been used occasionally to treat some breast or prostate cancers.

Procedure

Using either an anterior (transperitoneal) or a posterior (lumbar) approach, the surgeon explores the adrenal glands. The anterior approach offers better visualization of both glands. If the surgeon finds a tumor, he either resects it or removes the involved adrenal gland.

To remove a pheochromocytoma, the surgeon carefully excises the affected adrenal gland as well as adjacent areolar tissue (often the site of recurring tumors), and he palpates the abdominal organs for other tumors.

Complications

Hemorrhage, shock, hypotension, hypertension, and hyponatremia can complicate the patient's recovery from surgery. However, improved use of medications such as phenoxybenzamine or metyrosine and propranolol to prepare the patient before surgery has dramatically decreased the risk of postoperative complications.

Care considerations

Before surgery

• Make sure the patient understands the procedure and the preparation that is required for surgery.
• If surgery is performed to remove a pheochromocytoma, the doctor may prescribe medication 1 to 2 weeks before surgery. Metyrosine serves to block catecholamine synthesis, and phenoxybenzamine and propranolol control hypertension and tachycardia.
• On the morning of surgery, administer glucocorticoids to the patient with adrenal hyperfunction to prevent adrenal insufficiency during surgery.

After surgery

• Monitor vital signs during and after surgery. After surgery, closely assess vital signs for evidence of shock resulting from hemorrhage.
• Monitor serum levels of sodium and potassium, and observe the patient closely for signs and symptoms of adrenocortical insufficiency – lethargy, apathy, nausea, hypoglycemia, hyponatremia, and hyperkalemia. Monitoring serum potassium levels is especially important for the patient who had primary aldosteronism before surgery and who's receiving spironolactone, a potassium-sparing diuretic, for control of postoperative hypertension.
• Observe the dressing for excessive bleeding, and correlate findings with vital sign readings. For example, a blood-soaked dressing and a very rapid pulse could indicate an early stage of shock. Any wound drainage or fever should be reported to the patient's doctor immediately.
• Observe for postoperative hypertension. This is especially important because handling of the adrenal glands

during surgery stimulates catecholamine release, particularly after surgery for removal of a pheochromocytoma. Paradoxically, many patients develop hypotension, but it responds promptly to restoration of fluid balance.

• Analgesics are administered for pain, and replacement steroids are given. Glucocorticoids from the adrenal cortex are essential to life and must be replaced to prevent adrenal crisis.

Home care instructions

• Teach the importance of taking prescribed medication as directed. The patient who's had a unilateral adrenalectomy should understand that medications may be discontinued in a few months when his remaining gland resumes function. However, after a bilateral adrenalectomy, the patient must understand that lifelong medication is necessary because his body no longer has a glucocorticoid source.

• Because the adrenal gland also regulates sodium and potassium, the patient will need mineralocorticoid replacement, commonly with fludrocortisone acetate (Florinef).

• Teach the patient to recognize the signs of adrenal insufficiency, and emphasize how it can progress to adrenal crisis if not treated. Tell the patient to promptly report such adverse reactions as weight gain, acne, headaches, fatigue, and increased urinary frequency to the doctor. Advise the patient to take the prescribed steroid with meals or antacids to minimize gastric irritation.

• Make sure the patient understands that sudden withdrawal of steroids can precipitate adrenal crisis; therefore, continued medical follow-up is vital to provide appropriate adjustment of steroid dosage during stress or illness.

• Tell the patient who had adrenal hyperfunction to expect reversal of the physical signs of his disease over the next few months. However, warn him that these physical improvements don't mean that steroid medications can be discontinued.

• If the patient's surgical wound isn't completely healed, provide wound care instructions. Advise him to keep the incision clean, to avoid wearing clothing that may irritate the incision, and to follow his doctor's instructions regarding application of ointments or dressings. Tell him to report fever or any increased drainage, inflammation, or pain at the incision site.

• Urge the patient to wear a medical identification bracelet or carry a card to ensure adequate care in an emergency.

ADRENERGICS

Adrenergic drugs, also called sympathomimetic agents, stimulate the sympathetic nervous system. These agents' relative selectivity of action is the primary determinant of their clinical usefulness and can predict the most likely adverse reactions.

Adrenergics affect alpha- and beta-receptors in almost all body systems. Some adrenergics affect all types of alpha- and beta-receptors; others exert more selective effects. For example, the bronchodilating adrenergics exert a direct effect on the $beta_2$-receptors in the lungs, causing bronchodilation and vasodilation. Another group stimulates alpha-receptors and causes vasoconstriction, decongestion, and pressor effects. Adrenergics that stimulate $beta_1$-receptors in the heart cause increased myocardial contractility, conduction velocity, and heart rate.

The bronchodilating adrenergics include *isoproterenol, isoetharine,* and several other drugs. Isoproterenol has limited clinical use because of its adverse cardiac reactions, which result from its $beta_1$-stimulating effects. It can be given sublingually, by inhalation, or by infusion. Isoetharine, which can be given by inhalation, causes fewer adverse reactions than isoproterenol. Other beta₂-selective drugs—*terbutaline, metaproterenol,* and *albuterol*—can be given orally or by inhalation.

The alpha-stimulating adrenergic nasal decongestants include *oxymetazoline, phenylephrine,* and *pseudoephedrine.*

Adrenergic agents that stimulate beta₁-receptors in the heart include *isoproterenol, dopamine, norepinephrine,* and *dobutamine.*

Epinephrine may be administered I.V., S.C., or I.M. I.V. administration of this drug produces an almost immediate response; S.C. or I.M. administration produces effects in 3 to 5 minutes.

Purpose

• To relax bronchial smooth muscle, resulting in decreased airway resistance and, at times, increased vital capacity
• To cause vasoconstriction, relieving nasal congestion
• To produce an inotropic effect on the heart, resulting in increased cardiac output
• To reverse the effects of severe anaphylactic reactions.

Indications

Adrenergics that stimulate beta₁-receptors in the heart are used in the management of shock to treat hypoperfusion in normovolemic patients and in patients unresponsive to infusions of whole blood or plasma-volume expanders.

Applied to the nasal mucosa, the alpha-stimulating adrenergic nasal decongestants provide a rapid decongestant effect. However, tolerance may develop and rebound congestion may occur after chronic use.

Epinephrine helps reverse the effects of severe anaphylactic reactions. It stimulates alpha- and beta-adrenergic receptors within the sympathetic nervous system. Although epinephrine is no longer widely prescribed as a bronchodilator and decongestant because of its severe adverse reactions, it is the drug of choice for treating acute anaphylactic reactions.

Epinephrine should be given with extreme caution to patients with chronic obstructive pulmonary disease who have developed a degenerative cardiac disorder. It should also be given cautiously to elderly patients and to those with hyperthyroidism, angina, diabetes mellitus, or hypertension.

Adverse reactions

The type and severity of adverse reactions to adrenergics depend on the medication's specificity for the type of receptor stimulated. Medications that predominantly stimulate alpha-receptors, such as phenylephrine, produce adverse reactions related to alpha-stimulation. These reactions include peripheral and visceral vasoconstriction, with reduced blood flow to vital organs; decreased renal perfusion; tissue hypoxia; and metabolic acidosis. Bradycardia and decreased cardiac output may also occur. Adverse central nervous system (CNS) reactions include restlessness, anxiety, weakness, nervousness, and dizziness. Tremor, respiratory distress, and pallor or blanching of the skin are also related to alpha stimulation.

An adrenergic, such as isoproterenol, that produces predominant beta stimulation causes adverse cardiovascular reactions that include tachycardia, cardiac arrhythmias, and anginal pain, which are related to beta stimulation. The beta-adrenergics may also produce nervousness, restlessness, insomnia, anxiety, tension, fear, or excitement.

Additionally, epinephrine can cause severe hypertension when combined with tricyclic antidepressants and certain antihistamines, such as diphenhydramine or chlorpheniramine. Less severe reactions include headache, dizziness, palpitations, and anxiety.

Care considerations

• Review the patient's drug regimen for possible interactions. For example, concurrent use of an adrenergic and a beta blocker reduces the adrenergic's bronchodilating effect and may lead to bronchospasm. Other sympathomimetics, monoamine oxidase inhibitors, and tricyclic antidepressants can potentiate adrenergic effects.

• When administering epinephrine or terbutaline I.M. or S.C., pull back on the syringe before injection and check for blood to ensure that the needle isn't in a vein. After injection, massage the site to counteract possible vasoconstriction.

• Monitor the patient's respiratory function to assess his response to therapy. Measure the patient's forced expiratory volume in 1 second (FEV_1). An increase of 15% or more in his FEV_1 suggests that improvement will occur. However, increased airway resistance may indicate an allergic response to the drug or its preservatives.

• Monitor the patient for increased blood pressure and heart rate, even if you're giving a $beta_2$-selective drug. Report any such increases to the doctor, and reduce the dosage as ordered.

• When administering epinephrine, monitor the patient's vital signs every 5 minutes and keep resuscitation equipment available. Provide oxygen, if necessary. If the patient's blood pressure rises sharply, notify the doctor. He'll probably order rapid-acting vasodilators (such as nitrites) or alpha-adrenergic blocking agents to counteract epinephrine's pressor effects.

• Because several concentrations of epinephrine are available, carefully check the label before administering the drug. Use a tuberculin syringe for accuracy.

• Tremors, an annoying and common adverse effect of adrenergics, may reduce patient compliance. If the patient develops a severe hand tremor that interferes with his daily activities, reduce the dosage as ordered.

• If the patient is taking an adrenergic nasal decongestant, observe for excessive CNS stimulation and ask about headaches. If they occur, reduce the dosage as ordered.

Home care instructions

• Explain that long-term use of adrenergics can reduce their effectiveness. Advise the patient to report any reduced response. Warn against changing the dosage without the doctor's approval.

• If the patient is taking an inhalant bronchodilator, provide written directions for its use. Tell him to take his pulse, to assess for adverse reactions according to the amount of drug used, and to notify the doctor if the resting heart rate increases more than 10 beats/minute after starting treatment. Warn the patient against using any over-the-counter inhalants without the doctor's approval because these products usually contain epinephrine.

• Teach the patient who will be using a nebulizer how to clean and troubleshoot any equipment. Explain that the nebulizer can be a source of infection if it is not thoroughly rinsed and air-dryed between treatments.

• Instruct the patient who is taking an adrenergic that doesn't contain a preservative to store it in the refrigerator and, if appropriate, in a light-resistant container. Advise him not to use it if the color changes.

• If the patient is taking a nasal decongestant, warn him not to exceed the recommended dosage because headache and CNS stimulation may result. Explain that habitual use can cause rebound congestion with mucosal fullness and edema. Advise him to instill nose drops in the lateral head-down position to reduce the risk of swallowing the drug. If he is using an inhaler,

tell him to close one nostril and inhale through the open one.
- Explain that anaphylactic reactions are triggered by certain allergens, including drugs such as penicillin and local anesthetics, foods such as eggs and shellfish, and stinging insects such as bees and wasps.
- Instruct the patient to watch for signs of an allergic reaction – flushing, itching, hives, shortness of breath, wheezing, and chest tightness. If the patient has an anaphylaxis kit, show him and a family member how to inject epinephrine into the lateral thigh or the deltoid muscle and how to massage the injection site to counteract vasoconstriction and increase absorption. Instruct them to rotate sites if more than one injection is needed. Tell them to call for help immediately after injecting the epinephrine.
- Tell the patient who has an anaphylaxis kit to regularly inspect the epinephrine solution for precipitates or discoloration. If the solution isn't clear, the patient should discard it and ask his doctor for a new prescription. To prevent drug deterioration, advise the patient to store epinephrine in a cool, dark place – but to keep it accessible.
- Show family members how to position the patient for optimal oxygenation. They should also be prepared to correctly perform cardiopulmonary resuscitation.

AMINOGLYCOSIDES

The aminoglycosides include *amikacin, gentamicin, kanamycin, neomycin, netilmicin, streptomycin,* and *tobramycin.* These antibiotics are used primarily to treat severe gram-negative infections caused by *Pseudomonas, Escherichia coli, Proteus, Klebsiella,* and *Enterobacter.*

The aminoglycosides are not well absorbed from the GI tract; therefore, they must be given parenterally for systemic effect. They are given I.M. or I.V. for severe urinary tract, bone, joint, and pleural infections. They can be given intrathecally for central nervous system (CNS) infections and can be applied topically or given by inhalation.

Purpose
- To treat severe gram-negative infections caused by susceptible organisms. These drugs act directly on the ribosomes of pathogens; by binding directly to the 30S ribosomal subunit, they inhibit protein synthesis.

Indications
Amikacin, a semisynthetic derivative, combats urinary tract infections resistant to other aminoglycosides. Gentamicin is used for gram-negative sepsis. Given intrathecally for meningitis, it's also used with carbenicillin for severe *Pseudomonas aeruginosa* infections. Neomycin, the most toxic aminoglycoside, can be given orally for profuse diarrhea caused by *E. coli* or for preoperative bowel antisepsis. It's used topically in eye, ear, and skin infections. However, because of neomycin's potential toxicity, it isn't given parenterally. Kanamycin effectively combats many gram-negative infections. It's used for intestinal infections, for preoperative bowel antisepsis, and for intraperitoneal and wound irrigation. It may be given as an aerosol for respiratory infections. Netilmicin is used parenterally in severe staphylococcal and gram-negative infections. Streptomycin, a primary treatment for tuberculosis, may be administered with other antitubercular agents, but the emergence of resistant organisms has diminished its efficacy. Streptomycin is also used to treat bacterial endocarditis resulting from *Haemophilus influenzae,* tularemia, bubonic plague, and cholera. Closely related to gentamicin and possibly causing less nephrotoxicity, tobramycin treats meningitis and neonatal sepsis. It may also be used

Preventing aminoglycoside toxicity

Because aminoglycosides can compromise auditory and renal function, certain precautions are appropriate before, during, and after therapy. And, if the patient is taking a muscle relaxant, it's necessary to promptly recognize any neurotoxic effects. Be especially alert for aminoglycoside toxicity when treatment lasts longer than 7 days.

Before therapy
• Evaluate the patient's renal function. Check urinalysis findings, creatinine clearance, blood urea nitrogen (BUN), and serum creatinine levels.
• Evaluate the patient's hearing using the results from audiometric tests.

During therapy
• Keep the patient well hydrated to avoid renal irritation.
• Because ototoxicity can occur even at therapeutic aminoglycoside levels, monitor for tinnitus or vertigo, which indicates vestibular injury (more common with gentamicin and streptomycin). Also monitor hearing loss or high-frequency loss with audiometric tests (more common with kanamycin and neomycin). Ototoxic effects will probably require discontinuation of the drug.
• Monitor for early signs of nephrotoxicity, such as decreased urine output. Supportive laboratory findings include casts, albumin, or red or white blood cells in the urine; decreased or increased creatinine clearance; and elevated BUN levels. Any of these changes signals a need for dosage reduction or discontinuation of the drug.
• The patient who's also taking a muscle relaxant should be monitored for signs of neurotoxicity, such as apnea or depressed respirations.

After therapy
• Continue to monitor auditory and vestibular function for 4 weeks after treatment ends; the onset of hearing loss may be delayed.

with penicillins to combat *Pseudomonas.*

Although oral aminoglycosides are used for preoperative bowel sterilization, they shouldn't be given to patients with intestinal obstructions. Aminoglycosides must be given cautiously with other ototoxic, neurotoxic, or nephrotoxic drugs, or with general anesthetics, muscle relaxants, or diuretics.

Adverse reactions

Oxotoxicity and nephrotoxicity are the most serious complications of aminoglycoside therapy (see *Preventing aminoglycoside toxicity*). Ototoxicity involves both vestibular and auditory functions and usually is related to persistently high serum drug levels. Damage is reversible only if detected early

and if the drug is discontinued promptly.

Aminoglycosides may cause nephrotoxicity, which is usually reversible. The incidence of reported adverse reactions ranges from 2% to 10%. The damage results in tubular necrosis. Nephrotoxicity usually begins on the 4th to 7th day of therapy and appears to be dose-related.

Neuromuscular blockade results in skeletal weakness and respiratory distress similar to that seen with the use of neuromuscular blocking agents.

Oral aminoglycoside therapy most often causes nausea, vomiting, and diarrhea. Less common reactions include hematologic reactions and transient elevation of liver function values.

Parenterally administered forms of aminoglycosides may cause local reactions: vein irritation, phlebitis, and sterile abscess.

Care considerations

• To ensure adequate blood levels and avoid toxicity, monitor serum aminoglycoside levels frequently. Draw trough levels just before giving a dose and peak levels 30 to 60 minutes after giving it.

• Recognize that prolonged administration of aminoglycosides can cause ototoxicity and nephrotoxicity. Observe for optic neuritis, blurred vision, joint pain, nausea, rash, and signs of superinfection.

• Concurrent use of ethacrynic acid or furosemide increases the risk of ototoxicity.

• Aminoglycosides act synergistically with antipseudomonal penicillins.

Home care instructions

• Stress the importance of immediately reporting signs of ototoxicity or nephrotoxicity.

• Make sure that the patient is adequately hydrated to reduce the risk of nephrotoxicity.

AMPUTATION

Amputation, the partial or complete removal of a body part or organ, may be performed as an elective surgical procedure in severe disease such as malignant bone tumors, or it can occur traumatically as the result of an accident. In traumatic amputation, surgery is required to care for the resulting wound.

As an elective surgical treatment, amputation is performed to preserve function in the remaining body part or, at times, to prevent death. In most cases, amputation is really a reconstructive surgery that attempts to improve the patient's quality of life by relieving symptoms and improving function. (See *Levels of amputation*, pages 16 and 17.)

Purpose

• To remove all or part of a severely diseased or traumatized body part or organ.

Indications

Elective surgical amputation may be necessary because of progressive peripheral vascular disease, complications of diabetes mellitus, congenital deformity, malignant tumors, frostbite, gangrene, or septic wounds. Peripheral vascular disease is the cause of most lower extremity amputations.

Common causes of traumatic amputation include crush and thermal injuries, power tool and motor vehicle accidents, gunshot wounds, and household injuries.

Procedure

The two basic forms of surgical amputation are the closed or flap technique — the most commonly performed type — and the open technique — a rarely performed emergency procedure. In either technique, the patient receives a general or a spinal anesthetic (or perhaps a local anesthetic for a finger or toe amputation).

The *closed or flap technique* is appropriate when there is no evidence of infection. In this procedure the surgeon cuts the tissue to the bone, leaving enough tissue to cover the stump. Then, after the bone is removed, the skin flap is sutured over the bone stump; small drains may be inserted to promote wound healing.

The *open technique*, commonly indicated for an infected septic wound, consists of two separate operations. First, the surgeon makes an incision through the bone and all the tissue, leaving the wound open to drain and sometimes applying traction. After bed rest and antibiotic therapy resolve the

Levels of amputation

To determine the best level of amputation, the surgeon takes several facts into consideration. He wants to save as much of the limb as possible while maintaining an adequate blood supply for healing. He tries to avoid muscle imbalances and choose an amputation level that permits him to construct a functional stump.

AMPUTATION LEVEL	DESCRIPTION
Upper extremity	
Shoulder disarticulation	Rarely performed, this disabling and traumatic operation disconnects the arm at the shoulder.
Above the elbow	The surgeon removes the arm at least 1½" (3.8 cm) above the elbow. He tries to save as much length as possible to preserve arm strength.
Elbow disarticulation	Excellent level for amputation. (Difficulties once experienced in fitting prosthetic devices at this level have been overcome by modern prosthetic techniques.)
Below the elbow	The forearm is removed at about 7" (17.8 cm) below the elbow or at the junction between the middle and the lower third of the forearm.
Wrist disarticulation	The surgeon removes the hand at the wrist. A prosthesis fits easily at this level.
Fingers	Removal of one or more fingers at the hinge or condyloid joints requires careful stump construction so that the prosthesis won't interfere with the function of the remaining fingers.
Lower extremity	
Hemipelvectomy	In this disabling and rare procedure, the surgeon removes the leg and half of the pelvis.
Hip disarticulation	In this procedure, performed rarely except for cancer, extensive injuries, or gangrene, the surgeon removes the leg and hip.
Above the knee	The surgeon removes the leg from 3" (7.6 cm) above the knee to ensure enough stump tissue to provide control for a prosthesis.
Knee disarticulation	After the surgeon removes the patella, he brings the quadriceps over the end of the femur or, in the Gritti-Stokes amputation, fastens the patella to a cut surface between the condyles.

Levels of amputation (continued)	
AMPUTATION LEVEL	**DESCRIPTION**
Lower extremity (continued)	
Below the knee	Ideally, the surgeon removes the leg 5" (12.5 cm) to 7" below the knee to provide an adequate base for a prosthesis.
Ankle	Removing the foot at the ankle (Syme's operation) usually leaves a suitable stump for weight-bearing.
Foot	Imbalance and deformity can result from an amputation of the toes or the foot below the ankle. Therefore, the surgeon tries to salvage muscle and skin to provide flap covering.

infection, the surgeon completes the repair and constructs a stump.

Complications

Complications that may follow amputation include hemorrhage (the most life-threatening complication), severe pain, infection, hematoma, necrosis, wound dehiscence, skin irritation from dressings or drainage, contractures, neuromas, and phantom sensations. (See *Understanding phantom sensations*, page 18.)

Care considerations

Before surgery

• Provide emotional support. Loss of a body part can be emotionally devastating to the patient. Discuss the type and level of amputation.

• Teach and encourage the patient to perform range-of-motion and strengthening exercises before and after surgery to maintain muscle strength and tone, prevent contractures, and promote mobility and independence.

• Before lower extremity amputation, especially leg amputation, prepare the patient for ambulation by teaching him transfer techniques and reinforcing the physical therapist's instructions. The sooner the patient gets out of bed after surgery, the better his chances for successful rehabilitation.

• If appropriate, help the patient plan for the disposal of the amputated part in accordance with his religious beliefs.

After surgery

• Check vital signs and dressings frequently to detect any sign of hemorrhage. Keep a tourniquet at the bedside. If massive hemorrhage occurs, apply the tourniquet, elevate the leg, and notify the doctor immediately.

• Protect the wound from contamination and change the dressings as necessary, noting the patency of the drain and the amount, character, and odor of drainage.

• Rewrap the stump three or four times a day. Maintain adequate tension on the bandage to reduce edema and shape the stump to fit a prosthesis. When changing the bandage, observe the stump for redness, swelling, necrosis, increased skin temperature, drainage, and dehiscence.

• Provide analgesics and other pain-control measures (such as the use of transcutaneous electrical nerve stim-

Understanding phantom sensations

Phantom sensations — sensations in the missing limb as if the limb were still part of the patient — are a real, not an imagined, complication of amputation. Patients describe these sensations as an itching, a tingling or, most often, as a pain that is acute, crushing, cramping, burning, or throbbing.

No one knows exactly what causes phantom sensations, but one theory holds that remaining nerve tracks still send messages to the brain. According to another theory, suppressed anger, denial, depression, and grief over the amputation contribute to the sensation.

Phantom sensations usually feel more severe in the immediate postoperative period and generally subside with time. However, exacerbations and remissions of phantom itching and tingling can occur for years.

Phantom sensations have been treated with analgesics, anti-inflammatory drugs, distraction, early ambulation, transcutaneous electrical nerve stimulation, nerve block, and psychotherapy.

ulation units, heat application, or whirlpool) if ordered.
• Help the patient change position every 2 hours. Avoid positions that would encourage contractures. For example, don't let the stump hang over the edge of a bed or chair for a prolonged time, and don't place pillows under it that will cause joint flexion.
• Provide the patient and family with information about available prostheses. If this was not done before surgery, arrange for a consultation with the prosthetist and a meeting with a well-adjusted amputee.
• Encourage the patient and family to engage the full support of the rehabilitation team. Make sure the patient understands the role of the doctor,

nurse, psychologist, physical therapist, prosthetist, and social services.
• Encourage a positive outlook but, if necessary, provide referral for psychological counseling to help the patient adjust to his loss.
• Provide referral to social services, as necessary, to help the patient deal with life-style changes and financial, family, and social problems after discharge.

Home care instructions
• Instruct the patient to watch for and report any signs of infection, such as fever and chills, and to carefully check the amputation site for swelling, redness, skin changes (rashes, blisters, or abrasions), excessive drainage, and increased pain.
• Teach the patient how to care for the stump or wound according to the facility's protocol or doctor's preference. Emphasize that meticulous stump care can speed healing.
• Teach the patient how to apply a stump dressing. Explain that as the wound heals, he'll need to change the dressing less often.
• Teach the patient how to wrap the stump or apply a stump shrinker. Be sure the patient understands the potential for impaired circulation if this is not done correctly.
• If the patient gets a prosthesis before discharge from the hospital, teach him how to care for it.
• If the patient will require additional help at home, make appropriate referral to a home health care agency.

ANALGESICS, NONNARCOTIC

The nonnarcotic analgesics include the nonsteroidal anti-inflammatory drugs (NSAIDs), salicylates, and *acetaminophen*. The NSAIDs include *ibuprofen, indomethacin, naproxen, naproxen sodium, ketorolac, diclofenac,* and *sulindac*; salicylates include *aspirin, choline salicylate, magnesium salicylate,* and *sodium salicylate*. All these agents produce antipyretic and analgesic effects; they also produce anti-inflammatory effects. Because all these drugs have different chemical structures, they vary in onset of action, duration of effect, and method of metabolism and excretion.

Purpose
• To reduce pain
• To reduce fever.

Indications
Nonnarcotic analgesics treat mild-to-moderate pain. If combined with opioid analgesics, they can also relieve moderate-to-severe pain while allowing a reduced opioid dosage. Unlike the opioid analgesics, these drugs don't cause dependence. They are commonly used to treat postoperative and postpartum pain, headache, myalgias, arthralgias, and dysmenorrhea. These agents do not alter the course of the underlying disease.

Acetaminophen may be used in place of aspirin or NSAIDs in peptic ulcer or bleeding disorders. But long-term, high-dose use of acetaminophen may lead to hepatic damage.

NSAIDs shouldn't be used in patients with aspirin sensitivity—especially in those with the triad of allergies, asthma, and nasal polyps—because of the risk of bronchoconstriction or anaphylaxis. Some NSAIDs are also contraindicated in patients with renal dysfunction, hypertension, GI inflammation, or ulcers. Because aspirin prolongs bleeding time, it's contraindicated in hemophilia and other bleeding disorders. Aspirin shouldn't be given with anticoagulants or other ulcerogenic drugs, such as corticosteroids, and should also be avoided in patients scheduled for surgery within 1 week. Acetaminophen is contraindicated in patients with a hypersensitivity to the drug.

Adverse reactions
Adverse reactions to salicylates primarily involve the GI tract and commonly include dyspepsia, heartburn, epigastric distress, nausea, and abdominal pain. Aspirin is usually considered the salicylate most likely to cause adverse GI reactions.

In certain sensitive patients, usually those with rhinitis, nasal polyps, and asthma (the aspirin triad), aspirin may induce bronchospasm with or without angiospasm. Aspirin also may cause adverse hematologic reactions. Chronic salicylate intoxication may cause tinnitus, hearing loss, dim vision, headache, dizziness, confusion, lassitude, drowsiness, sweating, hepatotoxicity, renal damage, hyperventilation, and tachycardia.

Adverse reactions associated with the NSAIDs include GI irritation, hepatotoxicity, increased bleeding time, nephrotoxicity, and headache. GI irritation and bleeding occur more commonly with NSAIDs (except perhaps for ibuprofen and naproxen) than with acetaminophen.

Acetaminophen is usually well tolerated; sensitivity reactions, including rash, angioedema, or anaphylaxis, have been reported rarely. High doses of acetaminophen are associated with hepatic necrosis, which is potentially fatal.

Care considerations
• Before giving a nonnarcotic analgesic, check the patient's drug history for a previous hypersensitivity reaction, which may indicate hypersensitivity to a related drug.
• If the patient is taking an NSAID or a salicylate, ask about any GI irritation. If it occurs, the doctor may order a mucosal protectant medication such as misoprostol, or he may substitute another drug.
• During long-term therapy, report any abnormalities in renal and liver function studies. Also monitor hematologic studies and evaluate complaints of

nausea or gastric burning. Be alert for signs of iron deficiency anemia, such as pallor, unusual fatigue, or weakness.

Home care instructions

• Instruct the patient who's taking an NSAID to immediately report rash, dyspnea, confusion, blurred vision, nausea, bloody vomitus, or black, tarry stools. These may indicate an overdose, hypersensitivity, or GI bleeding.
• Tell the patient taking an NSAID to avoid alcohol while taking the drug because it may increase the risk of GI ulcers and bleeding.
• To minimize GI upset, instruct the patient to take the drug with food or a full glass of milk. Afterward, he should remain upright for 15 to 30 minutes to reduce esophageal irritation. If he experiences gastric burning or pain, tell him to notify the doctor.
• Tell the patient who's taking acetaminophen to immediately notify the doctor about any signs of an overdose: nausea, vomiting, abdominal cramps, or diarrhea.
• Explain that some NSAIDs may cause prolonged bleeding time. Warn the patient to avoid injury, which could cause bleeding.
• Reassure the patient that tinnitus— a dose-related effect of aspirin and other salicylates—is reversible. However, if it persists, he should notify the doctor, who may reduce the dosage.
• Inform the patient taking NSAIDs that dizziness or drowsiness may occur. Warn the patient to avoid driving and other hazardous tasks that require alertness until his response to the drug is known.
• Advise the patient to take a missed dose as soon as he remembers. However, if the next dose is less than 4 hours away, he should skip the missed dose and resume his regular schedule. He should never double-dose.
• During prolonged use of any nonnarcotic analgesic, emphasize the need

for periodic blood tests to detect nephritis and hepatotoxicity.

ANALGESICS, OPIOID

Opioid (narcotic) analgesics, which include natural opium alkaloids and their derivatives and synthetic compounds, provide relief from moderate-to-severe pain.

Opioid analgesics can be classified as agonists or agonist/antagonists. Agonists, such as *morphine, codeine, hydromorphone, levorphanol, meperidine, methadone,* and *propoxyphene,* produce analgesia by binding to central nervous system (CNS) opioid receptors. Agonist/antagonists, such as *buprenorphine, butorphanol, nalbuphine,* and *pentazocine,* also produce analgesia by binding to CNS receptors. However, these drugs act as antagonists to other opioids, blocking narcotic effects and causing withdrawal symptoms in narcotic-dependent patients.

Narcotic analgesics can be given by various routes: oral, I.M., I.V., epidural, or intrathecal; the oral route is preferred for most patients. I.M. administration, though usually effective, can result in erratic absorption, especially in debilitated patients. For severe pain, I.V. administration may be chosen for its rapid onset and precise dosage control. Continuous I.V. infusion has been used successfully in some cancer patients (see the entry "Patient-controlled Analgesia").

Purpose

• To relieve acute and chronic pain by binding to CNS opioid receptor sites.

Indications

The opioid agonists may be the drugs of choice for severe chronic cancer pain. The agonist/antagonists, in contrast, have limited use in cancer because many are available only in parenteral forms. Moreover, high doses produce hallucinations and other psychotomimetic effects; in the narcotic-dependent patient, they may produce withdrawal symptoms.

Other indications for opioid analgesics include pain in acute myocardial infarction (MI), pulmonary edema, cough, and GI and urinary tract disorders. Opioid analgesics are also used as preanesthetics.

Opioid analgesics, which depress respiratory function, are contraindicated in severe respiratory depression and should be used cautiously in chronic obstructive pulmonary disease. Because they're metabolized by the liver and excreted through the kidneys, they should also be used cautiously in patients with hepatic or renal disorders. And because they increase intracranial pressure (ICP), they should be used cautiously, if at all, in head injury or in any condition that raises ICP.

Because opioid analgesics can lead to increased tolerance and physiologic and psychological dependence, they shouldn't be used for chronic pain in nonmalignant disorders.

Adverse reactions

Opioid analgesics can cause severe reactions, such as respiratory depression and increased ICP. They can also induce miosis, which, in patients with head injury, can mask pupil dilation, an important indicator of increased ICP. Other reactions include drowsiness, faintness, dizziness, palpitations, dry mouth, muscle tremor, flushing of the face and neck, hypertension, orthostatic hypotension, nausea, vomiting, sweating, constipation, and cough suppression. Prolonged use can lead to increased tolerance and physiologic and psychological dependence.

Care considerations

• Before giving an opioid analgesic, review the patient's medication regimen for use of other CNS depressants. Concurrent use of another CNS depressant enhances drowsiness, sedation, disorientation, and fear.

• During administration, check the patient's vital signs. Be alert for respiratory depression. If respiratory rate declines to 10 breaths/minute or less, call the patient's name, touch him, and instruct him to breathe deeply. If your attempts to rouse him fail or if you observe confusion or restlessness, notify the doctor and prepare to administer oxygen. If ordered, administer a narcotic antagonist, such as naloxone.

• If the patient experiences persistent nausea and vomiting during therapy with an opioid, the doctor may substitute another drug. Give the patient an antiemetic, if ordered.

• To help prevent constipation, administer a stool softener. Also provide a high-fiber diet and encourage fluids, as ordered. Regular exercise may also promote GI motility.

• Because opioid analgesics can cause postural hypotension, take precautions to avoid accidents. For example, keep the bed's side rails raised. If the patient is mobile, help him out of bed and assist with ambulation.

• Encourage the patient to practice coughing and deep-breathing exercises to promote ventilation and prevent pooling of secretions, which could lead to respiratory difficulty.

• Evaluate the effectiveness of the drug. Is the patient experiencing relief of pain? Does the patient need increased dosage because of persistent or worsening pain? Is tolerance to the drug developing? Remember that the patient should receive the smallest effective dose for the shortest time. However, opioid analgesics shouldn't be withheld or given in ineffective doses for fear of iatrogenic dependence. Psychological dependence occurs in less than 1% of hospitalized patients.

Home care instructions

• Tell the patient that the prescribed drug is most effective when taken before pain becomes intense.

• Advise the patient to consult his doctor if the drug becomes less effective in relieving pain. Warn against increasing the dose or the frequency of administration.

• Tell the patient to take a missed dose as soon as he remembers, unless it's almost time for the next dose. Warn the patient never to double-dose.

• Instruct the patient's family to notify the doctor immediately if they detect signs of an overdose: cold, clammy skin; confusion; severe drowsiness or restlessness; slow or irregular breathing; pinpoint pupils; or unconsciousness. Teach them how to maintain respirations until help arrives.

• Advise the patient to get up slowly from a bed or chair because the drug can cause postural hypotension.

• Tell the patient to eat a high-fiber diet, to drink plenty of fluids, and to take a stool softener, if prescribed.

• Warn the patient to avoid drinking alcohol because it enhances CNS depression.

• Tell the patient to contact the doctor before discontinuing the drug because a gradual dosage reduction may be necessary to avoid withdrawal symptoms.

ANESTHETICS, TOPICAL

The topical drugs *benzocaine, dibucaine, dyclonine, lidocaine, pramoxine,* and *tetracaine* anesthetize the skin and mucous membranes. They can be applied to the mucous membranes of the rectum, vagina, urethra, and bladder before invasive procedures.

Purpose

• To produce a local loss of sensation by temporarily blocking conduction of pain impulses.

Indications

Topical anesthetics provide relief from the pain caused by sunburn, minor burns, pruritus, and other dermatologic conditions. They're also used to suppress the gag reflex before endoscopy and to anesthetize the pharynx, larynx, and trachea before intubation.

Topical anesthetics are contraindicated in severe, extensive skin disorders that cause abraded or broken skin.

Adverse reactions

Topical anesthetics can cause central nervous system (CNS) and hypersensitivity reactions as well as such local reactions as contact dermatitis. They are less effective in infected areas.

Care considerations

• Before applying a topical anesthetic, ask if the patient has a history of hypersensitivity to the drug. If so, the doctor may substitute a different topical anesthetic.

• After applying the anesthetic, observe the patient for CNS reactions, such as drowsiness, blurred vision, or seizures. Report such reactions to the doctor.

Home care instructions

• Emphasize the importance of applying the topical anesthetic correctly to avoid toxic effects.

• Inform the patient using viscous lidocaine that it may make swallowing difficult. As a result, he should avoid eating or drinking for 1 hour after application to prevent aspiration and minimize the risk of bite trauma to the oral mucosa.

• Advise the patient to discontinue using the drug and to contact the doctor if his condition worsens; if it doesn't improve in several days; or if a rash, swelling, or an infection occurs.

ANGIOPLASTY, PERCUTANEOUS TRANSLUMINAL CORONARY

Percutaneous transluminal coronary angioplasty (PTCA), a method of revascularization, is an alternative to coronary artery bypass surgery. PTCA was first performed in 1977 and has rapidly become the procedure of choice for improving coronary perfusion in many patients with coronary artery disease (CAD). This procedure, which uses a tiny balloon catheter to dilate a narrowed coronary artery, is favored over bypass surgery in certain subsets of patients. Perhaps more than 50% of 300,000 PTCAs performed annually in the United States are performed for multivessel disease. The usual initial success rate is approximately 90% to 95%. In patients with single-vessel disease or refractory angina, PTCA has been proven to provide greater relief of symptoms than medical therapy. However, PTCA's effect on long-term survival and how it compares with coronary artery bypass grafting (CABG) and other revascularization methods are still unknown. Now, fewer than about 4% of PTCA patients require emergency coronary artery bypass surgery.

A recent advance—laser angioplasty—makes it likely that the number of patients who undergo angioplasty will continue to rise (see *Laser angioplasty*, page 24).

Major limitations of PTCA are a 1% to 4% rate of acute complications, including coronary dissection, acute vessel closure, myocardial infarction (MI), emergent CABG, and a 30% to 50% rate of re-stenosis 3 to 6 months after the procedure.

Recently, PTCA has also emerged as an alternative to peripheral bypass surgery for many patients with peripheral vascular disease of the lower extremities.

Purpose

• To improve coronary blood flow by enlarging the lumens of diseased coronary arteries.

Indications

PTCA is indicated for treatment of single and multivessel CAD, of CAD in which there are multiple lesions (more than one occlusion in a single artery), and of occlusions in saphenous grafts placed to bypass coronary arteries. PTCA is usually reserved for lesions with at least 60% narrowing of the vessel lumen diameter.

PTCA is also indicated as emergency therapy during the first 12 hours after the onset of pain in an MI, especially when thrombolytic therapy is contraindicated and during acute episodes of unstable angina.

PTCA is most effective in vessels with discrete areas of occlusion and is most suitable for lesions that are concentric, nonangulated, nonthrombotic, and accessible. PTCA is least effective for lesions that are long, calcified, ostial, tortuous, angulated, or bifurcated and is not recommended for vessels with highly diffused disease. Unless a cardiac support pump is available, PTCA should not be used to treat left main stem coronary artery stenosis because the associated risk of cardiovascular collapse is high. PTCA is rarely used in arteries that have been totally occluded for an extended period because such old lesions are tough and rigid and therefore difficult to dilate with the balloon. PTCA is also not recommended for long segmental lesions or orificial coronary stenosis.

Procedure

PTCA is performed in the cardiac catheterization laboratory under local anesthesia. The patient is awake but sedated and must lie flat on a hard ta-

Laser angioplasty

Laser angioplasty shows great potential for vaporizing arterial occlusion and may also be used to remove calcified plaques. Newer lasers that deliver energy in brief pulses have helped solve the problem of thermal or acoustic damage to local tissues. With laser angioplasty, which uses a pulsed beam, it's easier for doctors to dispatch the blockage without destroying the vessel wall.

Laser angioplasty, with other percutaneous techniques for coronary revascularization, allows cardiologists to treat lesions of complex morphology without the hazards of open-heart coronary artery bypass surgery. Laser angioplasty is most effective for treating diffuse disease; long, calcified, or ostial lesions; totally occluded vessels; and diseased saphenous vein grafts. Laser angioplasty is not effective against thrombotic lesions.

To perform the procedure, the doctor threads a laser-containing catheter into the diseased artery. When the catheter nears the occlusion, the doctor rotates the catheter, advancing it until the occlusion is destroyed. This procedure takes about 1 hour and requires only local anesthesia. For optimal results, most patients (about 50% to 70%) also undergo balloon dilatation both before and after laser angioplasty.

Laser angioplasty is complicated by a higher rate of coronary dissection and re-stenosis than occurs following balloon percutaneous transluminal coronary angioplasty (PTCA). Nursing care after laser angioplasty is similar to that after PTCA. It always requires application of pressure to the insertion site for at least 20 minutes after the catheter is removed.

The cardiologist begins the procedure by cleaning and anesthetizing the catheter insertion site. The doctor then inserts a guide wire into the femoral or brachial artery, using a percutaneous approach (the brachial artery may also be used with a cutdown approach). Under fluoroscopic guidance, the doctor threads the catheter into the coronary artery, confirms the presence of the lesions by angiography (radiologic examination of blood vessels after injection of a radiopaque contrast medium into an artery or vein), and then introduces a small, double-lumen, balloon-tipped catheter through the guide wire. After positioning the balloon tip in the occluded coronary artery, he repeatedly inflates it with 0.9% sodium chloride solution and contrast medium. The inflated balloon compresses the atherosclerotic plaque against the arterial wall, thereby opening the arterial lumen.

To confirm successful PTCA, a repeat angiogram is performed and the pressure gradient across the lesion may be measured. The catheter is left in the femoral artery for up to 24 hours to provide emergency access in case coronary occlusion develops. All patients receive I.V. heparin during PTCA: a large initial bolus (usually 10,000 units), followed by a maintenance infusion that continues while the femoral access shealth is in place.

Complications

PTCA avoids many of the risks of surgery, and its incidence of serious complications has steadily declined, but PTCA is not without risk. The most dangerous complication is arterial dissection during dilatation, which can lead to coronary artery rupture, cardiac tamponade, myocardial ischemia, MI, or death. Because of the procedure's potentially serious complications, the surgical team should be available in case coronary artery bypass becomes necessary.

ble during this time. He may be asked to take deep breaths to allow visualization of the radiopaque balloon catheter. The procedure takes about 1 to 4 hours to complete.

The most common complication of PTCA is acute closure that can occur soon after the procedure or re-stenosis that can occur up to 6 months later. Acute closure is the sudden narrowing of the vessel due to thrombotic reocclusion within 24 to 48 hours after PTCA. Re-stenosis is the subacute narrowing of the vessel by fibromuscular hyperplasia that occurs within 3 to 6 months after PTCA. Late re-stenosis affects up to half of PTCA patients. However, if angioplasty is repeated to treat re-stenosis, long-term success occurs in about 85% of cases.

Other complications of PTCA include coronary artery spasm, bleeding, allergic reactions to the contrast medium, and arrhythmias during catheter manipulation. MI and local reactions at the vascular access site may also occur. Infrequently, thrombi may embolize and cause a cerebrovascular accident.

Care considerations

Before the procedure

• Be sure the patient understands the procedure and the care required. He should expect to experience a hot, flushing sensation or transient nausea when the contrast medium is injected.
• All patients without allergy or other contraindications to aspirin should receive pretreatment with aspirin, which decreases the rate of acute closure after PTCA.
• Tell the patient to expect chest discomfort or pain for 1 to 3 minutes while the balloon is inflated within the coronary artery.
• Check the patient's history for allergies; if he's had allergic reactions to shellfish, iodine, or contrast medium, notify the doctor.
• Restrict the patient's food and fluid intake for at least 6 hours before PTCA.
• Palpate the bilateral distal pulses (usually the dorsalis pedis or posterior tibial pulses) and mark them with indelible ink so that you can locate them later.

After the procedure

• The patient is sent to the intensive care unit or recovery area for monitoring. He may receive I.V. heparin or nitroglycerin.
• For the 1st hour, monitor blood pressure, heart rate and rhythm, and respirations every 15 minutes. Also assess peripheral pulses distal to the catheter insertion site. If pulses are difficult to palpate because of the size of the arterial catheter, use a Doppler ultrasound stethoscope to hear them. Notify the doctor if pulses are absent.
• The patient will receive I.V. fluids to promote excretion of contrast medium and should therefore be monitored for signs of fluid overload.
• After the arterial catheter is removed (usually 6 to 24 hours after the procedure), apply direct pressure to the insertion site for 30 minutes or until the bleeding stops. Then apply a pressure dressing to avoid bleeding or hematoma.
• Commonly, cardiac enzymes (creatine phosphokinase [CPK] and lactate dehydrogenase [LDH]) are serially monitored for evidence of MI.

Home care instructions

• Instruct the patient to notify the doctor of any bleeding or bruising at the arterial puncture site.
• Explain the necessity of taking prescribed medications, and ensure that the patient understands their intended effects.
• Tell the patient to resume normal activity. Most patients experience increased exercise tolerance.
• Instruct the patient to return for medical follow-up, particularly if anginal symptoms recur.

ANGIOTENSIN-CONVERTING ENZYME INHIBITORS

The newest class of antihypertensive drugs, angiotensin-converting enzyme (ACE) inhibitors have rapidly gained popularity among clinicians, mainly for treatment of hypertension. These drugs include *captopril, enalapril, lisinopril,* and *ramipril.* However, because ACE inhibitors can cause severe adverse effects, they're generally reserved for patients who experience intolerable reactions from other antihypertensive drugs or fail to respond to them.

Purpose

• To lower blood pressure by decreasing arterial resistance and afterload, which reduces cardiac workload, and by curtailing aldosterone secretion, which reduces fluid retention.

Indications

ACE inhibitors are used alone or in combination with other drugs—especially thiazide diuretics—as the first step of antihypertensive therapy in patients with normal renal function. Captopril is also used for severe congestive heart failure in patients who don't respond to digitalis glycosides and diuretics.

ACE inhibitors are contraindicated in patients with impaired renal function. They should be used cautiously in patients with immune disorders (especially systemic lupus erythematosus) or immunosuppression because neutropenia may develop several weeks after therapy begins. ACE inhibitors should also be given cautiously to patients with volume depletion or severe hyponatremia because they can cause severe hypotension.

Adverse reactions

The most common adverse reactions to ACE inhibitors include headache, tachycardia, dysgeusia, and orthostatic hypotension. Most of these dissipate after a few days to weeks of therapy. Other adverse reactions include allergic reactions, angioedema, proteinuria, hyperkalemia, and a persistent, nonproductive cough.

Care considerations

• Before starting ACE inhibitor therapy, evaluate the results of hematologic and renal and liver function tests. If tests show abnormalities such as proteinuria or an elevated white blood cell (WBC) count, the doctor may need to reconsider the desirability of ACE inhibitor therapy.

• Check the patient's drug regimen for possible interactions. For example, using ACE inhibitors with other antihypertensives, ganglionic blocking agents, nitroglycerin, or probenecid increases the effects of ACE inhibitors and may cause additive hypotension, requiring blood pressure monitoring.

• Potassium-sparing diuretics and potassium supplements, which increase renin activity and decrease aldosterone secretion, may cause hyperkalemia when given in combination with ACE inhibitors. When combining these drugs, monitor the patient's serum potassium levels. Nonsteroidal anti-inflammatory drugs and salicylates can decrease the antihypertensive effect of ACE inhibitors; patients taking these drugs may require increased dosages of ACE inhibitors.

• If the patient is taking a diuretic or adhering to a sodium-restricted diet, watch for a precipitous drop in blood pressure about 3 hours after the initial dose of an ACE inhibitor. If this occurs, place the patient in a supine position and infuse 0.9% sodium chloride solution, as ordered.

• Monitor the patient's pulse rate and blood pressure, and frequently assess

for edema. Also check WBC count and differential periodically for changes.
• After several weeks of therapy, watch for neutropenia, marked by mild symptoms of infection.

Home care instructions
• Warn the patient never to interrupt or discontinue his prescribed medication regimen without medical approval.
• Tell the patient to take a missed dose as soon as possible, but never to double-dose.
• Because food interferes with absorption, instruct the patient to take the drug on an empty stomach or 1 hour before meals.
• Tell the patient to watch for and immediately report any signs of infection (such as fever and sore throat) or swollen hands or feet.
• Instruct the patient to report excessive sweating, vomiting, or diarrhea. Explain that the resultant volume deficit may lead to severe hypotension.
• Teach the patient to minimize the risk of dizziness or fainting by rising slowly from a sitting or lying position.
• Warn the patient to avoid potassium-containing salt substitutes and to limit intake of foods with a high potassium content, such as bananas.

ANTACIDS

Antacids can be divided into two classes: nonsystemic and systemic. Nonsystemic antacids consist of various combinations of aluminum, calcium, and magnesium salts; the most commonly used ones include *calcium carbonate, magnesium hydrochloride,* and *aluminum hydroxide.* All antacids work by binding with hydrogen ions in the gastric contents, resulting in an elevation of gastric pH. Nonsystemic antacids form salts in the GI tract and are only minimally absorbed. Systemic antacids, such as *sodium bicarbonate,* are absorbed and result in systemic alkalosis.

Antacids come in powder, tablet, and liquid forms. After ingestion, antacids begin to act almost immediately and exert their effects for 1 to 3 hours, depending on whether they were taken with food or another medication. They're distributed throughout the GI tract and are eliminated primarily in the feces.

Purpose
• To relieve GI upset, including dyspepsia and heartburn
• To help heal gastric ulcers
• To strengthen the mucosal barrier
• To help increase esophageal sphincter tone.

Indications
Antacids may be used to treat gastric hyperacidity, duodenal and gastric ulcers, gastric hypersecretory conditions, Zollinger-Ellison syndrome, systemic mastocytosis, gastroesophageal reflux, and stress-related upper GI mucosal damage.

Contraindications vary with the specific antacid, but all antacids are contraindicated in patients with any symptoms of undiagnosed GI or rectal bleeding, intestinal obstruction, or appendicitis. Calcium-containing antacids should not be used by patients with hypercalcemia, constipation, hemorrhoids, hypoparathyroidism, or sarcoidosis. Aluminum-containing antacids should not be used by patients with constipation, chronic diarrhea, gastric outlet obstruction, or hemorrhoids. Magaldrate should not be used by patients with severe renal function impairment, ulcerative colitis, colostomy, diverticulitis or ileostomy, chronic diarrhea, or gastric outlet obstruction. Magnesium-containing antacids are contraindicated in patients with severe renal impairment, ulcerative colitis, colostomy, diverticulitis, ileostomy, or chronic diarrhea. Sodium bicarbonate-containing antacids are contraindicated in patients with renal or hepatic impairment, congestive heart failure, edema, and toxemia of pregnancy.

Adverse reactions

Magnesium-containing antacids, which have a laxative effect, may cause diarrhea. In patients with renal failure, they may cause hypermagnesemia.

Aluminum-containing antacids can cause constipation, which may lead to intestinal obstruction. They may also cause aluminum intoxication, osteomalacia, and hypophosphatemia.

Calcium carbonate, magaldrate, sodium bicarbonate, and magnesium oxide may cause rebound hyperacidity and milk-alkali syndrome.

Sodium bicarbonate commonly causes gastric distention and flatulence. Metabolic acidosis may occur when it's given in large doses.

Care considerations

• Evaluate the patient's bowel function by recording the amount and consistency of stools. Notify the doctor of constipation or diarrhea; he may change the drug or reduce the dosage.
• During long-term therapy with aluminum-containing antacids, regularly monitor the patient's serum phosphorus levels and be alert for signs of hypophosphatemia, such as anorexia, weakness, and malaise.
• Monitor the patient taking calcium- or magnesium-containing antacids for signs of hypercalcemia or hypermagnesemia, as appropriate. Be especially aware of these imbalances in patients with impaired renal function.
• If the patient is taking a calcium-containing antacid or sodium bicarbonate, check for early symptoms of milk-alkali syndrome: headache, confusion, and anorexia. Monitor blood urea nitrogen, serum calcium, and creatinine for elevated levels.

• Check for possible interactions with antacids. Aluminum-, calcium-, or magnesium-containing antacids can form insoluble complexes with many drugs, such as quinolones or tetracyclines, thereby decreasing their bioavailability. Aluminum-containing antacids delay gastric emptying and slow the absorption of such drugs as indomethacin, warfarin, isoniazid, and barbiturates. Magnesium-containing antacids decrease the bioavailability of digoxin and can potentiate the anticoagulant activity of dicumarol. All antacids can cause the premature release of enteric-coated drugs in the GI tract; to prevent this, separate doses of antacids and enteric-coated drugs by at least 2 hours.

Home care instructions

• If the patient is taking a liquid antacid, instruct him to shake the suspension thoroughly before pouring. If he's taking antacid tablets, tell him to chew each tablet well before swallowing and to follow the dose with a full glass of water.
• Warn the patient not to take antacids indiscriminately and not to switch brands without his doctor's advice.
• Instruct the patient to keep a record of his bowel movements and to report any changes in his normal pattern.
• Advise the patient not to take antacids within 2 hours of taking any other medication.

ANTIADRENERGICS

The centrally and peripherally acting antiadrenergics include *clonidine, guanethidine, methyldopa, prazosin, terazosin,* and the *reserpine derivatives.* These drugs inhibit the effects of postganglionic sympathetic nerves to reduce the release of norepinephrine.

Purpose

• To lower blood pressure by blocking adrenergic stimulation of blood vessels.

Indications

Antiadrenergics are used in the treatment of hypertension. For maintenance therapy, these drugs pose the same obstacle to patient compliance as many other antihypertensives: their common adverse reactions may seem worse than living with untreated hypertension. The reserpine derivatives especially can produce more serious adverse effects. Many of these drugs interact with other prescribed or over-the-counter medications, making safe long-term therapy difficult. Close patient monitoring is required at the start of therapy to establish the correct dosage. (See *Comparing antiadrenergics*, pages 30 and 31, for further information.)

Adverse reactions

Common adverse reactions associated with these drugs include fatigue and drowsiness. The reserpine derivatives can cause mental depression. Guanethidine may cause dizziness, weakness, syncope, orthostatic hypotension, bradycardia, congestive heart failure, arrhythmias, nasal congestion, diarrhea, edema, weight gain, and inhibition of ejaculation.

Prazosin and terazosin commonly cause orthostatic hypotension and syncope when therapy begins (the "first-dose" effect). They may also cause weakness, tachycardia, and nasal congestion.

Methyldopa may cause hemolytic anemia, reversible granulocytopenia, sedation, dizziness, decreased mental acuity, orthostatic hypotension, dry mouth, nasal congestion, and hepatic necrosis.

Care considerations

• When the patient begins therapy, monitor his response to the drug and its dosage. Check for common adverse reactions.
• To check for postural hypotension, take the blood pressure while the patient is lying down and again after he's been standing for at least 10 minutes. (The doctor will also probably evaluate blood pressure after exercise.) Ideally, standing blood pressure will be in the normal range, and the patient won't experience any faintness, dizziness, fatigue, or weakness.
• Check the patient's legs and feet for edema caused by fluid retention.
• Review the patient's medications for possible interactions.

Home care instructions

• Emphasize the importance of taking the prescribed medication despite the absence of symptoms. Reassure the patient that adverse reactions usually diminish within 4 to 6 weeks; if they persist, he should contact the doctor for adjustment of dosage. Warn the patient not to discontinue the drug without the doctor's approval.
• To minimize postural hypotension, tell the patient to rise slowly from a lying or standing position, to avoid prolonged standing in one position, to use an air conditioner in hot weather, and to avoid alcohol, hot showers, and hot baths. Teach the patient to lie down or place his head between his knees if he feels dizzy, weak, or faint.
• Inform the patient that the drug may cause drowsiness and nasal congestion.
• To relieve dry mouth, suggest hard sugarless candy, ice chips, chewing gum, or frequent rinsing of his mouth with water. Also recommend using a soft toothbrush and waxed dental floss. The patient who wears dentures can remove them and rinse them two or three times a day to keep the gums moistened, but he should avoid mouthwashes containing alcohol because they can increase mouth dryness.
• Advise the patient to tell his dentist about his medication regimen because

Comparing antiadrenergics

clonidine

Indications
For essential, renal, and malignant hypertension

Interactions
Alcohol, barbiturates, and other sedatives increase hypotensive effects; monoamine oxidase (MAO) inhibitors, tolazoline, and tricyclic antidepressants reduce these effects. Paradoxical hypertension may occur with propranolol.

Special considerations
- Check blood pressure and pulse frequently, especially during dosage adjustment.
- Teach patient ways to avoid postural hypotension. Monitor for dry mouth, sedation, constipation, and signs of depression.
- Withdraw drug slowly to prevent rebound hypertension.

guanethidine

Indications
For moderate or severe hypertension

Interactions
Alcohol, levodopa, rauwolfia derivatives, and diuretics enhance hypotensive effects; tricyclic antidepressants, MAO inhibitors, oral contraceptives, phenothiazines, dopamine, and catecholamines diminish these effects. Sympathomimetics in over-the-counter (OTC) cough and cold products may bring on hypertension.

Special considerations
- Contraindicated in pheochromocytoma.
- Teach patient ways to minimize postural hypotension.
- Drug can cause transient urine retention; tell patient to report urinary hesitancy.
- Discontinue drug 2 to 3 days before elective surgery to reduce risk of vascular collapse during anesthesia.
- Warn patient to avoid OTC cough and cold products.

methyldopa

Indications
For sustained mild-to-severe hypertension

Interactions
Tricyclic antidepressants, phenothiazines, amphetamines, and norepinephrine may cause hypertensive effects. Sympathomimetics in OTC cough and cold preparations may produce similar effects.

Special considerations
- Contraindicated in renal disease.
- Draw serum sample before treatment begins to provide baseline hematologic status. Continue to monitor during therapy to detect hemolytic anemia.
- Watch for fever and hepatic changes, which could indicate a hypersensitivity reaction; if they occur, stop drug and call doctor.
- Monitor patient for sedative effects and signs of postural hypotension.
- Watch for signs of fluid retention. Give a diuretic, if ordered.
- Warn patient to avoid OTC cough and cold products.

Comparing antiadrenergics *(continued)*

prazosin, terazosin

Indications
For mild or moderate hypotension

Interactions
Postural hypotension and syncope may occur after the first few doses ("first dose" effect). Beta blockers may enhance these adverse effects. Coadministration of verapamil or nifedipine may produce an acute hypotensive effect.

Special considerations
• Monitor patient for signs of postural hypotension and syncope.
• Tell patient to use caution when driving or operating heavy machinery.
• Instruct patient to take the first dose at bedtime.
• Reduce dosage and then retitrate when adding a diuretic or other antihypertensive drug.

reserpine derivatives

Indications
For mild or moderate hypertension

Interactions
MAO inhibitors may cause excitability and hypertension. Catecholamines may prolong reserpine's action.

Special considerations
• Because of their adverse effects, reserpine derivatives are not first-line drugs, but they are used when cost is a factor. These drugs are inexpensive.
• Monitor patient for drug-induced depression. Look for anorexia, insomnia, and despondency; stop drug and notify doctor if symptoms occur. Depression can persist for months after drug discontinuation.
• Give drug with food or milk to decrease GI upset.
• Monitor for sedative effects.
• Watch for signs of fluid retention.
• Discontinue drug 2 to 3 weeks before elective surgery to reduce risk of vascular collapse during anesthesia.

dry mouth can promote tooth demineralization.
• Advise the patient to watch for signs of fluid retention, such as swollen ankles, and to weigh himself daily at the same time and on the same scale, and to notify his doctor of a weight gain of 3 lb (1.4 kg) or more. If the doctor has recommended a salt-restricted diet, explain how sodium contributes to hypertension and fluid retention.

ANTIARRHYTHMICS

Typically the treatment of choice for arrhythmias, these drugs fall into one of four major classes, each based on its electrophysiological effects on the heart or on its mechanism of action.
• Class I drugs act by sodium channel blockade, similarly to local anesthetics. Class I drugs have been further classified based on their ability to depress the rate of membrane depolar-

(Text continues on page 37.)

Comparing antiarrhythmics

DRUG AND INDICATIONS	SPECIAL CONSIDERATIONS
Class IA	
disopyramide Premature ventricular contractions (PVCs) and ventricular tachycardia	• Contraindicated in cardiogenic shock and second- or third-degree heart block. • Use cautiously in congestive heart failure (CHF), renal or hepatic disease or impairment, myasthenia gravis, acute angle-closure glaucoma, and conduction abnormalities. • Check apical pulse before administering; report a rate under 60 beats/minute or over 120 beats/minute. • Watch for hypotension, edema, and decreased urine output. • Increase patient's fiber and fluid intake to prevent constipation. • Report depression, fatigue, weakness, dizziness, or agitation.
moricizine hydrochloride Life-threatening arrhythmias	• Contraindicated in patients with preexisting second- or third-degree atrioventricular (AV) block; right bundle-branch block when associated with left hemiblock unless a pacemaker is present; cardiogenic shock; and in patients hypersensitive to the drug. Administer with extreme caution, if at all, to patients with severe hepatic deficiency and with extreme caution to patients with sick sinus syndrome. • Monitor serum electrolyte studies and electrocardiogram (ECG). Hypokalemia or hyperkalemia and hypomagnesemia may alter the effects of the drug. • Observe for adverse reactions, including dizziness, headache, fatigue, anxiety, blurred vision, asthenia, nervousness, paresthesia, sleep disorders, proarrhythmic events, ECG abnormalities (conduction defect, sinus pause, junctional rhythm, or AV block), CHF, palpitations, sustained ventricular tachycardia, chest pain, sinus bradycardia, sinus arrest, nausea, vomiting, GI upset, abdominal pain, dyspepsia, diarrhea, and dry mouth. • Observe for interactions. Cimetidine increases plasma levels and decreases clearance of moricizine. The PR interval lengthens when moricizine is administered with propranolol and digoxin. When administered with theophylline, theophylline clearance is increased and plasma levels are reduced.
procainamide Atrial tachycardia, junctional tachycardia, PVCs, and ventricular tachycardia	• Contraindicated in complete AV block. • Watch for severe transient hypotension during I.V. administration; monitor ECG and blood pressure continuously. • Check for possible interactions. Amiodarone, cimetidine, propranolol, quinidine, ranitidine, sodium bicarbonate, or trimethoprim may increase blood levels of the drug. Watch for toxicity. • Patients taking procainamide may experience enhanced muscle relaxation when given succinylcholine. • Rash, itching, or pain with breathing may indicate lupuslike reaction or allergy.

Comparing antiarrhythmics *(continued)*

DRUG AND INDICATIONS	SPECIAL CONSIDERATIONS

Class IA *(continued)*

quinidine
Atrial tachycardia

- Contraindicated in digitalis toxicity when AV conduction is grossly impaired, unless the patient has a pacemaker.
- Use with caution in myasthenia gravis.
- I.V. route can cause severe cardiovascular reactions.
- Check for possible interactions. Acetazolamide, antacids, or sodium bicarbonate may raise quinidine blood levels; barbiturates, phenytoin, rifampin, and nifedipine decrease quinidine's effect. Verapamil may cause hypotension; monitor blood pressure.
- Monitor complete blood count for signs of hemolytic anemia, thrombocytopenia, and agranulocytosis.
- Watch for vertigo, headache, and light-headedness. Restrict ambulation if necessary; report symptoms.
- Call doctor if signs of toxicity — diarrhea, nausea, fever, cinchonism, abnormal liver function tests, or tinnitus — develop.
- Watch for PVCs, severe hypotension, sinoatrial (SA) or AV block, ventricular fibrillation, tachycardia, aggravation of CHF, and ECG changes (especially widening of QRS complex, notched P waves, widened Q-T interval, and ST-segment depression).

Class IB

lidocaine
Ventricular fibrillation, ventricular tachycardia, and PVCs

- Given only in hospital. Continuous monitoring is required.
- Contraindicated in patients with hypersensitivity to amide-type local anesthetics, Stokes-Adams syndrome, or heart block. Use cautiously in patients with Wolff-Parkinson-White syndrome, CHF, or renal or hepatic impairment.
- Compare ECGs with baseline throughout therapy.
- Watch for signs of overdose, such as blurred or double vision, nausea, vomiting, tinnitus, mental status changes, and tremors; call doctor if they occur. Monitor blood levels.

mexiletine
PVCs and ventricular tachycardia

- Monitor pulse rate and rhythm and ECGs for worsening of arrhythmias; drug has paradoxical action in some patients. Also watch for hypotension, heart block, and torsade de pointes.
- Watch for and report central nervous system (CNS), musculoskeletal, and visual disturbances.

phenytoin
Digitalis glycoside-induced arrhythmias

- Contraindicated in patients with phenacemide or hydantoin hypersensitivity, bradycardia, SA or AV block, or Stokes-Adams syndrome. Use cautiously in presence of hepatic or renal dysfunction, hypotension, myocardial insufficiency, or respiratory depression; in elderly or debilitated patients; and in those receiving other hydantoin derivatives.

(continued)

Comparing antiarrhythmics *(continued)*

DRUG AND INDICATIONS	SPECIAL CONSIDERATIONS

Class IB *(continued)*

phenytoin *(continued)*

- Watch for interactions: Phenytoin's effects are diminished by alcohol, antacids, antihistamines, barbiturates, antineoplastics, CNS depressants, oxacillin, and reserpine. They are increased by aspirin, anticoagulants, anticonvulsants, cimetidine, phenothiazines, and sulfonamides. Lidocaine and propranolol cause additive cardiac depressant effects.
- To prevent precipitation of drug, do not mix with other drugs or solutions. Some clinicians may infuse phenytoin after mixing in 0.9% sodium chloride solution. Always use an in-line filter.
- To prevent "purple glove syndrome," do not administer phenytoin by I.V. push into veins in the patient's hand.
- To minimize nausea, give divided doses with or after meals, but don't administer phenytoin with tube feedings; decreased absorption may result.
- Adverse reactions include ventricular fibrillation, CNS effects (such as slurred speech and confusion), blood dyscrasias, hypocalcemia, toxic hepatitis, exfoliative dermatitis, hirsutism, and toxic epidermal necrolysis.

tocainide
PVCs and ventricular tachycardia

- Tocainide is similar to lidocaine but may be given orally. Contraindicated in patients who are hypersensitive to lidocaine or amide-type local anesthetics.
- Watch for interactions. Allopurinol increases blood levels of tocainide; propranolol may cause paranoia.
- See also special considerations for lidocaine.

Class IC

flecainide
Atrial and ventricular tachycardia and Wolff-Parkinson-White syndrome

- Assess for adverse reactions, including transient blurred vision, dizziness, and light-headedness; dosage may need adjustment.
- When given with propranolol, expect a slight increase in blood levels of both drugs.

propafenone hydrochloride
Life-threatening ventricular arrhythmias, such as episodic ventricular tachycardia

- Contraindicated in severe or uncontrolled CHF; cardiogenic shock; SA, AV, or intraventricular disorders of impulse conduction; sinus node dysfunction in the absence of pacemaker; severe bradycardia (50 beats/minute or less); marked hypotension; bronchospastic disorders; severe obstructive pulmonary disease; severe electrolyte imbalance; severe hepatic failure; and known hypersensitivity to the drug.
- Observe for adverse reactions, including anorexia, anxiety, ataxia, dizziness, angina, atrial fibrillation, bradycardia, bundle-branch heart block, CHF, edema, hypotension, increased

Comparing antiarrhythmics *(continued)*

DRUG AND INDICATIONS	SPECIAL CONSIDERATIONS

Class IC *(continued)*

propafenone hydrochloride *(continued)*

QRS duration, first-degree AV block, palpitations and intraventricular conduction delay, abdominal pain or cramps, constipation, diarrhea, flatulence, and nausea and vomiting.
- Check for possible interactions. When used with other antiarrhythmics, there is an increased potential for CHF. Cimetidine decreases the metabolism of propafenone. Propafenone may increase the serum levels of digitalis glycosides and oral anticoagulants. Propafenone slows the metabolism of propranolol and metoprolol. Quinidine slows the metabolism of propafenone.
- Monitor ECG and serum digoxin levels.
- Administer drug with food to minimize adverse GI reactions.

Class II

acebutolol
Same as propranolol; especially used for supraventricular arrhythmias, ventricular tachycardias, and the control and correction of PVCs

- Contraindicated in patients with AV block; may cause asystole.
- Watch for allergic reaction, bradycardia, breathing difficulty (especially in patients with predisposition to bronchospasm), and signs of CHF.
- Elderly patients may have increased or decreased sensitivity to the effects of the usual adult dose. In these patients, doses should total no more than 800 mg.
- Reduced dosage in patients with renal impairment.

esmolol
Rapid and short-term control of ventricular rate in atrial fibrillation or atrial flutter in perioperative, postoperative, or other emergency situations and in noncompensatory sinus tachycardia requiring intervention

- Contraindicated in overt cardiac failure, cardiogenic shock, second- or third-degree AV block, and sinus bradycardia with a heart rate less than 45 beats/minute.
- Watch for adverse reactions, including hypotension, confusion, redness or swelling at injection site, reduced peripheral circulation, drowsiness, flushing, pale skin, headache, nausea, and vomiting.
- Do not use with oral antidiabetic agents, insulin, hypotension-producing medications, monoamine oxidase inhibitors, phenytoin, reserpine, sympathomimetics, xanthines, and nondepolarizing neuromuscular blocking agents.
- Monitor blood pressure, ECG, and heart rate.

propranolol
Atrial fibrillation, atrial tachycardia, ventricular tachycardia, and Wolff-Parkinson-White syndrome

- Contraindicated in patients with AV block; may cause asystole.
- When Wolff-Parkinson-White syndrome is complicated by atrial fibrillation, propranolol may worsen arrhythmias; monitor ECGs.
- Watch for CHF, bronchospasm, hypotension, and bradycardia.

(continued)

Comparing antiarrhythmics (continued)

DRUG AND INDICATIONS	SPECIAL CONSIDERATIONS

Class III

amiodarone
Atrial fibrillation, atrial flutter, atrial tachycardia, PVCs, ventricular tachycardia, and Wolff-Parkinson-White syndrome

- Often effective for arrhythmias resistant to other drug therapy; however, adverse effects limit its use. Reactions are more prevalent at high doses; they disappear gradually after drug is discontinued but may linger for as long as 4 months. Photosensitivity is the most common one — recommend sunscreen. Other reactions include corneal microdeposits, altered liver and thyroid function, pneumonitis, and pulmonary fibrosis (most prevalent in patients taking more than 600 mg daily).
- To prevent nausea, divide loading dosage into three doses and give with meals. If necessary, divide maintenance dosage into two doses and give with meals.
- Watch for interactions: Bradycardia may occur with beta blockers, lidocaine, and calcium channel blockers.

bretylium
PVCs, ventricular fibrillation, and ventricular tachycardia

- Severe postural hypotension, the most common adverse reaction, limits drug use to emergencies in which immediate control of life-threatening arrhythmias is required and in which monitoring and resuscitation equipment is at hand. Contraindicated in digitalis glycoside toxicity. Monitor blood pressure, heart rate, and rhythm frequently; notify doctor of any significant change.
- To minimize postural hypotension, keep patient supine until tolerance develops and avoid sudden postural changes while patient is receiving bretylium. If patient's supine diastolic pressure falls below 75 mm Hg, administer prescribed norepinephrine, dopamine, or volume expanders.
- Watch for potentiation of antihypertensive medications.
- For ventricular fibrillation, give I.V. injections as rapidly as possible. Follow dosage directions carefully to minimize GI effects.
- When giving bretylium I.M., rotate injection sites to prevent tissue damage and inject no more than 5 ml at any one site.

Class IV

verapamil
Atrial fibrillation, atrial flutter, atrial tachyarrhythmias, angina pectoris, and hypertension

- Contraindicated in sick sinus syndrome, AV conduction disturbances, cardiogenic shock, and advanced CHF (unless it's secondary to atrial tachyarrhythmias).
- Not usually effective against ventricular arrhythmias but may slow ventricular response to atrial fibrillation or flutter.

Using atropine as an antiarrhythmic

Atropine — an alkaloid found in the deadly nightshade plant — is a drug of many faces. It's used as an adjunct to anesthesia; as an antispasmodic, bronchodilator, and mydriatic; and, ironically, as an antidote for certain types of poisoning. In cardiac care, atropine is given I.V., usually to treat bradycardia, escape rhythms, and heart block accompanying acute myocardial infarction (MI).

Atropine is so versatile because it blocks parasympathetic effects throughout the body. In the heart, it blocks the action of acetylcholine on parasympathetic receptors, thereby increasing heart rate, conduction velocity, and force of contraction. In addition to its use in MI, atropine often successfully reverses first-degree atrioventricular (AV) block and Mobitz I block, two arrhythmias that are associated with increased vagal tone. (Mobitz II block, by contrast, usually isn't related to vagal tone and therefore doesn't respond to atropine.) Atropine can sometimes control complete AV block, but a temporary or permanent pacemaker commonly offers a better solution. Finally, atropine is often used with epinephrine and intubation to treat asystole.

Administering atropine

Atropine is usually given rapidly to a cardiac patient for two reasons. First, it's commonly given in an emergency when every second counts. But a less obvious reason for infusing the drug rapidly is to overcome a paradoxical effect: Small doses may briefly lower rather than raise heart rate, probably as a result of central vagal stimulation. Although this effect is reversed once peripheral cholinergic blocking occurs, it can be life-threatening in a patient with bradycardia.

To a certain extent, giving atropine to a patient who has suffered an MI is a calculated risk; the drug may cause arrhythmias (including ventricular tachycardia and fibrillation) leading to myocardial ischemia, hypertension, or hypotension. And in many cases, differentiating the drug's effects from underlying disease is difficult, even impossible.

Other adverse reactions are less serious and subside when the drug is withdrawn; these include headache, drowsiness, depression, confusion, flushed dry skin, dry mouth, urine retention, blurred vision, photophobia, eye pain, and conjunctivitis.

---

ization and to slow membrane repolarization. For example, class IA drugs (*quinidine, procainamide, disopyramide,* and *moricizine*) moderately depress phase 0 depolarization, slow conduction, and prolong repolarization. Class IB drugs (*lidocaine, mexiletine, phenytoin,* and *tocainide*) minimally affect phase 0 depolarization and conduction, but usually shorten repolarization. Class IC drugs (*flecainide* and *propafenone*) markedly depress phase 0 depolarization and slow conduction, but have little effect on repolarization.

• Class II drugs are beta-adrenergic blockers and include *acebutolol, esmolol,* and *propranolol.* These bind to beta-receptor sites, blocking adrenergic stimulation of the heart.

• Class III drugs include *amiodarone* and *bretylium.* Their action is complex, but they may be thought of as drugs that prolong repolarization.

• Class IV drugs are calcium channel blockers. *Verapamil,* the only one widely used for arrhythmias, inhibits the influx of calcium into myocardial cells, then slows activity through the sinoatrial (SA) and atrioventricular (AV) nodes.

• Anticholinergics such as atropine are commonly used as antiarrhythmics but are not classified in this manner (see *Using atropine as an antiarrhythmic*). Atropine blocks vagal effects on the SA node, relieving severe nodal or sinus bradycardia and AV block and accelerating the heart rate by increasing AV conduction.

Purpose

• To treat or prevent atrial and ventricular arrhythmias, including those secondary to myocardial infarction or digitalis toxicity.

Indications

Antiarrhythmics are used to treat atrial and ventricular arrhythmias of various causes. Selecting the most effective drug and dosage, pinpointing the cause of the arrhythmia, and predicting how it will respond to a given drug is often difficult. Moreover, patients' reactions to various drugs may differ, depending on their age, condition, and other medical problems. Some may suffer severe, even life-threatening reactions, while others tolerate antiarrhythmics easily. Finally, certain antiarrhythmics have a narrow therapeutic index: The toxic dose isn't much greater than the therapeutic dose.

Contraindications to antiarrhythmic therapy depend on the type of arrhythmia and on the other drugs the patient may be taking. Digitalis glycosides, in particular, alter the effectiveness of many antiarrhythmics, and the combination of the two may cause severe complications, such as worsening of arrhythmias. Hepatic and renal insufficiency can also complicate therapy by decreasing metabolism and delaying the excretion of antiarrhythmics.

Adverse reactions

Most class I antiarrhythmics exhibit proarrhythmic effects. Therefore, all patients taking these drugs should be monitored for new or worsened arrhythmias. Drug-induced arrhythmias may be difficult to identify because they may mimic the underlying disorder. These drugs may also cause various

other reactions (see *Comparing antiarrhythmics,* pages 32 to 36, for details).

Care considerations

• When caring for a patient receiving an antiarrhythmic, regularly check pulse rate, rhythm, and blood pressure.
• Check the drug regimen for possible interactions and be alert for adverse reactions.

Home care instructions

• Warn the patient about possible cardiac complications, such as palpitations and changes in heart rate or rhythm. Instruct him to take his pulse every morning before getting out of bed and to call the doctor if the rate drops below 60 beats/minute or exceeds 100 beats/minute.
• Warn the patient about possible neurologic adverse reactions (confusion, dizziness, and fatigue), especially if he is taking amiodarone or disopyramide. Tell him to call his doctor if such symptoms occur and to avoid driving and other hazardous activities that require coordination and alertness.
• Advise the patient to report reactions, such as blurred vision, photophobia, rash, dyspnea, cough, pleuritic chest pain, fever, palpitation, dizziness, edema, or weakness.

ANTICOAGULANTS

By interrupting the normal clotting process, the anticoagulant drugs *heparin* and *warfarin* prevent or inhibit thrombus formation.

Purpose

• To prevent and treat thromboembolic disorders.

Indications

Anticoagulants help prevent and treat pulmonary emboli, deep vein thrombosis, and thrombus formation during myocardial infarction or after cardio-vascular surgery. In addition, heparin provides anticoagulant effects in patients with disseminated intravascular coagulation or atrial fibrillation and in those undergoing dialysis and cardio-pulmonary bypass procedures. Warfarin, used for rheumatic heart disease with valvular damage, may also be used for atrial arrhythmias that disrupt normal hemodynamics.

Occasionally, anticoagulants are given prophylactically in low doses after major abdominal or thoracic surgery. Most commonly, they're given to patients with a history of thromboembolism or those on prolonged bed rest to prevent venous thrombosis or pulmonary embolism.

Because anticoagulants carry a high risk of bleeding, they're usually contraindicated in patients with blood dyscrasias, open wounds, suspected intracranial hemorrhage, bacterial endocarditis, peptic ulcer disease, severe hepatic or renal disease, threatened abortion, or recent surgery involving the eye, brain, or spinal cord. In addition, warfarin is contraindicated in patients with vitamin K deficiency.

Anticoagulants should be used cautiously in female patients during menses and immediately postpartum and in patients with a drainage tube, hepatic or renal disease, alcoholism, hypertension, allergies, asthma, GI ulcers, or any other condition that increases the risk of hemorrhage.

Adverse reactions

Reactions to heparin include hepatitis, bleeding, thrombocytopenia, rashes, urticaria, hypersensitivity, and fever. Reactions to warfarin include nausea, cramps, bleeding, dermal necrosis, and fever.

Care considerations

• During heparin therapy, frequently monitor the patient's complete blood count to detect possible thrombocytopenia (which can cause arterial

thrombosis). Also regularly check the activated partial thromboplastin time (aPTT). Values that are one and one-half to two times higher than the control value indicate effective anticoagulation.

• If possible, administer I.V. heparin via an infusion pump, and check the rate frequently. If the patient is receiving a continuous infusion, you can obtain a serum sample for aPTT measurement 8 hours after therapy begins; if an intermittent infusion, obtain a sample at least 30 minutes before the next scheduled heparin dose to prevent falsely prolonged aPTT. For the same reason, be sure to obtain the sample from the unaffected arm. To minimize bleeding, apply pressure dressings over venipuncture sites and avoid I.M. injections of other drugs.

• If the patient is taking warfarin, frequently check prothrombin time (PT). Look for a PT of one and one-half to two times the control value; notify the doctor if PT exceeds two and one-half times the control, which may indicate an increased risk of bleeding. Monitor for serious adverse GI reactions, including anorexia, nausea or vomiting, diarrhea, and paralytic ileus.

• Throughout anticoagulant therapy, regularly observe the patient for bleeding gums, bruises, petechiae, epistaxis, melena, tarry stools, hematuria, or hematemesis. Notify the doctor if you detect any of these signs of bleeding; they may require adjustment or discontinuation of anticoagulant therapy and, possibly, protamine sulfate to reverse the effects of heparin or vitamin K_1 (phytonadione) to counteract the effects of warfarin.

• Check the patient's drug regimen for possible interactions (see *Anticoagulant alert,* page 40).

Home care instructions

Because heparin is administered parenterally and almost exclusively in a hospital setting, it doesn't require home

Anticoagulant alert

Both heparin and warfarin interact with a large number of other drugs. Typically, the result is an increased risk of bleeding, diminished anticoagulant action, or ulcerogenic effects.

Hazardous interactions

The risk of bleeding increases when heparin is given with dextrans, dipyridamole, piperacillin, and valproic acid. It also increases when heparin is given with aspirin, carbenicillin, cefamandole, chloroquine, hydroxychloroquine, moxalactam, nonsteroidal anti-inflammatory agents, or plicamycin. The drug's anticoagulant effect diminishes when used with antihistamines, digitalis glycosides, oral contraceptives, protamine, or tetracycline.

The risk of bleeding rises when warfarin is given with amiodarone, chloramphenicol, clofibrate, diflunisal, thyroid drugs, heparin, anabolic steroids, cimetidine, disulfiram, glucagon, inhalation anesthetics, metronidazole, quinidine, influenza vaccine, sulindac, sulfinpyrazone, or sulfonamides. The risk also rises with concurrent, prolonged acetaminophen therapy. What's more, fatal hemorrhage can occur several weeks after cessation of barbiturate therapy unless the warfarin dosage is reduced.

The risk of ulcerogenic effects increases when warfarin is used with ethacrynic acid, indomethacin, mefenamic acid, oxyphenbutazone, phenylbutazone, or salicylates.

Warfarin's effectiveness decreases when carbamazepine, ethchlorvynol, griseofulvin, haloperidol, paraldehyde, or rifampin is given concurrently. Similarly, its effectiveness diminishes when given with laxatives or diuretics.

care instructions. However, warfarin therapy requires these directions:

• Instruct the patient to take the prescribed dose at the same time each day.

• Emphasize the importance of regular follow-up tests to monitor warfarin levels.

• Teach the patient and family to watch for and immediately report signs of bleeding, including hematuria, tarry stools, bleeding from the nose or gums, bruises and petechiae, hematemesis, or increased menstrual flow.

• To minimize bleeding, advise the patient to use a soft-bristled toothbrush; to floss gently with waxed floss; and to shave with an electric razor instead of a blade. Advise the patient to inform the dentist about warfarin therapy before any dental work.

• Warn the patient to avoid over-the-counter drugs containing aspirin or other salicylates, and to never take any other drug without medical approval.

• Explain that vitamin K can interfere with warfarin's anticoagulant action, and advise the patient to keep his intake of vitamin K-containing foods consistent to prevent altered drug effects. Patients who have switched to fad diets (such as an all-lettuce diet) have experienced difficulties while taking warfarin. Explain that leafy green vegetables contain the highest amounts of vitamin K and that fruits, cereals, dairy products, and meats supply lower amounts.

• Warn the patient to avoid excessive alcohol consumption, which can increase the risk of bleeding.

• Advise the patient to wear a medical identification bracelet or carry a card that specifies the prescribed drug and its dosage.

ANTICONVULSANTS

Anticonvulsants include various drugs that depress abnormal neuronal discharges in the central nervous system (CNS), thus inhibiting seizure activity. Anticonvulsants are classified primarily in four groups: *barbiturate derivatives, benzodiazepine derivatives, hydantoin derivatives,* and miscellaneous agents (including *succinimide* and *oxazolinedione derivatives*).

Purpose

• To reduce the frequency or severity of seizures in idiopathic seizure disorder or seizures secondary to drugs, disorders, or traumatic brain injury.

Indications

Each anticonvulsant is used to treat specific seizure disorders. Frequently, these drugs are used in combination for complex or mixed seizure disorders.

Barbiturate anticonvulsants are long-acting CNS depressants that provide a useful adjunct to other anticonvulsants, such as the benzodiazepines or hydantoin derivatives.

The barbiturate anticonvulsants include *phenobarbital* and *primidone*. Phenobarbital can be given orally for long-term treatment of generalized tonic-clonic and focal seizures; the parenteral form can be used for emergency treatment of status epilepticus and seizures caused by eclampsia, meningitis, or tetanus. Not a true barbiturate, primidone has anticonvulsant activity, and it is metabolized to phenobarbital. It's used as primary or adjunctive treatment for generalized tonic-clonic, psychomotor, and focal seizures.

Used alone or with other anticonvulsants, the benzodiazepines *clonazepam, clorazepate,* and *diazepam* prevent seizures or reduce their frequency or severity. Clonazepam proves useful in treating absence, akinetic, and myo-clonic seizures; clorazepate provides adjunctive therapy for simple partial seizures. In the parenteral form, diazepam helps treat status epilepticus. In the oral form, it's used adjunctively for seizures.

Typically, the benzodiazepines are preferred over the barbiturate anticonvulsants because they're more predictable; produce fewer adverse effects at therapeutic doses; have less potential for dependence, abuse, and interaction with other drugs; and are less toxic in overdosage.

The hydantoin derivatives — *phenytoin* and *mephenytoin* — treat generalized tonic-clonic and complex partial seizures. Because of their effectiveness and minimal adverse reactions, these drugs are considered the first-line treatment for these seizures.

Phenytoin is typically the hydantoin derivative of choice. Unlike the other hydantoin derivatives, which are administered only orally, phenytoin may be given orally or I.V. It can also be used in status epilepticus and nonepileptic seizures, but it must be used cautiously in patients with cardiac disease. Because of potentially life-threatening blood dyscrasias, mephenytoin is used infrequently.

Succinimides are sometimes used to control absence seizures. *Ethosuximide,* the most commonly prescribed drug in the class, can be administered to both adults and children, and can be used in combination with other anticonvulsants. When used alone in mixed types of epilepsy, the succinimide anticonvulsants may increase the frequency of primary generalized tonic-clonic seizures in some patients.

The valproic acid derivatives may be used alone or in combination with other anticonvulsants to treat absence seizures and complex absence seizures, or used as adjunctive treatment in patients with multiple seizure types.

Carbamazepine, chemically related to the tricyclic antidepressants, is used to treat partial seizures with complex symptoms as well as generalized tonic-clonic and mixed seizures.

Barbiturate anticonvulsants are contraindicated in patients with a hypersensitivity to at least one of the drugs; in patients with porphyria, cardiac or hepatic dysfunction, respiratory disease with dyspnea or obstruction, or nephritis. They should be used cautiously in elderly or debilitated patients and in those with severe anemia, diabetes mellitus, hyperthyroidism, or hypoadrenalism. Prolonged use of these drugs can lead to blood dyscrasias, physiologic and psychological dependence, and tolerance. When taken with alcohol or other CNS depressants, barbiturates can cause excessive CNS depression and death.

Because benzodiazepine dependence occurs most commonly in patients with a history of alcohol and drug abuse, these drugs should be avoided in such patients if possible. They should be used cautiously in patients with suicidal tendencies or in those whose history suggests potential abuse. They're contraindicated in patients with known hypersensitivity to any benzodiazepine, during pregnancy, and in patients with hepatic disease or acute angle-closure glaucoma. They should be administered judiciously to patients with renal impairment, chronic respiratory disease, or chronic open-angle glaucoma. I.V. administration should be avoided in shock or coma or with respiratory depression.

Because hydantoin derivatives are metabolized in the liver and excreted by the kidneys, they're usually contraindicated in hepatic and renal disorders. They're also contraindicated in patients with hematologic disorders or hydantoin hypersensitivity. All the hydantoins should be used cautiously in elderly or debilitated patients and in those with hypotension, myocardial insufficiency, or respiratory depression.

Adverse reactions

Adverse reactions to barbiturate derivatives most commonly reflect CNS depression and may include drowsiness (the most common reaction), lethargy, vertigo, headache, and confusion. In patients with severe pain, in elderly patients, or in children, they may cause paradoxical excitement. Long-term use is associated with the development of tolerance and dependence. Other reactions to barbiturate derivatives may include respiratory depression leading to apnea and circulatory collapse (following overdose), laryngospasm, and bronchospasm. GI reactions include constipation or diarrhea, nausea, vomiting, and epigastric pain.

Benzodiazepine derivatives usually produce adverse CNS reactions that include drowsiness, ataxia, fatigue, confusion, weakness, headache, dizziness, vertigo, and syncope. Other adverse CNS reactions include euphoria, nightmares, and hallucinations. Psychological and physical dependence occur with long-term use and may result in withdrawal symptoms. Adverse GI reactions include dry mouth, taste alterations, anorexia, nausea, vomiting, constipation, and abdominal discomfort.

Hydantoin derivatives frequently produce adverse reactions that vary widely and may have serious consequences. Adverse CNS reactions are the most common and are usually dose-related. Ataxia, slurred speech, mental confusion, dizziness, insomnia, nervousness, twitching, drowsiness, and headache are possible. Nystagmus is dose-related and may be one of the first symptoms of toxicity. GI reactions are common and usually consist of nausea, vomiting, diarrhea, or constipation. Cardiovascular reactions usually follow I.V. administration of phenytoin and may include hypotension, ventricular fibrillation, and cardiovascular collapse.

Comparing serum levels of anticonvulsants

To evaluate the safety and effectiveness of anticonvulsant drugs, you need to monitor the patient's serum drug levels. This table, which presents therapeutic ranges, toxic levels, and information on the onset and duration of action for some common anticonvulsants, helps evaluate the patient's response to his drug regimen.

DRUG	THERA-PEUTIC RANGE (mcg/ml)	TOXIC LEVEL (mcg/ml)	SERUM HALF-LIFE	TIME TO REACH STEADY STATE
carbamazepine	4 to 12	≥ 12	10 to 25 hr	4 to 6 days
clonazepam	0.03 to 0.06	≥ 0.08	19 to 48 hr	4 to 6 days
ethosuximide	40 to 100	≥ 150	30 to 60 hr	4 to 8 days
phenobarbital	10 to 30	≥ 35	50 to 120 hr	14 to 21 days
phenytoin	10 to 20	> 20	18 to 22 hr	5 to 7 days
primidone	5 to 12	≥ 15	3 to 12 hr	2 to 3 days
valproic acid	50 to 100	> 100	8 to 15 hr	2 to 3 days

Valproic acid has been associated with hepatic failure.

Most anticonvulsants, including succinimide derivatives, carbamazepine, and oxazolidinedione derivatives, have been associated with aplastic anemia or agranulocytosis.

Care considerations

Anticonvulsants require careful monitoring of dosage for toxicity (see *Comparing serum levels of anticonvulsants*). Each group requires specific additional precautions as listed below.

For barbiturates

• When administering I.V. barbiturates, carefully monitor the patient's vital signs, especially respirations. Watch for signs of toxicity: respiratory depression, bradycardia or tachycardia, oliguria, hypotension, lowered body temperature, and decreased level of consciousness. Because overdose can be fatal, keep resuscitation equipment available in case of respiratory or cardiac arrest.

• In early stages of treatment the patient may experience lethargy, drowsiness, confusion, decreased attention span, and slurred speech; an elderly or young patient may develop paradoxical hyperexcitability. Typically, these reactions occur when the dosage is being gradually increased to achieve optimum seizure control and subside after the patient develops tolerance, usually within 3 weeks. To prevent injury, assist the patient with ambulation and raise the side rails of his bed.

• During early therapy, watch for systemic or local dermatologic reactions, such as facial edema, purpura, urticaria, and skin rash or blisters. Such reactions may require discontinuing the drug or reducing its dosage.

• Monitor for anorexia or nausea. Encourage the patient to maintain a well-balanced diet even if he doesn't feel like eating. Because fluid loss from vomiting can affect serum barbiturate concentrations, monitor intake and output and ensure adequate hydration.

• Check the patient's medication history for medications that may potentiate barbiturate effects—monoamine oxidase inhibitors, valproic acid, and diazepam—and for rifampin, which may decrease barbiturate levels.

• During long-term barbiturate therapy, monitor hematologic status carefully to detect blood dyscrasias.

For benzodiazepines

• I.V. administration can cause apnea, hypotension, bradycardia, or cardiac arrest, particularly in elderly or severely ill patients and in those with limited pulmonary reserve or unstable cardiovascular status. Therefore, keep resuscitation equipment on hand when using the I.V. route. After I.V. administration, check for redness, pain, or swelling at the injection site.

• Monitor for drowsiness, dizziness, light-headedness, feelings of clumsiness or unsteadiness, and confusion, especially in elderly or debilitated patients, children and infants, and patients with hepatic disease or low serum albumin levels. Daytime sedation may occur even when the patient takes the drug at bedtime; this reaction occurs during the early stages of therapy and subsides within a few days. Impose safety precautions during this period.

• Observe for adverse GI reactions, such as anorexia, nausea, excessive thirst, and constipation or diarrhea. Giving the drug with food may reduce or eliminate these reactions.

• During long-term therapy, regularly monitor hepatic and renal function tests and blood counts, especially for the patient with liver or kidney impairment. Check for concurrent use of cimetidine, which may slow clearance of clorazepate and diazepam.

• Because abrupt withdrawal may precipitate status epilepticus, make sure the patient takes all of his scheduled medication.

For hydantoin derivatives

• While the patient builds therapeutic levels of the prescribed hydantoin de-

rivative, watch for common reactions: drowsiness, dizziness, rash, urticaria, ataxia, nausea or vomiting, insomnia, visual disturbances, hirsutism, and blood dyscrasias. Motor disturbances, drowsiness, and dizziness typically subside after the first few days of therapy. Until they do, impose safety precautions to protect the patient from falls. Reducing dosage of the hydantoin derivative may ease some persistent adverse reactions. To ease nausea and vomiting, give the drug with or after meals.

• Carefully monitor the patient's serum drug levels and physical status (including his level of seizure activity) to determine the safety and effectiveness of therapy. Pay special attention to toxic effects in elderly patients, who tend to metabolize hydantoin derivatives slowly; they may benefit from lower dosage.

• Check the patient's medication history and diet for possible interactions with the prescribed hydantoin derivative. Folic acid, dexamethasone, and tube feedings of Osmolite or Isocal may decrease absorption of a hydantoin derivative; anticoagulants, cimetidine, antihistamines, diazepam, salicylates, and sulfonamides may increase the drug's effect.

• Infuse I.V. phenytoin at a rate of less than 50 mg/minute in adults to prevent hypotension, arrhythmias, and cardiac arrest.

For succinimides

• Perform periodic blood counts. Notify the doctor of unexplained fever, bruising, or joint pain. Blood dyscrasias associated with succinimides may be fatal.

• Periodically review urinalysis and liver function studies.

• Observe for nausea, vomiting, epigastric and abdominal discomfort, drowsiness, and dizziness.

For valproic acid derivatives

• Observe for hemorrhage, bruising, or a disorder of hemostasis-coagulation. If these occur, the dosage should

be reduced or the therapy withdrawn. Monitor bleeding time and blood counts, including platelets.
• Monitor for nonspecific symptoms, such as a loss of seizure control, malaise, weakness, lethargy, facial edema, anorexia, jaundice, and vomiting. These symptoms may precede serious hepatotoxicity. Notify the doctor if any occur. Liver function tests must be performed before beginning therapy and at frequent intervals thereafter, especially during the first 6 months of therapy.
• To ease adverse GI reactions, have the patient take the drug with food.
• Use with extreme caution in children under age 2, in children with congenital metabolic disorders or mental retardation, and in patients with organic mental syndrome.

For carbamazepine
• Obtain complete blood count, platelet and reticulocyte counts, and serum iron levels weekly for the first 3 months, then monthly. If bone marrow depression develops, the drug should be discontinued. Obtain urinalysis, blood urea nitrogen, and liver function tests every 3 months. Periodic eye examinations are also recommended.
• Tell the patient to inform the doctor immediately of fever, sore throat, mouth ulcers, or easy bruising.
• Observe for signs of anorexia or subtle appetite changes, which may indicate excessive blood levels.
• Never discontinue the drug suddenly when treating seizures or status epilepticus. Notify the doctor immediately if adverse reactions occur.
• Tell the patient to take the drug with food to minimize GI distress.

Home care instructions
• Warn the patient to avoid hazardous activities requiring alertness and good coordination until he has adjusted to therapy.
• Warn that coma and death can result from using alcohol or other CNS depressants with barbiturates.

• Instruct the patient to follow the prescribed medication schedule closely. He should take a missed dose right away if he remembers it within 1 hour or so. Otherwise, he should omit the missed dose and return to the regular dosing schedule. He should never double-dose.
• Tell the patient never to break, crush, or chew extended-release capsules, but to swallow them whole.
• Warn the patient not to stop taking the drug abruptly without his doctor's approval; seizures and delirium may result.
• Emphasize the importance of regular physical examinations and blood tests to evaluate the safety and effectiveness of therapy with hydantoin derivatives, carbamazepine, succinimides, or valproic acid.
• Advise the patient to wear a medical identification bracelet or carry a card that specifies the name and dosage of the prescribed anticonvulsant drug.
• Explain the need to report any increased bruising or bleeding, which may indicate a blood dyscrasia, if the patient is taking carbamazepine, succinimides, or hydantoin derivatives.

ANTIDIARRHEALS

Antidiarrheals (antiperistaltic agents) reduce the fluidity of the stool and the frequency of defecation. The three most commonly prescribed antidiarrheals are *loperamide, diphenoxylate with atropine sulfate,* and *opium derivatives (paregoric).*

Purpose
• To treat acute, mild, or chronic stages of nonspecific diarrhea
• To relieve diarrhea by prolonging the transit of intestinal contents by inhibiting motility.

Indications
By inhibiting peristalsis, these drugs help to control acute or chronic diar-

rhea resulting from laxative abuse, malabsorption disorders, food or drug reactions, and infectious and inflammatory conditions.

Because antidiarrheals decrease intestinal motility, they're contraindicated in patients with conditions involving colonic stricture or stenosis (such as ulcerative colitis); in such patients, the drugs could precipitate acute intestinal obstruction or toxic megacolon. Antidiarrheals are also contraindicated in patients with diarrhea resulting from ingestion of a toxic substance because they inhibit elimination of toxins from the GI tract. Because they are opium derivatives, these drugs are contraindicated in patients with a history of opioid dependence. Paregoric's potential for physical dependence is well-known. Both loperamide and diphenoxylate, which are chemically related to meperidine, also carry a risk of central nervous system (CNS) depression and possibly opioid dependence.

Adverse reactions

Antidiarrheals that contain atropine may cause dryness of the skin and mucous membranes, flushing, hyperthermia, tachycardia, and urine retention, especially in children. Other reactions may include nausea, vomiting, dry mouth, dizziness, drowsiness, and hypersensitivity reactions.

Care considerations

• Carefully observe for adverse CNS reactions, ranging from dizziness and confusion to stupor and hallucinations. These effects are especially common and severe in children, elderly patients, and patients with impaired renal or hepatic function.
• If the patient is taking an opium derivative, also watch for nausea and vomiting.
• Frequently measure abdominal girth, and auscultate for bowel sounds. Abdominal distention and decreased or absent bowel sounds may herald the

development of acute intestinal obstruction, such as paralytic ileus or toxic megacolon. Notify the doctor of any abnormal findings.

Home care instructions

• Warn the patient never to exceed the prescribed dosage; doing so could produce sedation, euphoria, and other CNS effects. Explain that prolonged overuse could lead to dependence.
• Instruct the patient to keep an accurate record of the amount and consistency of all stools and to notify the doctor if no improvement occurs within 48 hours of starting drug therapy or if he experiences fever.
• Tell the patient to maintain adequate fluid intake during treatment. Explain that, contrary to popular belief, high fluid intake doesn't contribute to diarrhea. Rather, it helps replace the large amounts of fluid lost in diarrhea.
• If diphenoxylate is prescribed for a young child, advise parents that this drug can mask signs of fluid and electrolyte depletion. Instruct them to make sure the child maintains a high fluid intake and to watch for and report signs of dehydration: lethargy, low-grade fever, poor skin turgor, mucous membrane dryness, decreased urine output, and excessive thirst.
• Tell the patient to immediately report any abdominal pain or discomfort, bloody stools, or constipation.

ANTIEMBOLISM STOCKINGS

Antiembolism stockings help decrease the risk of deep vein thrombosis (DVT). The stockings compress superficial leg veins and the soleus muscle, thereby promoting venous return by forcing blood into the deep venous system instead of allowing it to pool in the legs and form clots. Antiembolism stockings can provide equal pressure over the entire leg or a graded pressure that is highest at the ankle and decreases to the knee or thigh. Graded pressures range from 18 mm Hg at the ankle to 8 mm Hg at the upper thigh.

These stockings should not be used on patients with dermatoses or open skin lesions, gangrene, severe arteriosclerosis or other ischemic vascular diseases, pulmonary or any massive edema, recent vein ligation, or vascular or skin grafts. (See *Understanding IPC stockings* and also the entry "Pneumatic Compression, Intermittent.")

Purpose

• To decrease the risk of DVT by decreasing venous stasis.

Indications

This treatment is usually indicated for patients at high risk for developing DVT. This includes patients with a previous history of DVT or blood disorders, cardiovascular or respiratory disease, cancer, diabetes, obesity, sepsis, stroke, inflammatory bowel disease, varicose veins, decreased mobility, or surgery involving the thigh or calf, pelvis, or abdomen; those who have had total hip or knee replacement; those with hip fractures, multiple injuries, or pelvic and spinal injuries; as well as those who are underweight and over age 40.

For patients with chronic venous problems, intermittent pneumatic compression (IPC) stockings may be

Understanding IPC stockings

For patients with chronic venous disease and those at risk for deep venous disease, intermittent pneumatic compression (IPC) stockings may be used during surgery and the postoperative period. These stockings are actually knee- or thigh-length cuffs connected to a pump and hoses. Wrapped from the ankle to the knee or thigh on each leg, the cuffs imitate normal leg pumping action by sequentially inflating and deflating a series of air cells from the ankle toward the trunk. This milking action propels blood toward the heart, preventing congestion in venous muscle sinuses and valve pockets and preventing backflow. Cuff pressures range from 35 to 55 mm Hg. The cuffs are foam-lined and adjustable to prevent skin irritation. After a few minutes of use the patient probably won't be aware of the pressure changes.

During treatment, evaluate the patient's skin color, temperature, sensation, and ability to move. Remove the cuffs and notify the doctor if the patient experiences numbness, tingling, or leg pain.

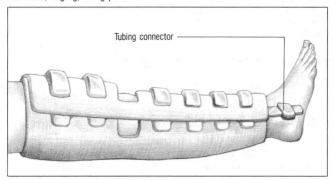

Tubing connector

Guide for applying antiembolism stockings

Antiembolism stockings are usually applied in the morning before getting out of bed.

To apply antiembolism stockings
- Lightly dust the ankle with talcum powder to ease stocking application.
- Insert your hand into the stocking from the top, and grab the heel pocket from the inside. Turn the stocking inside out so that the foot section is inside the stocking leg.
- Hook the index and middle fingers of both hands into the foot section. Ease the stocking over the toes, stretching it sideways as you move it up the foot. (Suggest that the patient point his toes to help ease the stocking on.)

- Insert the index and middle fingers into the gathered stocking at the ankle, and ease the stocking up the leg to the knee.

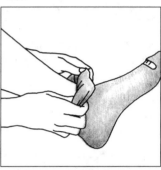

- Stretch the stocking toward the knee, front and back, to distribute the material evenly. The stocking should fit snugly and remain unwrinkled.

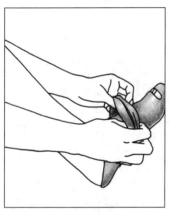

- Center the heel in the heel pocket. Then, gather the loose material at the ankle and slide the rest of the stocking up over the heel with short pulls, alternating front and back.

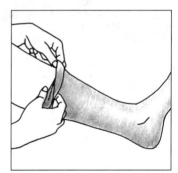

ordered during surgery and postoperatively.

Procedure

Antiembolism stockings are applied by nursing personnel, the patient, or a caregiver as medically indicated. Many doctors order application of stockings before surgery. The stockings are worn continuously until the risk of developing DVT has diminished. Studies have demonstrated that increased venous return persists for 30 minutes after removal of the stockings, possibly related to venous tone produced by the compression. (See *Guide for applying antiembolism stockings*.)

Follow the appropriate directions below for the length of stocking you are applying.

For a knee-length stocking

• Make sure the top of each stocking is below the crease at the back of the knee. If the top of the stocking sits in the crease, it can put pressure on the vein and decrease circulation to the leg.
• Repeat the steps to apply the second stocking.

For a thigh-length stocking

• Keep the leg extended and stretch the rest of the stocking over the knee. Then flex the patient's knee, and pull the stocking over the thigh until the top is 1″ to 3″ (2.5 to 7.6 cm) below the gluteal fold.
• Stretch the stocking from the top, front and back, to distribute the fabric evenly over the thigh.
• Gently snap the fabric behind the knee to eliminate gaps that could reduce pressure.
• Repeat the steps to apply the second stocking.

For waist-length stockings

• Extend the stockings to the top of the thigh and then over the gluteal muscles to the waist.
• Place the adjustable belt that accompanies the stockings around the waist to help hold them in place.

Complications

Obstruction of arterial blood flow (characterized by cold and bluish toes, dusky toenail beds, decreased or absent pedal pulses, and leg pain or cramps) or increased venous congestion can occur if the stockings roll down, producing a tourniquet effect. This can be avoided by proper measuring, application, and wearing of the stockings. Less serious complications are allergic reactions or skin irritations.

Care considerations

Before therapy

• Measure the patient's legs as specified by the manufacturer. Improperly fitted antiembolism stockings are not effective. Caution must be used with patients who have circulatory problems in or extreme deformities of their legs.
• Inspect the condition of the legs before applying the stockings. Apply the stockings to clean, dry legs. Powder may be applied beforehand to ease application if the patient is not allergic to it.
• Instruct the patient about the application, care, and purpose of the stockings. The stockings are to be worn in bed and while walking to provide continuous protection against thrombosis.

During therapy

• Evaluate the legs daily or every 4 hours for patients with faint pulses or edema. Such evaluation should include skin color, temperature, pulses, sensation, swelling, and mobility. If complications occur, remove the stockings and notify the doctor immediately.
• The stockings should be removed at least once a day to inspect and wash the legs.
• Be alert for an allergic reaction because some patients cannot tolerate the sizing in new stockings. Laundering new stockings before applying them decreases this risk.
• Launder the stockings as needed with warm water and a mild soap or according to the manufacturer's instructions. Inspect them for torn areas or loss of elasticity, and replace them as needed. It is helpful to order two pairs so that the patient can wear one pair while the other is being laundered.

Home care instructions

• Inform the patient and caregiver of the importance of wearing the stockings at all times until the patient's ac-

tivity level is back to normal or the doctor says they are no longer needed.
• Teach the patient or a caregiver how to apply the stockings correctly. Have the patient or caregiver demonstrate applying them and taking them off. These instructions should include the care and inspection of the stockings and how to order additional pairs if needed.

ANTIEMETICS

Antiemetics are generally categorized in one of these three groups: dopamine antagonists, anticholinergics, and miscellaneous agents.

Purpose
• To prevent or control nausea and vomiting.

Indications
Dopamine antagonists, such as the phenothiazines, help control vomiting that results from GI upset, radiation sickness, or cancer chemotherapy. They act by blocking the chemoreceptor trigger zone (or vomiting center) in the central nervous system (CNS). The dopamine antagonist *metoclopramide* is commonly used to prevent the nausea and vomiting that typically accompany cancer chemotherapy.

The anticholinergics, such as *dimenhydrinate* and *meclizine,* help control vomiting that results from vestibular disturbances, such as motion sickness.

Miscellaneous drugs include the cannabinoids and serotonin antagonists. The cannabinoids, such as *dronabinol,* can control refractory chemotherapy-induced nausea and vomiting. These drugs are derived from the marijuana plant *(Cannabis sativa);* many of their adverse effects are similar to the adverse CNS effects of marijuana. Serotonin antagonists, such as *ondansetron,* block the actions of serotonin on the gut as well as in the CNS. Ondansetron is used to treat chemotherapy-induced nausea and vomiting and is also used preoperatively.

Typically, the antiemetics prove most effective when administered prophylactically. Because these drugs produce sedation, they should be used cautiously in patients who are taking other CNS depressants. The dopamine antagonists can also cause extrapyramidal symptoms, especially if taken for a prolonged period.

Metoclopramide is contraindicated in GI obstruction because it stimulates GI motility. The phenothiazines have the opposite effect on peristalsis, and so should be used cautiously in patients with impaired GI motility. Because the phenothiazines may induce transient leukopenia, they're contraindicated in patients with bone marrow depression.

Adverse reactions
Phenothiazines, when used as antiemetics, primarily produce sedation, hypotension, and extrapyramidal effects. Adverse anticholinergic reactions typically include dry mouth, blurred vision, constipation, and urine retention.

The cannabinoids may cause euphoria, muddled thinking, or psychotic episodes. They also have a high abuse potential. Ondansetron is typically well tolerated, but it may cause headache in some patients.

Care considerations
• During therapy, carefully assess the patient's cardiovascular status; metoclopramide can produce transient hypertension, and phenothiazines and cannabinoids may cause tachycardia and orthostatic hypotension.
• If the patient is taking a phenothiazine, assess for signs of blood dyscrasias, such as fever, sore throat, and weakness. Also, check the results of hematologic studies for evidence of blood dyscrasias.

• Watch for constipation and urine retention.
• Check the patient's drug regimen for possible interactions. For example, if he's taking a phenothiazine, concurrent use of anticholinergics increases anticholinergic activity. Antacids interfere with phenothiazine absorption, and the two shouldn't be given within 2 hours of each other. Barbiturates may decrease the effects of phenothiazines.

Home care instructions

• Warn the patient to avoid alcohol and over-the-counter preparations such as cough and cold remedies or sleeping pills, which cause CNS depression.
• Instruct the patient to promptly report chest pain, palpitations, or persistent headache.
• Because antiemetics usually cause dizziness or drowsiness, tell the patient not to drive or perform any task requiring alertness until his response to the drug has been determined.
• Instruct the patient to minimize orthostatic hypotension by rising slowly from a sitting or lying position and by avoiding sudden bending or reaching.
• Advise the patient who experiences dry mouth to chew sugarless gum, suck hard candy, or rinse with a mouthwash that doesn't contain alcohol.
• If the patient experiences phenothiazine-induced photosensitivity, advise him to apply a sunscreen and wear protective clothing when outdoors.
• Because antacids inhibit absorption of oral phenothiazines, instruct the patient to separate doses of both drugs by at least 2 hours.

ANTIFUNGALS

Drugs used to treat systemic fungal infections include *flucytosine, nystatin, miconazole, amphotericin B, ketoconazole, fluconazole,* and *griseofulvin.* These drugs treat many types of fungal infections, which include *Tinea* (ringworm of nails, skin, and hair); oral, intestinal, and systemic candidiasis; and cryptococcosis, coccidioidomycosis, histoplasmosis, and *Trichophyton.* These severe, life-threatening fungal infections are common among immunocompromised patients with acquired immunodeficiency syndrome; they are also related to compromised immunity resulting from cancer chemotherapy.

Purpose

• To treat a wide range of fungal infections.

Indications

Amphotericin B is useful in the treatment of central nervous system (CNS), pulmonary, cardiac, renal, and other systemic fungal infections. It is effective against blastomycosis, histoplasmosis, cryptococcosis, candidiasis, sporotrichosis, aspergillosis, phycomycosis (mucormycosis), and coccidioidomycosis. Fluconazole is given orally or I.V. to treat various systemic fungal infections. Flucytosine is effective, usually in combination with amphotericin B, in the treatment of systemic candidiasis, cryptococcosis, and aspergillosis. Griseofulvin is used systemically in the treatment of *Tinea capitis* and other *Tinea* infections that do not respond to topical agents. Ketoconazole is given orally to treat a wide variety of systemic fungal infections previously susceptible only to parenteral agents. Miconazole is given I.V. to treat systemic coccidioidomycosis, candidiasis, cryptococcosis, and paracoccidioidomycosis. It is also used locally to treat vaginal fungal infections. Nystatin is used to treat oral, GI, and vaginal infections caused by *Candida albicans* and other *Candida* organisms. It is also used locally to treat vaginal infections.

Contraindications and cautions vary depending on the drug. Flucytosine should be used with extreme caution in patients with impaired hepatic or renal function or bone marrow depression. Fluconazole is contraindicated in patients hypersensitive to the drug and should be used cautiously in patients hypersensitive to other antifungal azole compounds. Amphotericin B should be used cautiously in patients with impaired renal function. Griseofulvin is contraindicated in porphyria or hepatocellular failure; it should be used cautiously in penicillin-sensitive patients because this drug is a penicillin derivative.

Adverse reactions

Adverse reactions occurring with antifungals may include GI reactions (nausea, vomiting, diarrhea, and anorexia) and hematologic reactions (anemia, leukopenia, thrombocytopenia, bone marrow suppression, and granulocytopenia). Other adverse reactions include Stevens-Johnson syndrome, hepatotoxicity, cardiac arrhythmias, hypokalemia, azotemia, renal impairment, thrombophlebitis, fever, headache, dizziness, rash, photosensitivity, superinfection, gynecomastia, and pruritus.

Care considerations

• Nystatin is essentially nontoxic and is very well tolerated. The other antifungals, however, must be used with caution because drug interactions and precautions for use vary with the antifungal used. Typically, drugs that interact with the systemic antifungals include oral anticoagulants, phenytoin, antacids, histamine-2 (H_2) receptor antagonists, and corticosteroids.
• Treatment with amphotericin B requires a test dose to determine patient tolerance before the full therapeutic dose. Most patients show some intolerance to amphotericin B even at a subtherapeutic dose, so monitor these patients closely for adverse reactions. A general toxic reaction that includes

fever, headache, nausea, vomiting, and malaise is common.
• To prevent local thrombophlebitis, heparin may be added to the amphotericin B infusion or administered on alternate days.
• Hydrocortisone or diphenhydramine are often given before or with amphotericin B to help decrease the severity of adverse reactions.
• Ketoconazole requires an acidic environment for absorption. Some patients may require the administration of dilute hydrochloric acid to achieve the proper stomach pH. Check with a pharmacist for proper instructions for administration.
• Monitor for the adverse reactions to antifungal agents: pruritus, rash, nausea, vomiting, and headache.
• Pregnant patients should not take ketoconazole because it may cause kernicterus in the neonate.
• Ketoconazole may interfere with the metabolism of other drugs, such as tetracycline, thereby increasing the risk of toxicity. Therefore, tell the patient to check with the doctor or pharmacist before taking other drugs.

Home care instructions

• Instruct the patient about possible adverse reactions and tell him to promptly report persistent fever, chills, headache, nausea, and vomiting.
• Tell the patient that he may take aspirin, acetaminophen, antihistamines, or antiemetics before each infusion to minimize adverse reactions to amphotericin B.
• Instruct the patient to promptly notify the doctor of decreased urination, which may result from renal impairment associated with amphotericin B.
• Advise the patient to follow instructions for all laboratory tests as scheduled to avoid any hematologic, renal, or hepatic complications.
• Advise the patient to take ketoconazole with food.

• Tell the patient who is also taking an H_2-receptor antagonist to take ketoconazole dose 2 hours before the other drug.

ANTIHISTAMINE ANTIPRURITICS

Most antihistamines are thought to block the physiologic action of histamine at the peripheral histamine-1 receptor sites. Histamine is the humoral compound that causes symptoms associated with allergic reactions. Antihistamines compete with histamine for receptor sites (by the process of competitive inhibition).

The antihistamine antipruritics include *tripelennamine, diphenhydramine, hydroxyzine, chlorpheniramine, methdilazine, trimeprazine, meclizine, cyproheptadine, astemizole,* and *terfenadine.*

Purpose

• To offer symptomatic relief of pruritic dermatoses.

Indications

Antihistamine antipruritics are used to treat mild, uncomplicated urticaria or pruritus resulting from allergic dermatoses. Although they don't cure the underlying disorder, they help to break the scratch-itch cycle and thus promote healing.

Contraindications to therapy include known hypersensitivity to antihistamines, stenosing peptic ulcer, and bladder neck obstruction. Although these drugs seem to be safe when taken during pregnancy, they should be used cautiously, if at all, in the first trimester. They shouldn't be used during lactation.

Adverse reactions

Sedation and drowsiness, the major adverse reactions to most systemic antihistamines, are magnified when these drugs are combined with central nervous system (CNS) depressants, such as barbiturates, alcohol, anticonvulsants, or muscle relaxants. The chemical structures of astemizole and terfenadine prevent them from entering the CNS. They are known as the "nonsedating" antihistamines.

When used with monoamine oxidase (MAO) inhibitors, antihistamines can cause anticholinergic effects, such as tachycardia, constipation, and urine retention, and adverse CNS effects. Increased anticholinergic effects may occur when antihistamines are used with tricyclic antidepressants.

In children and elderly patients, most antihistamines may cause paradoxical restlessness and hyperactivity. Children are especially prone to toxicity.

Care considerations

• Before administering an antihistamine, check the patient's drug regimen for concurrent use of CNS depressants, MAO inhibitors, or tricyclic antidepressants. Potential for adverse interactions with these drugs may require dosage adjustment or withholding of the antihistamine.
• If the patient is taking the nonsedating antihistamine terfenadine, he should avoid concomitant use with drugs that may block its metabolism, such as ketoconazole or erythromycin and its derivatives.
• Observe children for signs of toxicity, such as hallucinations, incoordination, tonic-clonic seizures, flushing, and fever. Notify the doctor of such signs immediately; toxicity can cause cerebral edema, deepening coma, and respiratory collapse in 2 to 18 hours.
• Expect some sedation in most patients taking systemic antihistamines. If these effects are distressing or interfere with daily activities, dosage may be adjusted or another antihistamine substituted. However, sedation can be useful if the patient has itching that interferes with sleep.

• Monitor the patient for excessive dryness of the mouth, nose, and throat. Continuing mouth dryness may lead to tooth decay, gum disease, or thrush; dehydration of the nose and throat may predispose him to upper respiratory tract infections. If he reports excessive dryness, notify the doctor.

Home care instructions

• Emphasize the importance of adhering to the prescribed drug regimen.
• Tell the patient to check with his doctor before taking any over-the-counter drug.
• Alert parents to adverse reactions that may occur in children taking systemic antihistamines, such as nightmares and hyperactivity. For all patients, briefly describe other possible reactions, such as sedation, blurred vision, painful or difficult urination, dizziness, rash, sore throat, or fever. Tell the patient to stop taking the drug and notify the doctor immediately if such reactions occur.
• To prevent excessive sedation, tell the patient not to make up any missed doses. Also warn him not to increase the dosage without first checking with the doctor because severe toxicity may result.
• Instruct the patient to take the drug with food or a glass of water or milk to minimize GI upset.
• Recommend sugarless candy or gum to relieve mouth dryness.
• If the patient is using a topical antihistamine, warn him not to apply it to damaged skin.
• Tell the patient to avoid driving and other hazardous activities that require alertness until the drug's CNS effects are known.

ANTIHYPERTENSIVE VASODILATORS

The antihypertensive vasodilators *hydralazine* and *minoxidil* treat severe hypertension that proves unmanageable with maximum therapeutic doses of diuretics and adrenergic blocking agents. Oral hydralazine, used alone or with other antihypertensives, treats essential hypertension. When given parenterally, hydralazine lowers blood pressure rapidly.

Purpose

• To lower blood pressure.

Indications

Because hydralazine usually lowers diastolic pressure more than systolic pressure, it isn't considered a primary treatment for essential hypertension. It should be used cautiously in patients with hypersensitivity to other antihypertensives, rheumatic heart disease, cerebrovascular accident (CVA), coronary artery disease, aortic aneurysm, renal failure, mitral valve disease, or myocardial infarction (MI).

The potent vasodilator minoxidil treats severe refractory hypertension. This drug directly dilates arteriolar vessels, thereby decreasing peripheral vascular resistance and profoundly lowering both systolic and diastolic pressure. Because minoxidil spurs adrenal secretion of catecholamines, it's contraindicated in pheochromocytoma. It's also contraindicated in pulmonary hypertension associated with mitral stenosis, CVA, malignant hypertension, drug hypersensitivity, pericardial effusion, renal failure, and coronary insufficiency. Typically, minoxidil isn't given to patients who have recently experienced MI because it precipitates angina and tachycardia.

Adverse reactions

Adverse reactions to the antihypertensive vasodilators may include angina pectoris, arrhythmias, diarrhea, flushing, sweating, anxiety, rapid or irregular heartbeat, depression, dry mouth, headache, nausea, palpitations, sodium retention, systemic lupus erythematosus-like syndrome (weakness, joint pain, pruritus, blisters, rash, sore throat, and fever), tachycardia, vomiting, and weight gain.

Other reactions include numbness and tingling in the extremities, dependent edema, and lymphadenopathy. Additionally, up to 80% of patients receiving minoxidil develop hypertrichosis—the elongation, thickening, and darkening of hair on the temples, eyebrows, forehead, and sideburn areas. This extra hair typically appears within the first 6 weeks of therapy but disappears 1 to 6 months after discontinuation of the drug.

Care considerations

• If the patient is taking hydralazine, observe closely for adverse reactions, especially if the daily dosage exceeds 200 mg. Severe reactions may require discontinuation of therapy.
• Check the patient's drug regimen for concurrent use of diuretics, monoamine oxidase (MAO) inhibitors, or epinephrine. Concurrent use of hydralazine with diuretics (particularly diazoxide) or MAO inhibitors can increase hypotensive effects; carefully monitor blood pressure. Concurrent use of hydralazine with epinephrine may cause tachycardia and hypotension.
• During long-term hydralazine therapy, periodically monitor the patient's complete blood count, lupus erythematosus cell preparation, and antinuclear antibody determinations.
• If the patient is taking minoxidil, frequently check his apical pulse and blood pressure. Fluid retention occurs in almost all patients receiving the drug; give loop diuretics, if ordered. Observe for dependent edema and enforce a sodium-restricted diet, as ordered. Weigh the patient daily and report any rapid gain of 3 lb (1.4 kg) or more. Note and report other adverse reactions.
• Check the patient's drug regimen for possible interactions. Concurrent use of minoxidil with diuretics and other antihypertensives may produce profound hypotension; guanethidine is especially dangerous and should be discontinued before beginning therapy, if possible. Epinephrine or norepinephrine may cause excessive cardiac stimulation, resulting in tachycardia, angina, and congestive heart failure.
• If the patient is taking either of these drugs, frequently check blood pressure and pulse.

Home care instructions

• Warn the patient not to discontinue taking the drug without the doctor's approval.
• Instruct the patient to take his pulse for 1 minute every morning before getting out of bed, and to call the doctor promptly if his pulse rate is above 100 beats/minute or below 60 beats/minute, if the rhythm is abnormal, or if he experiences pain.
• Tell the patient to notify the doctor immediately of dyspnea, dizziness, fainting, swollen feet or hands, chest pain, easy bruising, joint pain, or a rash.
• Tell the patient to weigh himself weekly at the same time of day, on the same scale, and wearing the same amount of clothing. Also tell him to promptly report a weight gain of 3 lb or more.
• Instruct the patient to take the drug with food to increase absorption.
• Tell the patient to limit his salt intake, as recommended by the doctor.
• Reassure the patient who experiences hypertrichosis from minoxidil that this effect will disappear after the drug is discontinued, although it may take several months. Advise female patients to remove unwanted hair with depilatory creams.
• To avoid hypotension and dizziness, instruct the patient to change positions slowly, avoid standing in one position for longer than a minute, and to avoid

hot baths and showers, strenuous exercise, and alcohol consumption.

ANTI-INFECTIVES, TOPICAL

Topical anti-infective drugs are effective against bacterial, viral, and fungal growths. These commonly used drugs include *acyclovir, bacitracin, chloramphenicol, ciclopirox, econazole, erythromycin, gentamicin, haloprogin, ketoconazole, miconazole, mupirocin, neomycin, nystatin, tetracycline,* and *tolnaftate.* These drugs can be prescribed alone or in combination. Many topical anti-infectives are available without a prescription.

Purpose
• To prevent infection in minor skin abrasions, cuts, and scratches
• To treat skin infections, such as those caused by gram-positive or gram-negative organisms (for example, *Staphylococcus* or *Pseudomonas*).

Indications
The topical antiviral ointment acyclovir is used to treat initial episodes of genital herpes and in limited non-life-threatening mucocutaneous herpes simplex virus infections in the immunocompromised patient. Acyclovir is for cutaneous use only and should not be applied to the eye.

The bactericidal drugs (bacitracin, gentamicin, and neomycin) and bacteriostatic drugs (chloramphenicol, chlorotetracycline, erythromycin, mupirocin, and tetracycline) are used to treat local bacterial infections caused by susceptible organisms.

Silver sulfadiazine, a drug with a broad antimicrobial spectrum, is used to treat or prevent wound infections in burn patients. It is contraindicated in patients with compromised hepatic or renal function.

Topical antifungal drugs (miconazole, econazole, ciclopirox, tolnaftate, ketoconazole, clotrimazole, haloprogin, and nystatin) are effective against dermatophytoses, such as *Tinea, Epidermophyton, Candida, Trichophyton,* and yeasts. These antifungals may be formulated as aerosol powders or spray solutions, topical powders, creams, or gels.

All the antifungal preparations have similar effects, and the choice of drug and vehicle is largely a matter of preference. The powder form offers some advantages for treating moist skin areas where its drying effect can help promote healing. When bacterial overgrowth complicates the infection, the doctor may choose a combination product.

Adverse reactions
All topical anti-infectives may cause burning, local rashes, pruritus, and hypersensitivity reactions. When applied to abraded areas, some (especially neomycin and chloramphenicol) may cause systemic toxicity.

Topical antifungals have low toxicity and are unlikely to cause hypersensitivity reactions. Percutaneous absorption is virtually nonexistent unless the preparation is applied to damaged skin. Adverse reactions are rare and usually mild. They may include overgrowth of nonsusceptible organisms, skin irritation, photosensitivity, edema, erythematous vesicular eruptions, hives, pruritus, stinging, peeling, blistering, maceration, and angioedema.

Care considerations
• Because these drugs are generally safe and effective and are commonly prescribed for outpatients, care considerations are minimal. However, watch for signs of hypersensitivity, such as skin irritation, that weren't present before application of the drug.
• Evaluate the patient's response to therapy. Improvement of severe fungal

infection may take up to 3 weeks. However, if the condition appears worse, the diagnosis and treatment should be reevaluated.

• Because of the potential risk of ototoxicity and nephrotoxicity, neomycin should be used with caution in patients with extensive skin abrasions or burns. In these situations, more absorption will occur.

Home care instructions

• Show the patient how to apply the medication. The specific procedure will depend on the type of medication prescribed. Typically, a ½″ (1.3 cm) ribbon of cream is used for every 4 in² of body surface; aerosols are sprayed onto the affected area from a distance of 6″ to 10″ (15 to 25 cm); spray solutions are released from a distance of 4″ (10 cm) to 6″; and topical powders are dusted lightly onto the affected area and gently rubbed in.

• Tell the patient to keep the affected areas clean and dry for maximum drug effectiveness. Instruct him to clean crusted or oozing lesions before applying the drug and to treat these areas frequently.

• Warn the patient not to expect immediate improvement, but to inform the doctor if the infection worsens or if he notes any evidence of new blistering, burning, peeling, or swelling, or excessive redness.

• Emphasize the need to continue the full course of treatment even if symptoms have cleared within a few days. Explain that symptoms of infection will reappear if the drug is discontinued prematurely.

• Tell the patient to return for a culture after completion of therapy to check for any remaining infection or overgrowth of new fungi or bacteria.

ANTILIPEMICS

Antilipemic drugs include *cholestyramine, clofibrate, colestipol, dextrothyroxine, gemfibrozil, lovastatin, niacin, pravastatin, probucol,* and *simvastatin.* Antilipemics counteract high concentrations of lipids in the blood. They do this by lowering levels of cholesterol, triglycerides, or both, to different degrees. Reduction of serum lipid levels, particularly cholesterol levels, may reduce the risk of coronary artery disease and myocardial infarction (MI).

Purpose

• To provide adjunctive treatment for severe primary hyperlipidemia that does not respond to dietary restrictions, weight loss, or exercise.

Indications

Several types of antilipemics are currently in clinical use. The choice of drug depends on the type of hyperlipidemia. Excessive cholesterol levels can be treated with bile acid sequestrants (cholestyramine or colestipol) or cholesterol synthesis inhibitors (clofibrate, dextrothyroxine, gemfibrozil, lovastatin, niacin, pravastatin, probucol, and simvastatin). Other antilipemics alter both cholesterol and triglyceride levels.

Lovastatin, pravastatin, and simvastatin are specific inhibitors of 3-hydroxy-3-methylglutaryl-coenzyme A (HMG-CoA) reductase, an enzyme in the biosynthetic pathway for cholesterol. They reduce both normal and elevated low-density lipoprotein (LDL) cholesterol concentrations. The effects of these changes in lipoprotein levels, including reduction of serum cholesterol, on cardiovascular morbidity or mortality have not been clearly established.

Cholestyramine and colestipol, bile acid sequestrants, lower LDL and serum cholesterol levels. Serum triglycerides may increase up to 20% during the first weeks of treatment, then return to pretreatment levels. These resins can only be used prophylactically; they can't remove fatty deposits that are already present. Although they reduce the incidence of nonfatal MI, they haven't been shown to lessen the risk of other cardiovascular disorders.

Adverse reactions

The bile acid sequestrants may cause constipation and GI upset, worsen peptic ulcer disease and malabsorption states, increase the risk of hyperchloremic acidosis in patients with impaired renal function, and must be used with caution in patients with biliary obstruction or atresia because bile acids are diminished or absent in such patients.

Clofibrate is associated with nausea, rash, weakness, and weight gain.

Nicotinic acid (niacin) most commonly causes cutaneous flushing, which may diminish over time or be relieved with prostaglandins. Niacin also causes headache, nausea, abdominal pain, rash, and exacerbation of ulcers. The sustained-release formulas may minimize flushing, but they increase GI discomfort and may be associated with hepatic damage.

Adverse reactions to lovastatin are usually GI related – diarrhea, constipation, and flatulence. This drug may also increase hepatic enzyme levels. Lovastatin has also caused rash, visual disturbances, and myositis in some patients.

Care considerations

• Monitor serum cholesterol level to evaluate drug effects.
• Monitor serum transaminase levels every 4 to 6 weeks in patients receiving the HMG-CoA reductase inhibitors. If levels rise to three times the upper limit of normal and are persistent, discontinue the drug.

• In patients receiving the bile acid sequestrants, inhibited absorption of calcium and vitamins A and D (which are fat-soluble) may require administration of supplements.
• Observe for adverse reactions, especially in patients with peptic ulcer disease, malabsorption, or impaired renal function.

Home care instructions

• Give the patient dietary guidelines and encourage increased intake of high-fiber foods to help combat constipation caused by the bile acid sequestrants. If constipation persists, the doctor may decrease dosage or prescribe a stool softener.
• To prevent esophageal irritation or blockage in patients taking the bile acid sequestrants, instruct the patient to take large amounts of water, fruit juice, soup, or pulpy fruits.
• Explain that heartburn, nausea, indigestion, and abdominal pain usually diminish during continued treatment with the bile acid sequestrants.
• Tell the patient taking a bile acid sequestrant to take a missed dose as soon as possible; however, he shouldn't double-dose.
• Advise the patient to take bile acid sequestrants either 1 hour before or 2 hours after meals. The HMG-CoA reductase inhibitors may be taken with meals. Lovastatin should be taken with the evening meal.

ANTIMANICS

The drugs *lithium carbonate* and *lithium citrate* act as mood stabilizers, reducing the severity or frequency of manic episodes. Under proper supervision, lithium may prevent up to 80% of manic and depressive episodes. Episodes that occur during lithium therapy are usually less severe and shorter than those that might occur without such therapy.

The mechanism of action is not fully understood; however, lithium may replace sodium ions and alter neuronal membrane conductance.

Purpose
• To prevent or control mania.

Indications
Lithium salts are used to treat acute manic or hypomanic episodes of bipolar disorders and to prevent their recurrence.

Because lithium salts have a narrow therapeutic margin, they are contraindicated if regular determinations of blood levels can't be made. They are also contraindicated in renal or cardiac dysfunction and during pregnancy because of possible teratogenic effects. Lithium therapy should also be used cautiously in patients with a history of fluid retention and in those who use diuretics or follow low-salt diets.

Adverse reactions
Lithium produces various central nervous system reactions; most commonly, these include lethargy, fatigue, muscle weakness, headache, mental confusion, and hand tremor, which occur in up to 50% of patients. Restlessness, stupor, blackouts, coma, seizures, exacerbation of psychotic symptoms, and hyperexcitability may also occur.

GI reactions are also common at the start of therapy but tend to be mild and reversible. These reactions include nausea, vomiting, bloating, anorexia, diarrhea, or abdominal pain and may signal lithium toxicity. Weight gain may be seen in 25% of patients.

Polyuria and polydipsia may develop in up to 50% of patients; polyuria may cause dry mouth. A diabetes insipidus-like syndrome has been observed. Serum electrolyte abnormalities are possible.

Hypothyroidism may require thyroid supplementation. Cardiac arrhythmias, bradycardia, and other reversible changes may occur. Lithium toxicity parallels serum concentration and produces these adverse reactions in greater severity.

Care considerations
• Check blood lithium levels 8 to 12 hours after the first dose and then every 2 to 3 days until the dosage is reduced (usually when the patient's manic symptoms abate). Thereafter, check drug levels weekly for the 1st month and then monthly. Therapeutic levels are 0.6 to 1.2 mEq/liter. Levels above 1.5 mEq/liter are usually associated with toxic effects. Draw blood samples before the morning dose to avoid spuriously high readings. Watch for symptoms of toxicity: drowsiness, slurred speech, twitching, increased tremors, vomiting, and staggering. If any occur, lithium should be discontinued.
• If the patient is also receiving haloperidol during initial lithium therapy, observe for extrapyramidal symptoms.
• Review the patient's medication regimen for other possible interactions. Diuretics that increase renal reabsorption of lithium can lead to toxicity. Carbamazepine, probenecid, indomethacin, methyldopa, and piroxicam potentiate lithium's effect; in contrast, aminophylline, sodium bicarbonate, and sodium chloride, which promote excretion of lithium, decrease its effect.
• Monitor the patient's electrocardiogram (ECG); serum electrolyte levels; and thyroid, renal, and hematologic studies during therapy. Lithium can cause reversible ECG changes, arrhythmias, hypotension, and leukocytosis. Prolonged use can cause renal toxicity and suppress thyroid hormone levels, requiring replacement therapy. Watch for thyroid enlargement or unusual fatigue or weakness.
• Check the diabetic patient's blood glucose levels regularly. Lithium may cause transient hyperglycemia, requiring increased dosage of a hypoglycemic drug. Tell the patient to re-

port nausea, polyuria, increased thirst, mild weakness, and hand tremors.

Home care instructions

• Tell the patient that lithium produces its full effects 1 to 3 weeks after the start of therapy.
• Emphasize the importance of returning for regular lithium level tests. Warn the patient and family that lithium toxicity can occur. If it occurs, tell the patient to omit one dose and call his doctor for further instructions. Tell the patient not to stop the drug abruptly.
• Unless the doctor prescribes the sustained-release form, tell the patient to take lithium at regular intervals. The patient may take a missed dose within 2 hours of the prescribed time, but he should not make up the dose after that nor double the next dose.
• If the patient experiences persistent hand tremors, the doctor may have him take most of the daily dose at bedtime. Also, instruct the patient to reduce caffeine intake.
• Advise the patient not to take any over-the-counter drugs without first checking with his doctor.
• Instruct the patient to drink about ten to twelve 8-oz glasses (2,500 to 3,000 ml) of fluid daily and to avoid excessive salt intake, which enhances lithium excretion and reduces the drug's effectiveness. Also warn against taking sodium-containing antacids.
• If the patient experiences GI upset, suggest taking lithium with a glass of water after meals or snacks.
• Tell the patient to contact his doctor if vomiting, diarrhea, or excessive perspiration occurs. Excessive loss of body fluids can require lithium dosage adjustment. For this reason, advise against strenuous exercise, particularly in hot weather.
• Inform the patient that lithium causes weight gain. Advise him to weigh himself daily. If he gains weight, teach him how to reduce his caloric intake while maintaining adequate nutrition.

ANTIMYASTHENICS

The antimyasthenics, also called cholinesterase inhibitors, include *neostigmine*, *ambenonium*, *edrophonium*, and *pyridostigmine*. Edrophonium (Tensilon) has a very short duration of action and is only used as a diagnostic agent. Neostigmine has the next shortest duration of action. Slower-acting pyridostigmine may produce fewer and less serious adverse effects than neostigmine. Even slower-acting ambenonium provides an alternative for patients with hypersensitivity to the bromide ion in neostigmine and pyridostigmine. However, this drug possesses the greatest potential for toxicity.

Selecting a specific antimyasthenic and its dosage depends on clinical experience, the patient's response, and the route of administration. With any drug or dosage, the oral form is preferred to treat recurrent myasthenic symptoms. The I.V. route may be used to treat myasthenic crisis or to alleviate swallowing difficulty.

Purpose

• To treat myasthenic symptoms by inhibiting the destruction of acetylcholine, thus increasing muscle strength
• To aid in diagnosis of myasthenia gravis (edrophonium).

Indications

The antimyasthenics are the treatment of choice for relieving myasthenic symptoms.

Neostigmine and pyridostigmine are used as antidotes for nondepolarizing neuromuscular blocking agents used in surgery. Neostigmine is sometimes used for the prevention and treatment of postoperative nonobstructive urine retention and ileus.

Because the antimyasthenics can constrict the bronchi and cause breathing problems, they should be administered cautiously in patients with asthma, pneumonia, or atelectasis and in all postoperative patients. Typically, these drugs are contraindicated in patients with arrhythmias, intestinal or urinary tract obstruction, or urinary tract infection.

Adverse reactions

Drug toxicity and myasthenic crisis are adverse reactions associated with the antimyasthenics. Signs of drug toxicity may include headaches, weakness, diaphoresis, abdominal pain, nausea and vomiting, diarrhea, excessive salivation, and bronchospasm. Myasthenic crisis is marked by bradycardia, difficulty breathing or swallowing, blurred vision, diarrhea, nausea or vomiting, excessive salivation, and weakness.

Care considerations

• Carefully monitor the patient's vital signs, especially his respirations. Keep atropine injection and resuscitation equipment available in case of respiratory arrest. To help identify the most effective dose, document the patient's muscle strength, ease of swallowing, and respiratory effort after each dose.
• Throughout therapy, watch for signs of drug toxicity or underdosage, which can cause myasthenic crisis. Inform the doctor of any adverse reactions to help distinguish between drug toxicity and myasthenic crisis.
• Check the patient's drug regimen for possible interactions. For example, concurrent use of aminoglycosides, anesthetics, lidocaine, polymyxin, lincomycin, quinidine, or procainamide may antagonize antimyasthenic effects. The antihypertensives guanethidine and trimethaphan may worsen myasthenic symptoms. Atropine and related compounds may reduce or prevent some adverse effects of antimyasthenics and may mask initial signs of toxicity. Concurrent use of other cholinesterase inhibitors, particularly edrophonium, can cause rapid toxicity.

Home care instructions

• Tell the patient and family caregiver the signs of drug toxicity and myasthenic crisis. Instruct them to report any such signs immediately.
• Allow the patient some control in determining his drug dose and schedule. To maximize the drug's effectiveness, encourage the patient to schedule his largest doses before usual periods of fatigue, such as the late afternoon and before meals, and to schedule rest times for such periods.
• Teach the patient how to evaluate and record variations in muscle strength. Instruct him to keep a diary of these variations, correlated to the time of day and medication schedule, to help the doctor evaluate therapy.
• During adjustment to therapy, have the patient take the drug with food or milk to minimize GI distress. Explain that scheduling a dose 30 minutes before meals may help alleviate dysphagia.
• Because even a minor respiratory infection can aggravate myasthenic symptoms, instruct the patient to avoid contact with all persons with infections.
• Advise the patient to wear a medical identification bracelet or carry a card indicating his condition and current drug regimen.

ANTIPSYCHOTICS

Antipsychotics (also called major tranquilizers and neuroleptics) are used to help control the symptoms of psychoses and may help patients become more receptive to psychotherapy. The major classes of antipsychotics include the *phenothiazines*, the *butyrophenones*, the *thioxanthenes*, the *dihydroindolones*, and two classes of *dibenzoxazepines*, the *dibenzodiazepines* and the *diphenylbutylpiperidines*.

Purpose

• To relieve psychotic symptoms
• To provide sedation.

Indications

Antipsychotics treat a wide variety of disorders, including schizophrenia, organic psychoses, and the manic phase of bipolar disorders. They're also used for acute psychotic symptoms, such as paranoia, hostility, combativeness, hallucinations, and persistent delusions. Some of these agents also may be used as antiemetics.

Adverse reactions

Patients receiving antipsychotics require careful monitoring for compliance and adverse reactions. Major reactions vary depending on the drug class, but may include excessive sedation, extrapyramidal symptoms (dystonic movements, torticollis, and parkinsonian symptoms), orthostatic hypotension with reflex tachycardia, fainting, dizziness, and arrhythmias; GI reactions such as nausea, dry mouth, vomiting, abdominal pain, and gastric irritation; ocular and visual changes; skin eruptions; photosensitivity; anticholinergic effects; leukopenia; and agranulocytosis (particularly seen with clozapine).

Neuroleptic malignant syndrome is a rare but life-threatening disorder that can accompany therapy with antipsychotics. This syndrome is characterized by respiratory distress, fever, hypertension or hypotension, incontinence, rigidity, and weakness. Other signs include pallor, fatigue, and arrhythmias. With early recognition of the syndrome, fatalities have decreased to about 4%.

Care considerations

• Carefully observe the patient for adverse reactions. Extrapyramidal symptoms are most common with the piperazine phenothiazines: haloperidol, thiothixene, molindone, and loxapine. Sedation is most common with chlorprom-azine, triflupromazine, or piperidine phenothiazines. Orthostatic hypotension occurs with chlorpromazine and thioridazine; anticholinergic effects, such as dry mouth, occur with promazine, triflupromazine, and thioridazine.

• Reassure the patient who experiences extrapyramidal symptoms that they are typically reversible. If ordered, administer an antiparkinsonian drug, such as diphenhydramine or benztropine. These symptoms usually subside within 3 months; if they persist, the doctor may discontinue the antipsychotic or reduce its dosage. However, if the patient experiences an acute dystonic reaction, administer diphenhydramine or benztropine I.M. or I.V., as ordered, and maintain airway clearance and adequate hydration.

• During prolonged therapy, watch for tardive dyskinesia, a potentially irreversible syndrome characterized by rhythmic, involuntary movements of the tongue, face, mouth, jaw, and extremities. If you detect this syndrome, notify the doctor immediately.

• If the patient experiences excessive sedation, take appropriate safety precautions, such as raising the side rails of the bed and assisting with ambulation.

• Monitor the patient's blood pressure to detect orthostatic hypotension. If it occurs, advise him to rise slowly from a sitting or lying position to avoid dizziness or light-headedness.

• If the patient experiences dry mouth, suggest hard candy or sugarless gum. To relieve constipation, increase the patient's fluid intake and provide a stool softener. Help the patient select low-calorie foods to combat weight gain and to maintain adequate nutrition.

• Be alert for neuroleptic malignant syndrome.

• Because antipsychotics can cause leukopenia and agranulocytosis, monitor complete blood count and differential count throughout therapy. Because these drugs can cause hepatic impair-

ment, observe for jaundice and check the results of liver function studies.
• Check also for tachycardia or electrocardiographic changes, which can require dosage adjustment.
• Review the patient's medication regimen for possible interactions. Barbiturates, for example, may reduce the therapeutic effect of phenothiazines. Lithium, commonly used with haloperidol during early treatment of acute manic episodes, may cause irreversible neurotoxicity with continued use.

Home care instructions

• Instruct the patient to make up a missed dose if he remembers within 2 hours of the scheduled administration time. If more than 2 hours elapse, advise him to omit the dose and take the next scheduled dose. Warn against doubling the next dose.
• Advise the patient to report a sore throat, fever, or weakness immediately. These symptoms may indicate blood dyscrasias.
• Caution the patient against driving or performing hazardous tasks that require alertness until predictable response to the drug is established.
• Warn the patient against excessive exposure to the sun to reduce the risk of phototoxicity.
• If the patient is receiving an antipsychotic that can cause orthostatic hypotension, such as chlorpromazine, suggest that he rise slowly from a lying or sitting position.
• If the patient takes antacids and a phenothiazine, instruct him to separate doses of these drugs by at least 2 hours.
• If the patient takes a liquid phenothiazine, warn him against skin contact with the drug because it may cause contact dermatitis.
• Tell the patient to avoid alcohol because it can cause additive sedation.
• Warn the patient to check with the doctor before discontinuing any antipsychotic. Patients are usually weaned

gradually; abrupt withdrawal may cause nausea, vomiting, trembling, and dizziness.
• Tell the patient taking clozapine to schedule weekly blood tests to identify potential life-threatening toxicity (leukopenia and agranuloytosis).

ANTISPASMODICS

Flavoxate and *oxybutynin* inhibit smooth-muscle spasm in the urinary tract.

Purpose

• To exert a direct spasmolytic effect on the smooth muscles of the urinary tract (flavoxate)
• To increase bladder capacity (oxybutynin)
• To provide local anesthetic and mild analgesic effects.

Indications

Antispasmodics are widely used to relieve contractions in neurogenic bladder and to provide symptomatic relief of dysuria, urinary frequency and urgency, nocturia, incontinence, suprapubic pain, and bladder and ureteral spasm in various urologic disorders.

Because of their spasmolytic effects, these drugs should be given cautiously to patients with suspected glaucoma, pyloric or duodenal obstruction, intestinal lesions or ileus, or urinary tract obstruction. For information on another drug used to treat neurogenic bladder, see *Treating urine retention with bethanechol*, page 64.

Adverse reactions

Adverse reactions include constipation; urine retention; visual disturbances such as eye pain, blurred vision, and photophobia; tachycardia; fever; rash; pruritus; urticaria; and mental confusion, such as memory loss and paradoxical excitement.

Treating urine retention with bethanechol

A potent cholinergic drug, bethanechol is widely used to treat urine retention caused by neurogenic bladder. It's also used to relieve acute postoperative and postpartum nonobstructive retention. Typically the initial treatment for these disorders, bethanechol may preclude the need for invasive measures, such as bladder drainage or permanent urinary diversion.

Administration tips
Because bethanechol is highly potent, it requires careful administration and monitoring of the patient's response. It's usually given orally in high doses (up to 100 mg) to relieve urine retention; S.C. test doses may be administered to determine the minimal effective dose. The drug should never be given I.M. or I.V.; doing so could precipitate hypotension, severe abdominal cramps, bloody diarrhea, and even shock, circulatory collapse, or cardiac arrest.

When giving bethanechol, monitor the patient's vital signs, noting especially his respiratory rate and pattern. Have atropine available and be prepared to provide respiratory support if needed. Watch closely for signs of drug toxicity, such as abdominal cramps and diarrhea, especially during S.C. administration.

Care considerations

• Review the patient's drug regimen for possible interactions. Concurrent use of anticholinergics, for instance, enhances the effects of both drugs.
• Periodically monitor vital signs during therapy, watching especially for tachycardia and fever. Notify the doctor if these signs occur.
• Observe for signs of drug hypersensitivity, such as rash, pruritus, and urticaria. If these develop, discontinue the drug and alert the doctor, who may reduce the dosage or substitute another drug.
• Monitor intake and output to assess the drug's effectiveness and detect urine retention. Encourage adequate fluid intake to help prevent retention and constipation.
• Assess for visual disturbances, such as eye pain, blurred vision, and photophobia; these may require ophthalmologic evaluation. Report any changes in mental status, such as confusion, memory loss, and paradoxical excitement. Elderly patients are especially susceptible to these effects.

Home care instructions

• Tell the patient to take oxybutynin or flavoxate with milk or food to help reduce GI upset. (The patient can take it with water on an empty stomach if he doesn't experience any discomfort.)
• Tell the patient taking oxybutynin or flavoxate that if he misses a dose, he should take it as soon as possible. However, if it's almost time for the next dose, he should omit the missed dose. Warn the patient never to double-dose.
• Because antispasmodics can cause dizziness or drowsiness, advise the patient against hazardous activities that require alertness, coordination, and clear vision until response to the drug has been determined.
• Warn the patient against using alcohol and other central nervous system (CNS) depressants, which can increase the drug's sedative effects.
• Because antispasmodics interfere with perspiration and thermoregulation, tell the patient to avoid prolonged exercise or strenuous activity, especially in hot weather, to prevent drug-induced heatstroke.
• Suggest sugarless gum, hard candy, or ice chips to relieve dry mouth and

throat. Tell the patient to report excessive dryness that lasts longer than 2 weeks.

• Instruct the patient to report any eye problems, such as blurred vision, pain, or abnormal sensitivity to light. Advise wearing sunglasses when outdoors.

• Tell the patient to report rash, flushing, hives, adverse CNS reactions (dizziness, drowsiness, anxiety, impaired coordination, agitation, or hallucinations), difficulty breathing, shortness of breath, or a rapid or irregular pulse.

• Explain to the patient that he can minimize constipation, another common adverse reaction, by increasing intake of fluids and high-fiber foods.

ANTITUSSIVES

Antitussives (codeine, dextromethorphan, diphenhydramine, hydrocodone, and hydromorphone) suppress cough by central mechanisms.

Purpose
• To relieve nonproductive cough.

Indications

Antitussives are used to provide symptomatic relief of cough due to various causes, including viral upper respiratory infections. These drugs effectively suppress a dry, nonproductive cough, which can tire a patient and interfere with sleep or daily activities. Antitussives may also be used to suppress coughing in patients at risk for pneumothorax, tussive syncope, or rib fractures.

The opiate antitussives, such as codeine phosphate and hydrocodone, effectively suppress coughing. However, their use is limited because of the potential for toxicity and abuse and the range of adverse effects, from GI upset to central nervous system (CNS) depression. The nonopiate antitussives, dextromethorphan and diphenhydra-

---

Alternatives to antitussives

Not every patient with a cough needs an antitussive. An expectorant, which liquefies secretions and promotes their expulsion, may be more useful when the patient has pneumonia, bronchitis, cystic fibrosis, or tuberculosis. The following expectorants are commonly used.

Acetylcysteine
This mucolytic is usually given by nebulization through a face mask or mouthpiece. It helps treat acute and chronic bronchopulmonary diseases. Acetylcysteine is contraindicated in patients with reactive airways because it may cause bronchospasm.

Guaifenesin
A common ingredient in over-the-counter cough preparations, guaifenesin liquefies secretions and promotes expectoration but can cause drowsiness and GI upset.

Terpin hydrate
This elixir liquefies secretions and promotes expectoration. The recommended dosage shouldn't be exceeded because of terpin hydrate's high alcohol content.

---

mine, are common ingredients in over-the-counter cough and cold preparations.

Opiate (narcotic) antitussives are not intended for chronic use and are not recommended in chronic obstructive pulmonary disease because even slight respiratory depression may have a harmful effect. They must be used cautiously in children and in patients with CNS disorders. In some cases, patients with a cough require an expectorant rather than an antitussive. (See *Alternatives to antitussives*.)

Adverse reactions

The opiate antitussives may cause CNS depression, dizziness, seizures, constipation, nausea and vomiting, palpitations, hypotension, pruritus, and hypersensitivity reactions. The nonopiate antitussives are associated with sedation, hypersensitivity reactions, dizziness, and constipation.

Care considerations

• At the start of therapy, carefully monitor CNS response to prevent accidents caused by dizziness and drowsiness. As needed, raise the side rails of the patient's bed, provide assistance with ambulation, and impose safety precautions.
• Ask the patient about adverse GI reactions, such as nausea.
• If the patient is taking an opiate antitussive, observe him for diaphoresis and light-headedness. If these signs occur with dizziness and nausea, the doctor may need to reduce the dosage.
• Observe for rash, pruritus, or urticaria, which may signal a hypersensitivity reaction. If any of these reactions occur, discontinue the drug and notify the doctor.
• Encourage fluids and a high-fiber diet because opiates may cause constipation.
• Monitor the patient's drug regimen for possible interactions. For example, using dextromethorphan with a monoamine oxidase (MAO) inhibitor can cause high fever, rigidity, laryngospasm, or bronchospasm. Using an opiate antitussive with narcotic analgesics, tranquilizers, sedatives, hypnotics, tricyclic antidepressants, or MAO inhibitors increases CNS depression.

Home care instructions

• Advise the patient to take the drug with food or milk to help prevent GI upset, to take the syrup form undiluted, and not to drink liquids afterward.
• Warn the patient that antitussives cause drowsiness. He should avoid driving and other hazardous activities that require alertness until CNS reactions are known.

• Recommend sugarless hard candy, ice chips, or sugarless gum to relieve dry mouth.
• Encourage the patient to drink about eight 8-oz glasses (2,000 ml) of fluid daily to thin secretions and ensure hydration. Suggest the use of a vaporizer at night to minimize the drying effects of room air. Recommend hot tea with honey and lemon, other hot beverages, and hard candy or lozenges to help relieve cough.
• If the patient is taking an opiate antitussive, tell him to avoid oversedation by not exceeding the recommended dosage. Emphasize that long-term use can lead to dependence.

ANTIVIRALS, SYSTEMIC

Systemic viral infections are generally treated using oral or I.V. antiviral therapy. The antivirals include *acyclovir, amantadine, didanosine (ddI), foscarnet, ganciclovir, ribavirin, vidarabine, zalcitabine (ddC),* and *zidovudine (AZT).*

Purpose

• To treat viral infections by inactivating the virus, inhibiting viral replication, or modifying the host response to infection.

Indications

Each antiviral is used for the treatment of a different viral infection.

Acyclovir is used to treat herpes simplex virus type 1 and type 2 and varicella-zoster (shingles) infections. Amantadine is used for the treatment or prophylaxis of influenza A virus. Ganciclovir is used to treat cytomegalovirus retinitis in immunocompromised patients, particularly those with acquired immunodeficiency syndrome (AIDS). Ribavirin is used most often in infants and children with respiratory syncytial virus. Vidarabine is used to treat herpes simplex virus encephalitis, neonatal herpes simplex virus infections, and herpes zoster in immunocompromised patients. Oral zidovudine has become a mainstay in the treatment of patients with human immunodeficiency virus (HIV) infection, AIDS-related complex, or AIDS. Didanosine and zalcitabine are usually reserved for AIDS patients who are unresponsive to or unable to tolerate treatment with zidovudine. The I.V. preparation of zidovudine is used to treat patients with HIV infections who have a history of *Pneumocystis carinii* pneumonia or an absolute CD4 + T-lymphocyte count below 200/mm³ before therapy. Foscarnet is indicated for the treatment of cytomegalovirus retinitis in patients with AIDS. Treatment with this drug requires monitoring of renal function and reduced dosage in patients with renal impairment.

Acyclovir should be given with caution to patients with dehydration, preexisting renal impairment, severe hepatic function impairment, neurologic abnormalities, or prior neurologic reactions to cytotoxic medications. Amantadine should be used cautiously in patients with seizure disorders, congestive heart failure, peripheral edema, hepatic disease, mental illness, eczematoid rash, renal impairment, orthostatic hypertension, and cardiovascular disease, and in elderly patients. Ganciclovir should not be administered if the patient's absolute neutrophil count is below 500/mm³ or his platelet count is below 25,000/mm³; dosage should be reduced in patients with renal function impairment. Ribavirin is contraindicated in women who are or may become pregnant during treatment; it should be used cautiously in ventilator-dependent patients because the drug may precipitate in the ventilator apparatus, causing a malfunction. Vidarabine should be used cautiously in patients with hepatic or renal dysfunction and in patients with restricted fluid intake. Zidovudine should be given with caution if the patient is also receiving acyclovir because

lethargy and fatigue may occur. Other drugs that interact if they are given concurrently with zidovudine include cotrimoxazole, acetaminophen, cytotoxic drugs, pentamidine, dapsone, flucytosine, amphotericin B, and probenecid.

Adverse reactions

Adverse reactions associated with I.V. administration of acyclovir include inflammation or phlebitis at the injection site and adverse central nervous system (CNS) reactions, such as headache, encephalopathic changes, lethargy, obtundation, tremors, confusion, hallucinations, agitation, seizures, and coma. GI symptoms associated with oral administration include nausea and vomiting. Skin rash or hives can occur regardless of the administration route. When administered with probenecid, blood levels of acyclovir may increase.

Common adverse reactions associated with amantadine include irritability, insomnia, light-headedness, difficulty concentrating, anorexia, nausea, nervousness, and livedo reticularis (purplish red, netlike, blotchy marks on the skin). Elderly patients with age-related decline in renal function may have increased sensitivity to the adverse reactions to amantadine.

Common adverse reactions to didanosine include headache, diarrhea, nausea, vomiting, and abdominal pain. The most serious adverse reactions include pancreatitis (which may be fatal) and peripheral neuropathy. Similarly, the most common toxic response associated with zalcitabine is peripheral neuropathy; the major life-threatening toxic response is pancreatitis.

Ribavirin causes little or no systemic toxicity, so adverse reactions are few. Some reactions include anemia, conjunctivitis, eyelid rash, or erythema, and worsening of the patient's respiratory state.

Adverse reactions associated with administration of vidarabine include tremor, dizziness, hallucinations, confusion, ataxia, anorexia, and nausea. Concurrent use with allopurinol reduces the metabolism of vibarabine and increases the risk of adverse CNS reactions.

Reactions to zidovudine include severe bone marrow depression (resulting in anemia), granulocytopenia, and thrombocytopenia.

The major dose-limiting effect of ganciclovir is myelosuppression. Other more common reactions are neutropenia and thrombocytopenia.

Care considerations

For acyclovir

• I.V. infusion must be administered over at least 1 hour to prevent renal tubular damage.

• Notify the doctor if the serum creatinine level does not return to normal within a few days.

• Ensure that the patient is adequately hydrated during acyclovir infusion.

• Keep in mind that encephalopathic changes are more likely in patients with neurologic disorders or in those who have had neurologic reactions to cytotoxic drugs.

For amantadine

• For best absorption, give the drug after meals.

• Elderly patients are more susceptible to neurologic adverse reactions. Administer the drug in two daily doses rather than a single dose to reduce their incidence.

• If insomnia occurs, have the patient take the drug several hours before bedtime.

• If orthostatic hypotension occurs, instruct the patient not to stand or change positions too quickly.

For didanosine and zalcitabine

• Peripheral neuropathy is a major adverse reaction to didanosine therapy; therefore, monitor the patient for distal numbness, tingling, or pain in the feet or hands.

• Pancreatitis may occur in as many as 9% of patients taking didanosine; it occurs in less than 1% of patients taking zalcitabine. Observe the patient for such signs as abdominal pain, nausea, or vomiting; elevated amylase, lipase, and serum bilirubin; or elevated white blood cell (WBC) count. If they occur, pancreatitis must be ruled out and the drug should be discontinued.

For foscarnet

• Monitor renal function and maintain adequate hydration throughout therapy.

• Observe the patient for adverse reactions, including fever, nausea, vomiting, anemia, diarrhea, headache, and seizures.

• Monitor serum electrolyte levels, especially calcium, magnesium, potassium, and phosphorus.

For ganciclovir

• The dosage should be reduced in patients with renal dysfunction.

• Infuse the drug I.V. over at least 1 hour because increased toxicity will result if given too quickly.

• Ensure that the patient is adequately hydrated during therapy.

• Obtain neutrophil and platelet counts every 2 days during twice-daily dosing (and at least weekly thereafter) to monitor for neutropenia and thrombocytopenia.

For ribavirin

• Administer ribavirin aerosol by the Viratek Small Particle Aerosol Generator (SPAG-2) only.

• To reconstitute this drug, use sterile water – not bacteriostatic water. The water used to reconstitute the drug should not contain any antimicrobial agent.

For vidarabine

• Monitor hematologic tests, such as hemoglobin, hematocrit, WBC count, and platelet count during therapy. These may be decreased by vidarabine therapy. Also monitor renal and liver function studies.

• Vidarabine administration requires a large volume of fluid for preparation and administration, so be alert for fluid overload.

• Patients with impaired renal function may need dosage adjustment.

For zidovudine

• The patient's complete blood count should be monitored every 2 weeks for the first 8 weeks of therapy to detect anemia or granulocytopenia.

• Periodically perform liver function tests to monitor for hepatotoxicity (rare).

Home care instructions

• Tell the patient receiving acyclovir to avoid sexual contact during therapy while herpes lesions are present. Explain that this medication does not cure herpes. Also tell the patient not to share the medication.

• Instruct the patient receiving amantadine to report adverse reactions to the doctor, especially dizziness, depression, anxiety, nausea, and urine retention. Also tell the patient to take the drug after meals for the best absorption.

• Monitor blood urea nitrogen, serum creatinine, WBC and differential, platelet count, serum bilirubin, serum alanine aminotransferase and serum aspartate aminotransferase if the patient is receiving ganciclovir.

• Be sure the patient receiving oral zidovudine, didanosine, or zalcitabine understands that these drugs do not cure HIV infection. Urge the patient to report any health changes to the doctor. Also reemphasize that the patient should avoid sexual contact or use a latex condom.

• Explain to the patient receiving zidovudine that it is important to take this medicine every 4 hours around the clock. Tell him to set an alarm clock to be certain that he will wake up to take the doses. Asymptomatic patients may take doses every 4 hours while awake.

• Tell the patient to take doses of didanosine at least 2 hours after taking

ketoconazole, dapsone, tetracycline, or quinolone antibiotics.

APPENDECTOMY

Appendectomy is the surgical removal of an inflamed vermiform appendix. Commonly performed as an emergency procedure, this surgery aims to prevent imminent rupture or perforation of the inflamed appendix. When completed before the onset of such complications, appendectomy is generally effective and uneventful. After an uncomplicated appendectomy, the patient can be discharged on the day of surgery. If perforation or rupture occurs before appendectomy, however, a localized right lower abdominal quadrant abscess, a pelvic abscess, or generalized peritonitis can occur. If an abscess occurs, the appendectomy is postponed for 6 to 12 weeks, during which antibiotics are administered to control the infection. If peritonitis occurs, an appendectomy is performed to remove the source of the infection.

Purpose

• To remove an inflamed appendix.

Indications

Appendectomy is indicated for acute appendicitis.

Procedure

An appendectomy is usually performed under general anesthesia but may be done under spinal or local anesthesia. To remove the appendix, an incision (McBurney, muscle-splitting or gridiron, or Rockey-Davis or transverse incision) is made over the point of tenderness in the right lower abdominal quadrant, and the appendix is exposed and removed. After removal, the surgeon ligates the base of the appendix, places a purse-string suture in the cecum, removes excess tis-

Laparoscopic appendectomy

Laparoscopic appendectomy is a new technique for removal of the appendix. In this procedure, the surgeon inserts a trocar and laparoscope through a small incision under the umbilicus and confirms the clinical diagnosis. With the help of transabdominal illumination by a light source inserted through the laparoscope, he makes another small abdominal incision to allow insertion of a second trocar. The surgeon detaches the appendix, using instruments inserted through the trocars, and then removes it from the abdominal cavity through a trocar without contaminating the incisions.

   This technique is believed to be relatively safe, simple, and quick. If the surgeon is skilled in laparoscopic procedures, laparoscopic appendectomy can be performed in about 10 minutes. Other advantages of this procedure include the absence of a large scar, reduced risk of thermal injury to surrounding organs, and easily achieved hemostasis.

sue and fluid from the abdomen, and closes the incision. (For an alternative approach to this procedure, see *Laparoscopic appendectomy*.)

   The incision usually heals without drainage. However, drains are used if an abscess is discovered, or if rupture occurred or is imminent.

Complications

Potential complications of appendectomy include peritonitis, which has a 10% mortality rate; pelvic or lumbar abscess; subphrenic abscess; paralytic ileus; and wound infection.

Care considerations

Before surgery

• Because it's commonly an emergency, appendectomy usually allows little time for preoperative teaching. If time permits, reassure the patient that the surgery will relieve his pain and won't interfere with normal GI function.
• Administer antibiotics as ordered to prevent infection.
• As appropriate, insert an I.V. line and administer I.V. fluids to replace lost fluids and maintain fluid balance.
• Position the patient in Fowler's position to reduce pain, but avoid using analgesics because they can mask the pain that heralds rupture.

• Don't administer heat, cathartics, or enemas because these measures can trigger rupture of the appendix.
• Insertion of a nasogastric tube to decompress the stomach and reduce nausea and vomiting is necessary if there is suspicion of or potential for paralytic ileus.

After surgery

• Place the patient in Fowler's position immediately after recovery from anesthesia to decrease the risk of infecting the upper abdomen by exposure to contaminated peritoneal fluid.
• Encourage ambulation within 12 hours of surgery.
• Encourage coughing, deep-breathing, and frequent position changes to prevent pulmonary complications.
• After an uncomplicated appendectomy, encourage the patient to gradually resume oral foods beginning on the day of surgery.
• If drains were inserted during surgery, monitor the type and amount of drainage.
• Throughout recovery, monitor for signs of peritonitis. Observe for continuing pain and fever, excessive wound drainage, hypotension, tachycardia, pallor, weakness, and other signs of infection and fluid and electrolyte loss. If peritonitis develops, emergency

treatment may include GI intubation, parenteral fluid and electrolyte replacement, and antibiotic therapy.

Home care instructions

• Instruct the patient to watch for and immediately report fever, chills, diaphoresis, nausea, vomiting, or abdominal pain and tenderness.
• The patient who is discharged after an uncomplicated appendectomy on the day of surgery should understand that he must return to have the sutures removed from the incision on the 5th or 7th postoperative day. If an appointment has not been made, remind him to call the doctor's office to schedule one.
• Emphasize the importance of medical follow-up to monitor healing and detect any developing complications.

ARRHYTHMIA CATHETER ABLATION

Catheter ablation is a new procedure for treatment of symptomatic sustained arrhythmias. It involves placing a special large-tipped electrode catheter inside the heart through the arterial or venous system and using direct current (DC) or radiofrequency (RF) energy to disrupt abnormally conducting tissue pathways. Presently, RF energy is the preferred method of ablation because it can deliver a more localized and discrete focus of energy with fewer complications.

Ablation is most effective for treatment of supraventricular tachycardia (SVT); results have been less consistent for treatment of ventricular tachycardia (VT). Catheter ablation is not indicated for patients in whom the arrhythmia focus (origin) cannot be precisely located nor when multiple foci are present. Because extensive electrical mapping is required, patients

must be hemodynamically stable during the arrhythmia.

Purpose

• To completely eliminate sustained arrhythmias
• To control arrhythmias in patients in whom previous drug and other therapy has been unsuccessful.

Indications

Catheter ablation is indicated for treatment of atrial, atrioventricular (AV) nodal, bypass tract, and ventricular arrhythmias where the site of origin of the arrhythmias is accessible and identifiable by precise catheter mapping.

Ablation for SVT has been reserved for patients not responsive to or intolerant of antiarrhythmic drugs, but is being used more often as first-line therapy to avoid the need for lifelong drug treatment.

VT ablation is indicated for drug-refractory patients who are not candidates for surgery or an implantable defibrillator and in some patients where the ventricular arrhythmia's exact site of origin can be localized. Improvement in technique and catheter design as well as development of new energy systems may make ablation the treatment of choice for a larger number of patients.

Procedure

Catheter ablation is performed in the electrophysiology or cardiac catheterization laboratory. Multiple electrode catheters are placed percutaneously into the femoral, brachial, internal jugular, or subclavian veins and through the femoral artery if access to the left heart is required. Catheters are guided under fluoroscopy to the right atrium, bundle of His, right ventricle, or coronary sinus. VT ablation may require placing a catheter into the left ventricle; some SVT ablations require left atrial catheterization. Electrocardiograms (ECGs) are recorded from surface ECG leads and intracardiac leads during normal sinus rhythm, during pacing, and after induction of the arrhythmia to identify the precise location of the arrhythmia focus. This area is then ablated as follows.

RF energy slowly heats the tissue and results in a well-demarcated area of necrosis less than 5 mm wide. Energy is delivered through the catheter for 20 to 30 seconds or up to 2 minutes, if needed. This can be repeated several times. It is done with the patient awake or lightly sedated and causes only minimal chest wall discomfort.

DC electrical shocks, performed less commonly, uses a standard defibrillator. DC shocks produce a larger area of damage, destroying the arrhythmia focus along with normal surrounding tissue. They also stimulate skeletal muscle and nerves, necessitating general anesthesia. Early experience with catheter ablation used DC energy to destroy the bundle of His or AV nodal area, eliminating drug-refractory SVT that was dependent on AV conduction. DC energy also induced complete heart block, requiring permanent pacemaker implantation.

Cryoablation, freezing with nitrous oxide, is performed primarily in the operating room, often with endocardial resection. Laser ablation and microwave ablation are currently under investigation.

Complications

Complications may include the risks associated with catheterization — venous or arterial damage, thrombosis, pericardial tamponade, cardiac perforation, and death. Possibly, the scar tissue created by ablation will become a new arrhythmia focus. Normal conduction tissue may be damaged by ablation, resulting in heart block. The overall risk of this procedure is low; however, complications are more likely with DC ablation.

Care considerations

• During and after ablation, patients should be monitored by telemetry for recurrence or worsening of arrhythmia or occurrence of heart block. Placement of a temporary or permanent pacemaker may be required.
• Monitor vital signs; be alert for signs of pericardial tamponade, such as hypotension, shortness of breath, and distended neck veins.
• Evaluate puncture sites for bleeding or hematoma formation.
• Check serum electrolytes, especially potassium and magnesium, for abnormalities that can predispose the patient to arrhythmias. Creatine phosphokinase levels may be determined to assess myocardial damage.
• Give the patient predischarge instructions appropriate to individual needs. Teaching should include instructions for antiarrhythmic drug or device therapy.

Home care instructions

• Follow-up care will vary, depending on the results of the ablation. Instruct the patient as appropriate. Tell the patient that follow-up electrophysiologic testing may be required, especially if symptomatic arrhythmias recur.
• Emphasize the importance of compliance with antiarrhythmic drug or device therapy, if applicable.

ARTHROCENTESIS

Arthrocentesis involves insertion of a needle into the joint space to aspirate synovial fluid or blood or to instill corticosteroids or other anti-inflammatory drugs. It also may be performed to obtain a specimen for diagnostic testing.

Arthrocentesis is most commonly performed on the knee, less often on the elbow, shoulder, or other joints. It's often combined with two related procedures: arthroscopy, which allows endoscopic visualization of the joint, and arthrography, an X-ray showing joint tissue and structure.

Purpose

• To relieve the pain, distention, and inflammation resulting from accumulation of fluid within a joint
• To administer local drug therapy, usually corticosteroids, especially when systemic routes are contraindicated or have been unsuccessful
• To obtain a specimen for laboratory analysis
• To aid the differential diagnosis of arthritis, particularly rheumatoid arthritis.

Indications

Arthrocentesis is commonly used as an adjunctive treatment for orthopedic problems or disorders, such as joint trauma or septic arthritis. As a diagnostic aid, arthrocentesis is indicated when an infection or other inflammatory arthropathy (such as rheumatoid arthritis) is suspected.

Arthrocentesis is contraindicated if the patient has bacteremia, if there is any local infection around the joint structure, or if the skin around the site is not intact. The presence of bacteremia contraindicates this procedure because insertion of the needle almost always causes some capillary breakage and leakage of blood into the joint fluid, which contaminates the joint fluid. This procedure is also contraindicated in the weight-bearing joints of patients with osteoarthritis, except in rare cases, because the benefits for these patients are transient and frequent injections result in joint destruction.

Procedure

Throughout the procedure, the joint must be kept motionless. Depending on the approach used and the site, the joint is stabilized in extension or flexion. Using sterile technique, the doctor prepares the site and injects or sprays a local anesthetic at the site. He then inserts the appropriate needle and aspirates at least 10 to 15 ml of synovial fluid. To administer medication into the joint, the needle is left in place while the fluid-filled syringe is detached and replaced by the drug-filled syringe. Then the drug is injected.

Complications

Although rare, complications of arthrocentesis may include joint infection, damage to the articular cartilage, hemorrhage leading to hemarthrosis (accumulation of blood within the joint), tendon rupture, and temporary nerve palsy.

Care considerations

Before the procedure

• Make sure that the patient understands the procedure.
• Inform the patient that a local anesthetic will be given, but he may feel some pain as the needle is introduced into the joint space.
• If the patient is having arthrocentesis to withdraw a sample of synovial fluid for glucose analysis, restrict food or fluids for the prescribed length of time (usually 6 to 12 hours) before the procedure.
• Check the patient's history for hypersensitivity to iodine compounds, such as povidone-iodine, and to lidocaine and other local anesthetics. If hypersensitivity exists, the patient should not receive a local anesthetic containing this agent. Also note if the patient is taking an anticoagulant, a corticosteroid, or any nonsteroidal anti-inflammatory drugs because these drugs can increase the risk of bleeding into the joint during and after the procedure.

After the procedure

• Monitor the puncture site for excessive bleeding. If this occurs, apply a pressure dressing and notify the doctor.

• Elevate the affected limb and apply ice or cold packs to the joint for 24 to 36 hours to decrease pain and swelling.

• Assess for signs of infection, such as fever or increased joint pain. Report such signs promptly, and prepare to initiate antibiotic therapy as appropriate.

• To minimize the risk of infection, keep the puncture site clean and handle dressings and linens carefully, using universal precautions.

Home care instructions

• Advise the patient to resume normal activities as appropriate. However, the patient should avoid overusing the affected joint for several days, to prevent increased pain, swelling, or stiffness.

• Instruct the patient to immediately report increased pain, redness, swelling, or fever; explain that these signs may indicate infection, which requires prompt medical attention.

• Emphasize the importance of follow-up appointments to evaluate the effectiveness of treatment.

ARTHROSCOPY

Arthroscopy is a surgical procedure that uses a specially designed fiber-optic tubular instrument called an arthroscope for visual examination of the interior of a joint. The procedure is performed under local, spinal, or general anesthesia, depending on the anticipated length and complexity of the procedure.

Arthroscopy is most commonly used to examine the knee but is increasingly being used for other joints (the shoulder, elbow, ankle, wrist, and hip). Arthroscopy is a useful diagnostic aid only after a thorough clinical workup and conservative treatment have failed to remedy the joint problem.

Purpose

• To perform joint surgery

• To monitor the progression of a disease

• To detect and diagnose meniscal, patellar, condylar, extrasynovial, and synovial diseases.

Indications

General indications for arthroscopy include the removal of loose fragments, synovectomy, the lysis of adhesions, and diagnostic viewing.

Arthroscopic knee surgery is indicated for resection of plicae, shaving of the patella, meniscus repair, and repairs of anterior and posterior ligaments.

Shoulder arthroscopy is indicated for synovial biopsy, bursectomies, stabilization of dislocations, relief of impingement syndrome, and correction of glenoid labrum, biceps tendon, and rotator cuff tears.

Elbow arthroscopy is indicated for the evaluation or debridement of osteochondritis dissecans of the capitellum and radial head. This procedure is typically used for evaluating fractures of the capitellum, radial head, or olecranon.

Ankle arthroscopy is indicated for lateral ligamentous reconstruction and osteochondritis dissecans of the talus. Arthroscopy is used infrequently in the wrist and hip joints, but use at these sites to aid diagnosis and visualization and to remove loose fragments is growing.

Procedure

This procedure is performed in the operating room under local or general anesthesia. After inserting a large-bore needle into the joint, the surgeon injects sterile 0.9% sodium chloride solution to distend the joint and then introduces the arthroscope into the joint through a small incision in the skin. The surgeon then empties the joint of blood and debris using arthroscopic irrigation and suction. When the joint is clear, the surgeon examines the articular cartilage and ligaments for abnormalities. The surgeon may then make a small incision at another place on the extremity and use this new entry site to insert small instruments to facilitate manipulation of anatomic structures and to allow certain repairs—for example, of a torn meniscus. These small incisions cause little or no scarring.

When the examination and procedure is completed, the arthroscope is removed and the joint is irrigated. Adhesive strips are applied over incision sites and a compression bandage is applied over the surgical site.

Complications

Arthroscopy rarely causes complications. The most common complications are infection and thrombophlebitis, but even these occur in fewer than 1% of patients. Hemarthrosis (blood in the joint cavity), stiffness, and delayed wound healing may occur. Vascular damage leading to loss of the limb is possible when arthroscopic instruments damage arteries, but this is exceedingly rare. There also is a small risk of instrument breakage within the joint.

Care considerations

Before surgery

• Describe the arthroscopy procedure and reinforce the doctor's explanation.
• Explain expected outcomes and the usual rehabilitative course.
• Teach the patient and family how to perform the prescribed postoperative exercises, as appropriate.
• Remind the patient to report any skin abrasions on the affected extremity or any new medical problems.

After surgery

• Monitor vital signs and perform circulatory and neurovascular assessments of the affected limb.
• Apply an ice pack to the affected extremity.

• The patient is typically discharged from the same-day surgical department several hours after the recovery room time is complete. After a more extensive procedure such as arthrotomy, the patient may stay overnight in the hospital, primarily for pain control.

Home care instructions

• Tell the patient that he may begin to resume a normal diet with clear liquids; if no nausea develops over several hours, he may progress to a regular diet. Tell the patient to avoid alcoholic beverages for at least 24 hours, avoid driving and other hazardous tasks that require alertness and good coordination, and take prescribed medications as directed. Explain that medications will decrease the pain, allowing easier participation in prescribed exercises.
• Activity restriction varies as recommended by the surgeon. However, any prescribed exercises should be considered as important as the surgery itself. Make sure the patient understands the importance of these exercises and how to perform them correctly. In some cases, the patient may begin physical therapy as early as 2 days after surgery. Active or passive-assistive exercises may require the help of family members.
• If ordered, tell the patient to keep the affected extremity elevated. Ice may be applied postoperatively for 24 to 48 hours.
• Tell the patient to keep the dressing clean and dry and not to change it. The dressing will be changed by the surgeon during the first postoperative follow-up visit.
• The patient should inform the surgeon of any loss of sensation, coldness, blueness, swelling, or rash, or if the dressing is uncomfortable or tight.

ATHERECTOMY

Atherectomy is the mechanical extraction of atherosclerotic plaque from the coronary arteries via a transluminal extraction catheter. The disposable catheter has a cutting head that rotates at 750 revolutions/minute to slice away or pulverize the plaque. The excised plaque is suctioned out of the artery to prevent embolism and subsequent infarction.

Patient selection for coronary atherectomy is based on an electrocardiogram (ECG), a treadmill stress test, cardiac enzyme levels, and angiography to determine the site and extent of the lesions. Proximal lesions are more likely than distal lesions to be treated with atherectomy because of the device's limitations.

Purpose
• To restore oxygenated blood flow to the myocardium
• To relieve angina
• To prevent myocardial infarction.

Indications
Atherectomy is indicated for patients who have angina that is unresponsive to medical therapy and who are candidates for percutaneous transluminal coronary angioplasty (PTCA) or coronary artery bypass grafting (CABG). If complications such as perforation occur during the procedure, immediate CABG or PTCA is necessary.

For patients who have had CABG, atherectomy is an alternative if venous grafts have less than a 50% reocclusion rate. (Venous grafts are thicker than native coronary arteries, so perforation is less likely than when atherectomy is performed in the actual coronary artery. Also, venous grafts may not open as well with angioplasty, so atherectomy is truly a viable option. Atherectomy is not recommended if the

internal mammary arteries were used as grafts.)

Contraindications include lesions at vessel bifurcations or side branches, lesions that may be angular in shape or located in an angle of a vessel, vessels that have developed aneurysms, ulcerated lesions, severely calcified lesions, and occlusions that resist passage of a guide wire.

Procedure
Atherectomies are performed in the cardiac catheterization laboratory with the open-heart surgical team on standby in case CABG becomes necessary. The doctor performs the procedure; however, nurses and cardiovascular technicians assist and are involved in monitoring the patient and in setting up for the procedure.

At the start of the procedure, the patient receives several medications. These may include I.V. nitroglycerin, which is titrated throughout the procedure to keep systolic pressure above 90 mm Hg; sublingual nifedipine to ensure maximal coronary artery dilation and reduced afterload; heparin to prevent thrombogenesis, which may occur because atherectomy is an invasive process; and an I.V. infusion of dextran 40 to prevent platelet aggregation.

To place the atherectomy device in the coronary artery, the doctor performs a femoral arterial puncture and inserts an arterial sheath into the femoral artery. Next, he inserts a guide wire through the sheath, advancing it through the lesion. When the guide wire is in place, the cutting head of the atherectomy device with suction attached is advanced over the guide wire and positioned against the lesion. The cutting head with suction is then activated, the lesion is excised, and plaque and other debris and blood are immediately suctioned out to prevent embolism and subsequent infarction. During the procedure, 0.9% sodium chloride solution is continuously infused into the affected coronary artery to prevent collapse.

Periodically, the atherectomy procedure is evaluated by angiography. If the lesion is not reduced by about 20% to 30%, or if atherosclerotic material has not been suctioned out, larger blades can be inserted because the guide wire remains in place. (See *New ways to cut plaque*, page 78.)

Complications

The most common complication from atherectomy is chest pain. Other common complications include vagal reactions, intimal injury, reocclusion, hematoma, and bleeding at the sheath site.

Rare but more serious complications include vessel perforation, cardiac tamponade, myocardial ischemia, embolization of debris, and vessel wall dissection.

Care considerations

Before the procedure

• Instruct the patient to take 325 mg of aspirin and 75 mg of dipyridamole the day before the procedure. The patient should bathe and shampoo twice with an antiseptic antimicrobial skin cleaner on the day before surgery.

• Reinforce the doctor's explanation of the procedure as necessary. Explain what will occur in the cardiac catheterization laboratory. Because a contrast medium will be used for the angiography, it's important to find out if the patient has any allergies to contrast medium or to shellfish or iodine – for example, to povidone-iodine solution.

• On the morning of surgery, start an I.V. infusion (using a large-bore I.V. catheter) of dextrose 5% in water (D_5W), running at a keep-vein-open (KVO) rate or as ordered.

• Premedicate the patient with an antianxiety agent such as diazepam and an antihistamine such as diphenhydramine, as appropriate. A patient with hypersensitivity to the contrast medium will need premedication with a corticosteroid to limit the severity of his immunologic response.

After the procedure

• Immediately after the procedure is completed and the sheath withdrawn, cover the site with a pressure dressing and apply pressure for at least 20 minutes.

• After returning to the nursing unit, the patient requires care and monitoring similar to that after PTCA. Obtain an ECG and coagulation profile and check vital signs every 15 minutes for the first hour. Maintain the KVO line with D_5W and continue the nitroglycerin infusion for 4 to 24 hours to keep the patient pain-free. Assess the arterial line for accuracy, and assess the bilateral puncture sites in the groin at least once an hour for hematoma and bleeding.

• Because the patient will be receiving heparin, some oozing can be expected. However, if signs of volume depletion occur, blood or fluid replacement may be necessary.

• Keep the patient on bed rest for 24 hours after the atherectomy. Patients typically stay in a cardiac monitoring area for several days.

• Before discharge, the patient should be evaluated with a multiple-gated acquisition scan (MUGA) to assess ventricular wall motion, ejection fraction, and cardiac output. If the MUGA is within normal limits, the patient will be discharged for follow-up by the referring doctor. Typically, a cardiac catheterization is performed in 6 months to assess for re-stenosis.

Home care instructions

• Supply the patient with detailed instructions about prescribed medications. The patient is likely to continue medications that decrease platelet aggregation and provide optimal coronary artery dilation. Explain the importance of taking these medications exactly as prescribed.

New ways to cut plaque

A recently improved method of cutting away and removing plaque, directional coronary atherectomy (DCA) employs a bullet-shaped probe, called the *Simpson Coronary AtheroCath*, that has an opening on one side of the casing. Atherectomy's benefits include less vascular trauma, lower risk of emergency by-pass surgery, decrease in re-stenosis, and greater safety and predictability. Some patients may undergo atherectomy and angioplasty.

Using a guide wire, the doctor inserts the catheter into the narrowed vessel lumen.

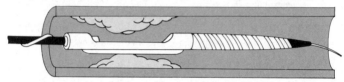

He inflates the balloon to force the open side of the catheter against the opposite vessel wall. This squeezes the atheromatous plaque into the casing chamber.

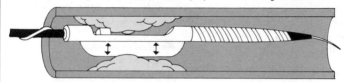

A tiny, rotating cup shaves off the plaque that projects into the chamber.

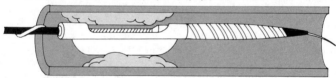

Then, the doctor rotates the AtheroCath and excises more plaque until serial angiograms show improved blood flow.

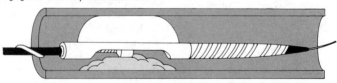

Variations on this procedure include the following:
- The *Kensey catheter* pulverizes plaque with tiny bits of water from a rotating tip.
- The *Auth-Richie Rotablater* uses a rotating tip studded with diamond chips to remove plaque.
- The *Tim Fischell device* is pulled through the stenotic area rather than pushed through it, obliterating plaque as it passes.

• Because the rate of re-stenosis can be as high as 25%, tell the patient to notify the doctor promptly of any anginal episodes.

• Give the patient instructions about coronary artery disease risk factors and make sure he understands how to reduce them.

• Consultation with the dietitian can help patients who need guidance in identifying high-fat foods. If weight reduction is necessary, the dietitian can help the patient develop an individualized diet plan.

• Be sure the patient understands the importance of regular exercise to increase high-density lipoprotein and decrease low-density lipoprotein levels.

• Encourage regular medical checkups to monitor progress.

AUTOTRANSFUSION

Autotransfusion (also called autologous transfusion) is a procedure for reinfusing a patient's own blood. It can be performed after trauma, preoperatively, intraoperatively, or postoperatively. Autotransfusion has become popular in recent years because of the acquired immunodeficiency syndrome (AIDS) crisis. Autotransfusion eliminates the danger of transmitting such blood-borne infections as AIDS and hepatitis from a blood donor to a blood recipient. It also greatly reduces the possibility of a transfusion reaction.

Moreover, autotransfusion conserves blood bank supplies and provides an available source of compatible blood, saving time otherwise spent on typing and crossmatching. This feature is especially important in treating trauma, where seconds may count. Unlike banked blood, autologous blood has a near-normal temperature and pH, a high oxygen-carrying capacity due to high levels of 2,3-diphosphoglycerate, and normal clotting factors.

Another positive feature of autologous blood transfusion is its possible acceptance by patients whose religious beliefs prohibit the transfusion of a donor's blood.

Purpose

• To correct hemodynamic imbalance through reinfusion of the patient's own blood.

Indications

Autotransfusion can be used for traumatic injuries, most commonly hemothorax. It can also be used after primary injury to the lungs, liver, chest wall, heart, pulmonary vessels, spleen, kidneys, and inferior vena cava, and to the iliac, portal, and subclavian veins. However, use of autotransfusion after abdominal vascular injuries is much less common because of the increased risk of fecal contamination.

Preoperative autotransfusion is indicated primarily for the patient with a rare blood type who will undergo major surgery, for the patient in whom isoimmunization may complicate future transfusion needs, or for a patient who fears exposure to blood-borne infection, such as AIDS or hepatitis, if blood must be transfused after surgery.

Intraoperative autotransfusion is performed most often during thoracic and cardiovascular surgery, but can also be used during hip resection, spinal fusion, liver resection, and ruptured ectopic pregnancy.

Postoperative autotransfusion is indicated to retrieve blood lost during cardiac surgery. A new method of autotransfusion has recently been developed for use after orthopedic surgery such as reconstructive procedures of the hip, knee, and spine. (See *Orthopedic autotransfusion*, pages 80 and 81.)

Contraindications include fecal or urinary contamination of blood lost from hemorrhage, which makes the patient susceptible to bacterial growth, leading to sepsis, coagulopathies, and

Orthopedic autotransfusion

Orth-evac allows postoperative collection of shed blood for reinfusion from patients who have undergone orthopedic procedures. It is a sterile, single-use system with wound drains that are inserted in the operating room at the end of the procedure.

To use the system, wound drains are connected to the Orth-evac bag using the Y-connector. If suction is required, tubing can be attached to the top of the bag at the suction port. Source vacuum must be set at a minimum of −110 mm Hg; the Orth-evac unit itself automatically regulates the vacuum applied in the wound to a safe, low-constant level. Gravity drainage can be accomplished by placing the unit below the wound site.

According to American Association of Blood Banks standards, blood collected in the Orth-evac bag must be reinfused within 6 hours of the beginning of collection.

To reinfuse the blood, clamp the drainage tubing, remove the Orth-evac collection bag from the support frame, and invert the bag so the spiked port is pointing up. Insert a microaggregate filter into this port, and attach a reinfusion set to the filter. While keeping the bag inverted, simply squeeze the bag to expel any air; then continue squeezing to prime the filter with blood. The bag can now be turned right side up and the reinfusion begun, following hospital policy for blood infusion.

Although the Orth-evac can be used for any major orthopedic surgery where blood loss is expected, it is especially important in patients undergoing joint revisions or surgery after major orthopedic trauma because blood loss is significantly greater in these patients.

The Orth-evac system should not be used in the presence of coagulopathy; malignant tumors; renal failure; wound infection; irrigation of the wound with substances such as povidone-iodine, which is not suitable for I.V. use; or the use of an absorbable gelatin sponge (such as Gelfoam) because it will cause clotting in the autotransfusion system.

microemboli. Autotransfusion is not recommended for patients with coagulation defects, malignant tumors, or respiratory infection, or for patients with traumatic wounds over 4 hours old because blood degradation occurs rapidly beyond that time. Patients with a hemoglobin (Hb) level below 11 g/dl should not plan to be preoperative autologous donors.

Procedure

Two methods of preoperative autotransfusion include collection of blood for later reinfusion and hemodilution. In the first method, blood for reinfusion is obtained several weeks before the planned surgery. The patient comes to the blood donor center, and the blood is removed from a vein in the antecubital space and stored until it's needed by the patient. In the second method, hemodilution, the patient's blood is withdrawn immediately before surgery and an equivalent volume of fluid is replaced with an I.V. crystalloid solution. The collected blood is reinfused as needed during or after surgery.

Intraoperative blood salvage is performed solely during surgery. The surgeon uses a suction catheter to remove

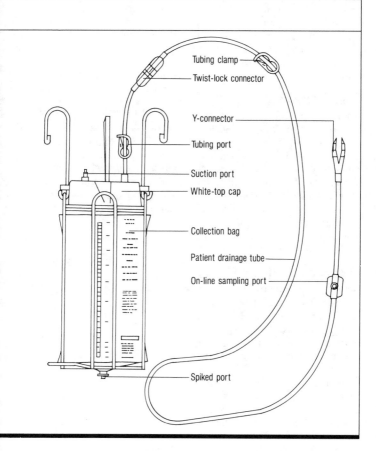

blood and debris from the surgical field and mixes it with a dilute solution of an anticoagulant. This aspirate is then filtered and placed in a rotating bowl (semicontinuous centrifuge), which removes the anticoagulant, the debris, and nearly all other blood components except the red blood cells (RBCs). The RBCs are then washed, mixed with 0.9% sodium chloride solution, and pumped into a bag for reinfusion. The blood is then reinfused I.V. as needed.

For postoperative or posttraumatic autotransfusion, the doctor inserts a #36 to #40 French chest tube and connects the tube to an autotransfusion device that provides an underwater seal, closed drainage, and suction. This procedure collects blood from the chest cavity for reinfusion while simultaneously relieving compression of the lungs and allowing their reexpansion. When sufficient blood has been collected for reinfusion, the blood collection bag is removed from the autotransfusion device, a microemboli filter is attached, and the blood is transfused into the patient in the typical way.

When this procedure is used postoperatively, the chest tube is inserted near the end of surgery; when performed for trauma, the chest tube is inserted as soon as possible after injury.

Whether the intraoperative, traumatic, or postoperative technique is used, the blood must be reinfused within 6 hours from the start of retrieval.

Complications

Autotransfusion has several potential complications, such as air embolism, which may result from faulty monitoring; coagulopathy; enteric contamination; sepsis; hemolysis; thrombocytopenia; and, if citrate phosphate dextrose was used to prevent clotting, citrate toxicity. Occasionally, autotransfusion causes transient hemoglobinuria as a result of trauma to the RBCs during collection.

Care considerations

Before the procedure

• Preoperative donation requires the doctor's written permission.

• The preoperative donor takes a daily supplement of iron, starting 1 week before the first donation and continuing to hospital admission.

• The date when a patient begins to donate his blood preoperatively varies, depending on the blood bank's storage conditions. A hospital staff member or the doctor notifies the patient of the start date for donation.

• Explain the appropriate procedure for blood collection and reinfusion to the patient before the procedure.

• The autotransfusion device should be set up according to the manufacturer's directions before the beginning of postoperative or posttraumatic autotransfusion.

During and after the procedure

• Monitor the volume of blood collected and reinfused.

• Monitor the patient's respiratory and cardiac status.

• Monitor the patient for signs of hemorrhage if drainage is more than expected, and notify the doctor. Further surgery or a repeat of the procedure may be necessary.

• Monitor laboratory data, particularly Hb and hematocrit levels, coagulation profile, and calcium levels, for significant changes.

• Observe for complications. If any occur, notify the doctor immediately.

Home care instructions

• If the chest tube site did not heal before discharge, instruct the patient about proper incision care.

• Teach the patient the signs of infection—fever, pain at the insertion site, and redness—about which he should contact his doctor.

B

BALLOON VALVULOPLASTY

Balloon valvuloplasty is a procedure used to enlarge the orifice of a stenotic heart valve. First performed in 1979 on children with congenital heart disease, it has been performed on thousands of adults and children in the United States. In most cases, this procedure results in improved valve function with relief of transvalvular obstruction. Balloon valvuloplasty provides curative results with less than 30% incidence of re-stenosis. Nevertheless, the treatment of choice for valvular heart disease is still often surgical — either valve replacement or commissurotomy — because balloon valvuloplasty leaves residual stenosis, and re-stenosis rates are as high as 75% in adults with stenotic aortic valves.

Purpose

• To enlarge the valve orifice and improve mobility of valve leaflets, thereby correcting valve stenosis.

Indications

Balloon valvuloplasty may be used to treat patients with valve stenosis. It is the procedure of choice for children with congenital aortic stenosis, young adults with mitral stenosis not associated with highly calcified valves, and patients with coarctation of the aorta. Balloon valvuloplasty offers a palliative alternative for patients who are poor candidates for surgery.

Procedure

Typically, the patient is awake during the procedure, which may take up to 4 hours. Under local anesthesia, the doctor performs valvuloplasty in a cardiac catheterization laboratory. After preparing and anesthetizing the catheter insertion site, the doctor inserts a catheter into the femoral artery (for left heart valves) or the femoral vein (for right heart valves or a transseptal approach to the mitral valve), then passes the balloon-tipped catheter through this catheter and, guided by fluoroscopy, slowly threads it into the heart. After positioning the deflated balloon in the valve opening, he repeatedly inflates it with a solution containing 0.9% sodium chloride and a contrast medium. The pressure of the inflated balloon causes the valve leaflets to split apart, allowing them to open and close freely and widening the valve's orifice.

Throughout the procedure, the doctor asks the patient to take deep breaths (to allow visualization of the catheter) and to answer questions about how he is feeling.

Once valve function is improved, the balloon-tipped catheter is removed. The other catheter is left in place for 6 to 12 hours in case the procedure must be repeated.

Complications

Balloon valvuloplasty can have serious complications. It can worsen valve insufficiency by misshaping the valve so that it doesn't close completely. Another serious complication is embolism, which can result if pieces of the calcified valve break off and travel to the brain or lungs. Valvuloplasty can also severely damage the delicate valve leaflets, requiring immediate surgery to replace the valve.

Other complications include bleeding and hematoma at the arterial puncture site, arrhythmias, myocardial ischemia, myocardial infarction, cardiac tamponade, cardiac perforation, and circulatory defects distal to the catheter entry site.

Care considerations

Before the procedure

• Reinforce the doctor's explanation of the procedure for both the patient and family, including the patient's role in the procedure and its risks, alternatives, and expected outcome. Be sure the patient knows why his cooperation during the procedure is important.
• Tell the patient to expect insertion of an I.V. line to provide access for medications. Also tell him that his groin area will be shaved and cleaned with an antiseptic before the procedure and that he'll feel a brief stinging sensation when the local anesthetic is injected.
• Assess bilateral distal pulses, color, temperature, and sensation in the patient's extremities to serve as a baseline for posttreatment comparisons.
• Restrict food or fluids for at least 6 hours before the procedure or as ordered.

After the procedure

• Continuously monitor arterial lines and the patient's electrocardiogram.
• Keep the patient's affected leg straight and elevate the head of the bed 20 to 30 degrees to prevent excessive hip flexion and migration of the catheter.
• Ensure that the sandbag remains in place over the insertion site to minimize bleeding until the catheter is removed.
• Provide adequate I.V. fluids (100 ml/hour) to aid excretion of the contrast medium. Be alert for signs of fluid overload: distended neck veins, atrial

and ventricular gallops, dyspnea, pulmonary congestion, tachycardia, hypertension, and hypoxemia. The patient may also receive I.V. heparin or nitroglycerin.
• Monitor vital signs frequently (usually every 15 minutes for the first hour, every 30 minutes for 2 hours, and then hourly for the next 5 hours). Also assess peripheral pulses distal to the insertion site and the color, temperature, and capillary refill time of the affected extremity. (Use a Doppler ultrasound stethoscope if necessary, and notify the doctor promptly if the pulses are absent.)
• Observe the insertion site for hematoma and ecchymosis or hemorrhage. If bleeding occurs, apply direct pressure and notify the doctor.
• Auscultate regularly for murmurs, which may indicate worsening valve insufficiency.
• After the doctor removes the femoral catheter, apply direct pressure over the puncture site for at least 30 minutes. Then apply a pressure dressing.

Home care instructions

• Tell the patient or caregiver that the patient can resume normal activity.
• Advise the patient to notify the doctor promptly of any bleeding or increased bruising at the puncture site or any recurrence of symptoms of valvular insufficiency, such as breathlessness or decreased exercise tolerance.
• Emphasize the need for regular medical follow-up visits.

BARBITURATE COMA

Barbiturate coma is a treatment method that uses high I.V. doses of a short-acting barbiturate (such as pentobarbital or thiopental) to produce coma. Barbiturate coma is typically induced only when cases of sustained or acute episodes of increased intracranial pressure

(ICP) have not responded to such conventional treatment as surgical decompression, osmotic diuretics, fluid restriction, steroids, hyperventilation, and cerebrospinal fluid drainage.

Purpose

• To reduce the patient's cerebral metabolic rate and cerebral blood flow, thereby relieving persistently increased ICP and preventing brain tissue damage.

Indications

Barbiturate coma is indicated for patients with acute ICP elevation above 25 to 30 mm Hg, persistent ICP elevation above 20 mm Hg, or rapidly deteriorating neurologic status that's unresponsive to other treatments.

Procedure

Before inducing barbiturate coma, the doctor establishes a reliable neurologic baseline via an EEG, a computed tomography scan and, possibly, brain stem auditory-evoked response testing. Barbiturate coma should only be induced in an intensive care setting. The patient is placed on mechanical ventilation, ICP monitoring, central venous pressure (CVP) monitoring, pulmonary artery pressure monitoring, and cardiac and intra-arterial pressure monitoring. The patient also requires an indwelling urinary catheter and nasogastric tube.

As soon as the tests are completed and the monitoring equipment is in place, the doctor induces the barbiturate coma according to the hospital's policy. This is done by administering a loading dose of the barbiturate and then establishing an hourly maintenance dose that will keep the barbiturate at the level required to decrease ICP.

When the patient's ICP has stabilized within acceptable limits, usually in 24 to 36 hours, or if the patient shows signs of progressive neurologic impairment, therapy is discontinued. Withdrawal from barbiturate therapy should occur over 24 hours to several days because abrupt withdrawal can cause seizures.

Complications

Barbiturate coma carries some serious risks, related mainly to the small margin between therapeutic and toxic doses: A high dose is needed to induce coma, but toxicity can produce severe, possibly fatal, central nervous system and respiratory depression. Even a therapeutic dose can cause such complications as hypotension and arrhythmias; abrupt withdrawal may cause seizures or delirium. In addition, these patients are also susceptible to infection and such complications of immobility as pressure ulcers and contractures.

Care considerations

Before therapy

• Provide clear explanations to the patient's family. Convey a positive outlook, but don't guarantee the therapy's success. Because barbiturate coma is a last resort to reduce ICP and save the patient's life, prepare them for the possibility that the patient may die or, if he survives, may have permanent neurologic impairment.

During therapy

• Evaluating neurologic function is impossible while the patient is in a drug-induced coma, but it is both possible and necessary to monitor the patient's ICP, electrocardiogram, CVP, and arterial pressure. Notify the doctor promptly of increased ICP, arrhythmias, or hypotension. Also monitor serum barbiturate levels and EEG results.

• Provide supportive care during therapy. This includes providing adequate ventilation because the patient's respiratory function is severely compromised; maintaining adequate hydration, fluid and electrolyte balance, and adequate nutrition (by parenteral nutrition, if necessary); and providing meticulous skin care, range-of-motion exercises, and regular repositioning. Also provide emotional support to the patient's family.

• Watch for sporadic elevations in ICP and for adverse reactions to barbiturate withdrawal as the barbiturates are discontinued. Notify the doctor and place the patient in a quiet, darkened room if you observe tremors, agitation, delirium or hallucinations, incoordination, or seizures.

After therapy

• As the patient emerges from the coma, watch for signs of returning neurologic function. Begin by checking for the presence of a gag reflex and for response to painful stimuli, then work up to a complete neurologic evaluation. Remember, however, that only after withdrawal is complete and the patient is fully conscious can you begin to determine the extent of neurologic impairment.

Home care instructions

• Barbiturate coma is induced only under well-controlled conditions in an intensive care setting.

BATHS, THERAPEUTIC

Balneotherapy, or a therapeutic bath, provides dermatologic treatment to large skin areas and also promotes relaxation. Four types of therapeutic baths are commonly used: antibacterial, colloidal, emollient, and tar. (For agents used, see *Comparing therapeutic baths*.)

Purpose

• To clean the skin, loosen or remove crusts or scales, and relieve pruritus
• To deliver topical medications or hydrate the outermost layer of the skin to allow penetration of topical medications.

Comparing therapeutic baths

TYPE	AGENTS	PURPOSE
Antibacterial	• Acetic acid • Hexachlorophene • Potassium permanganate • Povidone-iodine	To treat infected eczema, dirty ulcerations, furunculosis, and pemphigus
Colloidal	• Aveeno colloidal oatmeal • Aveeno colloidal oatmeal, oilated • Starch and baking soda	To relieve pruritus and to soothe irritated skin; indicated for any irritating or oozing condition, such as atopic eczema
Emollient	• Bath oils • Mineral oil	To clean and hydrate the skin, indicated for any dry skin condition
Tar	• Bath oils with tar • Coal tar concentrate	To treat scaly dermatoses, sometimes in combination with ultraviolet light therapy; loosens scales and relieves pruritus

Indications

Therapeutic baths help treat psoriasis, atopic eczema, exfoliative dermatitis, bullous diseases, and pyodermas.

Procedure

The patient soaks in a medicated bath, in water at approximately 97° F (36° C) for 20 to 30 minutes.

Complications

Complications are uncommon but can include dry skin, pruritus, scaling, and fissures, depending on the medication added to the bath and how long the patient soaks in it.

Care considerations

Before therapy

• Explain the purpose of the bath to the patient and answer any questions. Tell the patient that for safety reasons you must leave the door unlocked. Tell the patient to call if he feels weak or dizzy. Point out the location of the call bell.
• Make sure the tub and tub area are clean and a soiled dressing bin is available.
• Make sure the room is warm enough, and close the windows if necessary.
• Place the bath mat in the tub and run the bath. Use the bath thermometer to ensure correct water temperature.
• Carefully measure and add the ordered medication to the bath to achieve the proper dilution. Mix the water and medication well to prevent a sensitivity reaction.
• Ensure the patient's privacy during the bath; for example, by hanging an OCCUPIED sign on the door.

During therapy

• Position the patient comfortably by placing folded towels underneath his head and, if he is short, by placing a bath stool in the tub so that he can brace his feet. Making the patient comfortable is important because balneotherapy should promote relaxation.

• For safety reasons, instruct the patient not to stand in the tub.
• Check on the patient frequently during the bath. If the patient is old or debilitated, stay with him throughout the bath.

After therapy

• Assist the patient out of the tub.
• To prevent chills, instruct the patient to dry off quickly by patting gently with a towel until the skin is damp dry. Apply topical medications immediately because they're absorbed easily when the skin is damp.
• Note any improvement or reaction. If necessary, help the patient dress and escort him to his room.

Home care instructions

• Provide the patient with instructions and outline safety precautions. Explain that therapeutic agents may make the tub slippery and that a bath mat is necessary.
• Inform the patient that overly hot water can increase pruritus and scaling, and advise him to check water temperature with a bath thermometer.
• Explain that the average home bathtub holds 150 to 200 gallons of water. The patient should measure the prescribed medication accordingly and mix the water well to prevent a reaction to the medication.
• If the patient has dry skin, mention that soap is drying. Explain that normal skin requires bathing only every other day, with soap applied only to the underarms, groin, and bottoms of the feet.
• Remind the patient that friction during or after the bath can damage his skin. Unless the patient is being treated for psoriasis, advise washing with bare hands instead of a washcloth. Tell the patient with psoriasis to loosen crusts with a washcloth, but only after soaking for 15 or 20 minutes. Instruct all patients to gently pat themselves dry with a clean towel, leaving the skin slightly damp.

• Tell the patient to report any increase in pruritus, oozing, erythema, or scaling to the doctor, and encourage regular follow-up visits.

BEHAVIOR THERAPY

Behavior therapy assumes that problem behaviors are learned and, through special training, can be unlearned and replaced by acceptable ones. Unlike psychotherapy, behavior therapy doesn't attempt to uncover the reasons for problem behaviors. In fact, it de-emphasizes the patient's thoughts and feelings about them. The goal is to unlearn destructive or unproductive behaviors that result from faulty learning and to enhance effective social and adaptive behaviors. This type of therapy requires a motivated patient willing to work at positive change and a cooperative caregiver who must understand and respond consistently to specified behaviors.

Behavior therapy can change a negative behavioral pattern through various techniques, such as positive or negative reinforcement, shaping, modeling, punishment, or extinction.

Purpose

• To eliminate problem behaviors or replace them with more appropriate and acceptable behaviors
• To remove or reduce behavioral excesses, such as compulsive behaviors and rituals
• To reduce behavioral deficits, such as memory impairment or limited social skills.

Indications

Behavior therapy is indicated for many types of maladaptive behaviors, including phobias, smoking, alcoholism, and temper tantrums, and for certain somatic disorders, such as migraine headaches and hyperactive bowel syndrome. It is suitable for adults or children and can be used for individuals or groups of patients with a similar maladaptation.

Procedure

The behavioral therapist, who may be a psychologist, specially skilled nurse, or other specially educated individual, works with the patient to identify the specific behavior creating the problem. The analysis is based on the person's strengths, deficits, culture, and environmental influences. Therapy goals are mutually determined by the patient and the therapist. Once goals have been identified, the therapist — after considering additional factors, such as the patient's age and family status — decides which behavioral therapy or therapies to use. (For more information, see *Types of behavior therapy*.)

Positive reinforcement increases the likelihood of a desirable behavior being repeated by promptly praising or rewarding the patient when he performs it. By contrast, negative reinforcement involves the removal of a negative stimulus only after the patient provides a desirable response. Punishment discourages problem behavior by inflicting a penalty, such as temporary removal of a privilege. Although difficult to sustain, extinction is a technique that simply ignores undesirable behavior — provided, of course, that the behavior isn't dangerous or illegal. Another technique — shaping — initially rewards any behavior that resembles the desirable one. Then, step-by-step, the behavior required to gain a reward becomes progressively closer to the desired behavior. Modeling provides a reward when the patient imitates the required behavior. Relaxation techniques include muscle relaxation, biofeedback, and self-hypnosis.

Complications

Occasionally, a technique or a therapy prompts an undesired behavioral change.

Types of behavior therapy

Behavior therapy is a broad term that includes assertiveness training, desensitization, flooding and implosion, positive conditioning, social skills training, and token economy.

Assertiveness training
Using the techniques of positive reinforcement, shaping, and modeling, assertiveness training aims to reduce anxiety through improved communication. It teaches the patient acceptable ways to express feelings, ideas, and wishes without feeling guilty or demeaning others. The patient learns how to make requests in a frank way and how to refuse unacceptable or unreasonable requests. Assertiveness training is often helpful to patients who feel inhibited and unable to express their feelings.

Desensitization
The treatment of choice for phobias, desensitization slowly exposes the patient to something he fears. It's most successful when used with other psychological treatments because phobias typically reflect unresolved conflicts. Desensitization is also used to treat other problems that produce fear of failure or embarrassment, such as frigidity or impotence. In practice, desensitization teaches the patient to use deep-breathing or another relaxation technique when confronting a staged series of anxiety-producing situations. During desensitization, the patient requires reassurance and practices relaxation techniques. Monitor his response to each anxious situation and emphasize that he needn't proceed to the next stage until he feels ready.

Flooding and implosion
Flooding and implosion therapy can provide rapid relief of phobias such as travel phobias. It is also used to treat obsessive-compulsive disorder and behavior problems such as compulsive hoarding. Like desensitization, it involves direct exposure to an anxiety-producing situation. Unlike desensitization, it doesn't employ relaxation techniques. Instead, it assumes that anxiety and panic can't persist and that confrontation helps the patient to overcome fear.

Positive conditioning
Building on the principle of desensitization, this therapy attempts to gradually instill a positive or neutral attitude toward a phobia. Used effectively for patients with sexual problems, positive conditioning first introduces a pleasurable stimulus by associating other pleasurable experiences with it. Next, the therapist introduces the phobia stimulus along with the pleasurable one. Gradually, the patient develops a positive response to the phobia.

Social skills training
Using shaping and modeling techniques, this therapy helps patients develop or regain skills for forming relationships. Commonly used for institutionalized, acutely ill, and mentally retarded patients, its success depends on consistent reinforcement.

Token economy
Also called operant conditioning, this treatment reinforces acceptable behavior with rewards (tokens), which the patient can use as currency for some privilege or object. The therapist can also withhold or rescind tokens as punishment or to avert undesirable behavior. This therapy is often effective treatment for those with behavioral problems who do not respond well to verbal therapy techniques.

Care considerations
Before therapy
• Counsel the patient about what behaviors need changing, the goals of therapy, and the techniques used to accomplish them. Make clear what is expected of the patient and what he can expect from the health care staff.
During therapy
• Monitor the patient's response throughout therapy, reinforcing acceptable behaviors and discouraging unacceptable ones.
• If unacceptable behaviors persist, inform the therapist. He may need to try another technique.
After therapy
• Review the initial goals and the patient's progress during treatment.
• Be sure that follow-up appointments have been made with the patient's therapist to ensure continual effectiveness of the therapy.

Home care instructions
• If appropriate, teach the patient's family the basic techniques used to correct the problem behaviors. Encourage them to reinstitute the therapy if problem behaviors recur.
• Recommend an outpatient therapist to help reinforce desirable behaviors and to respond to the patient's and family's questions.
• If an appropriate support group is available, recommend that the patient join to build a strong, supportive network with his peers.

BENZODIAZEPINES

The benzodiazepines *flurazepam, quazepam, temazepam,* and *triazolam* produce hypnosis. They are more predictable and produce fewer adverse effects at therapeutic doses than barbiturates. They have less potential for dependence, abuse, and interaction with other drugs, and they're usually less toxic than barbiturates after overdosage.

Although benzodiazepines are effective and safe for short-term therapy, long-term use can result in psychological and physiologic dependence. And when taken in large doses with alcohol or other central nervous system (CNS) depressants, the benzodiazepines can produce severe CNS depression and death.

Purpose
• To produce a hypnotic effect by interfering with neural transmission through the reticular activating system, limbic system, thalamus, and hypothalamus.

Indications
The benzodiazepines are used to treat insomnia associated with difficulty falling asleep, frequent nocturnal awakenings, and early-morning awakening. They're preferred over barbiturates for such sleep problems.

Because benzodiazepine dependence occurs most commonly in patients with a history of alcohol or drug abuse, these drugs should be avoided in such patients, if possible. They should also be used cautiously in patients with suicidal tendencies or in those whose history indicates that they may increase drug dosage on their own. Benzodiazepines are contraindicated in patients with known hypersensitivity to any drug in the benzodiazepine family and in patients with hepatic disease or acute angle-closure glaucoma. They should be administered judiciously to patients with renal impairment, chronic respiratory disease, or chronic open-angle glaucoma.

Adverse reactions
Benzodiazepines usually produce adverse reactions that are extensions of their pharmacologic effects. These include drowsiness, dizziness, lightheadedness, unsteadiness, and confusion. Be especially alert for these re-

actions in elderly or debilitated patients and in those with hepatic disease or low serum albumin levels.

GI adverse reactions may include loss of appetite, dry mouth, abdominal discomfort, taste alterations, nausea, excessive thirst, and constipation or diarrhea.

Although uncommon, potentially serious psychiatric or behavioral adverse reactions can include confusion, suicidal ideation, agitation, hyperexcitability, hallucinations, delirium, aggression, sleepwalking, or other bizarre or abnormal behaviors. In some cases, amnesia about the behavior can occur. Benzodiazepines should be discontinued if behavioral reactions occur.

Care considerations

• Watch for common adverse reactions during benzodiazepine therapy. Typically, these reactions occur during the early stages of therapy and subside within a few days. During this period, protect the patient from injury—for example, raise the side rails and assist with ambulation.
• Watch for GI reactions.
• Check the patient's drug regimen for use of other sedatives and hypnotics, opioid analgesics, antihypertensives, monoamine oxidase inhibitors, or cimetidine, which may enhance the CNS depressant and hypotensive effects of benzidiazepines.
• These drugs should only be used for short-term therapy (4 weeks or less).

Home care instructions

• Warn the patient never to increase the dose of a benzodiazepine on his own even if he feels the drug isn't working effectively. Doing so will increase his risk of drug overdose or dependence. Explain that the drug's effects may not be apparent for 1 or 2 days.
• Discuss common, reportable adverse reactions, such as dizziness, drowsiness, lethargy, impaired coordination, and confusion.

• Instruct the patient to avoid activities that require alertness and coordination, such as driving, until his response to the drug has been determined.
• To prevent GI distress, advise taking the drug with meals.
• Explain that benzodiazepines accentuate the effects of alcohol and other CNS depressants—possibly causing severe CNS depression and even death. As a result, the patient should avoid these substances during therapy.
• Tell the patient to avoid smoking. Although the mechanism of interaction is unclear, tobacco apparently speeds the metabolism of benzodiazepines, thereby reducing their effectiveness.
• Explain that after the patient stops taking the drug, his body may take some time to adjust to withdrawal—from a few days to 3 weeks, depending on the dosage and the duration of therapy. Tell him to notify his doctor if he experiences extreme irritability, nervousness, incoordination, or weakness. Alert him to the possibility of rebound insomnia, which should persist for no more than 2 or 3 nights.
• Encourage the patient to seek alternative therapy to deal with the underlying cause of insomnia and to explore nonchemical sleep aids, such as biofeedback and progressive relaxation therapy.

BETA-ADRENERGIC BLOCKERS

By inhibiting the sympathetic response to beta-adrenergic stimulation and depressing renin output, beta-adrenergic blockers (also called beta blockers) decrease heart rate, conduction velocity, cardiac output, and myocardial contractility.

Beta blockers can be classified into two groups. The selective beta blockers—*acebutolol, esmolol, atenolol,* and *metoprolol*—act primarily on beta-receptors in the heart (beta$_1$-receptors). The non-selective beta blockers — *labetalol, nadolol, pindolol, propranolol,* and *timolol* — inhibit both beta$_1$-receptors and beta$_2$-receptors, which are found in skeletal muscle, blood vessels, and bronchioles. Beta blockers can be further classified by their ability to stimulate beta-adrenergic receptors, an ability known as intrinsic sympathomimetic activity (ISA), or beta-agonist activity. In general, the higher a drug's ISA, the less it lowers cardiac output and produces dangerous adverse reactions, such as bradycardia and bronchoconstriction. Pindolol has the highest ISA of all beta blockers, followed by acebutolol and timolol; the other beta blockers have low ISAs.

Purpose

• To relieve hypertension
• To help prevent angina and infarction by reducing myocardial oxygen requirements
• To control arrhythmias by reducing adrenergic stimulation.

Indications

These drugs are used primarily to control hypertension, either alone or in combination with other drugs (such as diuretics) in the treatment of hypertension. They may also be used to reduce the frequency of angina attacks, to control tachycardia and other arrhythmias, and to minimize damage (and possibly lower mortality) in acute myocardial infarction. They may be given prophylactically to lower the risk of reinfarction.

Typically, both selective and nonselective beta blockers are contraindicated in patients with heart block, cardiogenic shock, or congestive heart failure (CHF) and in patients with hypersensitivity to one of the drugs. Because nonselective beta blockers may inhibit bronchodilation from beta$_2$ stimulation, they shouldn't be given to patients with obstructive respiratory disorders, such as bronchial asthma, allergic rhinitis or other respiratory allergies, chronic obstructive pulmonary disease, or bronchospasm. All beta blockers — but particularly acebutolol, atenolol, and pindolol — should be administered carefully to patients with impaired renal or hepatic function; generally, such patients should receive reduced dosages. Beta blockers can mask signs of hypoglycemia, such as diaphoresis and tachycardia, and so should be used cautiously in diabetes mellitus. Because these drugs can reduce the heart's ability to respond to reflex stimuli, beta blocker therapy should be withdrawn before surgery.

Adverse reactions

Common reactions include cardiovascular disturbances, such as bradycardia, hypotension, and CHF, and central nervous system (CNS) disturbances, such as fatigue, lethargy, and dizziness. These CNS effects occur most commonly with propranolol and metoprolol because these drugs have moderate lipid solubility and thus can more readily penetrate into the CNS.

Severe reactions to beta blockers can cause the patient to feel worse during therapy. As a result, noncompliance with the prescribed drug regimen may be an important problem during beta blocker therapy.

Care considerations

• Always check the patient's apical pulse for 1 minute before administering a beta blocker. If the rate is below 60 beats/minute or over 100 beats/minute, withhold the drug and notify the doctor.
• Monitor the patient's blood pressure throughout therapy, and report severe hypotension immediately — it may require dosage adjustment or reevaluation of therapy.
• Monitor the patient for signs of developing CHF: pulmonary congestion, dyspnea, unexplained weight gain, pe-

ripheral edema, and distended neck veins. Weigh the patient daily to assess for fluid retention.

• If the patient has a history of respiratory disorders, watch closely for adverse pulmonary effects, such as airway constriction and dyspnea. Report any such effects to the doctor immediately.

• If the patient has diabetes, assess regularly for symptoms of hypoglycemia that aren't masked by beta blockers, such as diaphoresis, hunger, and fatigue. Because the combined effects of insulin and beta blockers may promote hypoglycemia, the diabetic patient may need readjustment of prescribed medication or diet.

• Check the patient's drug regimen for possible interactions. For example, concurrent use of beta blockers and catecholamine-depleting drugs such as reserpine can cause severe hypotension. Monitor blood pressure and heart rate in a patient taking both drugs. Interactions with digitalis glycosides or verapamil can depress cardiac conduction and possibly lead to heart block; watch for and immediately report significant electrocardiogram changes. Theophylline derivatives and beta blockers have antagonistic effects; observe the patient for bronchospasm and regulate doses carefully.

• To minimize withdrawal symptoms, beta blocker therapy should be discontinued gradually—ideally, over 1 to 2 weeks. As the drug is discontinued, watch the patient for withdrawal symptoms. Promptly report diaphoresis, palpitations, severe headache, chest pain, malaise, or tremors.

Home care instructions

• Teach the patient about his disease and how beta blocker therapy works. Stress the importance of taking the drug exactly as prescribed, even if he feels worse. Emphasize that he should never change the dosage or stop taking the drug without consulting his doctor.

Explain that abrupt withdrawal may cause angina, rebound hypertension, or other severe reactions.

• If the patient takes one dose daily, instruct him to take a missed dose if he remembers within 8 hours of the scheduled administration time. If the patient takes two or more doses a day, he should take a missed dose as soon as he remembers but should never double-dose.

• Advise the patient to take propranolol or metoprolol with food to increase absorption. Other beta blockers can be taken without regard to meals.

• Instruct the patient to check his pulse for 1 minute before taking his prescribed dosage. Explain that if his pulse rate is below 60 beats/minute or above 100 beats/minute, he should call his doctor immediately and not take the drug until the doctor tells him to do so.

• Tell the patient to weigh himself at least once a week at the same time of day, on the same scale, and while wearing the same amount of clothing. Advise the patient to notify the doctor if he gains 3 lb (1.4 kg) or more.

• Tell the patient to report difficulty breathing, wheezing, coughing, depression, dizziness, rash, fever, or swollen hands or feet.

• Reassure the patient who develops symptoms of an allergic reaction, such as rash, fever, sore throat, or pharyngitis, that these symptoms are usually mild and transient.

• If the patient has diabetes, explain that beta blockers can mask some signs of hypoglycemia, including low blood pressure and tachycardia. As a result, the patient should be alert for other symptoms of hypoglycemia: hunger, sweating, and fatigue.

• Because beta blockers may cause dizziness, weakness, and fatigue, warn the patient to avoid overexertion or known sources of stress until response to the drug has been established.

• Tell the patient who experiences visual disturbances or CNS effects to avoid driving and other hazardous tasks that require visual acuity, mental alertness, and coordination; tell him to report these effects to the doctor.

• To prevent orthostatic hypotension, advise the patient to avoid prolonged standing or sudden rising.

• Explain that beta blockers may produce symptoms of peripheral vascular insufficiency, such as numbness, tingling, and coldness in his fingers and toes. To minimize these symptoms, the patient should avoid prolonged exposure to cold temperatures.

• Instruct the patient to limit salt intake, as ordered, to minimize fluid retention.

• Warn against ingestion of alcohol, which can raise blood pressure.

• Encourage the patient to stop smoking because tobacco can reduce the effectiveness of beta blockers.

BIOTHERAPY

Biotherapy is defined as treatment with drugs derived from biological sources or affecting biological responses. It involves the use of drugs known as biological response modifiers (BRMs). Used mostly in cancer treatment, BRMs work to modify the interaction between tumor and host, ultimately leading to a therapeutic outcome. Although several BRMs have received approval from the Food and Drug Administration (FDA), many remain under clinical investigation. They can be used alone, in combination with chemotherapy, or with other BRMs.

How BRMs work against tumors is not fully understood; these drugs may have more than one mode of antitumor activity. According to their known modes of action, these drugs are classified into the following major groups:

• Drugs that augment, modulate, or restore the host's immunologic mechanisms

• Drugs that have direct (cytotoxic or cytostatic) antitumor activity

• Drugs that possess other biological effects, such as those that affect differentiation or maturation of cells or that interfere with a tumor's ability to metastasize.

Purpose

• To eradicate or control disease
• To detect or quantify disease
• To lessen adverse effects from other therapies, such as chemotherapy or radiation therapy.

Indications

The indications for these drugs are as numerous as the many different types of BRMs (see *Biological response modifiers: An overview*). The indications described below are for the FDA-approved BRMs.

Interferon alfa, the first BRM to gain FDA approval, is typically indicated in hairy cell leukemia and acquired immunodeficiency syndrome (AIDS)-related Kaposi's sarcoma; *interferon alfa-2b* (Intron A) is also indicated in chronic hepatitis (non-A, non-B/C) and hepatitis B. Intron A and interferon alfa n-3 (Alferon N) are used to treat condyloma acuminata. *Interferon gamma-1b* (Actimmune) is approved for the treatment of chronic granulomatous disease; *muromonab-CD3* (Orthoclone OKT-3), for the treatment of acute allograft rejection in renal transplant patients; *sargramostim*, or *granulocyte-macrophage colony stimulating factor, GM-CSF* (Leukine, Prokine), to accelerate myeloid recovery in patients with non-Hodgkin's lymphoma, acute lymphoblastic leukemia, and Hodgkin's disease after autologous bone marrow transplant; *filgrastim*, or *granulocyte colony stimulating factor, G-CSF* (Neupogen), to decrease the incidence of infection in neutropenic patients with non-myeloid cancers after antineo-

Biological response modifiers: An overview

DRUG AND BIOLOGICAL EFFECTS	INDICATIONS	ADVERSE REACTIONS
Colony-stimulating factors		
epoietin alfa (erythropoietin) *Epogen, Procrit* Stimulates the production of erythrocytes from progenitor cells in bone marrow	Treatment of chronic anemia in end-stage renal disease; treatment of anemia caused by antiretroviral therapy in patients who are carriers of the human immunodeficiency virus (Procrit only); treatment of the anemias associated with cancer chemotherapy (Procrit only)	Drug usually well tolerated; headache, hypertension, nausea and clotting of the vascular access device may occur; rare reactions include vomiting, tachycardia, hyperkalemia, shortness of breath, and diarrhea
filgrastim (granulocyte colony stimulating factor; G-CSF) *Neupogen* Stimulates the production of neutrophils from progenitor cells in bone marrow	Decreases the incidence of infection in patients with nonmyeloid cancers receiving antineoplastic agents that are associated with neutropenia and fever	Drug usually well tolerated, although bone pain and erythema at the injection site may occur; rare reactions may include reversible elevations in uric acid, lactate dehydrogenase, and alkaline phosphatase
macrophage colony-stimulating factor (M-CSF) Stimulates the production of monocytes and macrophages from progenitor cells	Investigational in the treatment of cancers	Not well defined, although mild thrombocytopenia and decreased serum low-density lipoprotein cholesterol may occur
sargramostim (granulocyte-macrophage colony stimulating factor; GM-CSF) *Prokine, Leukine* Stimulates the production of neutrophils, eosinophils, and monocytes/macrophages from progenitor cells in bone marrow	Acceleration of myeloid recovery in patients with non-Hodgkin's lymphoma, acute lymphoblastic leukemia, and Hodgkin's disease undergoing autalogous bone marrow transplantation	Mild constitutional symptoms, bone pain, fatigue, and erythema at injection site

(continued)

Biological response modifiers: An overview *(continued)*

DRUG AND BIOLOGICAL EFFECTS	INDICATIONS	ADVERSE REACTIONS
Interferons		
interferon alfa-2a *Roferon A* **interferon alfa-2b** *Intron A* Antiviral, antiproliferative, and immunomodulating effects	Hairy cell leukemia; acquired immunodeficiency syndrome (AIDS)-related Kaposi's sarcoma. Intron A is also indicated for chronic hepatitis (non-A, non-B/C) and condyloma acuminata	Common reactions include fatigue, anorexia, neutropenia, elevated liver enzymes, constitutional or flulike symptoms (fever, myalgia, headache, chills, and arthralgia); rarely, GI distress, rash, pruritus, and partial alopecia
interferon alfa-n3 *Alferon N* Antiviral, antiproliferative, and immunomodulating effects	Condyloma acuminata	Common reactions include fatigue, anorexia, neutropenia, elevated liver enzymes, constitutional or flulike symptoms (fever, myalgia, headache, chills, and arthralgia); rarely, GI distress, rash, pruritus, and partial alopecia
interferon gamma-1b *Actimmune* Antiviral, antiproliferative, and immunomodulating effects	Reduces the frequency and seriousness of infections. Chronic granulomatous disease	Occasional (dose-related) hypotension. Common reactions are the same as for interferon alfa: rash, diarrhea, nausea, and vomiting
Interleukins		
aldesleukin (interleukin-2; IL-2) *Proleukin* Supports the growth and maturation of T cells; stimulates cytotoxic T cells; induces the release of other lymphokines; stimulates antibody production	Treatment of metastatic renal cell cancer	Common reactions include constitutional symptoms, GI effects, skin changes, elevated liver enzymes, capillary leak syndrome leading to hypotension, occasional cardiac arrhythmias, pulmonary edema and renal dysfunction, and mental status changes (lethargy, somnolence, confusion, agitation)
interleukin-3 (IL-3; multipotential colony stimulating factor) Stimulates myeloid, erythroid, megakaryocytic and basophilic cells	Preliminary investigational uses include the treatment of myelodysplastic syndromes	Mild constitutional symptoms

Biological response modifiers: An overview *(continued)*

DRUG AND BIOLOGICAL EFFECTS	INDICATIONS	ADVERSE REACTIONS
Miscellaneous		
muromonab-CD3 *Orthoclone OKT-3* A murine monoclonal antibody to the CD3 receptor of human T cells	Treatment of acute allograft rejection in renal transplant patients	Potential expected reactions include allergic reactions, dyspnea, pruritus, fever, chills, chest pain, vomiting, wheezing, nausea, diarrhea, tremor, infections, and pulmonary edema
tumor necrosis factor (TNF) A protein that selectively targets transformed cells and causes necrosis of tumor cells; involved in the pathogenesis of infections, inflammation, and injury; acts as mediator of endotoxic shock	Investigational treatment of cancers; treatment of AIDS	Common reactions include fatigue, constitutional symptoms with severe chills, hypotension, and anorexia; rarely, hyperglycemia, hypertriglyceridemia, anemia, neutropenia, and elevated liver enzymes

plastic therapy; *epoetin alfa,* or *erythropoietin* (Epogen, Procrit) for the treatment of chronic anemia in end-stage renal disease. Procrit is also used to treat the anemia caused by zidovudine in the treatment of patients who are human immunodeficiency virus-positive and is now indicated for anemia in patients with cancer who are receiving chemotherapy. *Aldesleukin,* or *interleukin-2, IL-2* (Proleukin) is used to treat adults (age 18 and older) with renal cell cancer. Other indications for these drugs are investigational.

Adverse reactions

Adverse reactions and complications of BRMs are numerous and varied. They vary according to the drug used, the dosage, route, and the patient's physical status as well as the type and extent of the disease. Common complications include fatigue, anorexia, constitutional symptoms, and hematologic changes. Rare complications include severe hypotension, allergic reactions, and excessive weight gain. Typically, the majority of adverse reactions are reversible when drug therapy is discontinued.

Care considerations

• Biotherapy is generally administered by a nurse and should be administered according to the health care facility's policies and procedures for mixing, transport, administration, and disposal. BRMs do not directly affect the deoxyribonucleic acid in cells and are therefore not considered genotoxic substances, but many facilities hold that they require special handling.

• Biotherapy can be administered in the hospital, ambulatory care, office or clinic, or home setting.
• Most biotherapy drugs are given by the I.V., S.C., or I.M. route. The dosage, route, and schedule depend on the patient's type of cancer.

Before therapy

• Perform a thorough baseline assessment, including a physical examination, evaluation of critical laboratory values, current medications, chronic illnesses, and prior therapies. Assessment of psychosocial factors, including a baseline mental status examination and evaluation of social support systems and the patient's perception of treatment goals, should also be performed.
• Administer premedications, such as antiemetics and acetaminophen, as ordered.
• Evaluate the need for special emergency equipment.
• Verify written informed consent for treatment with investigational drugs.

During therapy

• Monitor continuously for adverse reactions. Observe for flulike symptoms, such as fever, headache, myalgias, and arthralgias. Other effects may include fatigue, anorexia, and hematologic changes.
• Initiate interventions to manage adverse effects and document how relief was obtained.
• Provide emotional support to the patient.

Home care instructions

• Teach the patient and caregivers expected adverse reactions and intervention management, reportable signs and symptoms and, when applicable, skills for self-administration of medication.
• Evaluate the patient for adherence to outpatient regimen.

BLADDER RESECTION, TRANSURETHRAL

A relatively quick and simple procedure, transurethral resection of the bladder (TURB) involves insertion of a cystoscope through the urethra and into the bladder to remove lesions. Tissue samples can then be collected for evaluation. (The procedure can also be performed using a Yag laser, although laser use precludes tissue collection.)

When used to remove superficial tumors, TURB may need to be performed as frequently as noninvasive recurrences are identified. A typical schedule might involve treatment every 3 months for the first 2 years, every 6 months for the next 3 years, and annually thereafter.

Purpose

• To remove superficial tumors or papillomas from the bladder wall
• To relieve bladder-neck fibrosis
• To fulgurate bleeding sites.

Indications

TURB is most commonly performed to treat small, superficial, low-grade bladder cancer and to obtain a biopsy of suspicious lesions. It may also be used to remove benign papillomas in the bladder or relieve fibrosis of the bladder neck.

This treatment should not be used to remove large or infiltrating tumors or for metastatic bladder cancer but to collect a specimen to determine its degree of infiltration.

Procedure

After general or spinal anesthesia is administered, the patient is placed in the lithotomy position. Then the doctor introduces a cystoscope into the urethra and passes it into the bladder. Next, he fills the bladder with a clear, nonconducting irrigating solution, lo-

Understanding TURB

In transurethral resection of the bladder (TURB), the doctor inserts a cystoscope through the urethra into the bladder to remove small superficial lesions.

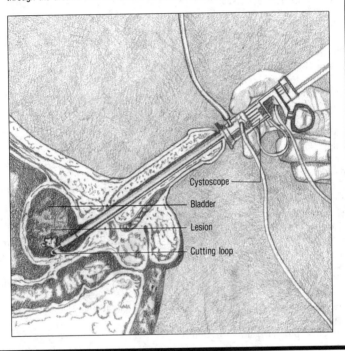

Cystoscope

Bladder

Lesion

Cutting loop

cates the lesion, and positions the cystoscope's cutting loop in place. He turns on the electric current, which runs through the loop, to cut or cauterize the lesion. Finally, he removes the cystoscope (see *Understanding TURB*).

Complications

Potential complications include hematuria, urine retention, bladder perforation, and urinary tract infection. The risk of complications can be reduced by careful monitoring and meticulous care of the indwelling urinary catheter.

Care considerations
Before surgery
• Explain the procedure to the patient and the care that he'll receive after TURB. Tell him that he will be awake if spinal anesthesia was administered for the procedure, that he should have little or no discomfort afterward, and that posttreatment effects, such as hematuria and a burning sensation during urination, should subside quickly. Also tell him that he may have painful bladder spasms, but that these can be relieved with analgesics.

After surgery
• Maintain catheter patency, and monitor for possible complications.

• Ensure that the patient has an adequate fluid intake; provide meticulous catheter care and irrigation as ordered. Intermittent or continuous bladder irrigation may be ordered. The doctor's preference usually determines the type of irrigation. Typically, if bleeding was minimal, the doctor orders intermittent manual irrigation; if bleeding was moderate to severe, the doctor may choose continuous bladder irrigation to avoid breaking the sterile urine drainage system and exposing the patient to possible urinary tract infection.

• Monitor urine output, amount, and color. Notify the doctor if an obstruction that will not clear with irrigation develops, if frank bleeding occurs, and if the patient does not void within 6 hours after TURB.

• Expect slight hematuria immediately after the procedure, but if hematuria seems excessive, observe the patient for signs of shock, such as increased pulse and respiratory rate, hypotension, pallor, and diaphoresis.

• Evaluate the patient for signs of bladder perforation: abdominal pain and rigidity, fever, and decreased urine output despite adequate hydration. If a perforation is suspected, notify the doctor and hold all fluids.

• Carefully determine the level and location of any pain the patient is experiencing. Administer antispasmodics for bladder spasm and analgesics for pain from any source, as ordered.

• If necessary, prepare the patient for tests such as intravenous pyelography, cystoscopy and biopsy, cystography, and bone scan, which may be required to further evaluate his condition.

Home care instructions

• Inform the patient that slight hematuria is normal for several days after TURB. However, bleeding or hematuria that lasts longer should be reported to the doctor.

• Advise the patient to drink plenty of water (about ten 8-oz glasses daily) and to void every 2 to 3 hours while gross hematuria persists to reduce the risk of clot formation, urethral obstruction, and urinary tract infection. Emphasize that he shouldn't ignore the urge to void.

• Instruct the patient to report urinary frequency and urgency and dysuria, commonly occurring signs of a lower urinary tract infection. The patient may also experience fever, chills, or flank pain, which indicate an upper urinary tract infection.

• To promote healing and reduce the risk of bleeding from increased intra-abdominal pressure, advise the patient to avoid sexual or other strenuous activity, not to lift anything heavier than 10 lb (4.5 kg), and to continue taking a stool softener or other laxative until the doctor approves a change.

• Emphasize the importance of follow-up examinations to evaluate the need for repeat treatments. Explain that early detection and removal of bladder tumors through TURB may prevent the need for cystectomy.

BLADDER TRAINING

Bladder training is a conservative approach to treatment of urinary incontinence. Preferable to use of drugs and surgery, bladder training uses behavior therapy techniques such as pelvic muscle (Kegel) exercises to make the patient more aware of the lower urinary tract and relaxation to help the patient control the urge to void. Successful bladder training requires a strongly motivated patient with the ability to discern body sensations.

Biofeedback may be used to enhance bladder training and pelvic exercises. It uses sophisticated equipment that gives visual and auditory feedback to help patients identify and use their bladder muscles more effectively.

Note that indwelling urinary catheters, both internal and external, are a last resort in the treatment of incontinence. They should be used only when incontinence cannot be managed medically, surgically, through behavior modification, or by intermittent catheterization.

Purpose
• To establish a regular voiding schedule and achieve urinary continence.

Indications
Bladder training is indicated for managing urinary incontinence that results from neurologic or mechanical bladder dysfunction.

Procedure
Bladder training requires the joint efforts of the patient and caregivers.

A bladder training program begins by instructing the patient in muscle strengthening exercises to increase the strength of the pelvic floor muscles. Next, the patient establishes a voiding record, which serves as the basis for the toileting schedule. The schedule indicates times when the patient should try to empty the bladder. In the early phase of bladder training, the interval between toileting is usually 1½ to 2 hours. Then, as the patient progresses, the interval is gradually prolonged by 30 minutes until a goal (usually 4 hours) is reached. The established toileting schedule is maintained even if the patient has episodes of incontinence.

If the patient has an urge to void before the scheduled toileting time, he is encouraged to relax and perform pelvic muscle strengthening exercises. Once the urge has passed, the patient then moves slowly (to prevent incontinence) to the bathroom.

If the patient has difficulty initiating urine flow, he is instructed to either sit or stand with the thighs flexed and the feet and back supported. It is also helpful to massage the bladder or lean forward when sitting. These methods help initiate bladder emptying by increasing intra-abdominal pressure.

Complications
No complications are associated with bladder training.

Care considerations
Before therapy
• Explain the training program and ensure that the patient understands and is willing to cooperate.
• Just before the start of the program, perform a thorough medical history and assessment to obtain treatment for preexisting conditions known to contribute to incontinence. Assessment should include specific questions regarding the patient's voiding patterns.
• Instruct the patient to consume a high-fiber diet and to maintain an adequate fluid intake of about six to eight 8-oz glasses (1,440 to 1,920 ml) per day but to limit fluid intake in the evening. A high-fiber diet prevents fecal impaction, which can increase bladder pressure and cause overflow incontinence. Adequate hydration during bladder training helps by preventing the formation of concentrated urine, which irritates the bladder wall and precipitates urinary incontinence.
During therapy
• Maintain a record of the progression of the program. Be sure to document incontinent episodes.
• Encourage and support the patient as necessary. Watch for frustration, anger, or depression. If appropriate, suggest psychological counseling to help the patient learn to cope with such feelings.

Home care instructions
• Environmental assessment of the home for access to toilet facilities is necessary to promote and restore continence.

• Teach the patient and caregiver the importance of dietary fiber intake and its relationship to the bladder training program.
• Instruct the caregiver to maintain the toileting schedule, which is essential to the success of the program.

BLOOD TRANSFUSION

A homologous blood transfusion is an I.V. infusion of whole blood or blood products. Depending on the indication, it may include *whole blood, packed red blood cells (RBCs), platelets, fresh frozen plasma, cryoprecipitate,* or *granulocytes.*

Whole blood transfusion replenishes the volume, RBC, and oxygen-carrying capacity of the circulatory system. Packed RBCs consist of blood in which 80% of the plasma has been removed. Infusion of packed cells restores the patient's RBC mass and oxygen-carrying capacity, but doesn't replenish lost blood volume. Platelets, the smallest of the formed elements, are necessary for blood coagulation. Each unit of platelets is suspended in 30 to 50 ml of plasma; however, 6 to 10 units may be suspended in one transfusion bag for a single transfusion. Fresh frozen plasma (FFP) is the liquid portion of blood that is frozen within a few hours of collection. It contains all of the blood's protein coagulation factors. Cryoprecipitates contain the stable clotting factors. Granulocytes are the blood cells that help fight bacterial infection.

Purpose
• To treat hypovolemic shock by replacing blood lost from hemorrhage
• To help treat anemia and other hematologic conditions.

Indications
Whole blood is typically administered only when hemorrhage significantly decreases oxygen-carrying capacity.

Packed RBCs are used to treat symptomatic anemia. However, because RBCs survive for only a short time, they provide only temporary improvement unless the underlying cause of the anemia is corrected. Washed packed RBCs are commonly used for patients previously sensitized by transfusions because they are rinsed with a special solution that removes white blood cells (WBCs) and platelets, thus decreasing the chance of a transfusion reaction.

Platelets can be administered prophylactically and therapeutically, especially in patients with severe thrombocytopenia or leukemia or in those who are receiving cancer chemotherapy. Transfusion may not increase platelet counts in patients with idiopathic thrombocytopenic purpura, splenomegaly, disseminated intravascular coagulation, or antibody reactions because these conditions involve platelet destruction. However, such patients may receive platelet transfusion to treat severe hemorrhage.

FFP is primarily used to treat clotting factor deficiencies. Occasionally, FFP may be used as a volume expander and protein source instead of crystalloids, albumin, or plasma protein fraction.

Cryoprecipitate is primarily used to treat patients with stable clotting factor deficiencies. Rarely, granulocytes are transfused in granulocytopenic patients who have an infection that resists anti-infective therapy. They're usually used as a last resort for patients who need WBCs to recover from infection—for example, neonates, whose immune systems are still undeveloped.

Procedure
Depending on the severity of the patient's condition, transfusions are performed on an inpatient or outpatient

basis. The whole blood or blood product is administered I.V. through a special blood tubing that contains a filter to remove fibrin clots that may have formed after the blood was placed in the blood transfusion bag. Commonly, 0.9% sodium chloride solution is hung with the blood or blood component using a Y-type blood administration set. The solution is used to keep the vein open if the transfusion must be stopped or delayed.

Units of whole blood and most blood products should be administered within a 4-hour period because unrefrigerated blood can become contaminated with bacteria. Platelets and granulocytes are administered at a much faster rate, usually 1 to 2 ml/minute.

Complications

Blood transfusion carries the risk of serious complications, including transfusion reactions such as an acute hemolytic reaction or an allergic reaction. Transfusion reactions can occur during, immediately after, or up to 10 days after a blood transfusion but most often occur immediately after the transfusion begins or within an hour after it is completed (see *Recognizing transfusion reactions,* pages 104 and 105).

Another serious complication is the transmission of infectious diseases such as hepatitis C (non-A, non-B hepatitis), cytomegalovirus, and acquired immunodeficiency syndrome. Because of current techniques for testing donor blood for these diseases, such transmission is uncommon.

Certain complications—such as hypothermia, bleeding tendencies, and hemosiderosis—typically result from multiple or massive transfusions.

Care considerations
Before therapy
• Explain the procedure and ensure that the patient understands the risks involved.

• Obtain a blood sample for blood typing and crossmatching and send it to the laboratory.
• Review the doctor's orders for any medications that are to be administered before transfusion. If the patient has a history of blood transfusion reactions, give pretransfusion medications, such as acetaminophen and diphenhydramine, as ordered. Before transfusion of granulocytes, the patient may receive meperidine and diphenhydramine.
• Check for an adequate I.V. infusion site. If needed, perform venipuncture. Then begin infusing 0.9% sodium chloride solution at a keep-vein-open rate, about 10 to 20 drops/minute.
• When the whole blood or the blood component arrives, check the expiration date on the bag and observe its contents for abnormal color, clumping, gas bubbles, and extraneous materials. Return outdated or abnormal blood to the blood bank.
• To prevent a possibly fatal transfusion reaction, carefully check both the amount and the component ordered. Also compare the name and number on the patient's identification band with that on the compatibility slip. Verify ABO and Rh compatibility. Then, have another nurse double-check each of these steps.
• Take the patient's vital signs as a baseline just before starting the transfusion.

During therapy
• Monitor the patient's vital signs according to hospital policy—for example, every 5 minutes for the first 15 minutes, then every 30 minutes for the duration of the transfusion. Observe the patient closely for signs of an acute reaction. Observe carefully for fever and increased pulse rate, often the first signs of a transfusion reaction. The first 15 minutes of the infusion is the most critical time for a transfusion reaction. At any sign of a reaction, notify the doctor, stop the transfusion, and

Recognizing transfusion reactions

Transfusion reactions result primarily from ABO incompatibility, contaminated blood, or too-rapid infusion. The chart below lists transfusion reactions, common causes, and related signs and symptoms.

REACTION	CAUSE	SIGNS AND SYMPTOMS
Reactions from any transfusion		
Allergic reaction	• Antibodies to leukocytes or plasma proteins	• Itching, hives, fever, chills, nausea, vomiting, facial swelling, wheezing, laryngeal edema • May progress to anaphylaxis
Bacterial contamination	• Gram-negative organisms • Improper blood collection or storage	• Chills, fever, vomiting, abdominal cramping, diarrhea, shock, signs of renal failure
Febrile reaction	• Presence of antibodies to leukocytes or plasma proteins	• Fever, chills, headache, flank pain, and, rarely, hypotension
Hemolytic reaction	• ABO or Rh incompatibility • Intradonor incompatibility • Improper blood storage	• Shaking, chills, fever, nausea, vomiting, chest pain, dyspnea, hypotension, oliguria, hemoglobinuria, flank pain, abnormal bleeding • May progress to shock and renal failure
Hypervolemia	• Too-rapid or excessive blood transfusion	• Dyspnea, hypertension, pulmonary edema
Reactions from multiple transfusions		
Bleeding tendencies	• Low platelet count in stored blood, causing dilutional thrombocytopenia	• Abnormal bleeding and oozing from cut or break in the skin surface
Elevated blood ammonia level	• Increased level of ammonia ion in stored blood	• Forgetfulness, confusion
Hemosiderosis	• Increased hemosiderin (iron-containing pigment) from red blood cell (RBC) destruction, especially after receiving chronic transfusions	• Iron plasma level greater than 200 mg/dl

Recognizing transfusion reactions *(continued)*

REACTION	CAUSE	SIGNS AND SYMPTOMS
Reactions from multiple transfusions *(continued)*		
Hypocalcemia	• Citrate toxicity from rapid infusion of citrate-treated blood. Citrate binds with calcium, causing a calcium deficiency, or normal citrate metabolism is hindered by hepatic disease.	• Tingling in fingers, muscle cramps, nausea, vomiting, hypotension, cardiac arrhythmias, seizures
Hypothermia	• Rapid infusion of large amounts of cold blood which decreases myocardial temperature	• Shaking chills, hypotension, ventricular fibrillation • Cardiac arrest if core temperature falls below 86° F (30° C)
Increased oxygen affinity for hemoglobin	• Decreased level of 2,3-diphosphoglycerate in stored blood, causing an increase in the oxygen's hemoglobin affinity; when this occurs, oxygen stays in the patient's bloodstream and isn't released into the tissues	• Depressed respiratory rate, especially in patients with chronic lung disease
Potassium intoxication	• An abnormally high level of potassium in stored plasma caused by RBC lysis	• Intestinal colic, diarrhea, muscle twitching, oliguria, renal failure, ECG changes with tall, peaked T waves, bradycardia proceeding to cardiac standstill

keep the I.V. line open with 0.9% sodium chloride solution.
• Keep emergency equipment available for treating a severe hemolytic or anaphylactic reaction.
• Monitor intake and output during transfusion and for 8 hours afterward. Report decreased urine output to the doctor.
• Assess the needle insertion site often for redness or swelling. If necessary, change the infusion site.
• Monitor the infusion rate. If the rate is too slow, check the patency of the I.V. line and change the administration set (if the filter is clogged). If you're using a gravity-flow infusion, you can

raise the height of the bag or apply a pressure bag to increase the flow rate.

After therapy
• Take the patient's vital signs and compare them with the baseline.
• If transfusion is done on an outpatient basis, observe the patient for at least 2 hours after the transfusion if possible.

Home care instructions

• Teach the patient and caregiver the symptoms of a delayed transfusion reaction and of hepatitis: fever, headache, anorexia, nausea, vomiting, and abdominal pain. Warn them that these symptoms most often occur 3 to 10 days after transfusion and must be reported immediately.

• Instruct the patient receiving platelets not to use aspirin because it interferes with platelet function. Instead, recommend acetaminophen for pain relief or fever.

BONE GROWTH STIMULATION

Bone growth stimulation, also known as galvanic therapy, involves the application of a mild electric current to bone fracture fragments to help stimulate new bone growth and speed healing.

Three methods of electrical bone growth stimulation are currently used, one noninvasive method and two types of invasive bone growth stimulators, which are partially or fully implantable. Each of the three methods requires 3 to 6 months of therapy to be effective.

The invasive devices are direct current stimulators. They produce a fixed electrical field that runs a constant direct current into the fracture site to produce osteogenesis 24 hours a day. The noninvasive pulsating electromagnetic fields (PEMF) device stimulates, not by direct application of current, but rather with electromagnetic forces. These devices are applied for from 3 to 10 hours daily, depending on the manufacturer.

Selection of a bone growth stimulator depends on such factors as the fracture's type and location, the doctor's preference, and perhaps most important, the patient's ability to comply with treatment. The fully implanted system requires little or no patient intervention; the semi-implanted and PEMF systems require that the patient manage his own treatment schedule and maintain the equipment.

These devices should not be used if the gap in the fractured bone (the point of nonunion) is larger than half the diameter of the bone at the level of the fracture. They also are not effective if synovial pseudoarthrosis is present.

Purpose

• To electrically stimulate new bone growth in areas of fracture and speed healing.

Indications

Bone growth stimulation is reserved for patients with fractures that fail to heal within 6 to 9 months of injury (about 5% of all skeletal fractures).

Studies continue on new applications for this electrical treatment. Researchers hope eventually to use it to reverse osteoporosis and avascular necrosis and even to heal soft tissue injuries, such as pressure ulcers, bruises, and other skin ulcers.

Procedure

For invasive device

Before implantation of an invasive device, the patient receives spinal or general anesthesia.

The fully implantable direct current stimulator consists of a power generator (a small battery pack), titanium cathode, and lead wires. The cathode is implanted in the fractured bone and the generator in nearby deep muscle fascia. The generator is connected to the cathode by a lead wire that is tunneled through the subcutaneous tissue. The device runs 24 hours a day.

The semi-implantable percutaneous stimulator uses several Teflon-coated cathode pins, an external anode skin pad, and battery pack. Cathodes are implanted just inside the margin of each bone at the fracture site. The cathode wires are brought out to the skin surface, and the surgical area is covered with cast padding. The cathode wires are attached to the battery pack. The anode pad is applied to the skin and attached to the battery pack with a lead wire, and a non–weight-bearing cast is applied to the site over the battery pack.

For noninvasive device

The noninvasive PEMF device uses external wire coils and a generator to produce the therapeutic electric current. The patient is first fitted with a snug plaster cast. The doctor then measures the cast's circumference at the fracture site. This measurement guides the distance between the electromagnetic coils placed on either side of the injured area as well as the amount of voltage required for the generator. The coils are placed on the cast and are held in place with a Velcro strap or a cufflike transducer. X-rays confirm proper coil placement in relation to the fracture. (See *Two methods of stimulating bone growth*.)

Complications

Complications after implantation of the direct current stimulator or the percutaneous stimulator include infection and discharge at the implantation site. Few complications are seen with the PEMF device, probably because it does not require implantation.

Care considerations

Before therapy

• Explain the procedure. If the patient is receiving a percutaneous stimulator or a PEMF device, inform him that he will be responsible for managing his own schedule and maintaining the equipment.

• Assure the patient that there is no risk of electrocution.

• Instruct the patient in cast care. Tell the patient who will have a PEMF device that he cannot place any weight on the involved limb until healing is completed.

• If the patient has a lower extremity fracture, be sure that he understands that he will not be able to bear weight

Two methods of stimulating bone growth

Electrical bone growth stimulators may be invasive or noninvasive. An invasive system, shown below, involves placement of a spiral-like cathode inside the bone. A wire leads from the cathode to a battery-powered generator, also implanted in the local tissues. The patient's body completes the electrical circuit.

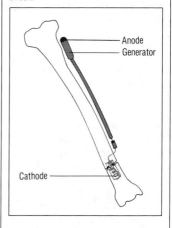

A noninvasive system, shown below, may include a cufflike transducer that wraps around the patient's limb at the level of the injury. Electric current penetrates the leg.

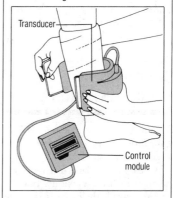

on the affected leg for the length of the therapy.

After therapy
• If the patient has an implanted or semi-implantable device, check vital signs and assess neurovascular status in the affected limb. Watch for signs of infection, such as fever and swelling, redness, tenderness, and discharge at or near the implantation site.
• Follow all the standard principles of cast care.
• For all types of devices, reinforce the doctor's instructions regarding weight-bearing restrictions.

Home care instructions
• Tell the patient to report any signs of infection at the treatment site.
• Make sure the patient understands how to care for the cast.
• As ordered, tell the patient when to expect weight-bearing on the affected leg. Typically, this will be after X-rays confirm complete healing.
• Emphasize the importance of regular follow-up examinations to evaluate therapy and healing.
• Instruct the patient using a PEMF device to wear the coils 3 to 10 hours a day, depending on the manufacturer, for intervals no shorter than 1 hour. Suggest that he wear the coils while sleeping to provide a long period of uninterrupted therapy. Also instruct him to test the unit regularly and to call the doctor if it doesn't work properly or if the generator alarm signals.

BONE MARROW TRANSPLANTATION

Bone marrow transplantation (BMT) is the infusion of fresh or stored bone marrow from a donor to a recipient. This treatment replaces diseased bone marrow with healthy bone marrow and thus may enable the patient to resume the normal production of blood cells.

Whether or not a patient receives BMT depends on the underlying disease, age, health status, and the availability of a histocompatible donor.

Types of BMT include *autologous*, *syngeneic*, and *allogeneic*. In an autologous BMT, marrow is procured from the patient, frozen, and stored for later use. After the patient receives chemotherapy or radiation therapy, the autologous marrow is returned to the patient. Autologous BMT may not be a treatment option for patients with diseased bone marrow.

Syngeneic BMT is the transplantation of bone marrow from an identical twin. When possible, it is the ideal option because the bone marrow of twins is histologically identical, yet free of disease.

Allogeneic BMT is the use of marrow from a histocompatible donor for transplantation. Donors for allogeneic BMT are usually siblings but may also be unrelated to the patient. Tissue typing is done to determine the histocompatibility of the recipient and donor. The tissue typing procedure tests for a specific set of antigen markers. If both the donor and the recipient have the same antigen markers, the bone marrow of the donor and the recipient are considered compatible. Other antigens exist but are not detectable at this time. Therefore, the tissue of the recipient and donor may not be perfectly matched, even though the bone marrow is considered compatible. For this reason the recipient requires immunosuppression after the transplantation.

Purpose
• To replace the bone marrow of patients whose marrow has been suppressed after preparative regimens that consist of marrow ablative chemotherapy, radiotherapy, or immunosuppressant therapy.

Indications

BMT is the treatment of choice for aplastic anemia and severe combined immunodeficiency disease. It is also used to treat acute leukemia, chronic leukemia, and lymphoma. In addition, BMT is being explored as a treatment for other hematologic diseases, such as multiple myeloma and selected solid tumors.

Procedure

To prepare a patient for BMT, high doses of chemotherapy – and sometimes total body irradiation – are given in an attempt to destroy diseased bone marrow and hidden cancer cells and to empty the marrow spaces to make room for healthy marrow. In a patient receiving an allogeneic BMT, chemotherapy is also given to suppress the patient's immune system so that the new marrow can begin to function.

Before the actual transplantation, bone marrow must be removed from the donor. This is known as bone marrow procurement or harvesting. After the marrow is obtained, it is administered to the recipient (see *Bone marrow procurement*).

On the day of the transplantation, the previously procured bone marrow is infused at the bedside, usually through a central venous catheter just as any blood product would be infused. Once in the central circulation, the transplanted bone marrow migrates to the bone marrow cavities where the new cells begin to grow and produce new blood cells (engraftment). Medications such as diphenhydramine and acetaminophen may be given before the infusion to prevent adverse reactions. Autologous bone marrow must be thawed immediately before infusion. Syngeneic and allogeneic bone marrow are infused immediately after procurement from the donor.

The rate of bone marrow infusion varies according to the volume of marrow obtained but may range from 1 to 4 hours. Engraftment after infusion of

Bone marrow procurement

The timing of bone marrow procurement is dependent on the type of bone marrow transplantation (BMT).

Bone marrow for autologous BMT is usually obtained at least 2 weeks before the day of the transplantation but can be obtained much sooner and preserved for long periods, even years. If necessary, the patient's bone marrow may undergo a process that removes or destroys cancer cells before it is frozen until the day of transplantation.

Bone marrow from syngeneic and allogeneic donors is removed from the donor on the day of transplantation and immediately given to the recipient.

In all cases, the marrow is collected from the donor in the operating room, under general or epidural anesthesia, through multiple bone marrow aspirations from the donor's iliac crest. The procurement procedure usually takes approximately 1½ to 2 hours to aspirate approximately 500 to 1,000 ml of marrow-containing stem cells. The marrow is filtered to remove bone and fat particles and other debris. It is mixed with heparin and a preservative to prevent coagulation and maintain viability of the marrow product. After the procedure, pressure dressings are applied to the donor sites and analgesics are given as needed.

the bone marrow may take from 10 days to 3 to 4 weeks.

Complications

The most common complications that may follow BMT include acute or chronic graft-versus-host disease (GVHD), bleeding, and infections. GVHD occurs only in allogeneic bone marrow transplant. (See *Common complications of bone marrow transplantation*, pages 110 and 111.)

Common complications of bone marrow transplantation

Graft-versus-host disease

Cause

T-lymphocytes in donor bone marrow attack specific target organs of the recipient

Special considerations

• Graft-versus-host disease (GVHD) occurs in about 50% of patients who receive allogeneic bone marrow transplantation (BMT).
• Disease does not occur in autologous or syngeneic BMT.
• GVHD may be acute or chronic: acute GVHD occurs 70 to 90 days after BMT; chronic GVHD occurs 90 days to years after BMT.
• Disease primarily affects the skin and mucous membranes, the GI tract, and the liver.
• Evaluate skin for rashes or erythema.
• Monitor intake and output.
• Notify doctor if abdominal cramps or diarrhea occur.
• Test stools for occult blood.
• Monitor liver function tests. Report any hepatomegaly, jaundice, and elevated liver enzymes.
• Administer medications to prevent or treat GVHD as ordered. Combination drug therapy with methotrexate and cyclosporine has recently been found to reduce the incidence and severity of GVHD.

Infection

Cause

Immunosuppression (allogeneic BMT patient) or lack of bone marrow capable of producing infection-fighting cells (autologous BMT patient)

Special considerations

• Risk of developing infection exists for at least 1 year after BMT.
• Pulmonary infections (most commonly viral infections, often with cytomegalovirus, but also with *Pneumocystis carinii)* occur most often after allogeneic BMT; may be fatal.
• Provide reverse (protective) isolation for the patient. Some patients are placed in laminar airflow or rooms with special air-filtering systems.
• Monitor the patient for signs of pulmonary and other infections every 4 to 8 hours.
• Perform cultures of urine, stool, throat flora, and blood routinely, according to hospital protocol.
• Administer prophylactic and therapeutic antibiotics as ordered.
• If possible, administer single donor platelet products to avoid exposing the BMT patient to multiple donors and thus increasing the possibility of infections.

Common complications of bone marrow transplantation *(continued)*

Bleeding

Cause
Prolonged thrombocytopenia, anemia, and altered liver function

Special considerations
- Risk of bleeding is lessened after patient's blood counts are self-sustaining, and they no longer require frequent transfusions.
- Monitor white blood cell, red blood cell, and platelet counts.
- Monitor vital signs frequently.
- Administer transfusions of blood products as ordered.

Care considerations

Before the procedure
- Reinforce the doctor's explanation as necessary. Answer the patient's and family's questions.
- Tell the patient that he'll first receive chemotherapy or radiation therapy, or both, to kill any residual cancer cells. He may also receive antibiotics to reduce the number of organisms typically present in the bowel.
- Before the transplantation, place the patient in reverse isolation to protect him from infection. Make sure that the patient understands that he will be very susceptible to infection after the procedure.

During the procedure
- Monitor the recipient for signs and symptoms of adverse reactions, and, if necessary, give ordered medications to relieve these symptoms. (Common adverse reactions are similar to blood transfusion reactions—fever, chills, pulmonary edema, dyspnea, hypertension or hypotension, hemolysis, and chest or back pain.)
- Monitor the patient's vital signs according to hospital policy—for example, every 15 minutes for 1 hour, every 30 minutes for 2 hours, and then every hour for 4 hours.
- Monitor the infusion rate carefully.

After the procedure
- Care after BMT focuses on monitoring the patient for effectiveness of therapy and occurrence of complications.
- Maintain reverse isolation. Ensure that all persons entering the patient's room wear sterile gowns, masks, gloves, and shoecovers. Explain that this is to prevent introducing infective organisms into the environment.
- Monitor the patient continuously for signs of complications.
- Monitor hematologic status at least daily. Until engraftment takes place, the patient's white blood cell count is zero and the red blood cell and platelet counts are drastically reduced. Administer platelet and blood cell transfusions, as ordered. These patients usually require frequent transfusion until blood cell counts are self-sustaining.

Home care instructions
- Provide information on protection from infection.
- Teach the patient or caregiver how to manage the central venous catheter.
- Teach the patient or caregiver how to administer medications correctly.
- Be sure the patient and caregiver know the signs and symptoms of complications. Tell them to report complications to the doctor promptly.

• Provide emergency phone numbers (doctor, ambulance, emergency squad) for the patient.

• Emphasize the need to keep follow-up appointments so that progress can be monitored and late-occurring complications can be identified and treated.

BOWEL OR ABDOMINOPERINEAL SURGERY WITH OSTOMY

An ostomy involves the resection of diseased colonic and rectal segments and the creation of an intestinal opening (stoma) on the abdominal surface. Fecal material that would normally pass through the bowel is excreted through the stoma and safely collected in a specially designed surgical appliance.

Several surgical approaches may be used to create an ostomy, also known as a colostomy, if it involves the large intestine or an enterostomy (ileostomy or jejunostomy) if it involves the small intestine.

An ostomy may be temporary or permanent. A temporary ostomy interrupts the intestinal flow to allow healing of inflamed or injured bowel segments. After healing occurs, usually within 10 weeks, an anastomosis of the divided segments restores bowel integrity and function.

Permanent colostomies typically accompany an abdominoperineal resection, which involves removal of the remaining colon, rectum, and anus.

Severe, widespread colonic obstruction or intractable inflammatory bowel disease may require total or near-total removal of the colon and rectum and creation of an ileostomy from the proximal ileum. A permanent ileostomy requires the patient to wear a drainage pouch over the stoma to receive the constant fecal drainage. In contrast, a continent (or Kock's) ileostomy doesn't require an external

pouch (see *Understanding Kock's pouch*). An ileoanal anastomosis eliminates the need for a permanent ileostomy, establishes an ileal reservoir, and maintains elimination through the anal sphincter. (See *Understanding ileoanal anastomosis*, page 114.)

Purpose

• To remove diseased colonic and rectal tissue and create a surgical opening, or stoma, through the abdominal wall for elimination of feces.

Indications

This surgery is commonly performed for inflammatory bowel disease, familial polyposis, diverticulitis, Hirschsprung's disease, rectovaginal fistula, and penetrating trauma. It is performed for advanced colorectal cancer if conservative surgery and other treatments fail or if the patient develops acute complications, such as obstruction, abscess, or fistula.

Procedure

This surgery is performed in an operating room, under general anesthesia. The type of ostomy depends on the nature and location of the problem. (See *Reviewing types of ostomies*, page 115, and *Types of ostomy surgery*, page 116.)

Complications

Common complications of ostomy include hemorrhage, sepsis, ileus, and fluid and electrolyte imbalance from excessive drainage through the stoma. Peritonitis can also complicate recovery. Rarely, the bowel may prolapse out of the abdominal cavity through the stoma and require surgery to reestablish it. Skin excoriation may occur around the stoma from contact with digestive enzymes in the drainage; irritation may result from pressure of the ostomy pouch. Excoriation occurs more commonly with an ileostomy because of the higher concentration of digestive juices in ileal drainage.

Understanding Kock's pouch

A continent ileal reservoir (Kock's pouch) may be an option for some patients with ulcerative colitis when conservative measures fail to relieve severe symptoms. This surgical procedure involves a proctocolectomy, which is the complete removal of the colon, rectum, and anus. However, instead of creating an ileostomy, the surgeon creates a reservoir from about 12″ (30 cm) of ileum. A nipple valve is created by pulling back the distal portion of the reservoir into the ileum, as in intussusception. The connecting segment of ileum is then brought out to the abdominal wall, and a stoma is formed. This procedure allows storage of fecal material in the reservoir for several hours. It is then removed by inserting a catheter through the external stoma into the reservoir. The main advantage is that it eliminates the need for wearing an external collection pouch. However, many patients experience malfunction of the nipple valve.

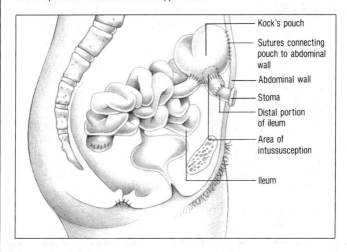

Kock's pouch

Sutures connecting pouch to abdominal wall

Abdominal wall

Stoma

Distal portion of ileum

Area of intussusception

Ileum

Care considerations

Before surgery

• If emergency surgery is necessary, briefly explain the procedure and prepare the patient for the postoperative physical changes.

• If emergency surgery isn't required, both the doctor and the nurse should provide a clear explanation of the surgery. If appropriate, include family members or caregivers in your discussion.

• Monitor fluid and electrolyte balance and nutritional status before surgery. If chronic bowel disease has seriously compromised the patient's condition, evaluate nutritional and fluid status for 3 to 4 days before surgery (if time permits). Typically, the patient will be receiving I.V. parenteral nutrition to prepare for the physiologic stress of surgery. Record the patient's fluid intake and output and weight daily, and watch for early signs of dehydration. Expect to draw periodic blood samples for hematocrit and hemoglobin determinations. Be prepared to transfuse blood if ordered.

• Tell the patient that analgesics will be provided for postoperative pain.

• Describe the type of ostomy the patient will have and explain how fecal

Understanding ileoanal anastomosis

An ileoanal anastomosis is a newer surgical procedure that may be an option for some patients with chronic ulcerative colitis or familial polyposis. This procedure involves a total abdominal colectomy and a mucosal proctectomy—removal of diseased colon and rectum. Then, the surgeon creates a reservoir by aligning about 20" (50 cm) of ileum into an "S" shape, opening that part of the bowel, and anastomosing adjacent walls to form a reservoir. The distal segment of the newly created reservoir is then anastomosed to the anus, and a temporary diverting loop ileostomy is created to permit healing below. This is usually closed a few months later. The patient should then have anal sphincter control over elimination. Bowel movements are less frequent after surgery; however, they may still number up to ten per day. Complications may include perianal skin irritation, stricture at the anastomosis site, and small-bowel obstruction.

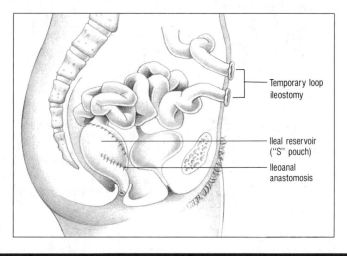

Temporary loop ileostomy

Ileal reservoir ("S" pouch)

Ileoanal anastomosis

matter drains through it. Use simple illustrations to facilitate your explanation. In this description, discuss selection and use of ostomy appliances. If possible, show the patient the actual appliances. Prepare him for the unpleasant odor and consistency of fecal drainage. This consistency varies from constant watery stools with an ileostomy to soft, semisolid stools with a colostomy in the descending colon.

• Inform the colostomy patient that he'll initially wear a pouch to collect fecal drainage. Point out that he may learn to control bowel movements by irrigating the colostomy. If he can learn

bowel control, he may not need to use a pouch.

• Reassure the patient that after becoming comfortable with ostomy management, he should be able to resume normal activity with few restrictions.

• Before surgery, try to arrange for a visit with an enterostomal therapist, who can provide more detailed information. If possible, also arrange for the patient to meet with former ostomy patients (from groups such as the United Ostomy Association) before surgery; these patients can share their personal insights into the realities of living with and caring for a stoma.

Reviewing types of ostomies

The type of ostomy depends on the patient's condition. Temporary ones, such as a double-barrel or loop colostomy, help treat perforated sigmoid diverticulitis, penetrating trauma, and other conditions in which intestinal healing is expected. Temporary ostomies are also used to bypass an unresectable intestinal tumor. Permanent colostomy or ileostomy typically accompanies extensive abdominal surgery, often for removal of a malignant tumor.

Permanent colostomy

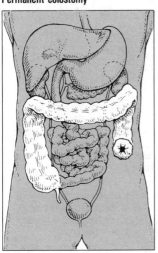

Loop colostomy

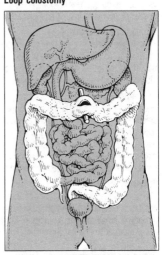

Double-barrel colostomy

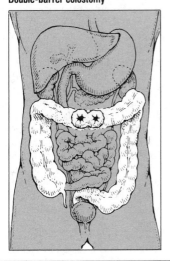

Ileostomy

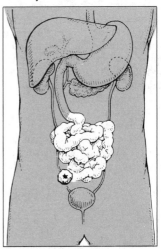

Types of ostomy surgery

Four types of ostomy surgery are described below.

Abdominoperineal resection

The surgeon makes a low abdominal incision and divides the sigmoid colon, then brings the proximal end of the colon out through another, smaller abdominal incision to create a permanent colostomy. Next, the surgeon makes a wide perineal incision and resects the anus, rectum, and distal portion of the sigmoid colon. After placing one or more sump drains in the abdomen and closing the abdominal wound, the surgeon either leaves the perineal wound open and packs it with gauze, or he may close it and place several Penrose drains in the closed wound.

Temporary loop colostomy

The surgeon brings a portion of intestine out through an abdominal incision, slips an ostomy bridge (a short plastic or glass rod) under the intestinal loop to support it on the outer abdominal wall, incises the intestine to create a temporary stoma, then closes the wound around the exposed intestinal loop.

Temporary double-barrel colostomy

The surgeon divides the colon and brings both ends through an abdominal incision to create a proximal stoma for fecal drainage and a distal stoma leading to the inactive bowel. After inserting abdominal sump drains, the surgeon closes the incision around the stomas. Later, when the intestinal injury has healed or the inflammation subsided, the loop or double-barrel temporary colostomy is discontinued, and the divided ends of the colon are anastomosed to restore bowel integrity.

Ileostomy

The surgeon resects all or part of the colon and rectum (proctocolectomy) and creates a permanent ileostomy by bringing a loop of the proximal ileum out through a small abdominal incision. Typically, the incision is located in the right lower quadrant between the midline and the right anterior iliac crest.

• If the patient is receiving long-term, low-dose corticosteroid therapy, continue to administer the drug to prevent rebound adrenocortical insufficiency. Explain that the drug will be withdrawn gradually after surgery. Also administer antibiotics, as ordered, to reduce intestinal flora.

After surgery

• In the immediate postoperative period, monitor intake and output and weigh the patient daily. Maintain fluid and electrolyte balance, and watch for signs of dehydration, such as decreased urine output, poor skin turgor, and electrolyte imbalance.

• Provide analgesics, as ordered. Be especially alert for pain in the patient who has had an abdominoperineal re-section because of the extent and location of the incisions.

• Note the color, consistency, and odor of fecal drainage from the stoma. If the patient has a double-barrel colostomy, check for mucus drainage from the inactive (distal) stoma. The type of ostomy surgery determines fecal drainage; typically, the more colon tissue that is preserved, the more closely drainage will resemble normal stool. For the first few days after surgery, fecal drainage probably will be mucoid (and possibly slightly blood-tinged) and mostly odorless. Report excessive blood or mucus content, which could indicate hemorrhage or infection.

• Observe the patient for signs of peritonitis or sepsis, caused by leakage of bowel contents into the abdominal cavity. Remember that patients receiving antibiotics or parenteral nutrition are at an increased risk for sepsis.

• Provide meticulous wound care, changing dressings often. Check dressings and drainage sites frequently for signs of infection (purulent drainage, foul odor) or fecal drainage. If the patient has had an abdominoperineal resection, irrigate the perineal area, as ordered.

• Regularly check the stoma and the surrounding skin for irritation and excoriation, which may result from contact with fecal drainage or from pressure caused by an overfilled or improperly fitted drainage pouch. Take measures to correct any such problems. Also observe the stoma's appearance. It should look smooth, cherry red, and slightly edematous; immediately report any discoloration or excessive swelling, which may indicate circulatory problems that could lead to ischemia and necrosis of the stoma. Also report any retraction or separation of the stoma from the skin edges.

• During the recovery period, encourage the patient to express his feelings and concerns. Reassure the patient who's anxious and depressed that these common postoperative reactions should fade with adjustment to the ostomy. Continue to arrange for visits by an enterostomal therapist, if possible.

Home care instructions

• The colostomy patient will need extensive home care instructions. Teach proper stoma care and drainage techniques, dietary modifications, and other long-term treatment measures.

• Teach the patient or caregiver how to apply, remove, and empty the pouch. When appropriate, provide instruction on how to irrigate the colostomy with warm tap water on a regular basis to gain some control over elimination. If appropriate, emphasize that continence can be achieved with dietary control and bowel retraining.

• Instruct the colostomy patient to change the stoma appliance as needed, to wash the stoma site with warm water and mild soap every 3 days, and to change the adhesive layer. These measures help prevent skin irritation and excoriation. If the patient has an ileostomy, instruct him to change the drainage pouch only when leakage occurs. Also emphasize meticulous skin care and use of a protective skin barrier around the stoma site.

• Discuss dietary restrictions (low-fiber diet) and suggestions (chew food well) to prevent stoma blockage, diarrhea, flatus, and offensive odor.

• Explain the need for maintaining a high fluid intake to help ensure fluid and electrolyte balance. Tell the patient that this is especially important in times of increased fluid loss; for example, during periods of hot weather or bouts of diarrhea.

• Warn the patient to avoid alcohol, laxatives, and diuretics, which will increase fluid loss and may contribute to an imbalance.

• Tell the patient to report persistent diarrhea through the stoma, which can quickly lead to fluid and electrolyte imbalance.

• If the patient has had an abdominoperineal resection, suggest sitz baths to help relieve perineal discomfort. Advise the patient to avoid intercourse until the perineum heals.

• Encourage all ostomy patients to discuss their feelings and questions about resuming sexual intercourse. Mention that the drainage pouch won't dislodge if the device is empty and fitted properly. Suggest avoiding food and fluids for several hours before intercourse.

• Remind the patient and family that depression is common after ostomy surgery. However, recommend counseling if depression is severe or persists.

BOWEL RESECTION AND ANASTOMOSIS

This surgical procedure removes diseased intestinal tissue and then reconnects (anastomoses) the edges of the remaining intestine. If large intestine is removed, the procedure is termed a colectomy; if small intestine is removed, it is termed an enterectomy. Whenever possible, the surgeon will perform resection with anastomosis to preserve bowel continuity. In some cases, particularly when there is not enough healthy tissue to anastomose, a temporary or permanent colostomy or ileostomy may be necessary. (See the entry "Bowel or Abdominoperineal Surgery with Ostomy.")

Unlike the patient who undergoes total colectomy or more extensive surgery, the patient who undergoes simple resection and anastomosis usually retains normal bowel function.

Purpose

• To remove diseased portions of the bowel and join the remaining segments to restore bowel integrity and function.

Indications

Bowel resection and anastomosis helps treat localized obstructive disorders, including diverticulosis (with an area of acute diverticulitis, stricture, or abscess formation), intestinal polyps, adhesions that cause bowel dysfunction, and malignant or benign intestinal tumors.

It's the preferred surgical technique for localized bowel cancer but not for widespread carcinoma, which usually requires creation of a temporary or permanent colostomy or an ileostomy. It may also be used to remove the diseased segment of the bowel in inflammatory disorders of the bowel, such as Crohn's disease or colitis, when medical intervention fails to control the disorder.

Procedure

The surgeon performs the procedure with the patient under general anesthesia. The abdominal incision site varies, depending on the site of the diseased tissue. Once the incision is made, the surgeon will excise the diseased portion of the colon and then anastomose the remaining healthy bowel segments to restore continuity. End-to-end anastomosis provides the most physiologically sound junction and is the quickest to perform, but it requires that the approximated bowel segments be large enough to prevent postoperative obstruction at the anastomotic site. Side-to-side anastomosis minimizes the danger of anastomotic obstruction, but this longer procedure may be contraindicated in some situations.

If surgery is performed for removal of a malignant tumor, the surgeon removes the associated blood vessels and lymphatic channels as well as the cancerous structures as a unit in order to prevent shedding of cancer cells and seeding of cancer cells into other peritoneal structures. The surgeon may irrigate the peritoneum with an anticancer agent as a further precaution and may also obtain a biopsy of the liver (the primary metastatic site) and abdominal lymph nodes in order to aid staging of cancer and guide continuing treatment.

Complications

Complications of bowel resection and anastomosis include bleeding from the anastomotic site, which can progress to hemorrhage and hypovolemic shock if severe; peritonitis and resultant sepsis; postresection obstruction, most often caused by development of adhesions; leakage of bowel contents at the suture line connecting the bowel segments; and other problems common to abdominal surgery, such as wound infection and atelectasis.

Care considerations
Before surgery

• Reinforce the surgeon's explanation of the proposed surgery and its attendant potential risks and complications. Answer the patient's and family's questions about the surgery and its effects on the patient's life-style.

• Discuss anticipated postoperative care measures. The patient will awaken from surgery with a nasogastric (NG) tube in place to drain air and fluid from the intestinal tract and prevent distention. Explain that the tube will be removed when peristalsis returns, usually within 2 to 3 days. Tell the patient to anticipate ambulation on the 1st day after surgery, which will promote return of peristalsis. Also prepare the patient to expect abdominal drains, an indwelling urinary catheter, and an I.V. line, which will provide fluid replacement.

• To reduce the risk of postoperative atelectasis and pneumonia, teach the patient how to cough and deep-breathe properly, and emphasize the need to do so regularly throughout recovery. Demonstrate incisional splinting to protect the sutures and reduce discomfort during coughing.

• Just before surgery, as ordered, administer antibiotics to reduce intestinal flora and laxatives or enemas to remove fecal contents.

After surgery

• For the first few days after surgery, monitor intake and output and weigh the patient daily. Maintain fluid and electrolyte balance through I.V. replacement therapy; check the patient regularly for signs of dehydration, such as decreased urine output and poor skin turgor.

• Keep the NG tube patent.

• To detect possible complications, monitor the patient's vital signs and closely evaluate his overall condition. Observe him closely for signs of complications: anastomotic leakage (low-grade fever, malaise, slight leukocytosis, abdominal distention and tenderness); hypovolemic shock (precipitous drop in blood pressure and pulse rate, peripheral vasoconstriction, respiratory difficulty, decreased level of consciousness, bloody stools); peritonitis or sepsis (abdominal pain of sudden or gradual onset, fever, vomiting, rapid and shallow respirations, abdominal tenderness and rigidity, wound drainage, diminished or absent bowel sounds); and postresection obstruction (abdominal distention and rigidity, absent or decreased bowel sounds, no passage of flatus or feces).

• Provide frequent mouth and tube care to prevent sepsis, which can result from "wicking" of colonic bacteria up the NG tube to the oral cavity.

• Provide meticulous wound care and change dressings often. Check dressings and drainage sites frequently for signs of infection (purulent drainage, foul odor) or fecal drainage. Also watch for sudden fever, especially when accompanied by abdominal pain and tenderness.

• When the patient regains peristalsis and bowel function, take steps to prevent constipation and straining during defecation, both of which can damage the anastomosis. Encourage adequate fluid intake, and administer a stool softener or laxatives, as ordered. Note the frequency and amount of all bowel movements as well as characteristics of the stools.

• Encourage regular coughing and deep-breathing to prevent atelectasis; remind the patient to splint the incision site during coughing.

Home care instructions

• Instruct the patient to record the frequency and character of bowel movements and to notify the doctor of any changes from normal pattern. Warn against using laxatives without the doctor's approval.

• Warn the patient to avoid abdominal straining and heavy lifting until the sutures are completely healed and the doctor allows unrestricted activity.

• Instruct the patient to maintain the prescribed semibland diet until the bowel has healed completely (usually 4 to 8 weeks after surgery). Urge the patient to avoid carbonated beverages and gas-forming foods.

• Because extensive bowel resection may interfere with absorption of nutrients from food, emphasize the importance of taking prescribed vitamin supplements.

BOWEL TRAINING

Bowel training attempts to establish a regular pattern of elimination through changes in diet and life-style supplemented as necessary by limited use of laxatives, enemas, or suppositories.

The success of a bowel-training program depends on the patient's ability and willingness to perform self-care and the presence of a strong support system of family or friends. This program requires considerable time and patience to be effective. It requires sensitivity to the patient's feelings of discomfort and embarrassment as well.

Purpose
• To help the patient establish a normal pattern of elimination.

Indications
Bowel training can correct constipation and, in some cases, bowel incontinence.

Procedure
Bowel training requires a regular schedule for defecation. Toileting should follow each meal so that attempts at defecation are made at about the same time each day. The patient should assume the normal position for defecation so that gravity can assist elimination. He should remain in this position for at least 10 minutes and no longer than 30 minutes. The patient can help stimulate a scheduled bowel movement by leaning forward to increase abdominal pressure or by applying direct pressure to the abdominal wall and massaging the abdomen from right to left.

In addition to a regular schedule for defecation, essential components of a bowel-training program include an adequate fluid intake (usually between 2,000 and 4,000 ml/day, unless contraindicated) to promote softer stools and help stimulate peristalsis, increased intake of dietary fiber to add bulk to the stools and stimulate peristalsis, and increase in the level of activity to stimulate and maintain intestinal motility. (See *Techniques to aid bowel training*.)

Complications
No complications are associated with bowel training.

Care considerations
Before therapy
• Evaluate the patient's overall condition before establishing an elimination schedule to ensure the patient's ability to withstand a prolonged and occasionally frustrating bowel-training program. This involves taking a complete bowel history that includes the patient's defecation patterns, use of laxatives, and regular dietary habits. It's essential to provide privacy and use a supportive tone of voice during this interview.

• After establishing the patient's cooperation and stamina, discuss the overall goal of the program, which is the establishment of a regular pattern of elimination based on individual needs and abilities.

• Explain the requirements of the program (defecation schedule, adequate fluid intake, increased dietary fiber, and increased activity).

Techniques to aid bowel training

If the patient needs additional help, the bowel-training program may also include mechanical stimulation, digital stimulation, or operative conditioning.

Mechanical stimulation through the use of stool softeners, enemas, laxatives, or glycerin suppositories may be needed early in the training program. However, after a routine is well-established, these aids should gradually be withdrawn so that the patient can defecate consistently without them.

Digital stimulation with a lubricated finger may be necessary to induce reflex constriction and promote elimination. For a patient with a spinal cord injury or other neurologic damage, it may be a necessary part of the training program. To perform this procedure, insert a lubricated finger of a gloved hand about ½″ to 1″ (1 to 2 cm) into the patient's rectum. Then gently rotate the finger for 30 to 60 seconds.

Operant conditioning may be necessary to improve muscle tone in an incontinent patient. To accomplish this, a specially skilled nurse or technician inserts a balloon attached to a monitor into the rectum and inflates it. The patient is instructed to contract his sphincter against the balloon pressure and to check his progress on the monitor. Another method of operant conditioning requires the insertion of measured amounts of water into the rectum. The patient then holds the water as long as he can in an effort to control the sphincter muscles. The patient holds the water for longer periods as he gains greater control of the sphincter muscles.

During therapy
• Be sure that all caregivers follow the program strictly. Consistency is crucial to success.
• Consult with other health care providers as necessary to eliminate any

barriers to successful training. For example, dental work may be required if bad teeth or poorly fitting dentures interfere with maintaining the prescribed diet.
• Provide encouragement and support as necessary.

Home care instructions
• Consult with caregivers to ensure access to clean, private toilet facilities.
• Instruct the patient never to ignore the urge to defecate.
• Teach the patient and caregivers about the dietary measures required by his bowel management program.
• Warn the patient against excessive ingestion of bran, which can impair iron absorption.

BREAST RECONSTRUCTION

Breast reconstruction is an option available to any woman who has had a mastectomy for breast cancer. Dramatic developments in plastic surgery make breast reconstruction more feasible, more appealing, and less costly than in the past. Health care insurance companies are covering the costs as rehabilitative surgery, rather than cosmetic surgery.

Reconstructive surgery can revive a woman's self-esteem and self-confidence, which may have been lost due to her mastectomy. Most women who choose to have breast reconstruction are satisfied with the cosmetic results. It eliminates artificial prostheses and restores a sense of well-being and wholeness even though reconstruction will not restore the sensation lost through mastectomy. Any surgery on the breast can damage the sensitive nerves in that area.

Breast reconstruction must be tailored to meet each woman's individual needs. Five types of reconstructive procedures are available; which one is appropriate depends on the type of mas-

Breast reconstruction methods

Review the breast reconstruction methods below. Be prepared to address the patient's questions and expectations about each procedure and its outcome.

Simple reconstruction without flap

This method of breast reconstruction requires insertion of the implant in a pocket created between skin and muscle. An incision of approximately 2″ (5 cm) is made along the lower border of the breast. If the mastectomy incision was low enough, it can be used again, leaving only one scar. The procedure takes 1 to 2 hours under general anesthesia.

Tissue expansion

The purpose of this procedure is to stretch the skin so that an implant that matches the opposite breast can be inserted. Under local or general anesthesia, an incision is made and the deflated tissue expander is inserted under the skin and muscle. (This can be done at the time of the mastectomy.) After its placement, the expander is filled with a small amount of sterile fluid. The procedure takes 1 to 1½ hours.

Over the next 8 to 12 weeks, the doctor will inject additional fluid once a week during an office visit. Gradually, the enlarged expander will stretch the tissue over it. When the tissue has stretched enough to hold the desired size implant, the surgeon removes the tissue expander and inserts the permanent implant. The last step can be done as an outpatient procedure under local anesthesia.

Latissimus dorsi flap

The latissimus dorsi flap or myocutaneous flap is a technique in which skin, subcutaneous tissue, and muscle are transferred to the mastectomy site from another body site. The area most often used is the latissimus dorsi muscle of the back—a broad, flat muscle covering one side of the back below the shoulder blade. This muscle is freed from the spine and pelvic bone and is tunneled under the skin forward to the chest wall, then positioned in place. This surgical procedure is dependable and successful. It takes 3 to 4 hours. It leaves a scar on the back and on the chest.

Rectus abdominis flap

This procedure requires the transfer of one of the rectus abdominis muscles—either the left or right muscle of the abdomen—with the overlying skin and a section of subcutaneous fat. The surgeon moves this flap to the breast area and contours it into the shape of a breast. The artery supplying blood to this muscle is also carried with the flap to the chest to ensure that the muscle will be viable.

Free flap

This new technique uses a wedge of tissue, including skin, fat, and a little muscle and a small artery and vein from the abdomen, buttock, or thigh, which is transplanted into the chest wall; the artery and vein are attached to existing blood vessels that had nourished the real breast tissue. Then, the tissue is shaped into a new breast that closely resembles the natural breast.

Nipple and areola reconstruction

Several weeks or months after reconstruction of the breast, women may elect to have surgery to create a nipple and areola. The surgery takes 1 to 2 hours.

The most common technique for reconstructing the areola is to use the skin from the upper inner thigh or skin from behind the ear. The nipple is formed from tissue from the newly created breast or by grafting a piece of nipple from the natural breast. Another technique creates the nipple and areola from vaginal skin. If the reconstructed areola is not dark enough, ultraviolet light may be used to improve the color match.

tectomy performed. (See *Breast reconstruction methods.*)

Simple breast reconstruction, without a flap, uses the woman's remaining tissue at the mastectomy site and requires a healthy pectoral muscle and an ample amount of good healthy skin. Skin that has been irradiated, is tight, or is too thin may not be suitable for this procedure.

Tissue expansion is indicated for women whose skin and muscle is of good quality but insufficient to cover an implant that will match the opposite breast.

The latissimus dorsi flap procedure is indicated for women whose skin is tight or thinning and for women whose remaining pectoral muscle is inadequate for other methods of breast reconstruction. Patients who need this type of reconstruction commonly have had radiation treatments or skin grafting.

The rectus abdominis flap procedure reduces and tightens the abdominal area much like a "tummy tuck." This is an appealing option for many women. It also can be used for patients who have had radiation treatments or skin grafting.

Free flap surgery, the newest technique, can be used for most women who have undergone mastectomy. This technique also provides the cosmetic advantage of a "tummy tuck" if the fatty tissue used in the reconstruction is taken from the abdomen.

Purpose

• To replace breasts removed by radical surgery for breast cancer and restore an acceptable body image.

Indications

Reconstructive breast surgery is indicated virtually for any woman who has had a mastectomy for breast cancer. However, some types of mastectomy or adjunctive treatments may require

---

Understanding breast implants

Breast implants used in breast reconstructive surgery are soft, fluid-filled sacs. They are round and shaped like a teardrop. Implants can be punctured by a sharp object, but under normal conditions are very durable. There are three types of implants.

Silicone gel implant
This implant, the focus of recent controversy about its safety, comes in a variety of sizes.

Inflatable implant
An empty silicone bag is inserted into the incision and filled by injecting 0.9% sodium chloride through a valve. This implant requires a smaller incision than a prefilled implant and can be filled to the volume needed for the best fit. Leakage may occur and requires replacement of the implant.

Double-lumen implant
This is a combination of an inner bag, containing silicone gel, surrounded by an outer bag, filled with 0.9% sodium chloride solution. The outer bag's size can be adjusted to achieve the appropriate size.

---

complicated reconstructive surgeries to achieve optimal results.

Procedure

Breast reconstruction involves creation of a pocket between skin and muscle for placement of a prosthetic implant. (See *Understanding breast implants.*)

Complications

All surgery entails risks or complications such as bleeding or infection. Special concerns during breast reconstruction are infection at the breast site, decreased blood circulation to the skin, and capsular contracture. The implant might have to be removed temporarily until any infection at the breast site clears. If circulation to the skin is insufficient, skin necrosis may occur, resulting in removal of the implant and skin grafting. After surgery, a fibrous capsule of scar tissue forms around the implant, causing the breast to look firm and spherical. Sometimes, this scar tissue causes the implant to be displaced. Capsular contracture occurs in about 25% of all implants. It can be corrected, but usually requires further surgery.

Infection and decreased blood circulation to the area are less likely if the reconstruction is not done immediately at the time of the mastectomy. Recent studies have shown that silicone implants have leaked and can possibly burst, causing the release of silicone into the surrounding breast tissue and resulting in pain and hardness in the tissue.

Care considerations
Before surgery
• Reinforce the doctor's explanation of the procedure. Answer the patient's questions.
• Prepare the patient for surgery according to hospital policy.
After surgery
• Monitor the drainage from drains inserted during surgery.
• Administer antibiotic therapy, as appropriate.
• Encourage early ambulation to decrease the risk of pneumonia or postoperative complications.
• Observe flap color and circulation to the affected upper extremity, and report any abnormalities to the doctor immediately.
• Provide psychological support to patient and caregivers.

Home care instructions
• Teach the patient or caregivers how to empty and care for drains.

• Instruct the patient how to regularly massage the implant as recommended by the doctor.
• Tell the patient to perform specified reconstruction exercises as advised by her doctor.
• Tell the patient to avoid swimming, tennis, bowling, or other strenuous exercises until her doctor approves return to unrestricted activity.
• Teach the patient how to perform breast self-examination. Explain that after reconstruction she should continue to examine her natural breast and the reconstructed breast once a month to note any change.

BRONCHODILATORS

Methylxanthine bronchodilators include *theophylline;* its soluble salts, *aminophylline* and *oxtriphylline;* and a related derivative, *dyphylline.* These drugs relax bronchiolar smooth muscle. As a result, they're used to treat bronchial asthma, chronic bronchitis, and emphysema. They also play an important role in treating acute respiratory conditions, such as status asthmaticus.

Aminophylline, the major I.V. preparation, provides rapid treatment of bronchoconstriction. Theophylline provides long-term control of asthma and other bronchospastic conditions. Both theophylline and its derivatives are available in varied oral, parenteral, and rectal forms, with different durations of action. Short-acting oral preparations, which require frequent doses, may present a patient compliance problem. However, newer sustained-release formulations can help overcome this by permitting daily or twice-daily dosing.

Purpose
• To prevent bronchospasm.

Indications

The methylxanthine bronchodilators are indicated for symptomatic relief of bronchial asthma, bronchospasm of chronic bronchitis, and emphysema.

These drugs are contraindicated in patients with a hypersensitivity to xanthine compounds, such as caffeine and theobromine, or with severe arrhythmias. They should be used cautiously in patients with liver disease, congestive heart failure (CHF), pulmonary edema, viral infection, or recent viral immunization because these conditions slow the rate of drug metabolism. Because the methylxanthines can increase the volume and acidity of gastric secretions, they should also be used cautiously in patients with peptic ulcer disease.

Adverse reactions

Reactions to the methylxanthines may include hypotension, arrhythmias, palpitations, GI distress (nausea and vomiting), and central nervous system (CNS) stimulation (headache, irritability). These reactions are dose-related and can often be avoided or controlled by careful dosage titration. Unfortunately, toxicity may occur abruptly, heralded by tachycardia, ventricular arrhythmias, or seizures. Milder symptoms don't always precede these severe toxic effects.

Care considerations

• Evaluate the effectiveness of therapy by monitoring respirations and by asking the patient if spasmodic coughing and chest tightness have subsided. Check pulmonary function studies, primarily the amount of air exhaled in the first second of a forced expiration after a full inspiration (FEV_1), for indications of increased airflow. Monitor the patient's vital signs and pulse quality.

• Watch the patient carefully for signs of GI toxicity, which may include bleeding, abdominal pain, diarrhea, nausea, and vomiting (possibly bloody).

Also watch for CNS effects (irritability, confusion, seizures, dizziness, insomnia, trembling, and headache). Observe the patient also for flushed skin, frequent voiding, rapid respiratory and pulse rates, and weakness. If any of these signs occur, stop the drug immediately and notify the doctor.

• If I.V. aminophylline is given, watch for rash and hives for up to 24 hours. Discontinue the drug if these signs of hypersensitivity occur. If no such signs occur, substitute an oral form when ordered. Typically, an oral dose is administered before discontinuing the infusion.

• Review the patient's drug regimen for possible interactions. Concurrent use of propranolol and nadolol with methylxanthines, for example, may cause bronchospasm; use of oral contraceptives, troleandomycin, erythromycin, and cimetidine may decrease hepatic clearance of methylxanthines; ephedrine and other bronchodilators can produce additive effects; primidone, rifampin, barbiturates, and phenytoin reduce serum methylxanthine levels.

• Monitor serum drug levels carefully, especially if the patient has CHF, liver disease, pulmonary edema, or another condition that can decrease drug metabolism. Depending on serum drug levels, the dosage may be reduced. Also monitor drug levels if your patient smokes because tobacco stimulates methylxanthine metabolism.

• Monitor therapy with methylxanthines (except for dyphylline) by assessing plasma theophylline levels because aminophylline and oxtriphylline release free theophylline into the bloodstream. Initially, evaluate serum levels at least 72 hours after the first dose. Then, measure peak serum levels 8 to 12 hours after the morning dose of a 24-hour preparation; 4 to 6 hours after the morning dose of a 12-hour preparation; 2 hours after the dose of a standard, rapidly absorbed preparation; or 30 minutes after an I.V.

loading dose. Serum theophylline levels should range from 10 to 20 mcg/ml. Levels below 10 mcg/ml are typically less effective, and levels above 20 mcg/ml are associated with toxicity. (Dyphylline is a chemical derivative of theophylline; its therapeutic levels are unknown.)

Home care instructions

• Instruct the patient to report signs of drug toxicity. Warn against exceeding the prescribed dosage.
• Tell the patient to take the drug with food and a full glass of water to reduce GI upset, and to avoid eating large amounts of charcoal-broiled foods because the hydrocarbons they contain can lower serum methylxanthine levels.
• Advise the patient to avoid smoking because this increases drug metabolism.
• Warn the patient not to dissolve, crush, or chew a sustained-release formulation.
• Advise the patient to take a missed dose as soon as he remembers unless the next dose is due; in that case, he should omit the missed dose and return to the regular schedule without double-dosing.
• Warn the patient not to change the drug brand or formulation (from a short-acting to a sustained-release preparation, for example) without consulting the doctor.
• Warn the patient not to ingest large amounts of caffeinated beverages or foods because they can increase CNS stimulation. Also warn against using over-the-counter drugs, such as cold and allergy remedies, that contain ephedrine and theophylline salts because of increased CNS stimulation.
• Tell the patient to notify the doctor of a cold or other viral illness because it may require dosage adjustment.

BRONCHOSCOPY

Bronchoscopy may be performed to remove an obstruction in the more distal airways. This procedure is performed with a metal or fiber-optic bronchoscope; it allows direct visualization of the trachea and the tracheobronchial tree through a slender, flexible tube with mirrors and a light at its distal end. Bronchoscopy can be performed on any patient even if an endotracheal (ET) or tracheostomy tube is in place.

Most often, a flexible fiber-optic bronchoscope is used because it's smaller, allows a greater viewing range of the segmental and subsegmental bronchi, and carries less risk of trauma than a rigid metal bronchoscope (see *How a flexible bronchoscope works*). A rigid metal bronchoscope is used to remove a foreign body, excise endobronchial lesions, and control massive hemoptysis.

When bronchoscopy is performed for diagnostic purposes, biopsy forceps, a brush, or a catheter may be passed through the bronchoscope to obtain specimens for cytologic and bacteriologic examinations.

Purpose

• To visualize and remove a foreign body or mucus from the tracheobronchial tree.

Indications

Bronchoscopy is indicated to remove foreign bodies, malignant or benign tumors, mucus plugs, or excessive secretions from the tracheobronchial tree. Bronchoscopy is also performed to inspect the tracheobronchial tree for asymptomatic cancer before chest surgery.

Procedure

Typically, the doctor perfoms bronchoscopy with a flexible fiber-optic

How a flexible bronchoscope works

Inserted through the patient's nostril and into the bronchi, the flexible fiber-optic bronchoscope has four channels (see enlargement). Two light channels (A) provide a light source; one visualizing channel (B) allows direct examination; and one open channel (C) can accommodate biopsy forceps, a cytology brush, an anesthetic, or oxygen as well as suctioning or lavage.

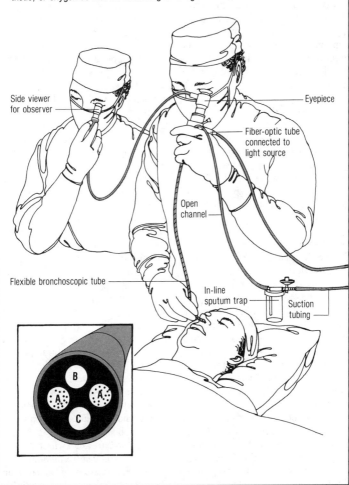

Side viewer for observer

Eyepiece

Fiber-optic tube connected to light source

Open channel

Flexible bronchoscopic tube

In-line sputum trap

Suction tubing

scope. The patient is placed in a sitting position and requested to hyperextend his neck, place his arms at his sides, and breathe through his nose.

A local anesthetic is sprayed into the patient's nose and mouth to suppress the gag reflex. (General anesthesia may be used for children or extremely apprehensive patients.)

After the anesthetic takes effect, the doctor introduces a lubricated bronchoscope into the upper airway. Once he visualizes the vocal chords, he instills lidocaine to continue suppression of the gag reflex and to anesthetize the vocal chords. The doctor then advances the bronchoscope through the larynx and into the trachea and bronchi, where he removes mucus, secretions, or a foreign body or withdraws a specimen for laboratory analysis. The bronchoscope is withdrawn after removal of the foreign body, mucus, or specimen.

Complications

A complication of a transbronchial biopsy is pneumothorax. Some rare complications of bronchoscopy include hypoxemia, hemorrhage (most likely to occur with biopsy), laryngeal edema or laryngospasm, bronchospasm, infection, and tracheal or bronchial perforation.

Care considerations

Before the procedure

• Explain the procedure. Be sure to explain that the patient will be able to breathe but will be unable to speak during the procedure. Emphasize that the airway won't be blocked and that oxygen will be administered through a nasal cannula, face-mask, or an ET tube if the patient will be intubated and receive general anesthesia. Warn the patient of the unpleasant taste of the local anesthetic.

• Withhold food and fluids for 6 to 12 hours before the procedure. If appropriate, tell the patient that food, fluids, and oral drugs will also be withheld for about 2 hours after the procedure, until the gag reflex returns.

• Just before the procedure, evaluate the patient's condition, check the medical history for hypersensitivity to the anesthetic, and obtain baseline vital signs and, possibly, arterial blood gas analysis. Administer a preoperative

sedative, as ordered, and check vital signs again. Begin an I.V. infusion, as ordered. Then administer the prescribed preoperative medication. Instruct the patient who wears dentures to remove them just before the procedure.

During the procedure

• Provide tissues and an emesis basin because excess fluid will cause coughing and gagging.

• After the bronchoscope is introduced into the upper airway, remind the patient not to speak because this will irritate his vocal chords.

• Administer ordered medications. The doctor may order medications such as atropine to decrease secretions and an I.V. barbiturate or narcotic to provide sedation or amnesia and relieve anxiety.

• Check the patient's vital signs frequently and monitor for signs of an adverse reaction to the sedative.

After the procedure

• As ordered, place the conscious patient in semi-Fowler's position; place the unconscious patient on his side, with the head of the bed slightly elevated to prevent aspiration.

• Check vital signs until the patient is stable.

• Closely monitor respiratory status by listening to breath sounds and watching for symptoms of respiratory difficulty, such as stridor and dyspnea resulting from laryngeal edema or bronchospasm. Also check for decreased breath sounds on one side, which may indicate pneumothorax. Promptly report any abnormal findings to the doctor, and prepare for a chest X-ray if ordered to confirm pneumothorax.

• Provide an emesis basin, and instruct the patient to spit out saliva rather than swallow it.

• Keep resuscitation equipment, an ET tube, a laryngoscope, and tracheotomy tray available in case of severe respiratory distress evidenced by bronchospasm, laryngospasm, or laryngeal edema.

• Anticipate blood-tinged sputum for up to several hours after the procedure. However, report prolonged bleeding or persistent hemoptysis to the doctor.

• Encourage the patient to rest quietly. Restrict all oral intake until after the gag reflex returns (usually in 2 hours). If the patient experiences hoarseness and a sore throat, provide medicated lozenges when allowed; advise the patient to refrain from talking in order to rest his vocal chords.

Home care instructions

• If bronchoscopy was performed on an outpatient basis or in the emergency room, tell the patient to promptly report any shortness of breath, pain, or prolonged bleeding.

• Advise the patient to avoid straining his voice, but reassure him that sore throat and hoarseness are temporary.

• Tell the patient to report signs of infection, such as fever or thick yellow sputum.

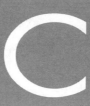

CALCIUM CHANNEL BLOCKERS

Calcium channel blockers block the entry of calcium into cardiac cells and smooth-muscle cells. Because extracellular calcium is necessary for cardiac and smooth-muscle contraction, these drugs can cause vasodilation, decrease heart rate, and lower blood pressure. The calcium channel blockers available in the United States belong to three different chemical classes; their pharmacologic properties are quite different. Although most agents are good vasodilators, *diltiazem* and *verapamil* are most effective at suppressing cardiac contractility and slowing atrioventricular (AV) nodal conduction.

Purpose

• To dilate coronary arteries, increasing blood flow to the myocardium and alleviating anginal pain
• To reduce afterload, decreasing coronary work load and oxygen consumption
• To dilate peripheral blood vessels, decreasing blood pressure
• To dilate cerebral vasculature and relieve vasospasm following a stroke, thereby preventing further neurologic damage
• To treat supraventricular and other arrhythmias.

Indications

Calcium channel blockers are used to treat vasospastic angina (Prinzmetal's or variant angina) and classic, stable angina pectoris. Bepridil, diltiazem, nicardipine, nifedipine, and verapamil are used to relieve angina. Diltiazem, felodipine, isradipine, nicardipine, sustained-released nifedipine, and verapamil are used to treat hypertension. Verapamil is used to treat arrhythmias. Nimodipine is used to alleviate cerebral artery spasm following subarachnoid hemorrhage.

Calcium channel blockers are contraindicated in patients with impaired cardiac contractility, impulse conduction, or impulse formation. Such disorders include sick sinus syndrome, severe hypotension, second- or third-degree heart block, advanced congestive heart failure (CHF), extreme bradycardia, cardiogenic shock, or severe left ventricular dysfunction. These drugs should be used cautiously in patients with impaired hepatic or renal function.

Adverse reactions

Serious adverse reactions to calcium channel blockers include dyspnea, coughing or wheezing, chest pain, syncope, irregular or rapid heartbeat, hypotension, peripheral edema, and bradycardia. Minor reactions, such as dizziness, headache, nausea, fatigue, constipation, flushing, or rash, may also occur. Bepridil has the potential to cause serious ventricular arrhythmias; therefore, its use should be reserved for patients in whom treatment with other antianginal agents has failed. Adverse reactions tend to occur most commonly with nifedipine and verapamil.

Hazards of using calcium channel blockers with other cardiac drugs

INTERACTING DRUG	EFFECT	NURSING ACTIONS
beta blockers	Severe bradycardia, increased atrioventricular (AV) conduction block, congestive heart failure (CHF)	• Because of additive myocardial depressant effects, don't give I.V. verapamil and beta blockers within 4 hours of each other. • To decrease the risk of CHF, gradually discontinue beta blockers before beginning nifedipine therapy, if possible. Monitor patients taking diltiazem or verapamil concurrently with beta blockers. Watch for peripheral or pulmonary edema, dyspnea, wheezing, and cough.
digitalis glycosides	Severe bradycardia, increased AV conduction block, digitalis toxicity	• Monitor serum digitalis glycoside levels carefully; verapamil and nifedipine raise these levels by 50% to 70%. (The degree of increase relates directly to the dose of calcium channel blocker.) • Assess for signs of digitalis toxicity: irregular rhythm, headache, blurred vision, halos around lights, green or yellow flashes, confusion, hallucinations, and GI upset.
quinidine	Severe hypotension, ventricular tachycardia, AV block, pulmonary edema, bradycardia	• Carefully monitor blood pressure and pulse rate.

Care considerations

• During I.V. infusion of calcium channel blockers, frequently monitor the patient's electrocardiogram (ECG), pulse rate, and blood pressure, and auscultate his lungs. Keep emergency equipment available. Check regularly for edema and weight gain.
• Continue to monitor for adverse reactions to calcium channel blockers.
• Review the patient's drug regimen for possible interactions. Concurrent use of digitalis, beta-adrenergic blockers, or quinidine causes severe effects (see *Hazards of using calcium channel blockers with other cardiac drugs*). Nitrates may accentuate hypotension, and disopyramide may aggravate CHF symptoms. As a precaution, don't administer disopyramide for 48 hours before or 24 hours after I.V. infusion of verapamil.

Home care instructions

• Instruct the patient who's taking diltiazem or verapamil to count his pulse rate for 1 minute before each dose and to notify his doctor if the rate is below 50 beats/minute. If he's taking verapamil, warn him to avoid alcohol, which may aggravate CHF symptoms.

• Tell the patient to watch for and report early signs of CHF: swollen hands or feet, lung congestion, or dyspnea.

• Instruct the patient to weigh himself once a week at the same time of day, on the same scale, and wearing the same amount of clothes. Advise him to notify his doctor of an overall weight gain of 3 lb (1.4 kg) or more.

• Tell the patient to swallow oral medication whole, without crushing or chewing it.

• Instruct the patient to take a missed dose as soon as he remembers, unless it's near the time for the next scheduled dose. In this case, he should omit the missed dose and resume his schedule with the next dose. Warn the patient never to double-dose.

• If a calcium channel blocker is prescribed for a patient on nitrate therapy for angina, instruct him to continue taking the nitrate as scheduled. Warn him that he may experience worsened anginal attacks for a few days. The patient who's taking nitroglycerin may increase its use during this period, as ordered.

• Tell the patient to take the drug with food to prevent GI upset.

• Explain that the patient can help prevent constipation, a possible adverse reaction, by eating plenty of vegetables and fresh or dried fruits. He may also take a mild laxative, if recommended by the doctor.

CALCULI BASKETING

When ureteral calculi do not progress readily during conservative management, removal with a basketing instrument is a treatment option. This procedure, called calculi basketing, avoids major surgery and helps relieve pain,

prevent infection, and restore the renal function threatened by the calculi's blockage of the ureter. The basketing instrument is inserted through a cystoscope or ureteroscope into the ureter to capture the calculus and is then withdrawn to remove it. However, because of the risk of ureteral perforation, basketing is generally contraindicated for removal of an excessively wide calculus or one located above the lower one-third of the ureter.

Purpose

• To remove obstructing ureteral calculi.

Indications

This treatment is indicated for patients with urinary calculi when a calculus is impacted in the ureter, the patient has unmanageable pain, or if there is threatened renal damage or suspected renal or systemic infection.

Procedure

The patient is placed in the lithotomy position on an X-ray table, and a lower abdominal X-ray is taken to locate the obstructing calculus. General or spinal anesthesia is then administered, as appropriate. After inserting a cystoscope or ureteroscope (which will also require a guide wire) into the urethra, the surgeon passes the special loop or basket catheter through the cystoscope or ureteroscope and into the ureter where the calculus is located. To understand how the calculus is caught and removed, see *Understanding calculi basketing*.

After removing the calculus, the surgeon typically inserts a ureteral catheter or stent to the level of the renal pelvis to drain urine into the bladder and, possibly, an indwelling urinary catheter to aid bladder drainage.

Depending on the location of the calculus, the surgeon may first perform a percutaneous nephrostomy (creation of an opening through the skin into

Understanding calculi basketing

In this technique for removing ureteral calculi, a basketing instrument housed within a catheter is inserted through a cystoscope or ureteroscope into the ureter and advanced to the calculus as shown here.

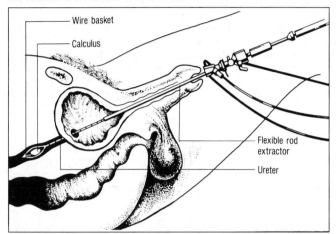

Once the apparatus is adjacent to the calculus, the surgeon pushes the wire basket through the rod and beyond the calculus, allowing the flexible wires to spread out within the ureter; he then slowly pulls back the wire basket to capture the calculus. Finally, the surgeon carefully withdraws the entire apparatus.

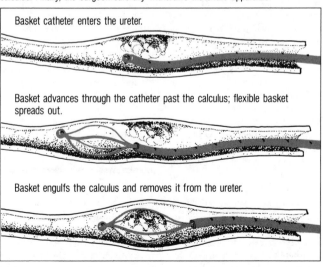

Basket catheter enters the ureter.

Basket advances through the catheter past the calculus; flexible basket spreads out.

Basket engulfs the calculus and removes it from the ureter.

the renal collecting system) and insert the cystoscope and the basketing instrument through this opening to remove the calculus. Percutaneous nephrostomy is also performed to maintain renal function and to drain infected urine until the calculus can be removed. After the calculus is removed, the percutaneous nephrostomy tube is left in place to ensure that the ureter is not blocked by blood clots or edema. The calculus is also examined and compared with the X-ray film to confirm that it has been totally removed.

Complications

When performed properly, basketing should cause few complications. Potential complications include infection, bleeding, ureteral perforation, and ureteral tearing or fistula formation. Occasionally, the calculi basket becomes impacted, requiring surgical removal.

Care considerations

Before surgery

• Prepare the patient for tests to determine the location of calculi and his renal status. Such tests typically include abdominal X-rays and intravenous pyelography.
• Observe the patient for such signs as fever, chills, and persistent flank pain, which reflect infection that may cause gram-negative bacteremia.
• Administer broad-spectrum antibiotics to prevent infection, as prescribed.

After surgery

• Monitor the patient's vital signs after the procedure.
• Observe urine drainage for color and clots; it should be blood-tinged at first, clearing within 24 to 48 hours. Notify the doctor of frank or persistent hematuria. Irrigate the indwelling urinary catheter as ordered. Check the drainage system for kinks or leaks.
• Administer I.V. fluids, as ordered, until oral fluids are well tolerated to maintain a urine output greater than 50 ml/hour; 30 ml/hour is the minimum acceptable urine output rate. Fluids increase urine output, prevent or minimize the chance of urinary tract infection, flush calculi fragments through the urinary tract, and preserve renal function.
• Observe and report any signs of septicemia, which may result from ureteral perforation during basketing. If infection is suspected, obtain blood and urine samples for laboratory analysis.
• Administer analgesics to control pain, as prescribed.

Home care instructions

• Teach the patient and family the importance of following prescribed dietary and medication regimens to prevent recurrence of calculi.
• To prevent recurrence, encourage the patient to drink at least 3 qt of water daily, in addition to all other fluid intake, unless contraindicated.
• Advise the patient to take prescribed analgesics as needed.
• Tell the patient to report signs and symptoms of recurrent calculi (flank pain, hematuria, nausea, fever, and chills) or acute ureteral obstruction (severe pain and inability to void) immediately.
• Encourage regular follow-up examinations to assess for formation of new calculi.

CALDWELL-LUC PROCEDURE

The Caldwell-Luc procedure, known also as the *radical antrum operation*, is a surgical means of gaining access to the maxillary sinus without altering the surrounding normal structures. It permits visualization of the antrum, facilitates sinus drainage, and allows access to infected sinuses when an intranasal approach isn't possible because of suppuration or inflammation. This treatment can be used alone or in conjunction with other treatments, such as ethmoidectomy.

Purpose
• To treat chronic sinusitis
• To ligate the maxillary artery in persistent epistaxis
• To close an oroantral fistula resulting from dental extraction or maxillary cancer
• To remove nasal polyps
• To obtain a tissue sample for histologic analysis.

Indications
This therapy is most commonly performed to treat chronic maxillary sinusitis that's unresponsive to other treatments. It may also be used to treat oroantral fistula, persistent epistaxis, and nasal polyps.

Procedure
Performed under local or general anesthesia, this treatment is usually well tolerated and causes little bleeding. The surgeon incises the mouth under the upper lip and above the level of the roots of the maxillary teeth, retracts the periosteum (thus exposing the fossa above the upper canine teeth), then incises the antrum wall. If the patient has sinusitis, the surgeon strips the diseased sinus lining and makes an opening between the nose and the antrum (an intranasal antrostomy) to improve drainage. When multiple sinuses are involved, this procedure may resolve infection by draining the upper sinuses. If necessary, a drainage tube is placed in the nose so the sinus can be irrigated.

If the patient has an antral lesion, the surgeon will take a tissue sample for histologic analysis and leave the maxillary mucosa intact. If the patient has persistent epistaxis, the surgeon will remove part of the posterior sinus wall, exposing the internal maxillary artery, and then ligate the artery.

The surgeon sutures the incision loosely or, occasionally, leaves it to heal spontaneously. If bleeding occurs, the surgeon may pack the maxillary sinus through the nose.

Complications
A potential complication of the Caldwell-Luc procedure is diminished sensation or numbness in the upper lip and gum for several months after the surgery.

Care considerations
Before surgery
• Explain the procedure to the patient.
After surgery
• Monitor for facial edema and bleeding from the incision site. Apply an ice pack as necessary to the upper lip.
• If the patient has packing in place, explain that the doctor will remove it within 48 hours. If a drainage tube is in place for irrigation, assist with irrigation and tell the patient that the tube will be removed in 3 to 4 days.
• Assess the patient's mouth frequently. Although bleeding is uncommon after this procedure, check for bright red blood at the back of the throat and in any drainage or emesis.
• Warn the patient not to brush his teeth, but rather to rinse the mouth gently with tepid 0.9% sodium chloride solution or dilute mouthwash.
• Encourage the patient to begin fluid intake 4 hours after surgery (unless he's nauseated) and then progress to a full soft diet, as ordered. Until the incision heals, the patient should avoid foods that require thorough chewing.

Home care instructions
• Tell the patient to expect some drainage from the nose for a few days after surgery and to monitor its amount, color, and odor. Advise the patient to notify the doctor of any bleeding or

foul smell or drainage that persists for more than 5 days.

• Instruct the patient to clean his teeth with gauze pads wrapped around his finger, supplemented by gentle mouthwashes.

• Warn against rubbing or bumping the incision. Tell the patient to plan menus for the next 2 weeks that don't require much chewing in order to avoid injuring the incision. Tell the patient who wears dentures to avoid inserting the upper plate for 2 weeks.

• Tell the patient to avoid vigorous activity and forcefully blowing his nose for 2 weeks. The patient should sniff gently to clear his nostrils.

CARBONIC ANHYDRASE INHIBITORS

The carbonic anhydrase inhibitors *acetazolamide, dichlorphenamide,* and *methazolamide* treat chronic open-angle, acute angle-closure, and secondary glaucoma. These drugs reduce intraocular pressure by diminishing the production of aqueous humor up to 60%. They also produce systemic acidosis, which adds to their ocular hypotensive effect.

Carbonic anhydrase inhibitors are commonly used with other antiglaucoma drugs, such as miotics and mydriatics, in ophthalmic emergencies. They may also be given with osmotic drugs, such as mannitol or urea. Although carbonic anhydrase inhibitors are administered orally, acetazolamide, the most widely used drug in this class, may also be given parenterally.

Purpose

• To reduce aqueous humor production, thus lowering intraocular pressure

• To prevent or treat acute mountain sickness.

Indications

Because they inhibit the enzymes necessary to produce aqueous humor of the eye, carbonic anhydrase inhibitors are useful in the treatment of glaucoma. They are also used as adjuncts in the treatment of certain seizure disorders, although tolerance to their anticonvulsant action develops very rapidly. Acetazolamide is used to prevent acute high-altitude sickness in mountain climbers attempting rapid ascent.

Carbonic anhydrase inhibitors should be used cautiously in patients with diabetes mellitus because the drugs may raise blood glucose levels, those with obstructive pulmonary disease because they may precipitate acute respiratory failure, and patients with impaired hepatic function because they may precipitate hepatic coma.

Adverse reactions

Carbonic anhydrase inhibitors may cause hypokalemia and hyperchloremic acidosis. Aplastic anemia, hemolytic anemia, and leukopenia may occur. Adverse reactions that may also occur include malaise, anorexia, weight loss, fatigue, weakness, nausea, vomiting, drowsiness, paresthesias, confusion, and, in infants, a failure to thrive. Diuresis may occur initially but commonly subsides with continued therapy or a change in dosage. With prolonged therapy, renal calculi may form.

Care considerations

• Because GI symptoms commonly occur with carbonic anhydrase inhibitors, give the drug with food.

• Assess for signs of central nervous system toxicity, such as confusion.

• As ordered, monitor the patient's intake and output, weight, and serum electrolyte levels.

Home care instructions

• Advise the patient to schedule doses at mealtimes, if possible, to minimize

GI distress. To prevent nocturnal diuresis, the patient should take the last dose no later than 6 p.m.

• Tell the patient to take a missed dose as soon as he remembers, unless it's within 2 hours of the next scheduled dose. In that case, he should omit the missed dose and maintain his regular schedule. Warn the patient never to double-dose.

• Tell the patient to report signs of hypokalemia, such as fatigue, muscle cramps, and increased thirst. If appropriate, tell him to eat high-potassium foods, such as bananas and avocados.

• Tell the patient to contact the doctor if he experiences depression, difficult or painful urination, lower back pain, sore throat, fever, or skin rash.

• Inform the patient that this drug may cause drowsiness. If it does, he should avoid driving or other hazardous activities that require alertness.

• Advise the patient not to store capsule or tablet forms of the drug in the bathroom because heat and moisture will cause them to decompose.

CARDIOPULMONARY RESUSCITATION

Cardiopulmonary resuscitation (CPR) is performed to support and maintain respiration and circulation when heart rate and breathing are failing or have stopped.

An individual can have respiratory arrest without cardiac arrest. However, if respiratory arrest is not corrected, cardiac arrest will soon follow. Rescue breathing is initiated for respiratory arrest; rescue breathing and chest compressions are initiated for cardiac arrest.

Recent studies have indicated that a new method using alternate chest and abdominal compressions (double thrust resuscitation technique) significantly improves cardiac output and blood flow to the brain and heart as compared to chest compressions alone. In one study, this new method improved survival by 18%. This method is currently under study and is not yet recommended for general use.

About two-thirds of sudden deaths due to coronary artery disease take place outside of the hospital and occur within 2 hours after the onset of symptoms. Many sudden deaths from coronary heart disease can be prevented by prompt recognition, early entry into the emergency medical service (EMS) system, initiation of CPR, early defibrillation, and early initiation of advanced cardiac life support measures.

The steps of CPR can be remembered easily by thinking of A, B, C—*Airway, Breathing,* and *Circulation.* However, as a result of the National Conference on Emergency Cardiac Care and Cardiopulmonary Resuscitation in February 1992, the new steps to follow for CPR are A, A, B, and C: The first A stands for *Access* into the EMS system. (For details, see *How to perform CPR,* pages 138 to 141.)

External chest compressions and rescue breathing may be ineffective in supporting life, even when properly performed. The timeliness of the initiation of CPR affects the outcome. Basic life support is usually successful if definitive care, such as defibrillation, can be performed within 8 to 10 minutes. If CPR or definitive care is delayed, irreversible neurologic damage or death can result. There are exceptions—a drowning victim who has been in cold water or someone who has suffered hypothermia, for instance. However, CPR should be initiated regardless of the suspected time interval from arrest.

Purpose

• CPR is performed to restore and maintain breathing and circulation and to provide oxygen and blood flow to

(Text continues on page 140.)

How to perform CPR

You can perform cardiopulmonary resuscitation (CPR) quickly in almost any situation without assistance or equipment. To follow the correct sequence for CPR, remember AABC: **A**ccess the emergency medical service (EMS) system, open the **A**irway, restore **B**reathing, and restore **C**irculation.

One-person adult CPR

If you're the only rescuer, follow this procedure for CPR on an adult.
• Gently shake the patient's shoulders and shout, "Are you okay?" This simple action ensures that you don't start CPR on a conscious person.
• Quickly scan the patient for major injuries, particularly to the head and neck.
• Access the EMS system for your area.
• Place the patient in a supine position on a hard, flat surface, such as the floor. If you suspect a head or neck injury, move the patient as little as possible to reduce the risk of paralysis. If you must move him, logroll him into a supine position, supporting the head and neck to avoid twisting the spinal column.
• Open the airway.
• If a neck injury is not suspected, use the head-tilt–chin-lift maneuver. Place one hand on the patient's forehead and the fingers of the other hand on the bony portion of the lower jaw near the chin. Gently push his forehead back and pull upward on the chin, making sure the teeth are almost touching.

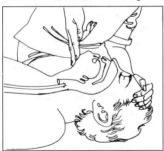

• If you suspect a neck injury, open the airway using the jaw-thrust maneuver. Curve your index fingers under the patient's jaw by his ears. With a strong,

steady motion, lift his jaw upward and outward. This maneuver opens the airway without moving the neck.

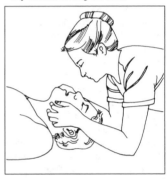

Restore breathing

• Keep the patient's airway open as you place your ear over his mouth and nose and look toward his feet. Listen for the sound of air moving, and watch for chest movement. You may also feel air on your cheek.

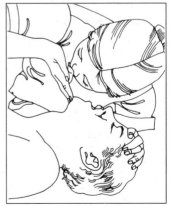

- If you detect signs of breathing and cervical trauma is not suspected, place the patient in the recovery position by rolling him onto his side to help protect the airway.
- If you don't detect breathing once you've opened the airway, begin rescue breathing. Pinch the patient's nostrils shut with the thumb and index finger of the hand you have on his forehead.
- Take a deep breath and cover the patient's mouth with yours, creating a tight seal. Give two full ventilations, taking a deep breath after each to allow enough time for his chest to relax and to prevent gastric distention. Each ventilation should last 1.5 to 2 seconds.

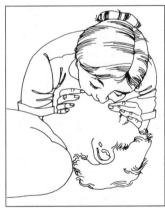

- If the first ventilation attempt doesn't work, reposition the patient's head and try again. If that doesn't work, suspect a foreign body (such as dentures) blocking the airway. If you see an object, follow the procedure for clearing a foreign-body airway obstruction.

Restore circulation
- Keep one hand on the patient's forehead so the airway remains open. With your other hand, palpate the carotid artery closer to you by placing your index

and middle fingers in the groove between the trachea and the sternocleidomastoid muscle. Palpatè the artery for 5 to 10 seconds.

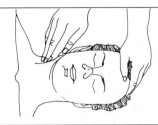

- If you detect a pulse, don't begin chest compressions. Instead, continue rescue breathing, giving 10 to 12 ventilations/ minute (or one every 5 seconds). Recheck the pulse every 2 to 3 minutes.
- If you don't detect a pulse and help hasn't arrived yet, start chest compressions. First, spread your knees apart for a wide base of support. Then, using the hand closer to the patient's foot, locate the lower margin of his rib cage.

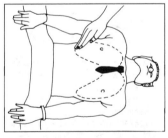

- Move your fingertips along the margin to the notch where the ribs meet the sternum. Place your middle finger on that notch and your index finger next to it. Your index finger should be on the bottom half of the patient's sternum, just above the xiphoid process.

(continued)

How to perform CPR   *(continued)*

- Put the heel of your other hand on the patient's sternum, next to your index finger. The long axis of the heel of your hand should align with the long axis of the sternum.

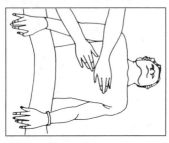

- Take your fingers off the notch, and put that hand directly on top of your other hand.

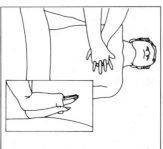

- Make sure your fingers don't rest on the patient's chest. Proper hand position keeps the force of the compressions on the sternum equal and reduces the risk of a rib fracture, lung puncture, or liver laceration.

- With your elbows locked, arms straight, and shoulders directly over your hands, you're ready to start chest compressions. Using the weight of your upper body, compress the patient's sternum 1½" to 2" (3.8 to 5 cm), delivering the pressure through the heels of your hands.

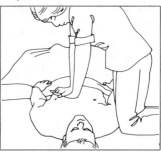

- After each compression, release the pressure and allow the chest to return to its normal position so that the heart can fill with blood. To prevent injuries, don't change your hand position during compressions.
- Give 15 compressions at a rate of 80 to 100 compressions/minute. Count "one and two and three and..." up to 15, compressing on the number and releasing on "and."
- After 15 compressions, give 2 ventilations. Then find the proper hand position again and deliver 15 more compressions. Continue this pattern for four full cycles.
- Palpate the carotid artery again. If you still don't detect a pulse, continue CPR in cycles of 15 compressions and 2 ventilations, beginning with ventilations.

the heart, brain, and other vital organs until more advanced methods can be instituted.

Indications

CPR is indicated in situations where either breathing or pulse is absent. Some common causes of respiratory and cardiac arrest are ventricular fibrillation, electric shock, drowning, drug

• Every few minutes, check for breathing and a pulse. If you detect a pulse but no breathing, give 10 to 12 ventilations/minute and monitor the pulse. If you detect both a pulse and breathing, monitor the patient's respirations and pulse closely. Don't stop CPR until respirations and a pulse return, you turn CPR over to someone else, or you become too exhausted to continue.

Child and infant CPR
Perform CPR on a child or an infant as you would on an adult, with the following key variations.

• If you discover an unresponsive child or infant and you are alone, continue your assessment and perform CPR for 1 minute, if indicated, before you activate the EMS system.

• Deliver rescue breaths at a rate of 20 breaths/minute for an infant or child, with each ventilation taking 1.5 to 2 seconds. Inflate a child's or an infant's lungs with smaller volumes of air at faster rates. You need two hands to maintain the airway for a child.

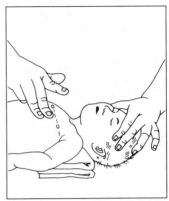

• When doing chest compressions, use the same landmarks as with an adult to find proper hand placement. (Because you need to give 100 compressions/minute, you don't have time to start at the notch and work upward; you need to visualize hand placement.) Give chest compressions with only one hand for a child (as shown at left) and two or three fingers for an infant (as shown above). Depress the sternum only 1″ to 1½″ (2.5 to 3.8 cm) for a child and ½″ to 1″ (1.3 to 2.5 cm) for an infant. Hand (finger) placement for an infant can be maintained because the other hand alone will keep the airway open; once correct hand placement is achieved, your fingers need not leave the infant's chest. You need to give at least 100 chest compressions/minute for an infant.

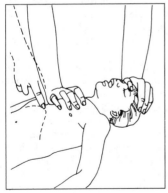

reactions or overdose, asphyxiation, allergic reactions, trauma, hypothermia, airway obstruction, or severe shock.

Procedure

CPR can be performed by any trained person. CPR training can follow American Heart Association or American Red Cross guidelines and recommendations. Both organizations teach by the same protocols, although different terminology is given for the course in which one is trained.

CPR includes rescue breathing, whereby the rescuer administers mouth-to-mouth breaths to the victim to provide oxygen to the lungs. Then the rescuer applies external chest compressions to help circulate the blood through the heart to vital organs of the body.

CPR may be administered to an adult by the one-rescuer or the two-rescuer technique; the principles are the same for both. Only one-rescuer CPR is taught to nonprofessional rescuers. Variations of the adult method are used for infants and children.

Complications

Even properly performed CPR can cause complications. The most common problem associated with rescue breathing is gastric distention, which is caused by giving too much air during ventilation. It can lead to vomiting, which then poses the risk of aspiration. Gastric distention is common in children. If vomiting occurs, turn the victim on his side and wipe out the mouth; then return him to the supine position and continue resuscitation measures.

Improper hand placement or strong compressions performed on a patient with frail bones may cause rib or sternal fractures. A fractured rib can puncture a lung and result in a tension pneumothorax. With this complication, air enters – but can't escape – the pleural space, building up positive pressure in the thoracic cavity and collapsing the lung. Bone fractures can also precipitate fat or bone marrow emboli.

Too-deep compressions can result in cardiac contusions and can lead to arrhythmias or excess fluid in the pericardial sac.

Incorrect positioning of the hands over the xiphoid process during compressions may break off the xiphoid

process and lacerate the highly vascular liver.

Care considerations

• Although the human immunodeficiency virus has not been proven to be transmitted by saliva, the Centers for Disease Control and Prevention's "Recommendations for Prevention of Human Immunodeficiency Virus" advise that the need for mouth-to-mouth resuscitation should be reduced as much as possible by keeping mouthpieces, resuscitation bags, or other ventilation devices available for immediate use in areas where the need for resuscitation is predictable. Because of this recommendation, mouth-to-mask rescue breathing is taught to all health care providers who are trained in two-rescuer CPR; furthermore, in health care facilities, masks are positioned at or near the bedside in case rescue breathing is necessary.

• If a patient collapses or suddenly becomes unconscious, call out for help, assess the patient for unresponsiveness as described in *How to perform CPR*, pages 138 to 141, and activate the EMS system.

• Check for breathing and pulse, and begin CPR only if the patient is not breathing and does not have a pulse. If the patient has a pulse but is not breathing, perform only rescue breathing, not chest compressions; frequently, establishing an adequate airway alone will resolve the situation. If the patient was eating or could have had a foreign object in his mouth immediately before breathing stopped, the airway may be blocked, and you may have to perform an abdominal thrust to clear the airway. Abdominal thrusts are performed only after the rescuer has been unsuccessful in delivering a breath and has tried repositioning the airway first (according to the guidelines for managing an obstructed airway). Keep in mind that patients can become unconscious or collapse and not require rescue breathing or chest compressions.

• If you're in a hospital, call out for help and begin CPR. If you're in a public location and another person is present, one of you may activate the EMS system while the other begins CPR.

• Perform CPR until someone arrives who can relieve you or help with resuscitation.

Home care instructions

• Recommend that family members or significant others who are living with a high-risk patient become trained in CPR.

CARDIOVERSION, SYNCHRONIZED

Cardioversion is the delivery of a synchronized electrical current to the heart muscle or myocardium. It is used in an attempt to convert a tachyarrhythmia, which is either unstable or refractory to medical management, to a normal sinus rhythm.

In cardioversion, unlike defibrillation, the electrical current must be discharged simultaneously with the peak of the R wave. The heart muscle cell is electrically unstable or vulnerable during the downstroke of the T wave. Discharge of the electrical current during a vulnerable period could precipitate an episode of ventricular fibrillation.

Purpose

• To restore the sinoatrial node as the primary pacemaker of the heart
• To convert tachyarrhythmias to a normal sinus rhythm.

Indications

Cardioversion may be used in an attempt to terminate ventricular tachycardia with a pulse or supraventricular tachyarrhythmias that are compromising cardiac output. This procedure may also be used to treat atrial fibrillation or atrial flutter.

Cardioversion is contraindicated in patients with chronic atrial fibrillation who have not received anticoagulant therapy for at least 3 weeks or those with digitalis toxicity or third-degree heart block.

Procedure

Synchronized cardioversion can be performed as an elective or emergency procedure. The patient is sedated with diazepam or another sedative, or he's given "light" anesthesia. In elective cardioversion, the nurse typically assists the doctor. In an emergency, many hospitals authorize specially skilled nurses to perform the procedure.

Cardioversion is performed with the use of a defibrillator; however, the synchronized button on the defibrillator unit must be activated. The patient is connected to the defibrillator's electrocardiogram (ECG) leads. It is important that the oscilloscope show a distinctive upright R wave that is high above the other waves, because discharge of electrical current on the T wave could precipitate ventricular fibrillation. Paddles are positioned as for defibrillation and then are charged to the desired energy level (according to the doctor's order or hospital protocol). The discharge buttons are pressed and held until all the current is released while forearm pressure is applied to each paddle. (The countershock will synchronize with the R wave and may not occur exactly when the discharge button is pressed.) To ensure safety, the operator should state "all clear" and check that no one is touching the patient or the bed before he or she discharges the current. If the first cardioversion doesn't correct the arrhythmia, the procedure may be repeated at a higher energy level.

Complications

Synchronized cardioversion may cause other arrhythmias. Emboli may be released to the circulation. Skin burns may result from the placement of the paddles if the conductive gel pads are dry or improperly placed.

Care considerations

Before the procedure

• Explain the procedure (as time permits depending on the situation).
• Monitor cardiac rhythm and vital signs and obtain cardiac rhythm tracings for baseline data.
• Obtain 12-lead ECG (optional) for baseline data.
• If warranted, check digitalis levels and potassium levels. Cardioversion performed on a hypokalemic patient can predispose to ventricular fibrillation.
• Initiate anticoagulation therapy as ordered. This may be started several days to months before elective cardioversion to reduce the risk of emboli.
• Ensure patent I.V. access in case emergency drugs are necessary.
• Ensure that a signed consent form has been obtained.
• Administer an ordered sedative to the conscious patient. Cardioversion may be extremely uncomfortable.
• Check that the patient receives nothing by mouth for the time ordered (ideally 8 to 12 hours before the procedure) to reduce the risk of emesis during cardioversion.
• Have emergency resuscitation equipment at the bedside.
• Ensure a safe work environment for the health care team.

During the procedure

• Turn off oxygen at the bedside to avoid a fire hazard.
• Place the patient in a supine position.
• Monitor cardiac rhythm. If ventricular fibrillation occurs, the operator needs to immediately turn off the synchronizer circuit and begin defibrillation.

After the procedure

• Ensure patency of the airway.
• Monitor cardiac rhythm, vital signs, peripheral pulses, and mental status. Compare with baseline.
• Document the procedure, the energy required for conversion, precardioversion and postcardioversion rhythms, and the patient's tolerance of the procedure.
• Observe for complications. Check the patient's skin for evidence of burns from the paddles.

Home care instructions

• Teach the patient and caregiver how to assess the pulse. Tell them that if the patient notices the onset of a tachyarrhythmia, they should notify the doctor immediately and call an ambulance if there is no one to drive them to the emergency department.
• If skin burns occur as a result of the cardioversion procedure, instruct the patient or caregiver how to care for them and how to observe for signs of infection.

CAROTID ENDARTERECTOMY

Carotid endarterectomy is a surgical procedure that removes atheromatous plaque from the carotid arteries to improve intracranial perfusion by increasing blood flow through the carotid arteries. Because carotid lesions commonly lead to stroke in both symptomatic and asymptomatic patients, this procedure may be considered a prophylactic treatment for stroke. Because it imposes significant surgical risks, patients should be carefully evaluated on a risk-versus-benefit scale. (See *Identifying level of risk in carotid endarterectomy*.)

Identifying level of risk in carotid endarterectomy

For patients being considered for carotid endarterectomy, a risk-versus-benefit ratio should be utilized. Patients identified as grade 1 have the lowest risk; those identified as grade 4, the highest risk.

Grade 1: Patients have a physiologic age under 70 with bilateral or unilateral focal carotid stenosis. Take into account medical risk factors that may make a patient appear older physiologically, such as alcohol abuse, cigarette smoking, diabetes, or hyperlipidemia. These patients have no fixed neurologic deficits and are considered neurologically stable.

Grade 2: These patients appear as grade 1 but have significant angiographic evidence of a high-grade stenosis. Medical risk factors in combination with angiographic evidence make these patients a higher risk for surgery.

Grade 3: These patients have significant risk factors, angiographic evidence of significant lesions, and such complications as coronary artery disease, myocardial infarction (within 6 months), blood pressure over 180/110, chronic obstructive pulmonary disease, severe obesity, or a physiologic age over 70.

Grade 4: These patients are neurologically unstable before surgery and represent the greatest risk. Neurologic instability includes a stroke in progress, frequent uncontrolled transient ischemic attacks, or multiple neurologic deficits from past cerebral infarctions.

Purpose

• To improve intracranial perfusion and alleviate symptoms of ischemia
• To prevent total carotid occlusion
• To remove a potential source of emboli
• To prevent stroke.

Indications

Carotid endarterectomy is indicated in patients who have experienced reversible ischemic neurologic deficit or a completed stroke. Patients who experience transient ischemic attacks, syncope, and dizziness may benefit greatly from carotid endarterectomy. Those who manifest high-grade asymptomatic or ulcerative lesions may also be good candidates for this procedure.

Patients who have concurrent coronary artery disease (CAD) and carotid disease may have both conditions repaired at the same time if they are neurologically stable and good candidates for surgery.

Carotid endarterectomy is contraindicated in patients with uncontrolled hypertension, chronic internal carotid artery occlusion, acute carotid artery occlusion with massive cerebral infarction, and permanent hemiplegia, and in those patients who are poor surgical risks. Patients who are not appropriate candidates for this surgery are treated instead with medical therapy, such as antiplatelet agents and warfarin sodium.

Procedure

During carotid endarterectomy, light general anesthesia may be used to allow accurate monitoring of brain waves by EEG during the surgery. The EEG, when used intraoperatively, continues from induction of anesthesia to extubation at the end of the procedure.

An incision is made along the anterior border of the sternocleidomastoid muscle or transversely in a skin crease in the neck. The common carotid artery, external carotid artery, and internal coronary artery are exposed at levels not involved in the disease. The carotid arteries are then clamped, and stump pressures are measured to evaluate the adequacy of collateral circulation. If cerebral perfusion (blood flow) is inadequate, a shunt that permits blood flow past the obstruction in the carotid artery is constructed. Shunts provide temporary bypass routes for blood flow to ensure adequate cerebral circulation during surgery.

When the carotid artery is stabilized, heparin is started to prevent thrombosis. The affected arteries are then incised and the plaque removed. The artery is then patched with an autogenous saphenous vein or prosthetic material and closed. If a shunt was used, it is removed before complete closure.

Complications

The most common problem after carotid endarterectomy is blood pressure lability; transient hypertension frequently results from manipulation of the carotid body. Another complication is the loss of carotid body function, which can be temporary or permanent. Normally, carotid body function causes blood pressure and ventilation to increase in response to hypoxia; however, the loss of carotid body function causes blood pressure and ventilation to decrease in response to hypoxia.

Postoperative respiratory distress, evidenced by labored respirations and stridor, can result from tracheal compression by a hematoma. Rarely, vocal cord paralysis arises from manipulation of the vagus nerve. Wound complications may also occur at the operative site.

Another uncommon complication is hyperperfusion syndrome, a sudden increase in cerebral blood flow. It can lead to ipsilateral vascular headaches, seizures, and intracerebral hemorrhage.

The most serious complication of carotid endarterectomy is perioperative stroke, which is thought to result from the embolization of debris during the dissection of plaque. Rethrombosis is possible and may be prevented by postoperative heparinization.

Care considerations
Before surgery

• Provide preoperative teaching to inform and reassure the patient and the family about the procedure.
• Discuss the location of the lesion. Explain the atherosclerotic process so the patient can modify risk factors after surgery.
• Explain and provide support for all preoperative diagnostic tests used to evaluate carotid disease: periorbital ultrasound, ocular pneumoplethysmography, carotid phonoangiography, computed tomography scan, and cerebral angiography. For the patient with concurrent CAD, preoperative diagnostic tests include an electrocardiogram (ECG), coronary angiography, and a treadmill exercise stress test.
• Before surgery, a radial arterial catheter is inserted to monitor arterial blood gas levels and blood pressure.
• Because wide fluctuations of blood pressure are common during this procedure, premix I.V. pressors and vasodilators so that they are ready for use if needed.
• Check that a baseline EEG is done preoperatively before the patient is anesthetized.
• Provide a tour of the critical care unit for the patient and family to prepare them for the postoperative course.
• Explain postoperative care, including the presence of I.V. lines, hemodynamic measuring devices, tubes, and monitoring equipment that will be connected to the patient.
• Tell the patient that analgesic medications will be available to control discomfort after the surgery.
• Tell the patient to expect that a nurse will routinely check his neurologic signs, including level of consciousness, orientation, extremity strength, speech, and

fine hand movements every hour; tell him this is not an indication that he is not doing well.

After surgery

• Monitor vital signs every 15 minutes for the 1st hour after surgery until the patient is stable. Lowered blood pressure and elevated heart rate and Cheyne-Stokes respirations could indicate cerebral ischemia.

• Perform a neurologic assessment every hour for the first 24 hours, including extremity strength, fine hand movements, speech, visual acuity, and orientation.

• Monitor intake and output hourly for the first 24 hours.

• Continuous cardiac monitoring should be performed for the first 24 hours. Afterward, the ECG should be checked for chest pain or arrhythmias because many patients undergoing this procedure have CAD as well.

Home care instructions

• Encourage the patient to lower any relevant risk factors, such as smoking, high lipid levels, and obesity.

• Provide referral to a home health care agency if the patient has experienced a stroke and needs follow-up care.

• Emphasize the importance of taking all prescribed medications. Explain proper administration, dosage, and adverse effects.

• Review any deficits — neurologic, sensory, or motor — that may have occurred during surgery and the need for medical follow-up.

• Review signs and symptoms of wound infection.

• Tell the patient to immediately report any new neurologic symptoms. (The rate of reocclusion may range from 1.5% to 23%.)

• Emphasize the importance of regular medical checkups.

CAROTID SINUS MASSAGE

Carotid sinus massage (CSM) is a non-invasive method for evaluating and terminating certain tachyarrhythmias. It involves manual stimulation of pressure receptors in the carotid artery, which in turn triggers a parasympathetic response and depresses heart rate and conductivity.

Patient response to CSM differs, depending on the type of arrhythmia involved. (This difference can be used diagnostically to help distinguish ectopic tachyarrhythmias from sinus tachycardia, but it limits CSM's usefulness as a treatment.) In patients with sinus tachycardia, the heart rate slows gradually during CSM and speeds up again afterward. In those with atrial tachycardia, the response to CSM is unpredictable: The arrhythmia may or may not terminate, or atrioventricular (AV) block may worsen. In patients with paroxysmal atrial tachycardia, reversion to sinus rhythm occurs about 20% of the time. In those with nonparoxysmal tachycardia and ventricular tachycardia, there's no response to CSM. In patients with atrial fibrillation or flutter, the ventricular rate slows because of increased AV block.

Purpose

• To slow the heart rate and terminate arrhythmias

• To distinguish ectopic tachyarrhythmias from sinus tachycardia.

Indications

CSM is indicated in patients with sinus, atrial, or functional tachyarrhythmias.

An absolute contraindication to CSM is the presence of a bruit close to the jaw line, which suggests arteriosclerotic plaques in the carotid artery. CSM should be used cautiously in elderly patients, in those receiving digitalis glycosides, and in those with heart block, hypertension, coronary artery disease, diabetes mellitus, or hyperkalemia. CSM should not be used in patients with digitalis toxicity, cerebrovascular disease, or previous carotid surgery.

Procedure

CSM may be performed by a doctor or specially prepared nurse. First, locate the patient's larynx with the tips of your index and middle fingers; then slide the fingers laterally into the groove between the trachea and the neck muscles. A strong pulse will be felt over the carotid artery. Follow the carotid artery to the bifurcation – the location of the carotid sinus area – by sliding the fingers to the angle of the mandible. Place four fingers medial to the pulsating artery. Press the artery against the underlying vertebrae and begin massaging it firmly in a circular motion (counterclockwise); massage for 3 to 5 seconds, *but no longer than 5 seconds*, because of the risk of asystole. The artery should be released as soon as the electrocardiogram (ECG) shows slowing of the heart rate. If a dangerous arrhythmia occurs, prepare to give emergency treatment. If the procedure has no effect, perform CSM on the other side, massaging both sides simultaneously.

Complications

CSM may cause ventricular standstill, ventricular tachycardia, or ventricular fibrillation. By worsening AV block, CSM can also cause functional or ventricular escape rhythms. Another potential complication is cerebral damage from inadequate tissue perfusion. If the carotid artery is totally occluded during CSM, decreased cerebral blood flow may cause a cerebrovascular accident (CVA). Also, compression of the carotid sinus may release endothelial plaque into the circulation, which can migrate and cause CVA.

Care considerations

Before therapy

• Explain the procedure and tell the patient to let you know if he feels lightheaded.
• Place the patient in a supine position, and insert an I.V. line if necessary.
• Obtain a rhythm strip using the lead that shows the strongest P waves.
• Auscultate both carotid sinuses. If you note bruits, inform the doctor and do not perform CSM.

During therapy

• Monitor the ECG throughout the procedure.
• Continue to watch the patient carefully for changes in neurologic status.

After therapy

• Check vital signs, watching especially for hypotension and bradycardia.
• Obtain a rhythm strip to document changes.
• Record the date and time of the procedure, who performed it, and why it was necessary.
• Document the patient's response, any complications, and treatment given.
• Continue cardiac monitoring for at least 4 hours to assess the effects of treatment and to watch for recurrence of arrhythmia.
• Assess neurologic status every hour for the first 4 hours to detect symptoms of CVA.

Home care instructions

• Show the patient how to take his radial pulse. Instruct him to take it for 1 full minute each morning, before getting out of bed, and whenever he experiences chest pain, palpitations, dizziness, or faintness.
• Warn the patient to report these signs as well as a heart rate less than 60 beats/minute or greater than 100 beats/minute promptly to the doctor.

CARPAL TUNNEL RELEASE

Carpal tunnel syndrome is a relatively common, painful disorder caused by compression of the median nerve within the carpal tunnel by the transverse carpal ligament.

This syndrome may develop after strenuous or repetitive use of the hands or may follow wrist injuries, such as fractures, dislocations, or bruises. Often, however, the patient has no history of significant trauma.

If rest, splinting, and corticosteroid injections fail to relieve carpal tunnel syndrome, surgery may be necessary to decompress the median nerve. This surgery involves sectioning the entire transverse carpal tunnel ligament and may include neurolysis as well. Surgical division of the transverse carpal ligament gives lasting relief from pain. However, muscle strength returns slowly, and complete recovery is unlikely if atrophy is pronounced.

Purpose
• To decompress the median nerve within the carpal tunnel, thereby relieving pain and restoring function.

Indications
A carpal tunnel release is indicated for patients who experience pain and loss of function of the affected wrist and hand, after noninvasive therapies have proven ineffective.

Procedure
The surgeon can choose from several techniques. Each involves complete transection of the transverse carpal ligament to ensure adequate median nerve decompression. This procedure is performed in the operating room, usually with a local anesthetic.

In one commonly used technique, the surgeon makes an incision around the thenar eminence of the wrist to expose the flexor retinaculum, which he then transects to relieve pressure on the median nerve. Depending on the extent of nerve compression, he also may have to free nerve fibers from the surrounding tissue.

Complications
This relatively simple surgery is generally risk-free, but certain complications may arise. These include hematoma formation, infection, painful scar formation, and tenosynovitis.

Care considerations
Before surgery
• As necessary, reinforce the surgeon's explanation of the surgery.
• Inform the patient that the affected arm will be shaved and cleaned.
• Prepare the patient for postoperative care, which will include a dressing in place for 1 to 2 days and analgesics for pain.
• Teach the patient rehabilitative exercises, such as range-of-motion exercises of the wrist and fingers, which will be recommended postoperatively if he can tolerate them.

After surgery
• Monitor vital signs, and carefully assess circulation as well as sensory and motor function in the affected arm.
• Keep the hand elevated to reduce swelling and discomfort.
• Examine the dressing for drainage or bleeding, which may indicate infection.
• Assess for pain and provide analgesics as needed.
• Report severe, persistent pain or tenderness, which may indicate tenosynovitis or hematoma formation.
• Encourage the patient to perform rehabilitative exercises daily to improve circulation and enhance muscle tone. If these exercises are painful, have the patient perform them with the wrist and hand immersed in warm water. (Have the patient wear a surgical glove if the dressing is still in place.)

Home care instructions

• Instruct the patient to keep the incision site clean and dry. Tell him to cover it with a surgical or rubber glove when immersing it in water for exercises or when bathing.
• Teach the patient how to change the dressing. Instruct him to do so once a day until healing is complete.
• Tell the patient to notify the doctor of redness, swelling, pain, or persistent or excessive drainage at the operative site.
• Encourage the patient to continue daily wrist and finger exercises. However, warn against overusing the affected wrist or against lifting any object heavier than a thin magazine.
• If the patient's carpal tunnel syndrome is work-related, suggest occupational counseling to find more suitable employment.

CATARACT REMOVAL

A cataract is a clouding or opacity of the normally transparent crystalline lens. Surgical removal of the cloudy lens is the treatment of choice. It can be removed by one of two techniques: intracapsular cataract extraction (ICCE) or extracapsular cataract extraction (ECCE).

Purpose

• To remove a cloudy lens that prevents light rays from reaching the retina.

Indications

Traditionally, cataract extraction was not performed until lens opacification seriously impaired vision. Currently, a cataract can be removed as soon as lens

---

Comparing methods of cataract removal

Cataracts can be removed by intracapsular or extracapsular techniques.

Intracapsular cataract extraction
In this technique, the surgeon makes a partial incision at the superior limbus arc and then removes the lens with either a specially designed forceps or a cryoprobe; the latter freezes and adheres to the lens, facilitating its removal.

Extracapsular cataract extraction
In this technique, the surgeon may use irrigation and aspiration or phacoemulsification. In the former approach, the surgeon makes an incision at the limbus, opens the anterior lens capsule with a cystotome, and exerts pressure from below to express the lens. He then irrigates and suctions the remaining lens cortex.

In phacoemulsification, the surgeon uses an ultrasonic probe to break the lens into minute particles, which are aspirated by the probe.

Intracapsular extraction

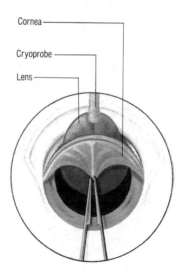

Cornea

Cryoprobe

Lens

opacification causes the patient to notice vision impairment.

Procedure

Cataract extraction may be done in the hospital as a short-stay procedure or in an ophthalmologist's office-based surgical facility.

Cataract surgery is generally performed under local anesthesia. The anesthetist usually places the patient in a state of conscious sedation, in which the patient is awake but has diminished motor activity and response to pain. The procedure can also be performed under general anesthesia.

The doctor will instill mydriatics into the eye to dilate the pupil and facilitate cataract removal. In ICCE, the entire lens is removed with an instrument called a cryoprobe. The cryoprobe freezes and adheres to the lens, facilitating its removal. In ECCE, the anterior capsule, cortex, and nucleus of the patient's eye are removed, leaving the posterior capsule of the eye intact. This technique may be carried out using manual extraction, irrigation and aspiration, or phacoemulsification. In phacoemulsification, the surgeon uses an ultrasonic probe to break the lens into minute particles, which are then aspirated by a probe. (See *Comparing methods of cataract removal*.)

Immediately after removal of the lens, the doctor may insert one of many types of lens implants.

After the procedure, the doctor will instill antibiotic medications before he dresses the eye with a patch and a shield.

Both the operative eye and the unoperated eye can work together after cataract surgery with lens implanta-

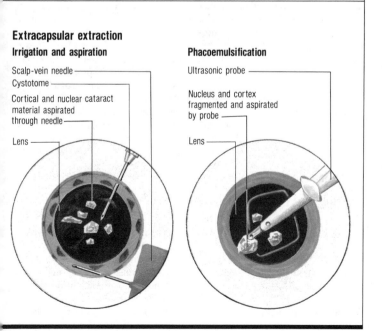

Extracapsular extraction
Irrigation and aspiration

Scalp-vein needle
Cystotome
Cortical and nuclear cataract material aspirated through needle
Lens

Phacoemulsification

Ultrasonic probe
Nucleus and cortex fragmented and aspirated by probe
Lens

tion. After the eye has healed (approximately 2 months), glasses for reading and any remaining astigmatism will be prescribed.

Complications

Secondary membrane opacification, the most common complication of cataract removal, involves the formation of a second membrane that becomes opaque and results in reduced vision. It can be easily corrected using the neodymium : yttrium - aluminum - garnet (Nd:YAG) laser and can be performed as an office procedure. Other complications include infection, retinal detachment, glaucoma, and hemorrhage.

Care considerations

Before surgery

• Explain the surgical procedure as well as preoperative and postoperative restrictions. Emphasize postoperative restrictions.

• Inform the patient that he'll receive medications that will dilate the eye and facilitate cataract removal, antibiotics to reduce the risk of infection, and a sedative for relaxation during the procedure.

• If ordered, perform an antiseptic facial scrub to reduce the risk of infection.

• Ensure that the patient has signed a consent form.

• Instruct the patient not to eat or drink after midnight the night before surgery.

• Encourage the patient to void before he's transported to the operating room.

After surgery

• If the procedure is performed in an ophthalmologist's surgical facility, the patient will be observed for 2 to 3 hours and sent home.

• Notify the doctor of severe pain, bleeding, increased drainage, or fever.

• Monitor vital signs according to the policy of the health care facility.

• Because of the change in the patient's depth perception, observe safety precautions; for example, keep the side rails of his bed raised and assist with ambulation.

• Maintain the eye patch, and have the patient wear an eye shield, especially when sleeping.

• Keep the patient's bed elevated 45 degrees or place two pillows under the patient's head.

Home care instructions

• Warn the patient to contact the doctor immediately if he notices sudden eye pain, bleeding, increased discharge, decreased vision, or if he sees light flashes or floaters. These may indicate complications.

• Instruct the patient to avoid activities that raise intraocular pressure and place pressure on the sutures: heavy lifting, bending, straining during defecation, or vigorous coughing and sneezing. Advise the patient to sleep on his back or on the unoperative side and to avoid strenuous exercise for 6 to 10 weeks.

• Explain that follow-up appointments are necessary to monitor the results of the surgery and to detect complications.

• Teach the patient or a family member how to instill eyedrops and ointments and how to change the eye patch. Stress the importance of continuing these medications as prescribed.

• Suggest that the patient wear dark glasses to relieve discomfort in bright light.

CATHETERIZATION

Urinary catheterization is the insertion of a drainage device into the bladder using aseptic technique. Catheterization may be intermittent or continuous. Intermittent catheterization drains urine that remains in the bladder after voiding or when the patient is unable to void naturally. An indwelling urinary catheter (also known as a Foley or retention catheter) provides continuous drainage of urine.

Purpose

• To remove urine from the bladder
• To irrigate the bladder or instill medications
• To obtain a urine specimen for laboratory analysis
• To allow accurate measurement of urine output
• To provide postoperative urine drainage.

Indications

Intermittent catheterization may be used postoperatively for patients with urinary incontinence to remove residual urine or for patients with urethral strictures, cystitis, prostatic obstruction, neurogenic bladder, or other disorders that interfere with bladder emptying. The patient may also perform this procedure at home if he has a chronic bladder disorder. (See *Self-catheterization*, pages 155 and 156.)

Indwelling catheterization is indicated to relieve bladder distention caused by such conditions as urinary tract obstruction and neurogenic bladder. It also allows continuous urine drainage in patients with a swollen urinary meatus related to surgery, local trauma, or childbirth. What's more, indwelling catheterization can provide accurate monitoring of urine output when normal voiding is impaired.

Procedure

The female patient is placed in the supine position, with her knees flexed and separated and her feet flat on the bed. The male patient is also placed in a supine position but with his legs flat and extended.

The patient's genitalia and perineum are cleaned with soap and water or an antiseptic solution to avoid introducing infection into the bladder.

Because this is a sterile procedure, the nurse will wear gloves throughout.

To accomplish intermittent catheterization, a nurse inserts a sterile straight catheter through the urethra into the bladder. This type of catheter is left in place only long enough to drain residual urine and is withdrawn when the urine flow stops.

If an indwelling urinary catheter will be used for continuous drainage of urine, a balloon at the proximal end of the catheter is inflated with sterile water to secure the catheter in place within the bladder. The catheter is connected to a collection bag that's positioned below the level of the bladder to enhance drainage and prevent urine reflux into the bladder, which can cause infection. The catheter is then secured in position to prevent traction on the bladder and to maintain the normal direction of urine flow.

Complications

Patients who have an indwelling urinary catheter are at risk for developing urinary tract infections or sustaining urethral trauma.

Care considerations

Before the procedure

• Thoroughly review the procedure with the patient.
• Reassure the patient that although catheterization may produce slight discomfort, it shouldn't be painful. Explain that you'll stop the procedure if he experiences severe discomfort.
• Assemble the necessary equipment and, if possible, arrange for someone to assist you with the procedure. Inspect the catheter for cracks or rough areas.

During the procedure

• Ensure privacy for the patient and adequate lighting to provide maximum visualization of the urinary meatus.
• Insert the catheter using sterile technique.

• Note the difficulty or ease of insertion, any patient discomfort, and the amount and nature of urine drainage. Notify the doctor if you observe hematuria or extremely foul-smelling or cloudy urine. During urine drainage, monitor the patient for pallor, diaphoresis, and painful bladder spasms. If these occur, clamp the catheter tubing and call the doctor. Also see *Combating catheter problems*, page 157, for guidelines on handling possible problems.
• Never force a catheter forward during insertion. If you encounter resistance, stop the procedure and notify the doctor, who may have to insert the catheter using size-graduated dilating instruments.
• Before you inflate the catheter balloon, observe for urine flow to ensure that you've inserted the catheter into the bladder and not left it in the urethral channel. If you can't elicit urine flow, palpate the bladder to check whether it's empty. If the bladder is empty, make sure you've advanced the catheter at least 3″ (7.6 cm) for a female and approximately 6″ to 7″ (15 to 18 cm) for a male before inflating the balloon to avoid any injury to the urethra.
• Do not use 0.9% sodium chloride solution to inflate the catheter because it can crystallize and cause incomplete deflation of the balloon, resulting in urethral trauma when the catheter is removed.

After the procedure
• Tape or strap the catheter to a female patient's thigh to prevent tension in the urogenital area. In males, secure the catheter to the thigh or lower abdomen. Attaching the catheter to the lower abdomen prevents pressure on the urethra at the penoscrotal junction, which can cause formation of urethrocutaneous fistulas.
• To maintain proper position of the drainage system, ensure that the tubing remains free of kinks.
• Throughout the course of treatment, provide catheter care at least once daily.

• Expect a small amount of mucus drainage at the catheter insertion site from irritation of the urethral wall, but notify the doctor of excessive, bloody, or purulent drainage.
• Monitor the patient's intake and output.
• Encourage adequate fluid intake (up to 3,000 ml/day, if necessary) to maintain continuous urine flow through the catheter and decrease the risk of infection and clot formation. Note the color and amount of urine drainage: Dark, concentrated urine may warrant increased fluid intake.
• To help prevent infection, avoid separating the catheter and tubing unless absolutely necessary. Use the collection port to secure specimens and instill medications. However, if you must separate the catheter and tubing, maintain strict asepsis and wipe the connection with an antiseptic solution before and after the procedure.
• Throughout treatment, remain alert for signs of urinary tract infection, including low-grade fever, possibly with chills; meatal or scrotal swelling and tenderness; flank pain; and cloudy, foul-smelling urine. Report these signs to the patient's doctor, and prepare to take samples for culture and sensitivity tests.
• Monitor for signs of catheter obstruction. Watch for decreased or absent urine output (less than 30 ml/hour); severe, persistent bladder spasms; urine leakage around the catheter insertion site; and bladder distention. If you suspect obstruction, try to clear it yourself. If you're unsuccessful, promptly notify the doctor.

Home care considerations
• Instruct the patient to drink at least 2 quarts of water daily, unless the doctor orders otherwise.
• Teach the patient how to minimize the risk of infection by performing daily periurethral care.

Self-catheterization

A patient with impaired or absent bladder function may learn self-catheterization for routine bladder drainage. Called intermittent self-catheterization, this procedure requires thorough and careful teaching. The patient will probably use clean technique for self-catheterization at home but must use sterile technique in the hospital because of the increased risk of infection.

Equipment

The patient needs the following: rubber catheter, washcloth, soap and water, gloves (sterile ones if using sterile technique), water-soluble lubricant, plastic storage bag. Optional: drainage container, paper towels, rubber or plastic sheets, gooseneck lamp, catheterization record.

The patient should keep a supply of catheters at home and use each catheter only once before cleaning it. When all but the last one have been used, the patient should boil the catheters for 20 minutes in a pan of water, drain the water, and store the catheters in the pan or a freshly laundered towel. The catheters will become brittle with repeated use and should be checked often. A new supply should be ordered well in advance.

The patient begins by trying to urinate into a toilet or, if he needs to measure urine quantity, into a drainage container. The patient should then wash his hands thoroughly with soap and water and dry them.

Female patient

A female patient begins by separating the labia as widely as possible with the fingers of her nondominant hand to obtain a full view of the urinary meatus. She will then use her dominant hand to wash the perineal area thoroughly with a soapy washcloth, using downward strokes. The area is then rinsed with the washcloth in downward strokes.

She then squeezes some lubricant onto the first 3″ (7.6 cm) of the catheter. Then, holding the catheter like a pencil about ½″ (1.3 cm) from its tip while

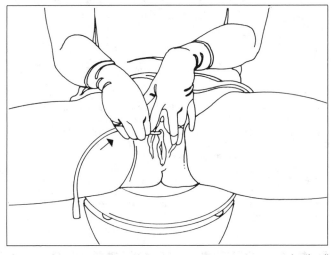

(continued)

Self-catheterization *(continued)*

keeping the vaginal folds separated, the patient inserts the lubricated catheter about 3″ into the urethra. Pressing down with her abdominal muscles will help to empty the bladder, allowing urine to drain through the catheter and into the toilet or drainage container.

When the urine stops draining, she slowly removes the catheter and then washes it with warm, soapy water, rinses it inside and out, and dries it with a paper towel.

Male patient

A male patient should thoroughly wash and rinse the end of his penis with soap and water, pulling back the foreskin if appropriate. He should keep the foreskin pulled back during the procedure.

Next, he squeezes lubricant onto a paper towel and rolls the first 7″ to 10″ (17.8 to 25 cm) of the catheter in the lubricant. This copious amount of lubricant will make the procedure more comfortable. He then uses his nondominant hand to hold his penis at a right angle to his body.

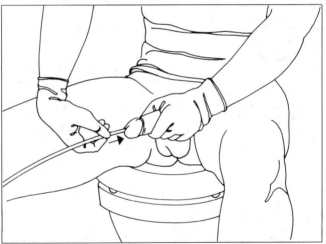

Then, holding the catheter like a pencil in his dominant hand, the patient slowly inserts it 7″ to 10″ into the urethra until urine begins to flow. He advances the catheter about 1″ (2.5 cm) farther, allowing all urine to drain into the toilet or drainage container. When the urine stops draining, he removes the catheter slowly and, if necessary, pulls the foreskin forward again. He washes, rinses, and dries the catheter as described above.

The timing of catherization is critical to prevent overdistention of the bladder, which can lead to infection. Intermittent self-catheterizations are usually performed every 4 to 6 hours around the clock (or more often at first).

Combating catheter problems

If the patient's indwelling urinary catheter won't drain, the following tips may help you find the cause of poor drainage and correct the problem.

First, help the patient into a different position — one that promotes drainage by the force of gravity. Then have him cough and bear down slightly. Often, this will be enough to clear the obstruction.

However, if the obstruction persists, you may need to irrigate the catheter. (Be sure to obtain the doctor's permission.) To irrigate the catheter, first clamp the drainage tubing behind the catheter's sampling port, and then inject 30 to 100 ml of sterile 0.9% sodium chloride solution through the port. Next, unclamp the tubing to allow the solution to flow back through the catheter, and check for clearing. *Caution:* To avoid painful bladder distention, don't inject more than 100 ml of irrigant at one time.

Check catheter placement to ensure that the balloon tip is still in the bladder. Gently push on the catheter to see if you can move it into the bladder; then pull back slightly to seat the balloon in the bladder. If the obstruction is still present, notify the doctor, who may order insertion of a new catheter.

If the catheter doesn't have an irrigation port, verify catheter placement before you irrigate. Also, remember to clean the area where the catheter and tubing are attached with antiseptic solution before you disconnect the system. Irrigate with 30 to 60 ml of sterile 0.9% sodium chloride solution, using a piston syringe. If resistance is met, stop and notify the doctor; otherwise, instill the solution and allow it to flow back freely.

• Stress the need for thorough hand washing before and after handling the catheter and collection system.
• Ensure that the patient who has an indwelling urinary catheter knows how to secure the tubing and the leg bag. Tell him to alternate legs every other day to prevent skin irritation. Instruct him to keep the leg bag or closed-system drainage bag lower than bladder level to facilitate drainage. Advise the patient to empty the bag when it's about half full, and teach him how to empty it. Also demonstrate how to apply a new bag.
• Tell the patient that he may take showers but should avoid tub baths while the catheter is in place.
• Instruct the patient to notify the doctor of urine leakage around the catheter. Also instruct him to report any signs of urinary tract infection, such as fever, chills, flank or urinary tract pain, and cloudy or foul-smelling urine.
• Teach the patient and family caregiver how to do intermittent catheterization

if ordered, and make sure they are comfortable with performing the procedure.

CEPHALOSPORINS

Chemically related to penicillin, cephalosporins are a group of semisynthetic, broad-spectrum antibiotics. They're useful in treating both gram-positive and gram-negative aerobic and anaerobic organisms.

Differences among individual cephalosporins relate to their bacterial sensitivity, duration of action, and routes of administration and excretion. The first-generation cephalosporins include *cefadroxil, cephalexin monohydrate, cefazolin, cephalothin, cephapirin,* and *cephradine.* The second-generation drugs, such as *cefaclor, cefamandole,* and *cefoxitin,* have expanded antibacterial activity against such gram-negative organisms as *Bac-*

teroides fragilis, which is resistant to many other antibiotics. Third-generation cephalosporins—*cefixime, cefoperazone, cefotaxime, ceftazidime, ceftizoxime,* and *ceftriaxone*—further expand the spectrum of antibacterial activity to include effectiveness against *Pseudomonas aeruginosa,* an organism resistant to all other cephalosporins. Many third-generation drugs also penetrate cerebrospinal fluid.

Purpose

• To treat infection caused by gram-negative and, to a lesser extent, gram-positive organisms
• To provide prophylaxis before surgery.

Indications

Specifically, cephalosporins combat infections of the skin, soft tissues, bones, joints, and urinary and respiratory tracts caused mainly by staphylococci, streptococci, *Escherichia coli, Proteus mirabilis,* and shigella. They may also be used prophylactically before cardiac, orthopedic, gynecologic, or bowel surgery.

Cephalosporins are contraindicated in patients with a previous anaphylactic reaction to cephalosporins or penicillins (possible cross-allergenicity). They should not be used concurrently with other nephrotoxic drugs and should be used cautiously in patients with renal impairment.

Adverse reactions

Hypersensitivity reactions range from mild rashes, fever, and eosinophilia to fatal anaphylaxis and are more common in patients with penicillin allergy. Hematologic reactions include positive direct and indirect antiglobulin test (Coombs' test), thrombocytopenia or thrombocythemia, transient neutropenia, and reversible leukopenia. Adverse renal reactions are most common in older patients, those with decreased renal function, and those taking other nephrotoxic drugs. GI reactions include nausea, vomiting, diarrhea, abdominal pain, glossitis, dyspepsia, and tenesmus. Local pain and irritation are common after I.M. injection. Bacterial and fungal superinfection results from suppression of normal flora. Disulfiram-type reactions occur when cefamandole, cefoperazone, moxalactam, cefonicid, or cefotetan are administered within 48 to 72 hours of alcohol ingestion.

Care considerations

• Be alert for signs of cephalosporin hypersensitivity.
• If administering a cephalosporin I.V., infuse it over at least 30 minutes; too-rapid infusion causes pain, vein irritation, and phlebitis. If administering a cephalosporin I.M., apply ice packs to the site before and after injection. If administering one orally, give it with food to reduce nausea, vomiting, or diarrhea.
• Check for signs of superinfection, a common complication of oral administration marked by diarrhea, vaginal itching, or sore mouth. Also monitor prothrombin time because some cephalosporins, such as moxalactam, can cause hypoprothrombinemia.
• For patients who require dialysis, administer cephalosporins *after* a treatment to prevent reduced drug effectiveness. If the patient is receiving probenecid, expect increased cephalosporin blood levels. Notify the doctor.

Home care instructions

• Instruct the patient to immediately report signs of an allergic reaction (rash, hives and, possibly, fever) or decreased urine output to his doctor.
• Tell the patient to take oral cephalosporins on an empty stomach unless doing so causes GI upset.
• Advise the patient to avoid alcohol. Some cephalosporins interact with it, causing flushing, nausea, and palpitations (disulfiram reaction).

• Instruct the patient to complete the full course of therapy (usually 7 to 10 days).

CEREBRAL ANEURYSM REPAIR

An aneurysm is an area of dilation or outpouching of a blood vessel wall. For cerebral aneurysm, surgical treatment is the only sure way to prevent initial rupture or rebleeding with subsequent bleeding into the subarachnoid space.

The surgeon can choose among several techniques for aneurysm repair, depending on the shape and location of the aneurysm. These techniques include clamping the affected artery, wrapping the aneurysm wall with a biological or synthetic material, or clipping or ligating the aneurysm. Clipping is the treatment of choice. (See *Techniques for repairing aneurysms*, page 160.)

The decision to perform surgery is based on many factors, such as the location of the aneurysm, the presence or absence of vasospasm, and the general condition of the patient.

Purpose

• To repair a cerebral aneurysm, thereby preventing possible rupture or rebleeding and stabilizing cerebral blood flow.

Indications

Surgical intervention may be performed to prevent initial rupture of a cerebral aneurysm or to stop bleeding associated with rupture.

Procedure

After cerebral arteriography has identified the location of the aneurysm and ruled out vasospasm, the surgeon will perform a craniotomy to expose the aneurysm. Because cerebral aneurysms usually occur in the internal carotid or middle cerebral artery, craniotomy is usually done in the suboccipital or subfrontal areas. The surgeon visualizes the aneurysm with the aid of a microscope and then carefully frees the aneurysm from the arachnoid tissue and wraps it with a biological or synthetic material. To clip the aneurysm, the surgeon opens a small, spring-loaded clip and slips it over the neck of the aneurysm or over its feeder vessel. (A large aneurysm may require more than one clip.) When the clip is in place, he releases it, letting it close to block blood flow to the aneurysm. The surgeon may simply leave the clip in place or may secure it with methyl methacrylate or a similar liquid agent that quickly solidifies around the clip and the aneurysm. He then ligates and removes the sac of the aneurysm. The surgeon then reverses the craniotomy procedure to close the incision.

Complications

The complications of cerebral aneurysm repair are similar to those of a craniotomy: infection, hemorrhage, respiratory compromise, and increased intracranial pressure (ICP). An additional risk is vasospasm, which can spread through the major cerebral vessels and cause ischemia and possible infarction of involved areas. The patient's surgical risk depends on his preoperative condition and the complexity of the required surgery.

Care considerations
Before surgery
• Explain the surgical procedure to the patient. A clipped aneurysm seals off the aneurysm from the cerebral circulation, preventing vessel rupture. If the aneurysm will be wrapped, explain that this technique supports the arterial wall.
• Monitor neurologic status, maintain a stress-free environment, and include other measures to prevent rupture or rebleeding and their complications, such as increased ICP and pulmonary

Techniques for repairing aneurysms

Using a metal spring clip, the surgeon can isolate a berry aneurysm (named for its shape) from the cerebral circulation. With other types of aneurysms, such as a fusiform aneurysm, the arterial wall is wrapped with biological or synthetic material for support.

Clipping a berry aneurysm

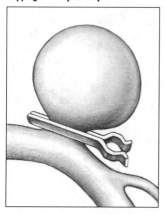

Wrapping a fusiform aneurysm

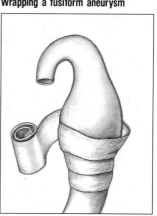

emboli. Provide emotional support to the patient and family.

• Record all assessment data, such as pupillary response, level of consciousness (LOC), and motor function, as a baseline for your postoperative evaluation. Immediately, report signs of bleeding, such as a new or worsening headache, renewed or increased nuchal rigidity, or decreasing LOC.

• Restrict the patient's activities and limit visitors. Explain the reasons for this to the patient and the family.

• Administer medications, as ordered. These may include anticonvulsants to prevent seizures, corticosteroids to prevent cerebral edema, stool softeners to prevent increased ICP caused by straining, and analgesics to relieve headache. If the patient is receiving I.V. fluids, monitor and record intake and output.

• Ensure that the patient has signed a consent form for surgery.

After surgery

• Monitor the patient's vital signs as well as his fluid and electrolyte balance and neurologic status.

• Notify the doctor of any change in the patient's neuromuscular status or of hemiparesis, worsening of an existing motor deficit, visual disturbances, seizures, or altered LOC.

• Encourage deep-breathing, but warn the patient that coughing and sneezing may cause problems. If you need to suction the patient, do so gently.

• Carefully turn the patient every 2 hours. As appropriate, encourage range-of-motion exercises every 2 hours. (If the patient can't perform active exercises, provide passive leg exercises more often than every 2 hours to help prevent thrombus formation.) Also apply anti-embolism stockings, elastic bandages, or intermittent pneumatic compression stockings (see *Understanding IPC stockings*, page 47).

• Provide good wound care. Make sure the dressing stays dry and in place, and that it's not too tight. Notify the doctor of excessive bloody drainage, indicative of cerebral hemorrhage, or clear yellow drainage, indicative of cerebrospinal fluid leak. Monitor for signs of wound infection.

• Encourage a quiet, calm environment to minimize anxiety and help lower ICP.

• Administer anticonvulsants as ordered, and maintain seizure precautions. As ordered, give corticosteroids to reduce cerebral edema, stool softeners to prevent straining (which may increase ICP), and analgesics to relieve pain.

Home care instructions

• Emphasize the importance of returning for scheduled follow-up examinations and tests.

• Explain that the patient can gradually resume normal activities.

• Teach the patient how to care for the wound, and tell him to evaluate the incision regularly.

• Inform the patient that he may wear a wig, hat, or scarf if he is self-conscious about his appearance.

• Remind the patient to continue taking prescribed medications, and tell him to report any drug reactions.

CEREBRAL STIMULANTS

Cerebral stimulants—such as *amphetamine sulfate, methylphenidate hydrochloride, dextroamphetamine sulfate,* and *pemoline*—are useful drugs for treating attention deficit disorder with hyperactivity (ADDH). They may be used alone or with psychological treatments and educational or social modifications.

Beginning 2 to 3 weeks after therapy starts, cerebral stimulants achieve a paradoxical calming effect in a child with hyperkinesia. This calming effect increases the child's attention span, curbs impulsiveness, and assists socialization. Relieving the distressing symptoms of ADDH also increases the child's amenability to adjunctive psychotherapy and educational modifications. Before the start of such treatment, the child should have a complete physical examination and have a detailed psychological history taken. During treatment, close supervision is required because of the potential for drug dependence.

The amphetamines were formerly used mainly as appetite suppressants (anorexigenics). However, the Food and Drug Administration has recommended that their use as anorexigenics should be limited to short-term weight control, and only as an adjunct to caloric restriction and behavior modification. Many experts feel that these drugs have no place in weight-control programs.

Purpose

• To produce a calming effect in children with ADDH

• To provide an analeptic effect in narcolepsy.

Indications

Cerebral stimulants may be used for short-term treatment of exogenous obesity. Dextroamphetamine and methylphenidate are therapeutic adjuncts in children with ADDH. Dextroamphetamine, amphetamine sulfate, and methylphenidate may be used to treat adults with narcolepsy.

Amphetamines are contraindicated in patients with symptomatic cardiovascular disease, hyperthyroidism, nephritis, angina pectoris, any degree of hypertension, arteriosclerosis-induced parkinsonism, certain types of glaucoma, advanced arteriosclerosis, agitated states, or a history of substance abuse.

Amphetamines should be used cautiously in patients with diabetes mellitus; in elderly, debilitated, or hyperexcitable patients; and in children with Tourette syndrome. Long-term therapy should be avoided when possible because of the risk of psychological dependence or habituation.

All cerebral stimulants are contraindicated in children under age 3. Methylphenidate and pemoline are also contraindicated in children under age 6 because of the increased risk of Tourette syndrome.

Adverse reactions

Cerebral stimulants commonly cause adverse central nervous system (CNS) reactions, such as restlessness, hyperactivity, talkativeness, and insomnia. Cardiovascular reactions may include tachycardia, palpitations, hypertension, or hypotension. GI reactions may include nausea, vomiting, cramps, diarrhea, anorexia, and weight loss. Prolonged administration of cerebral stimulants to children with ADDH may be associated with temporary decreased growth. Prolonged use may cause physical or psychological dependence.

Care considerations

• Observe the patient for signs of excessive stimulation: rapid pulse, hypertension, and nervousness. Such effects may require a reduced dosage.
• Because methylphenidate and pemoline may precipitate Tourette syndrome and amphetamine may intensify symptoms of this disorder, observe children receiving these drugs for tic, echolalia (patient repeats words addressed to him), coprolalia (use of foul language), and motor incoordination, especially at the start of therapy.
• During pemoline therapy, periodic liver function studies are recommended to monitor for hepatic dysfunction.
• If the patient has diabetes, regularly check the blood glucose level because cerebral stimulants may alter insulin

requirements. Also review the patient's medication regimen for possible interactions. Concurrent use of monoamine oxidase inhibitors, for example, could cause life-threatening hypertensive crisis. Antacids, acetazolamide, and sodium bicarbonate increase the effects of cerebral stimulants; phenothiazines and haloperidol decrease them.
• If a child is receiving long-term therapy, check height and weight regularly to detect growth retardation.

Home care instructions

• Inform the patient or parents to administer the drug at least 6 hours before bedtime to prevent insomnia and, if appropriate, after meals to reduce appetite suppression.
• Tell the patient to take a missed dose only if remembered more than 2 hours before the next scheduled dose.
• Warn the patient or parents to restrict hazardous activities that require alertness or good motor coordination until the patient's CNS response to the drug has been determined.
• Tell the patient to avoid coffee, chocolate, colas, and other caffeinated products. These substances enhance the effects of most cerebral stimulants.
• Warn the patient or parents against suddenly discontinuing the medication after long-term use. Acute rebound depression will occur unless the dose is decreased gradually.
• Remind the patient or parents that cerebral stimulants are addictive and should be stored in a secure location.

CERVICAL CONIZATION

Cervical conization, also referred to as cone biopsy, is the surgical removal of a cone-shaped portion of the uterine cervix for diagnostic and therapeutic purposes. Before development of colposcopic evaluation, conization was the method of choice for evaluating ab-

Performing cervical conization

These illustrations indicate the area that is removed during conization.

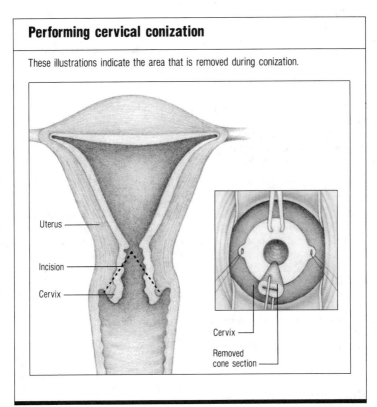

Uterus

Incision

Cervix

Cervix

Removed cone section

normal Papanicolaou (PAP) tests. It is currently performed less often and only in selected cases.

Purpose

• To remove a portion of the uterine cervix for diagnosis or treatment of cervical dysplasia.

Indications

Conization is most commonly indicated to remove a precancerous portion of the endocervix (inside the cervical canal) when there is positive dysplasia (abnormal development) noted during endocervical curettage.

Conization is also indicated when colposcopic examination is inadequate to rule out squamous cell carcinoma and when there is evidence of severe dysplasia and cancer in situ, especially if multiple lesions are present. (Laser carbon dioxide therapy may be used for lesser lesions, to retain optimum fertility, or for conditions such as chronic cervicitis, condylomata, and moderate dysplasia.)

Procedure

The procedure is performed in the outpatient department, and the patient receives general anesthesia. The surgeon uses a cold scalpel (cold knife) or a laser to cut a circular incision around the external opening of the cervix to remove a cone-shaped piece of tissue. A laser is believed to cause less bleeding of the operative site. The surgeon then sutures the site. (See *Performing cervical conization*.)

Complications

Potential complications include cervical perforation, heavy bleeding, infection, infertility, cervical stenosis, decreased cervical mucus, and premature labor in future pregnancies due to weakening of the cervix.

There seems to be a direct correlation between the size of the cone and the incidence of complications. The best method to decrease the incidence of complications is to limit the size of the cone.

Care considerations

• Because conization is performed on an outpatient basis, preoperative care must include patient teaching about complications and follow-up care.
• After surgery, monitor the patient's vital signs frequently for any indication of hemorrhage or shock.
• Provide a sanitary pad, and instruct the patient to monitor the amount and color of all vaginal drainage.
• Offer analgesics as needed.
• Provide emotional support relevant to the diagnosis.

Home care instructions

• Explain the importance of the patient's taking all prophylactic antibiotics (doxycycline for 5 to 7 days may be ordered).
• Instruct the patient to return for follow-up examination in 2 to 4 weeks.
• Tell the patient to immediately report any signs or symptoms of infection or excessive bleeding.
• Emphasize the importance of lifelong follow-up care. Current recommendations are for Pap tests every 6 to 12 months.
• Teach the patient that menstrual bleeding may be heavier, with brownish premenstrual discharge.
• Instruct the patient to maintain pelvic rest (avoiding intercourse, tampons, and douches) until after the postoperative visit.

CERVICAL SUTURING

Cervical suturing (cerclage) uses a purse-string suture to reinforce an incompetent cervix in order to maintain pregnancy. Typically performed between the 14th and 18th week of gestation, after the major risk of spontaneous abortion has passed, cervical suturing is indicated for patients with a history of premature delivery caused by an incompetent cervix.

Two cervical suturing procedures are commonly used. The *modified Shirodkar technique* involves threading and tying a Mersilene band around the internal cervical os of the uterus. *Cervical cerclage*, or the *McDonald procedure*, places a nonabsorbable suture around the cervix, high on the mucosa. Both techniques are successful in maintaining pregnancy for about 90% of patients.

Purpose

• To maintain closure of the internal cervical os until the pregnancy has reached term, preventing premature labor and delivery.

Indications

Cerclage is indicated when an incompetent cervix is confirmed. Some factors that predispose to cervical incompetence are previous second-trimester elective abortion, previous difficult delivery, trauma to the cervix, and cervical conization.

Cervical suturing is contraindicated if the patient has vaginal bleeding or uterine cramping, or if ultrasonography indicates that the fetus is not viable.

Procedure

Before the procedure, ultrasound examination is performed to verify that the fetus is viable. After fetal viability has been established, the patient will receive spinal or general anesthesia.

Cervical cerclage

In a patient with an incompetent cervix, the cervical canal partially dilates, allowing the membranes to prolapse. To help correct this defect and allow a pregnancy to continue, the doctor may perform cervical cerclage. In this procedure, he places a nonabsorbable suture (Mersilene) around the cervix beneath the mucosa to constrict the opening as shown here.

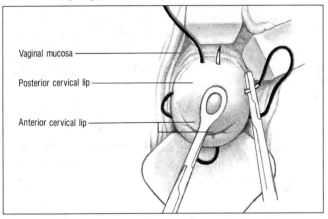

Vaginal mucosa

Posterior cervical lip

Anterior cervical lip

As shown in this cross section, the suture works much like the string in a drawstring bag. The key to this procedure's success is placing the suture high enough on the cervix so that it remains in place.

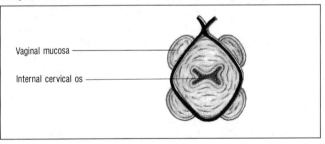

Vaginal mucosa

Internal cervical os

Then, if using the modified Shirodkar technique, the surgeon retracts the vaginal walls with an instrument and elevates the vaginal mucous membrane. After making an incision, the surgeon weaves a narrow nonabsorbable suture, such as Mersilene, around the internal cervical os of the uterus, tightens the suture to close the os, restores the vaginal mucosa to its original position, and sutures it in place, usually with an absorbable suture. For information on the McDonald procedure, see *Cervical cerclage*.

The sutures are allowed to remain in place until the pregnancy has reached full term, at which time the sutures are removed and labor is allowed to begin spontaneously.

Complications

Cervical suturing can cause complications such as preterm labor, hemorrhage, sepsis, or rupture of the amniotic membranes during the procedure. Occasionally, scarring and stenosis of the os occur as a result of suturing and render the cervix incapable of dilating after the suture is removed. When this happens, a cesarean delivery is necessary.

Care considerations

Before surgery
• Inform the patient that she'll receive anesthesia and that she will be hospitalized for 1 to 2 days.
• Briefly explain the procedure to the patient. Tell her that the suture will be surgically removed when pregnancy has reached full term, allowing labor to begin spontaneously.
• Ensure that the patient has signed a consent form.
• Perform a thorough obstetric history, and assess the patient to verify that the amniotic membranes have not ruptured and the cervix isn't effaced more than 50%.

After surgery
• Monitor the fetal heart rate after the procedure, as ordered, or at least every 30 minutes.
• Note the amount of blood on the perineal pad. Spotting is normal, but report any bright red blood immediately. Also report any uterine contractions, fever, or amniotic membrane rupture.
• Maintain bed rest for 24 hours, and increase the patient's activity afterward as appropriate.

Home care considerations

• Instruct the patient to immediately report uterine contractions, amniotic membrane rupture, vaginal bleeding, fever, or pain.
• Tell the patient to expect some spotting from the cervical incision for several days after the procedure, but to immediately report bright red blood or excessive bleeding to the doctor.
• Instruct her to change the perineal pad as needed or at least every 8 hours. Mention that she may find tiny pieces of suture on the pad. Reassure her that these come from the absorbable suture used to close the incision – not from the suture holding the cervix closed.
• Tell the patient to abstain from intercourse until she has had her postoperative checkup. Inform her that pelvic rest and bed rest may be prescribed for the remainder of the pregnancy.

CESAREAN SECTION

Cesarean section is an operative procedure in which the fetus is delivered by surgical incisions in the abdominal wall and uterus. It becomes necessary when vaginal delivery is unsafe for mother or fetus.

Several approaches may be used. The procedure of choice – lower segment cesarean delivery – involves a vertical or horizontal abdominal incision as well as an incision in the lower uterine segment. This characteristically leads to less maternal blood loss and a stronger uterine scar than the classic procedure, which involves vertical incisions in both the abdomen and uterus.

The current cesarean section rate is 25%. This represents both elective and unanticipated cesarean births.

Purpose
• To manage or prevent maternal or fetal complications resulting from conditions that make vaginal delivery hazardous or impossible.

Indications
The most common indication for cesarean delivery is cephalopelvic disproportion. This occurs when there is a spatial inadequacy of the maternal

pelvis in relation to the fetal head, which interferes with the fetus's negotiating the pelvic canal. Other indications for cesarean delivery include severe pregnancy-induced hypertension, maternal diabetes, placenta previa, fetal distress, premature separation of the placenta, breech presentation, prolapsed umbilical cord, previous uterine surgery, and an ineffective labor pattern caused by uterine dysfunction.

Procedure

To begin, the patient will receive general or regional (spinal or epidural) anesthesia. If both are contraindicated, local anesthesia may be given. Shaving and cleaning the incisional site may be performed in the operating room immediately before the operation.

The surgeon makes an abdominal incision, retracts the bladder, and makes an incision in the uterus. He then removes the retractor and delivers the fetal presenting part. Next, he suctions the infant's nose and mouth with a bulb syringe to clear the airway. Then he completes the delivery. After he clamps and cuts the umbilical cord, the surgeon transfers the infant to the neonatal team.

Next, the surgeon administers I.V. oxytocin to contract the uterus. This helps reduce blood loss and promotes delivery of the placenta. Then he closes the incision. Finally, the fundus is palpated and massaged to help contract the uterus because uterine relaxation may cause hemorrhage.

Complications

Maternal complications may include anesthesia reactions, infection, hemorrhage, wound dehiscence, and injury to pelvic or abdominal organs. Fetal complications may include hypoxia, acidosis, respiratory distress, and prematurity.

Care considerations

Before surgery

• Explain the procedure to the parents, and tell them what they should expect after the birth.
• Monitor maternal vital signs, labor status, and fetal heart rate.
• Prepare the patient for an I.V. infusion to provide hydration, fluid replacement, and access for medication.
• Inform the patient that she'll have an indwelling urinary catheter inserted to prevent bladder damage during surgery.
• Ensure that the patient has signed a consent form.
• If the patient's partner is allowed in the operating room, have him scrub or dress according to hospital policy.

After surgery

• Palpate the fundus to determine uterine relaxation. The uterus should be firm, indicating contraction. However, if the uterus is deviated to the left or is higher than the umbilicus, check the patency of the indwelling urinary catheter. This may indicate that the bladder is full and is displacing the uterus.
• Monitor the patient's vital signs. Be alert for signs that may indicate hemorrhage, shock, or infection.
• Record intake and output to help determine the rate of fluid replacement. After removal of the indwelling urinary catheter, check for dysuria and decreased output.
• Evaluate the lochia; initially, it will contain clots. Note the lochia's color (red for the first 3 or 4 days postpartum), amount (moderate is normal; a heavy discharge may indicate excessive bleeding), and odor (if unusual, suspect infection).
• If the patient received a spinal or an epidural anesthetic, explain that she'll experience tingling when sensation returns. If she received a spinal anesthetic, explain that she may have a headache. Measures to prevent such headache include adequate hydration

and lying flat in bed for 8 hours post-operatively.

• Check the dressing for bleeding and the wound for signs of infection and hematoma formation.

• To promote maternal-infant bonding, provide for early contact between the mother and her infant, if appropriate. Allow the patient to express any anger, guilt, or grief she may feel about not experiencing vaginal delivery or about the condition of her infant.

Home care instructions

• Tell the patient to immediately report hemorrhage, chest or leg pain (possible thrombosis), dyspnea, separation of the edges of the incision, and signs of infection (fever, difficult urination, or flank pain).

• Remind the patient to keep her follow-up appointment (usually in 4 weeks). At that time, she can talk to the doctor about contraceptive measures and resumption of intercourse.

• Have the patient check with her doctor before resuming an exercise program. Isometric exercises and walking will probably be permitted. Tell her to avoid strenuous exercises until after her postpartum checkup.

CHELATION THERAPY FOR LEAD POISONING

Chelation therapy is the administration of drugs that are used to bind with lead present in the body to facilitate its excretion and reduce its toxic effects. It is commonly used to treat lead poisoning. Lead poisoning is considered the most serious chronic childhood disease in children in the United States today. Chelation therapy may also be used to bind with other metals, such as iron, arsenic, and mercury.

Several medications are available for chelation therapy. Age, health status, presence of iron deficiency anemia or sickle cell disease, and the environment of the home and any additional addresses of the child are all factors that determine the use and method of chelation therapy.

Chelation therapy is not a permanent solution to the problem of lead poisoning. Only abatement of the housing unit in which the child lives or moving the family to lead-safe housing can be considered permanent treatment of the problem.

Purpose

• To increase excretion of lead from the body.

Indications

Children with blood lead levels of 40 mcg/dl or more are candidates for chelation therapy.

Chelation therapy using edetate calcium disodium (Calcium EDTA) is contraindicated in patients with severe renal disease and inadequate urine output. Dimercaprol should only be used in life-threatening situations, such as lead encephalopathy, in patients with normal levels of glucose-6-phosphate dehydrogenase (G6PD) because the drug may induce hemolysis in these patients.

Procedure
For dimercaprol
Dimercaprol is usually used with edetate calcium disodium and only in children with blood lead levels over 70 mcg/dl or those who are symptomatic (ataxia, vomiting, lethargy, coma, or seizures). This drug increases the excretion of lead in feces and urine. However, because the primary site of excretion is through the liver, dimercaprol can be used in patients with renal impairment. Dimercaprol is available in oil only and is administered I.M. Dosage depends on the lead level and the presence or absence of overt symptoms. The maximum dosage the patient can tolerate is given while the

patient is symptomatic and is titrated down as symptoms subside. *Caution:* Dimercaprol should not be used in patients allergic to peanuts or derivative products.

For edetate calcium disodium

This drug is used to treat children with lead levels of 40 mcg/dl or more. It can be given I.M. or I.V., but is typically given I.M. in young children. When administered I.M. with dimercaprol, edetate calcium disodium is given at a different site than dimercaprol. This injection is very painful and should be mixed with procaine hydrochloride. Continuous I.V. infusion of edetate calcium disodium is most effective and may be used in adults with lead poisoning.

Because it is a cardiac irritant, edetate calcium disodium should be administered slowly. Do not administer this drug by rapid I.V. infusion because deaths have been reported. In the patient with encephalopathy, it can be given around-the-clock to alleviate symptoms. Therapy is limited to 5-day intervals with a 2-day rest between treatments. If lead levels rebound to 40 mcg/dl or above, this may indicate a need for a repeated course of therapy. Edetate calcium disodium is not recommended for oral use because it enhances the absorption of lead from the GI tract and is itself poorly absorbed.

Edetate calcium disodium without dimercaprol may exacerbate symptoms in patients with very high lead levels; therefore, these two drugs should be used concurrently in symptomatic children and in children with high lead levels.

This drug can be used for outpatient treatment of lead poisoning, but the patient must return to the hospital or clinic to receive the medication.

For succimer

This recently approved drug is used to treat children with lead levels of 45 mcg/dl or more.

Succimer is water soluble and is absorbed readily by the GI tract and therefore may be administered orally. It produces lead diuresis.

When given on an outpatient basis, succimer can be administered by the parent. However, therapy should begin in a hospital setting (especially the first 5 days) until the child's housing is made lead-safe either through abatement or relocation.

For D-penicillamine

Although this drug is not yet approved by the Food and Drug Administration as a chelating agent for lead poisoning, some clinicians use it for this indication. It may be advantageous because it can be given orally for extended periods (weeks to months) and may be given on an outpatient basis, provided the patient complies with clinic visits and remains in lead-safe housing. D-penicillamine has been particularly useful as follow-up therapy after initial treatment of lead poisoning with dimercaprol or edetate calcium disodium.

Complications

The most common adverse effects of dimercaprol are mild febrile reactions, increased levels of hepatic transaminase, nausea with occasional vomiting, headache, mild conjunctivitis, lacrimation (tearing), rhinorrhea (runny nose), and excessive salivation.

Doses of edetate calcium disodium over 1,500 mg/m² of body surface area are nephrotoxic and may cause renal tubular necrosis. Impending renal failure is reversible once therapy is discontinued and the remainder of the drug is excreted. Cardiac arrhythmias may also occur, especially with rapid I.V. infusion.

Succimer can cause drowsiness, dizziness, paresthesia, nausea, vomiting, metallic taste in the mouth, flulike symptoms, and increased levels of hepatic transaminase.

D-penicillamine can cause renal failure, blood dyscrasias, and allergic reactions. Use this drug cautiously in patients with hypersensitivity to penicillin because cross-sensitivity may occur.

Care considerations

Before therapy

• Explain the procedure to the child and parents. If the parents will be administering the drug, make sure they are fully informed about drug administration and possible adverse reactions.

• Check the results of liver function tests as well as blood urea nitrogen (BUN) and creatinine levels before initiation of edetate calcium disodium therapy. If you note any abnormalities, delay therapy and notify the doctor.

• Make referrals to social services as needed. The child will need to be in lead-safe housing when receiving edetate calcium disodium because this therapy will increase GI absorption of lead if exposure to lead continues during treatment. All patients with lead poisoning must eventually have a lead-safe environment for permanent treatment.

During therapy

• Administer the drug as prescribed.

• Ensure adequate I.V. hydration and limit oral intake for the first 48 to 72 hours of dimercaprol therapy to minimize GI distress.

• Do not administer iron therapy to patients receiving dimercaprol therapy. Iron therapy must be delayed until dimercaprol therapy is completed because the combination of medications has an emetic effect.

• Do not mistakenly give edetate disodium as therapy for lead poisoning because it will cause tetany and possibly fatal hypocalcemia.

• Monitor intake and output, BUN, serum creatinine levels, and electrocardiograms in the patient receiving edetate calcium disodium to detect complications. Force fluids to ensure

adequate urine output and facilitate urinary excretion of lead.

After therapy

• Monitor for adverse reactions and response to therapy.

• Make certain that the patient is not discharged to a lead-contaminated environment.

Home care instructions

• Encourage follow-up visits to assess the patient's status and evaluate environmental circumstances.

CHEMOTHERAPY, CANCER

Cancer chemotherapy is the use of drugs designed to attack cells that are rapidly dividing and either kill them or render them incapable of further division. Cancer is many different diseases (over 200); therefore, it's necessary to use many types and combinations of chemotherapy drugs. These agents are classified according to their mechanism of action (see *Classes of chemotherapy drugs*). Treatment can consist of one drug type (single-drug chemotherapy) or multiple drugs (combination chemotherapy). It may be given as the sole treatment (primary treatment) or in combination with other methods, such as surgery or radiation therapy (multimodality treatment).

Purpose

• To eradicate cancer completely

• To control the cancer with the expectation that it will recur and progress in the future

• To alleviate symptoms caused by the cancer (pain, hypercalcemia).

Indications

Cancer chemotherapy is used for cancers that have the potential to—or have already—spread to other sites by means of the bloodstream or lymphatic system or by direct extension. These drugs

Classes of chemotherapy drugs

Chemotherapeutic drugs include alkylating agents, antimetabolites, antibiotic antineoplastics, and hormonal antineoplastics. These drugs destroy cancer cells by interfering with neoplastic cell growth and function. Chemotherapy is most effective during early stages of tumor growth when fewer cancer cells are present. In these early stages, the patient is not weakened and overwhelmed by the disease and is better able to combat the drug's toxic effects. Protocols for administering these drugs vary among facilities.

Alkylating agents

These drugs can inhibit cell division at any point in the cell cycle, but they're most effective in the late G phase and S phase. The alkylating agents include busulfan, carmustine, cisplatin, ifosfamide, and mechlorethamine. Used alone or with other drugs, alkylating agents act against chronic and acute leukemias, non-Hodgkin's lymphomas, multiple myeloma, melanoma, sarcoma, and cancers of the breast, ovary, uterus, lung, brain, testes, bladder, prostate, and stomach.

Antimetabolites

The first group of antineoplastic drugs designed specifically as antitumor agents, antimetabolites act during the entire cell cycle but are most effective during the S phase.

All antimetabolites interfere with deoxyribonucleic acid (DNA) synthesis. Azathioprine, mercaptopurine, and thioguanine inhibit purine synthesis. Cytarabine, floxuridine, and fluorouracil inhibit pyrimidine synthesis. Hydroxyurea inhibits ribonucleotide reductase, and methotrexate prevents reduction of folic acid to dihydrofolate reductase.

Antimetabolites are used to treat acute leukemia, breast cancer, GI tract adenocarcinomas, non-Hodgkin's lymphomas, and squamous cell carcinomas of the head, neck, and cervix.

Antibiotic antineoplastics

These antimicrobial drugs achieve their effects by binding with DNA. Unlike other anti-infective drugs, the antineoplastic antibiotics can inhibit the function of both normal and malignant cells. Except for bleomycin, which causes its major effects in the G2 phase, these drugs are cell-cycle-nonspecific.

Among these agents, bleomycin, dactinomycin, doxorubicin, mitomycin, and procarbazine are used mainly to treat carcinomas, sarcomas, and lymphomas. Daunorubicin is used to treat acute leukemias, and plicamycin is used to treat testicular cancer and hypercalcemia from various causes.

Hormonal antineoplastics

These drugs are especially useful in treating cancer because they inhibit neoplastic growth in specific tissues without directly causing cytotoxicity. Their mechanism of action is not completely understood.

Estrogens, such as chlorotrianisene and diethylstilbestrol, are used as palliative therapy for metastatic breast cancer in postmenopausal women and for men with advanced prostate cancer. Antiestrogens, such as tamoxifen citrate, are favored for advanced breast cancer involving estrogen receptor-positive tumors. Androgens, such as testolactone and testosterone, are indicated for prostate cancer and palliation of advanced breast cancer. The adrenocortical suppressant aminoglutethimide is used against advanced breast cancer. Progestins, such as medroxyprogesterone acetate, are used as palliative treatment for advanced endometrial, breast, and renal cancers. Corticosteroids, such as prednisone and dexamethasone, are useful in treating lymphatic leukemias, myeloma, and malignant lymphomas. Gonadotropin-releasing hormone analogs, such as leuprolide acetate, are used to treat advanced prostate cancer.

are also used to treat certain nonmalignant diseases, such as arthritis and lupus erythematosus.

Because most cancer chemotherapies lower blood counts, they are contraindicated in patients with blood counts below designated levels. Also, patients with fevers should not receive chemotherapy.

Procedure

Cancer chemotherapy can be administered in hospital, ambulatory care, office or clinic, or home settings. Treatments are scheduled to allow recovery of healthy tissues and thus minimize adverse reactions. These drugs are administered in various ways: I.M., I.V., S.C., intra-arterially, orally, topically, intracavitarily, intravesically, and intrathecally. I.V. administration may be peripheral or central. Administration by ambulatory infusion pumps is a new technique using portable, battery-operated pumps. Small enough to hook onto a belt, ambulatory infusion pumps allow the patient to continue his active daily life while receiving continuous chemotherapy.

Cancer chemotherapy drugs are administered by doctors or a chemotherapy-certified nurse according to health care facility, state, and national guidelines. Specific health care facility policies and procedures must be followed at all times for the mixing, transport, administration, and disposal of these drugs. Chemotherapy is administered according to specific protocols that recommend dose, intervals, duration of therapy, and route. Each protocol depends on the individual's cancer type, extent of the disease, and overall status.

Complications

The many toxicities of chemotherapy drugs put the patient at risk for hazardous complications. One common reaction, myelosuppression, leads to decreased numbers of circulating blood cells. When treatment produces a reduced white blood cell (WBC) count, known as leukopenia, the patient is at increased risk for infection; in some instances, colony-stimulating factors may be administered to stimulate the production of WBCs. When chemotherapy reduces the platelet count (thrombocytopenia), the patient is at increased risk for hemorrhage; when it reduces the red blood cells, the patient can develop anemia. The nadir (time of deepest reduction of blood counts) varies with each drug. Nursing interventions are scheduled according to expected nadirs.

Some chemotherapy drugs are vesicants and cause tissue damage if they leak outside the vein. Determining vein patency before and during administration is crucial. Other chemotherapy drugs cause psychological complications, such as depression and altered body image as a result of the disease process and the treatment.

Care considerations
Before therapy
• Determine the educational needs of the patient and family. Answer all questions, and provide explanations when there is evidence of patient misunderstanding or confusion regarding the disease process or treatment.
• Inform the patient and family how to reduce or control the adverse reactions of chemotherapy. (See *Managing common adverse effects of chemotherapy*.)
• Provide emotional support to the patient and family throughout therapy.
• Ensure that an informed consent has been obtained.
• Obtain a detailed medical and drug history.
• Perform a complete physical assessment. Be sure to include hematopoietic status, nutritional status, rehabilitation needs, and self-care abilities.
• Review the results of laboratory and nuclear imaging studies.

Managing common adverse effects of chemotherapy

ADVERSE EFFECT	NURSING ACTIONS	HOME CARE INSTRUCTIONS
Alopecia	• Reassure the patient that alopecia is usually temporary. • Tell the patient that he may experience discomfort before hair loss starts and that alopecia can affect all body hair. It may range from thinning to complete hair loss, and hair may regrow in a different color and texture. • Remember that hair loss is one of the most distressing effects of chemotherapy; it is a daily reminder of having cancer. Caregivers must address issues of body image and self-esteem. Some patients prefer to have their hair cut short to make thinning hair less noticeable.	• Advise the patient to wash his hair with a mild shampoo and avoid frequent brushing, combing, use of rollers, or permanent-waving. • Suggest wearing a hat, scarf, toupee, or wig. • Provide a list of local support services, such as those offered by the American Cancer Society and the Look Good-Feel Better program.
Anorexia	• Assess the patient's nutritional status before and during chemotherapy. Weigh him weekly or as ordered. • Explain the need for adequate nutrition despite loss of appetite.	• Encourage the patient's family to supply nutritional foods to help him maintain his weight. • Suggest that the patient eat small, frequent meals. Also advise use of high-calorie supplements.
Bone marrow depression (leukopenia, thrombocyto-penia, anemia)	• Establish baseline white blood cell (WBC) and platelet counts, hemoglobin level, and hematocrit before therapy begins. Monitor these studies during therapy. • Absolute neutrophil count (ANC) is used to determine the potential risk of infection. (ANC = WBC × neutrophil count ÷ 100). The normal range of ANC is 2,500 to 6,000 cells/mm³; an ANC > 1,000 cells/mm³ indicates low or mild risk; 500 to 1,000 cells/mm³, moderate risk; < 500 cells/mm³, high or severe risk. • Report an ANC below 2,000 cells/mm³ or a platelet count below 100,000 as required by the facility's guidelines.	• Instruct the patient to immediately report fever, chills, sore throat, lethargy, unusual fatigue, or pallor. • Warn the patient to avoid exposure to persons with infections for several months. • Explain that the patient and his family shouldn't receive immunizations during or shortly after chemotherapy because an exaggerated reaction may occur.

(continued)

Managing common adverse effects of chemotherapy *(continued)*

ADVERSE EFFECT	NURSING ACTIONS	HOME CARE INSTRUCTIONS
Bone marrow depression *(continued)*	• Monitor temperature orally every 4 hours, and regularly inspect the skin and body orifices for signs of infection. Observe for petechiae, easy bruising, and bleeding at all orifices and lines. Check for hematuria and tarry stools, and also monitor the patient's blood pressure. Be alert for signs of anemia. • Limit S.C. and I.M. injections. If these are necessary, apply pressure for 3 to 5 minutes after injection to prevent leakage or hematoma. Report unusual bleeding after injection. • Take precautions to prevent bleeding. Use extra care with razors, nail trimmers, dental floss, toothbrushes, and other sharp or abrasive objects. Avoid digital examinations, rectal suppositories, and enemas. Increase fluid intake to prevent constipation. • Administer vitamin and iron supplements, as ordered. Provide a diet high in iron.	• Tell the patient to avoid activities that could cause traumatic injury and bleeding. Advise him to report any episodes of bleeding or bruising to the doctor. • Tell the patient to eat high-iron foods, such as liver and spinach. • Stress the importance of follow-up blood studies even after completion of treatment.
Diarrhea and abdominal cramps	• Assess the frequency, color, consistency, and amount of diarrhea. Give antidiarrheals, as ordered. • Assess the severity of cramps, and observe for signs of dehydration (poor skin turgor, oliguria, irritability) and acidosis (confusion, nausea, vomiting, decreased level of consciousness), which may indicate electrolyte imbalance. • Assess for bowel perforation. • Encourage fluids and, if ordered, give I.V. fluids and potassium supplements. • Provide good skin care, especially to the perianal area.	• Teach the patient how to use antidiarrheals, and instruct him to report diarrhea to the doctor. • Encourage the patient to maintain an adequate fluid intake and to follow a bland, low-fiber diet. • Explain that good perianal hygiene can help prevent tissue breakdown and infection.
Nausea and vomiting	• Before chemotherapy begins, administer antiemetics, as ordered, to reduce the severity of these reactions. Continue antiemetics as needed.	• Provide an antiemetic plan for the patient and his family, including how and when to

Managing common adverse effects of chemotherapy *(continued)*

ADVERSE EFFECT	NURSING ACTIONS	HOME CARE INSTRUCTIONS
Nausea and vomiting *(continued)*	• Monitor and record the frequency, character, and amount of vomitus. • Monitor serum electrolyte levels, and provide total parenteral nutrition if necessary.	take the medication, what to report if the medication is ineffective, and an appropriate hydration and nutrition plan.
Stomatitis	• Before drug administration, observe for dry mouth, erythema, and white patchy areas on the oral mucosa. Be alert for bleeding gums or complaints of a burning sensation when drinking acidic liquids. • Emphasize the principles of good mouth care with the patient and his family. • Provide mouth care every 4 to 6 hours (while the patient is awake) with an appropriate solution as determined by the facility's guidelines. Avoid lemon or glycerin swabs because they tend to reduce saliva and change mouth pH. • Provide daily applications of fluoride gel. • Ask the dietitian to provide bland foods at medium temperatures.	• Instruct the patient to prevent trauma to the oral cavity by avoiding smoking, alcohol, spicy foods, and extremely hot or cold foods or liquids. • Teach the patient and his family how to do oral assessments daily and to report any changes promptly. • Encourage meticulous brushing and flossing, as appropriate. • If the patient has dentures, they should be left out as much as possible and cleaned several times a day.

• Develop a plan of care for managing symptoms and identifying long- and short-term needs.

During therapy
• Provide a relaxed environment.

After therapy
• Document the patient's response during therapy and his response to treatment.

• Monitor for adverse reactions. These reactions depend on the specific drug and its dose, the patient's physical and psychological status and his sensitivity to the drug, as well as the type of cancer and its extent. Adverse reactions include alopecia, myelosuppression, nausea, vomiting, stomatitis, and alterations in bowel function. Other reactions include fatigue, dermatologic reactions, and altered reproductive and sexual function. Adverse reactions can range from mild to severe; they can be acute, subacute, chronic, or long-term or latent, and they are drug-specific. It's important to remember that each patient is an individual and will react differently.

Home care instructions

• Be sure the patient understands the potential toxicities and interventions available to minimize or control them.

• Provide telephone numbers of resource persons the patient may call (doctor, nurse, and other health care workers) if concerns arise.
• Make appointments for follow-up laboratory studies and medical visits.
• Provide a plan of care for the patient's home needs, including rehabilitation, a safe home environment, interventions to minimize or prevent chemotherapy toxicity, and possible referrals to home health agencies.
• Provide a list of resources, such as the American Cancer Society and local support groups, for the patient and family.

CHEST DRAINAGE THERAPY

Chest drainage therapy is used to relieve the accumulation of air, fluid, or pus in the pleural space. A chest tube is inserted and connected to suction or a water-seal drainage system. This drainage system permits air and fluid to leave the chest and not be drawn back in during inspiration. As negative pleural pressure is restored, the lung can reinflate. When all of the air and fluid have been removed and the lung fully reexpands, the chest tube is removed and chest drainage is discontinued.

Purpose

• To remove air, blood, or pus from the pleural space, permitting lung reinflation
• To remove blood from the mediastinum after heart surgery.

Indications

Chest drainage therapy is indicated for patients with pneumothorax, hemothorax, chylothorax, empyema, or pleural effusion. All patients who have major lung surgery, except those having a pneumonectomy, will require chest drainage. Chest drainage is also used after heart surgery to drain blood from the mediastinum.

When a collapsed lung is not life-threatening, as with empyema, a related contraindication is prolonged prothrombin time. With a life-threatening collapsed lung, establishing chest drainage is often an emergency procedure and has no contraindications.

Procedure

Except for intraoperative insertions, the patient is awake during insertion of chest tubes and receives a local anesthetic. When the doctor inserts the chest tube into the desired location in the pleural space, the external end of the tube is connected to the chest drainage system. The proximal end is stablized by suturing the tube into place. Petroleum gauze and a dry sterile dressing are then applied. To prevent dislodgment, the chest tube should be taped to the patient's chest wall distal to the insertion site. All tube connections are taped, and suction is regulated as ordered.

A disposable water-seal drainage system is used most commonly. This compact, one-piece unit is composed of three compartments. The first compartment collects the fluid drained from the chest; the second compartment—the water-seal chamber—allows pleural air to escape but prevents the return of atmospheric air; and the third compartment controls suction. The amount of water in the third chamber determines the degree of suction.

Disposable waterless systems are also available. In these systems, no water is added to the suction-control chamber; instead, a screw-type valve or spring is used to regulate suction. (See *Managing problems of chest drainage*.)

Complications

Tension pneumothorax, a life-threatening complication, can result from an occluded or dislodged chest tube or

Managing problems of chest drainage

PROBLEM	NURSING INTERVENTIONS
Patient rolls over on drainage tubing, causing obstruction.	• Reposition patient and remove any kinks in the tubing. • Auscultate for decreased breath sounds and percuss for dullness, indicating fluid accumulation, or for hyperresonance, indicating air accumulation.
Dependent loops in tubing trap fluids and prevent effective drainage.	• Make sure chest drainage unit sits below patient's chest level. If necessary, raise the bed slightly to increase gravity flow. Remove kinks in tubing. • Monitor for decreased breath sounds and percuss for dullness.
No drainage appears in the collection chamber.	• If not draining blood or other fluid, suspect a clot or obstruction in the tubing. Gently milk the tubing to expel the obstruction if hospital policy permits. • Monitor the patient for lung tissue compression (atelectasis) caused by accumulated pleural fluid.
Substantial increase in bloody drainage occurs, indicating possible active bleeding or drainage of old blood.	• Monitor patient's vital signs. Look for increased pulse rate, decreased blood pressure, and orthostatic changes that may indicate acute blood loss. • Measure drainage every 15 to 30 minutes to determine if it occurs continuously or in one gush caused by position changes.
No bubbling is seen in the suction-control chamber.	• Check for obstructions in the tubing. Make sure connections are tight. • Check that suction apparatus is turned on. Increase suction slowly until you see gentle bubbling.
Loud, vigorous bubbling occurs in the suction-control chamber.	• Turn down the suction source until bubbling is just visible.
Evaporation causes the water level in the suction-control chamber to drop below desired -20 cm H_2O.	• Using a syringe and needle, add water or 0.9% sodium chloride solution through the resealable diaphragm on the back of the suction-control chamber.
Patient has trouble breathing immediately after a special procedure. The chest drainage unit is improperly placed on his bed, interfering with drainage.	• Raise the head of the bed and reposition the unit so that gravity promotes drainage. • Perform a quick respiratory assessment and take the patient's vital signs. Check to ensure that there's enough water in the water-seal and suction-control chambers.

(continued)

Managing problems of chest drainage (continued)	
PROBLEM	**NURSING INTERVENTIONS**
As the bed is lowered, the chest drainage unit gets caught under the bed; the tubing comes apart and becomes contaminated.	• Clamp the chest tube proximal to the latex connection tubing. • Irrigate the tubing using the sealed jar of sterile water or 0.9% sodium chloride solution kept at the patient's bedside. • Insert the distal end of the chest tube into the jar of fluid until the end is ¾″ to 1½″ (2 to 4 cm) below the top of the water. Unclamp the chest tube. • Have another nurse obtain a new closed chest drainage system and set it up. • Attach the chest tube to the new unit.

from a malfunctioning chest drainage system. Other complications may include lung puncture at time of chest tube insertion, bleeding, and infection.

Care considerations
Before therapy
• If time permits, explain the procedure to the patient and tell him that it will allow him to breathe more easily.
• Take the patient's vital signs to serve as a baseline.
• Ensure that the patient has signed a consent form.
• Administer a sedative, as prescribed.
• If warranted, obtain the equipment needed for chest tube insertion.
• Set up the water-seal drainage system according to the manufacturer's instructions, and place it at the bedside below the patient's chest level.

During therapy
• Assist with insertion of the chest tube, if warranted, and support the patient.
• Take the patient's vital signs immediately after chest tube insertion and frequently thereafter as warranted by the patient's condition.
• Prepare the patient for a chest X-ray to verify tube placement and to assess the outcome of treatment. As required,

arrange for daily X-rays to monitor his progress.
• Monitor for signs and symptoms of complications. Notify the doctor immediately about hypotension, a rapid thready pulse, severe dyspnea, anxiety, tachypnea, and tracheal deviation, all of which suggest a tension pneumothorax.
• Check the dressing to see that it's airtight, clean, dry, and intact.
• Check the tubing to be sure that it is patent, that all connections are taped, and that dependent loops are avoided.
• Check the collection chamber. Assess the drainage for amount, color, consistency, and rate of flow. Describe and record all drainage on the patient's intake and output sheet.
• Check the water-seal chamber. If the patient has a pneumothorax, anticipate bubbling here because air is being removed from the pleural cavity. When most of the air has been removed, the water-seal chamber should bubble only during forced expiration.
• Check the suction chamber. Make sure the water is bubbling and is filled to the ordered level.

After therapy
• After removal of the chest tube, make certain that an airtight, sterile petroleum dressing is applied to the site.

• Monitor for signs of respiratory distress.

Home care instructions
• Teach the patient with a recently removed chest tube how to clean the wound site and change dressings. Tell him to report any signs of infection.
• Emphasize the importance of keeping follow-up appointments.

CHEST PHYSIOTHERAPY

Chest physiotherapy is a collective term that includes coughing and deep-breathing exercises, postural drainage, and chest percussion and vibration. Together, these techniques aid elimination of secretions and reexpansion of lung tissue and promote efficient use of respiratory muscles. Chest physiotherapy is often combined with other treatments, such as suctioning, incentive spirometry, nebulizer treatments, and administration of expectorants and other drugs.

Successful treatment with chest physiotherapy produces improved breath sounds, improved partial pressure of oxygen in arterial blood, and increased sputum production and air flow.

Chest physiotherapy is contraindicated during active pulmonary bleeding with hemoptysis as well as during the posthemorrhage stage. Other contraindications include fractured ribs, an unstable chest wall, lung contusions, pulmonary tuberculosis, untreated pneumothorax, acute asthma or bronchospasm, pulmonary embolism, lung abscess or tumor, head injury, and recent myocardial infarction.

Purpose
• To mobilize pulmonary secretions (especially from peripheral lung areas)

• To increase clearance of tracheobronchial mucus and promote maximum ventilation.

Indications
Chest physiotherapy is useful for patients with secretions associated with bronchitis, cystic fibrosis, bronchiectasis, or pneumonia; a disease that causes neuromuscular weakness (Guillain-Barré syndrome, myasthenia gravis, tetanus); chronic obstructive pulmonary disease; a disease associated with aspiration (cerebral palsy or muscular dystrophy); or postoperative pain associated with impaired breathing (thoracic or abdominal incisions). It may also be used for patients with prolonged immobility.

Procedure
Chest physiotherapy is often performed for hospitalized patients by a respiratory therapist or a nurse. If such therapy is required after discharge, it can be performed by a family member (see *Mechanical percussion and vibration*, page 180).

Coughing is performed with deep-breathing exercises to help prevent obstruction by keeping the patient's airways clear and open. Coughing dislodges and removes secretions from the pulmonary tree; deep breathing that's performed after coughing increases air in the alveoli and makes the cough more effective.

Postural drainage should follow coughing and deep-breathing exercises to further clear the airways (see *How to perform chest physiotherapy*, page 183). Performed with percussion and vibration treatments, postural drainage is the sequential positioning of the patient so that gravity can drain the peripheral pulmonary secretions into the major bronchi or the trachea (see *Positioning patients for postural drainage*, pages 181 and 182). Secretions usually drain best when the bronchi are positioned perpendicular to the floor. The

Mechanical percussion and vibration

A mechanical percussion and vibration device may be used in the hospital and can also be used by a patient at home to self-administer chest percussion and vibration. Medicare-approved, this device uses directional stroking percussers, which loosen secretions and help move them in the desired direction. A separate pad can be attached to provide chest vibration, and small attachments are available for use with infants.

lower and middle lobe bronchi usually drain best in the head-down position; the upper lobe bronchi, in the head-up position. Chest X-ray results and chest auscultation findings determine which position the patient must assume for the most effective drainage.

In generalized pulmonary disease, drainage usually begins with the lower lobes, continues with the middle lobes, and ends with the upper lobes. In localized disease, drainage should begin with the affected lobes and then proceed to the other lobes to avoid contamination of uninvolved areas.

Percussion is performed by mechanically percussing the chest with cupped hands, a percussion cup, or a mechanical percussion and vibration device. This procedure mechanically dislodges thick, tenacious secretions from the bronchial wall so they can be expectorated or suctioned. If the patient has poor skin turgor, cover the area to be percussed with a gown, thin towel, or other soft clothing to prevent skin trauma.

Vibration is used during postural drainage, either with percussion or as an alternative to it for a patient who's frail, in pain, or recovering from thoracic surgery or trauma. Vibration increases the velocity and turbulence of exhaled air, loosens secretions, and propels them into the larger bronchi so they can be expectorated or suctioned.

Complications

Complications of chest physiotherapy are few. The head-down position used in postural drainage can impair respiratory excursion, which can result in hypoxia or postural hypotension. Vigorous percussion or vibration may cause rib fracture.

Care considerations

• Maintain adequate hydration to dilute and ease mobilization of secretions.
• Evaluate the patient's tolerance for chest physiotherapy and adjust the procedure as necessary. For example, an elderly or debilitated patient may require shorter sessions. Administration of supplemental oxygen may also increase a hypoxic patient's tolerance of chest physiotherapy.
• Observe the patient for fatigue because it diminishes his ability to cough and deep-breathe. The patient who quickly becomes fatigued benefits when therapy is divided into shorter sessions.
• To minimize discomfort, administer pain medication and wait for it to take effect before beginning therapy. For the same reason, surgical patients should splint their incision during therapy.
• Use suction if the patient has a diminished gag reflex or difficulty in expectorating secretions.
• Provide oral hygiene after therapy because secretions may taste foul or have an unpleasant odor.
• Ensure that adjunct therapy — such as intermittent positive-pressure breathing, or aerosol or nebulizer treatment — precedes chest physiotherapy.

Home care instructions

• Teach the patient and his family the appropriate techniques and positions,

Positioning patients for postural drainage

The following illustrations show you the various postural drainage positions and the areas of the lungs affected by each.

Lower lobes: Posterior basal segments
Elevate the foot of the bed 30 degrees. With the patient on his abdomen and his head lowered, position pillows under his chest and abdomen. Percuss his lower ribs on both sides of his spine.

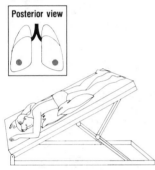

Lower lobes: Lateral basal segments
Elevate the foot of the bed 30 degrees. Instruct the patient to lie on his abdomen with his head lowered and his upper leg flexed over a pillow for support. Then have him rotate a quarter turn upward. Percuss his lower ribs on the uppermost portion of his lateral chest wall.

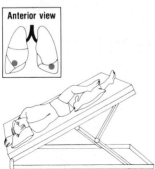

Lower lobes: Anterior basal segments
Elevate the foot of the bed 30 degrees. Instruct the patient to lie on his side with his head lowered. Then place pillows as shown below. Percuss with a slightly cupped hand over his lower ribs just beneath the axilla. *Note:* If an acutely ill patient experiences breathing difficulty in this position, adjust the angle of the bed to one he can tolerate. Then begin percussion.

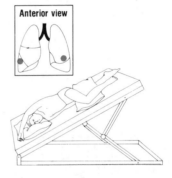

Lower lobes: Superior segments
With the bed flat, have the patient lie on his abdomen. Place two pillows under his hips. Percuss on both sides of his spine at the lower tip of his scapulae.

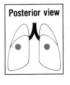
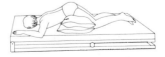

(continued)

Positioning patients for postural drainage *(continued)*

Right middle lobe: Medial and lateral segments

Elevate the foot of the bed 15 degrees. Have the patient lie on his left side with his head lowered and his knees flexed. Then have him rotate a quarter turn backward. Place a pillow beneath him. Percuss with your hand moderately cupped over the right nipple. In females, cup your hand so that its heel is under the armpit and your fingers extend forward beneath her breast.

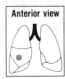

Anterior view

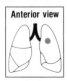

Left upper lobe: Superior and inferior segments (lingular portion)

Elevate the foot of the bed 15 degrees. Have the patient lie on his right side with his head lowered and knees flexed. Then have him rotate a quarter turn backward. Place a pillow behind him, from shoulders to hips. Percuss with your hand moderately cupped over his left nipple. In females, cup your hand so that its heel is beneath the armpit and your fingers extend forward beneath the breast.

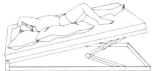

Anterior view

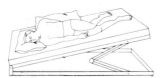

Upper lobes: Anterior segments

Make sure the bed is flat. Instruct the patient to lie on his back with a pillow folded under his knees, as shown below. Then have him rotate slightly away from the side being drained. Percuss between his clavicle and nipple.

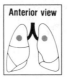

Anterior view

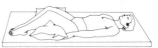

Upper lobes: Apical segments

Keep the bed flat. Have the patient lean back at a 30-degree angle against you and a pillow. Percuss with a cupped hand between his clavicles and the top of each scapula.

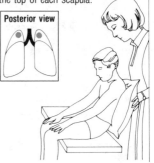

Posterior view

Upper lobes: Posterior segments

Keep the bed flat. Have the patient lean over a pillow at a 30-degree angle. Percuss and clap his upper back on each side.

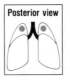

Posterior view

How to perform chest physiotherapy

As you review this guide, keep in mind that coughing and deep-breathing exercises are performed together and that they are followed by postural drainage, which is performed in conjunction with percussion and vibration.

Coughing
- Assume a comfortable upright position.
- Inhale deeply through the nose and exhale in three short huffs.
- Inhale deeply and cough three times with the mouth slightly open.
- Repeat the exercise two or three times.

Deep breathing
- Assume a seated or supine position with the head of the bed elevated. Put one hand on the middle of the chest and the other on the abdomen just below the ribs. This permits you to feel your diaphragm rise and fall.
- Inhale slowly and deeply, pushing your abdomen out against your hand to provide optimal distribution of air to the alveoli. Then, purse your lips and exhale. Contract your abdomen at the same time.
- Breathe this way for 1 minute and then rest for 2 minutes. Gradually progress to a 10-minute exercise period four times a day.

Postural drainage
- Assume the position that most effectively loosens and drains the area.
- Remain in each position for 10 to 15 minutes while another person performs percussion and vibration, as discussed below.

Percussion
- Have the person who will be percussed breathe slowly and deeply, using the diaphragm to promote relaxation.
- Cup your hands with your finger flexed and your thumb tight against your index finger. Percuss each lung segment for 1 to 2 minutes, rhythmically alternating your hands. Listen for a hollow sound to gauge the effectiveness of your technique.

Vibration
- Have the person who requires vibration inhale deeply and exhale slowly through pursed lips. While he exhales firmly, place your hands flat against his chest wall on the lung segment being drained. Position your hands side by side with your fingers extended.
- Vibrate the chest wall by quickly contracting and relaxing the muscles of your arms and shoulders to generate fine vibrations. Stop vibrating during inhalation. Vibrate during five exhalations over each lung segment.

and stress the importance of performing this therapy as directed.
- Arrange for the patient to obtain a percussion cup or a mechanical percussion and vibration device, if prescribed.
- Warn the patient and appropriate family members to avoid percussing over the spine, sternum, liver, kidneys, or the female breasts to prevent injury to internal organs.
- Emphasize the need to maintain adequate hydration.

CHOLINERGIC BLOCKERS

Typically used as an adjunct to histamine-receptor antagonists and antacids, the cholinergic blockers (also called anticholinergics or parasympatholytics) inhibit GI motility and prolong gastric emptying, thereby enhancing the effects of antiulcer drugs.

The cholinergic blockers used for GI dysfunction include the belladonna alkaloids *atropine* and *belladonna elixir;* the quaternary cholinergic blockers *anisotropine methylbromide, isopropamide iodide, methantheline bromide,* and *propantheline bromide;* and the antispasmodic *dicyclomine.* These drugs are usually given orally, although some of them can be given I.V. if the patient requires rapid symptomatic relief.

Antiparkinsonian agents include *benztropine, biperiden, procyclidine, glycopyrrolate, scopolamine,* and *trihexyphenidyl.* The choice of a specific antiparkinsonian agent depends on the patient's response and the drug's pharmacokinetic profile. For example, because both procyclidine and trihexyphenidyl have a direct antispasmodic effect on smooth muscle, they may be especially useful for the patient with muscle rigidity.

Because cholinergic blockers are not organ-specific, their widespread action increases the hazards of various adverse reactions. For example, administration of atropine to reverse severe bradycardia can dry oral and respiratory secretions.

Purpose

• To reduce gastric acid secretion and intestinal motility
• To relax GI smooth muscle
• To relieve parkinsonian and extrapyramidal symptoms
• To treat sinus bradycardia
• To prevent motion sickness
• To decrease secretions.

Indications

Certain cholinergic blockers may be used to help relieve peptic ulcer pain and to treat irritable and spastic colon, other functional GI disorders, and neurogenic bowel disorders. Other cholinergic blockers may be used instead of the naturally occurring belladonna alkaloids to treat Parkinson's disease. Used alone or with levodopa, these drugs are used to treat drug-induced extrapyramidal symptoms, such as tremors and akinesia. Atropine may be used to treat sinus bradycardia caused by drugs, poisons, or sinus node dysfunction. As preanesthetic medications, atropine, glycopyrrolate, and scopolamine are used to reduce salivary and respiratory secretions. Scopolamine may be used to prevent motion sickness.

Cholinergic blockers are usually contraindicated in patients with acute angle-closure glaucoma; tachyarrhythmias or any cardiovascular illness in which an increased heart rate could be hazardous; any obstructive GI or urologic disorder; severe ulcerative colitis; disorders of decreased GI motility, such as paralytic ileus, intestinal atony, and toxic megacolon; and myasthenia gravis. Cholinergic blockers shouldn't be used to treat gastric ulcers because the increased gastric emptying time can aggravate the ulcer. They should be used cautiously in infants, elderly patients, and patients with autonomic neuropathy, hyperthyroidism, hiatal hernia associated with reflux esophagitis, or hepatic or renal dysfunction.

Adverse reactions

Cholinergic blockers may produce adverse GI reactions (dry mouth, thirst, constipation, nausea, and vomiting); urinary symptoms (urinary hesitancy and urine retention); cardiovascular reactions (tachycardia, palpitations, and activation of angina); dermatologic reactions (hot, flushed skin); and visual changes (mydriasis, blurred vision, and photophobia). Because the belladonna alkaloids and antispasmodics are rapidly absorbed and readily cross the blood-brain barrier, they also cause central nervous system (CNS) reactions. In contrast, the quaternary cholinergic blockers, which don't readily cross the blood-brain barrier, cause negligible CNS reactions. Possible CNS reactions include headache, restlessness, ataxia, disorientation, hallucinations, delirium, confusion, insomnia, and coma with excessive dosage.

Care considerations

• When administering a cholinergic blocker, check the dosage carefully; even a slight overdosage can lead to toxicity. Expect to use lower dosages in elderly patients and children, who are most prone to toxic effects.
• Observe for adverse reactions and report them to the doctor, who may want to reduce the dosage. If you detect severe CNS effects, such as delirium or paralysis, immediately discontinue the drug and call the doctor. (Severe CNS effects are most common with belladonna alkaloids or antispasmodics.)
• During therapy with a cholinergic blocker, carefully monitor the patient's vital signs. Be alert for palpitations and tachycardia. Monitor intake and output and assess for signs of urine retention, such as bladder enlargement. To help prevent retention, have the patient void before taking the drug.
• Observe for signs of anhidrosis and hyperthermia; to reduce the risk of hyperthermia, keep the patient's room cool.
• Carefully check for GI effects, including nausea, vomiting or constipation, and abdominal pain and distention; such effects may indicate paralytic ileus.
• Ask the patient about visual changes. If any develop, take precautions to prevent accidents, such as assisting the patient with ambulation and removing furniture and other objects from his path.
• Review the patient's medication regimen for possible interactions. Concurrent use of antiparkinsonian agents with antihistamines, magnesium sulfate, or CNS depressants may cause excessive sedation. Concurrent use of cyclobenzaprine, haloperidol, monoamine oxidase inhibitors, phenothiazines, procainamide, or tricyclic antidepressants may intensify antimuscarinic effects and lead to paralytic ileus. Chlorpromazine may increase anticholinergic activity and actually aggravate parkinsonian symptoms.
• Because antacids and absorbent antidiarrheals may reduce the therapeutic effects of antiparkinsonian agents, give these drugs at least 1 hour before or after an antiparkinsonian agent.

Home care instructions

• Inform the patient of possible adverse reactions. Instruct him to report such effects immediately if they are severe.
• Warn the patient to avoid overexertion in hot or humid weather. Explain that the drug decreases sweating, thereby causing body temperature to rise and possibly leading to heatstroke. Teach him to watch for and report early signs of heatstroke: fever, confusion, and dry skin and mucous membranes.
• Emphasize the importance of immediately reporting any abdominal pain, distention, or constipation, which may signal paralytic ileus.
• Explain that the patient should avoid hazardous activities that require alertness and coordination until CNS response to the drug has been determined.
• Warn the patient to avoid alcohol and other CNS depressants, which increase these drug's sedative effects.
• Suggest alleviating dry mouth with frequent sips of water, ice chips, or sugarless gum or hard candy.

• Explain that these drugs may cause dizziness, confusion, and visual problems. Instruct an elderly patient's caregivers to remove objects that could cause him to fall, such as footstools and throw rugs.
• When taking cholinergic blockers to treat GI dysfunction, the patient should take the drug as prescribed, generally 30 minutes to 1 hour before meals or with meals.
• Warn the patient taking an antiparkinsonian cholinergic blocker never to stop taking the drug without the doctor's approval. Explain that abrupt withdrawal may cause sudden exacerbation of parkinsonian symptoms.
• Instruct the patient to follow the prescribed dosage schedule of the antiparkinsonian cholinergic blocker even if he feels the drug isn't working. Explain that therapeutic effects may not be apparent for several weeks.
• To help minimize gastric irritation caused by an antiparkinsonian cholinergic blocker, tell the patient to take the drug with or immediately after meals.

CHOLINERGICS

Cholinergics, including *carbachol* and *bethanechol*, are used to simulate the actions of acetylcholine at postganglionic neuroeffector sites. Also called parasympathomimetic agents, these drugs produce parasympathetic responses. They are not organ-specific. Thus, these drugs can produce a therapeutic effect at one site (for example, by preventing urine retention in the bladder) and annoying adverse reactions at another (for example, by causing excessive salivation).

Purpose

• To relieve GI and urinary tract atony
• To provide miosis (topical carbachol).

Indications

Bethanechol is used to treat paralytic ileus, postoperative abdominal distention, gastric atony or stasis and, possibly, congenital megacolon. It may also be used to treat postoperative or postpartum urine retention and, in certain cases, neurogenic bladder. Topical carbachol is used to treat glaucoma. Because of its short duration of action, acetylcholine is used only for perioperative miosis.

Adverse reactions

Cholinergics may cause dizziness, confusion, hallucinations, muscle weakness, nervousness, blurred vision, tearing, bronchospasm, bronchial constriction, nausea, vomiting, and belching. These drugs may precipitate asthma attacks in susceptible patients.

Clinical effects of overdose primarily involve muscarinic symptoms, such as nausea, vomiting, diarrhea, abdominal discomfort, involuntary defecation, urinary urgency, increased bronchial and salivary secretions, respiratory depression, skin flushing or heat sensation, and bradycardia; cardiac arrest has also occurred.

Care considerations

• Regularly monitor the patient's vital signs, especially his heart rate and respirations and fluid intake and output.
• Evaluate the patient for changes in muscle strength, and observe closely for adverse drug effects or signs of acute toxicity. Have atropine injection readily available.
• Impose safety precautions. The patient may become restless or confused or may experience blurred vision and need assistance with ambulation.
• Never give bethanechol I.M. or I.V; this could cause circulatory collapse, hypotension, shock, severe abdominal cramping, bloody diarrhea, or cardiac arrest.

Home care instructions

• If appropriate, teach the patient how to instill carbachol. Advise him to wash his hands before and after administering ointment or solution. Instruct him to apply light finger pressure to the lacrimal sac for 1 minute after instillation to reduce systemic absorption.

• Instruct the patient to stop using the drug immediately and contact the doctor if he develops excessive salivation, diarrhea, weakness, or other signs of toxicity.

• Reassure the patient using topical carbachol that the stinging and blurred vision caused by this drug usually diminish with continued use.

• Warn against driving after dark if the drug causes poor night vision.

• Explain to the patient with glaucoma that close medical supervision is vital during cholinergic therapy to monitor intraocular pressure.

CIRCUMCISION

Circumcision is the surgical removal of the foreskin from the glans penis. This procedure is commonly performed on infants; however, much controversy currently surrounds routine neonatal circumcision. Its proponents contend that circumcision helps reduce the risk of future penile cancer and of cervical cancer in female sexual partners and minimizes the risk of phimosis; they also believe that circumcision decreases the risk of urinary tract infections in men. However, in 1975, the American Academy of Pediatrics stated that there was no medical justification for routine circumcision. In 1989, however, the academy changed positions, stating that the procedure may have medical benefits as well as risks. Despite this controversy, circumcision remains the most commonly performed of all pediatric surgeries, largely because this procedure has significance in the Jewish faith.

Purpose

• To correct foreskin disorders
• To remove the foreskin for religious or cultural reasons.

Indications

Excision of the foreskin from the glans penis may be performed on an adult patient to treat phimosis (abnormal tightening of the foreskin around the glans) or paraphimosis (inability to return the foreskin to its normal position after retraction). Most commonly, circumcision is performed on neonates 1 to 2 days after birth or later, if performed for religious or cultural reasons.

In neonates, circumcision is contraindicated in infants who have bleeding disorders or ambiguous genitalia. It is also contraindicated in infants with hypospadias because the foreskin will be needed for later surgical reconstruction. If the mother is infected with human immunodeficiency virus (HIV), the doctor will delay circumcision until the neonate's HIV status is determined.

Procedure

The doctor can choose from several different procedures. For the neonate, he may use a Gomco clamp or plastic circumcision bell (Plastibell). The latter is used to control bleeding. If he's using a plastic bell, he slides the device between the foreskin and glans penis and then tightly ties a length of suture around the foreskin at the glans' coronal edge. The foreskin distal to the suture first becomes ischemic and then atrophic. After 5 to 8 days, the foreskin with the plastic bell attached will drop off, leaving a clean, well-healed line of excision.

Using a Gomco clamp, the doctor stretches the foreskin forward over the glans and applies the clamp on the penis distal to the glans. He then excises the foreskin and removes the clamp. After either procedure, sterile petroleum gauze is usually applied to the area.

If performing a sleeve resection, the preferred method for an adult patient, the doctor incises and dissects the inner and outer surfaces of the foreskin, then puts sutures in place to approximate the skin edges. Electrocoagulation may be used to control bleeding, if necessary, and a compression dressing may be applied. Alternatively, the doctor may use a clamp procedure for an adult patient as well.

Complications

Although circumcision is a relatively minor and safe operation, it can cause bleeding or, less commonly, infection and urethral damage, such as meatal stenosis or a urethral fistula. With application of the plastic circumcision bell, incomplete amputation of the foreskin may occur.

Care considerations
Before the procedure
• Review the procedure with the patient or his parents. Explain circumcision care. The adult patient is usually discharged the day of the procedure.
• Before circumcision to relieve a foreskin disorder, reassure the patient that surgery will not interfere with urinary, sexual, or reproductive function.
• Ensure that the patient or a responsible family member has signed the consent form.
• Make sure the neonate hasn't been fed for at least 1 hour before surgery to reduce the risk of vomiting.
• To assist with the procedure, prepare the necessary equipment. Remember to include a restraining board with arm and leg restraints for the neonate.
During the procedure
• Anesthesia is usually not administered to the neonate because of the risk of respiratory complications. However, some doctors now use local anesthesia

for the neonate to eliminate pain. In either case, assist with the procedure and ensure that the neonate is firmly restrained.
After the procedure
• Check for bleeding every 15 minutes for the 1st hour and every hour for the next 6 to 24 hours. Leave the neonate diaperless for 1 to 2 hours to check for bleeding and to reduce irritation.
• Control slight bleeding by applying pressure with sterile gauze pads. However, notify the doctor if bleeding is heavy or persistent.
• Periodically examine the suture line and glans penis for swelling, redness, or purulent exudate. Report any signs of infection, and obtain a specimen of the exudate for culture and analysis.
• Take the neonate to his parents as soon as possible after the procedure for the comfort and reassurance of both.
• Check for or encourage voiding after surgery. If the patient doesn't void within 6 hours, notify the doctor.
• Promote healing and enhance the patient's comfort. At each diaper change, apply antibiotic ointment, petroleum jelly or petroleum gauze. Position the patient on his abdomen for at least 12 hours.
• Diaper the neonate loosely to prevent irritation.
• As ordered, provide analgesics to relieve incisional pain. For the older patient, who is more subject to pain from pressure exerted on the suture line by an erection, apply a topical anesthetic ointment or spray as needed.

Home care instructions
• Teach the patient or his parents proper wound care, including (if appropriate) how to change a dressing. Tell them to watch for and report any renewed bleeding or signs of infection, such as swelling at the incision area or drainage. Inform them that a thin yellow-white exudate will normally form over the site within 1 to 2 days after the procedure; this should not be re-

moved because it protects the wound until healing occurs.

• Tell the adult patient that he can resume normal activities within 1 week and may resume sexual activity as soon as healing is complete, usually after 1 to 2 weeks. Explain that if barbiturate sleeping medication has been prescribed, its purpose is to suppress rapid eye movements during sleep and thereby prevent normal nocturnal erections. This will eliminate tension on the suture line.

• Encourage the use of prescribed analgesics to relieve discomfort.

• Inform the adult patient that the sutures will be absorbed and need not be removed, but that he should schedule a postoperative office visit with the doctor.

CLEFT LIP AND CLEFT PALATE REPAIR

Cleft lip and cleft palate are two congenital defects that may occur separately or together in various degrees of clefting. A cleft lip is formed when incomplete fusion of the maxillary and medial nasal processes occurs. The defect can range from a slight dimpling in the lip area to large bilateral clefts.

Cleft palate results from incomplete fusion of the palate. Cleft palate can range from a small unilateral groove on the uvula to bilateral clefts that can extend the entire length of the soft and hard palates. They may also involve the nasal cavity. (See *Variations in cleft lip and palate*, page 190.)

Surgical repair of a cleft lip is typically done within the first 3 months of life, although the type and degree of cleft may necessitate several operations to complete cosmetic closure. Optimal timing of cleft palate repair is individualized for each patient and usually occurs between ages 6 and 18 months. The goal is to repair the defect before faulty speech habits develop. Methods used to repair the defect may vary according to the degree of the defect and the doctor's preference.

Purpose
For cleft lip repair
• To restore the function and cosmetic appearance of the face and mouth
• To approximate the gums for teeth eruption.

For cleft palate repair
• To restore normal function of the hard and soft palate
• To improve speech patterns and eating ability
• To avoid hearing loss and fluid build-up within the ear related to displacement of the eustachian tubes
• To allow for normal development and eruption of the teeth.

Indications
Surgical repair of cleft lip and cleft palate is indicated for infants who are born with these defects.

Procedure
For cleft lip repair
Before closure of the cleft, the surgeon excises minimal amounts of lip tissue to preserve soft tissue and mucous membranes. Closure of the cleft is performed by one of three methods: rotation-advancement, interdigitation, or straight-line closure. The first two methods leave a zig-zag scar. Straight-line closure is rarely used because of the tendency of the suture line to retract, leaving a notching of the lip.

Bilateral cleft lip repair is almost always done in two stages, providing reduced tension on the closure sutures and improved accuracy of measurements for the second repair.

For cleft palate repair
Until palate closure is performed, a prosthesis is fitted to the infant to allow feeding, speech development, and reduction of respiratory tract infections. To repair the defect, the surgeon

Variations in cleft lip and palate

Cleft lip and cleft palate are genetic defects that occur alone or together in various degrees of severity. Cleft lip may range from a simple notch to a complete cleft; cleft palate, from partial to complete.

Unilateral incomplete

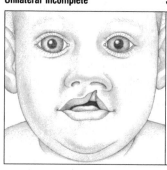

Soft palate only

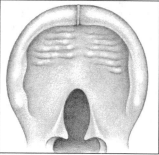

Unilateral complete

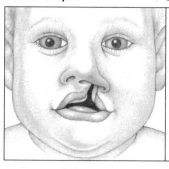

Unilateral complete

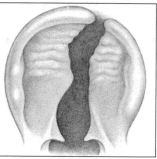

Bilateral complete

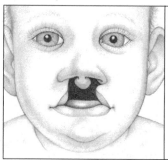

Bilateral complete

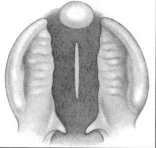

uses tissue adjacent to the defect to close the cleft. The repair may be done in one operation or may require several stages of repair, depending on the severity of the defect.

Complications

Hemorrhage, shock, and respiratory distress may complicate the immediate postoperative period. Respiratory distress may result from the surgically reduced airway or aspiration of blood or serous drainage secretions in the nasopharynx. A simple suture on the tongue may be used to assure that the tongue does not occlude the airway.

Care considerations

• Place the child on his side or abdomen to prevent aspiration of blood or serous drainage. Gentle suctioning of the nasopharynx may be indicated.
• Monitor vital signs for indications of hemorrhage and asphyxia.
• Apply elbow restraints to prevent the infant from disturbing the sutures, removing one restraint at a time at frequent intervals for exercise. Apply jacket restraints for infants who can roll over.
• Offer comfort measures to prevent crying, which causes tension on the suture line.
• After cleft lip repair, use only a fluid diet and administer with a medicine dropper or syringe into the side of the mouth. Breast-feeding or bottle feedings may be resumed 24 hours after surgery.
• After cleft palate repair, only a cup or the side of a spoon may be used; nothing should be put into the mouth. The diet should be fluid or semifluid.
• After feeding, clean the child's mouth with water.
• Keep the suture line clean and free from crust formation; clean the site with a dabbing rather than rubbing action.
• Apply petroleum jelly or topical antibiotic ointment, if prescribed.

• After cleft lip repair, inform the parents that the child will return from surgery with a butterfly adhesive restraint, Steri-Strips, or a curved metal bow taped down on both sides of the suture line over the lip (Logan clamp) to prevent tension on the suture line.

Home care instructions

• Teach the parents and caregivers about appropriate diet, feeding techniques, and care of the suture lines.
• Teach the parents the signs of ear infection.
• Discuss with the parents the use of restraints and the prevention of undue tension on the suture line related to crying.
• Advise the parents that the child may need additional referral to speech and hearing therapists, orthodontists, or reconstructive surgeons – depending on the degree of the defect and repair required.
• Refer the parents to support groups and other families whose children have had similiar defects for reassurance and exchange of information.
• Refer the parents for genetic counseling so they can understand their greater-than-normal risk for similar defects in future children.

CONTINUOUS POSITIVE AIRWAY PRESSURE

Continuous positive airway pressure (CPAP) is an adjunct to ventilation therapy. Positive pressure is applied to the airways, forcing the patient to exhale against positive airway pressure. Maintaining positive pressure in the lungs increases the functional residual capacity by distending collapsed alveoli. This improves oxygenation by decreasing intrapulmonary shunting. In nasal CPAP, used to treat obstructive sleep apnea, high-flow compressed air is directed into a mask that covers only the patient's nose.

The pressure supplied through the mask serves as a back-pressure splint, preventing the unstable upper airway from collapsing during inspiration.

CPAP may be delivered through an artificial airway or a mask by means of a ventilator or a separate high-flow generating system. To receive CPAP, the patient must have the ability to breathe spontaneously.

Purpose
• To improve oxygenation in acute respiratory disorders
• To prevent closure of upper airway passages in obstructive sleep apnea
• To prevent airway and alveolar collapse in neonates with respiratory distress syndrome
• To assist with weaning from mechanical ventilation.

Indications
Besides treating respiratory distress syndrome, CPAP has been used successfully to treat pulmonary edema, bronchiolitis, pneumonitis, viral pneumonia, and postoperative atelectasis. In mild to moderate respiratory disorders, CPAP provides an alternative to intubation and mechanical ventilation. It can also be used to help wean a patient from mechanical ventilation.

CPAP is contraindicated for patients with untreated hypovolemia caused by hemorrhage; dehydration; neurogenic, anaphylactic, or septic shock; or drug-induced decreased cardiac output or compromised circulation. In such patients, the extra pressure generated by CPAP would aggravate circulatory problems. CPAP is also contraindicated for patients with injury or disease affecting only one lung because therapy would magnify the difference in blood distribution and ventilation between the two lungs. Because mask CPAP can cause nausea and vomiting, it shouldn't be used in patients who are unresponsive or at risk for vomiting and aspiration.

Procedure
CPAP is usually performed by a respiratory therapist or a nurse, but health care facility policies vary. The patient with a tracheostomy or endotracheal tube will have the T-piece on the CPAP device connected to his airway. The ventilator will be set to CPAP, and the pressure setting will be adjusted to the desired centimeters of water (cm H_2O) — typically a total flow rate three to four times the patient's minute ventilation.

For mask CPAP, the cm H_2O setting is adjusted to exceed the patient's maximal inspiratory flow rate. The mask should be transparent and lightweight and should have a soft, pliable seal.

For mask CPAP used to prevent sleep apnea in an adult, the cm H_2O setting is adjusted as ordered. Typically, this is initiated at 5 cm H_2O and the pressure is gradually increased until apnea subsides (usually at 10 to 12 cm H_2O). If the patient is routinely hypoxemic when awake, his optimal CPAP level without oxygen will be determined, and then oxygen will be added to the CPAP circuit with sufficient flow to maintain at least 90% oxygen saturation.

Whichever delivery system is used, most patients can tolerate CPAP for only 12 to 36 hours. If CPAP therapy has been successful, it will be discontinued; if it hasn't been successful, positive-pressure ventilation may be required.

Complications
The main risks of CPAP and other types of positive-pressure mechanical apparatuses are pneumothorax, pneumomediastinum, and pneumopericardium. Patients with neurologic disorders are also at risk because CPAP can increase intracranial pressure. Other complications of CPAP include gastric distress, particularly if the patient swallows air during the treatment; this is most common when CPAP is delivered without intubation. Rarely, CPAP

causes barotrauma or lowers cardiac output.

Care considerations

Before therapy
• Explain the treatment to the patient or his caregiver.
• Obtain vital signs and lung sounds to provide a baseline.
• Obtain arterial blood gas levels and pulmonary function studies, as ordered, to serve as a baseline.
• If the patient will be receiving nasal CPAP for sleep apnea, assess for nasal congestion. If needed, have him use a nasal decongestant spray before you start CPAP.

During therapy
• If the patient is receiving CPAP for an acute condition, monitor heart rate, blood pressure, and urine output hourly.
• Continue to monitor the patient until he's stable at a CPAP setting necessary to maintain a partial pressure of oxygen in arterial blood greater than 60 mm Hg with a fraction of inspired oxygen of 50% or less.
• Check for decreased cardiac output, which may result from increased intrathoracic pressure.
• Watch closely for changes in respiratory rate and pattern. Uncoordinated breathing patterns may indicate severe respiratory muscle fatigue that can't be helped by CPAP. Such a patient may need mechanical ventilation.
• Check the CPAP system for pressure fluctuations. Because high airway pressures increase the risk of pneumothorax, monitor for chest pain and decreased breath sounds.
• Use oximetry, if possible, to monitor oxygen saturations, especially if you remove the CPAP mask to provide routine care.
• If the patient who's wearing a mask is stable and his condition permits, remove the mask briefly every 2 to 4 hours to provide fluids and mouth and skin care. As ordered, increase the length of time the mask is off as the patient's ability to maintain oxygenation without CPAP improves. Between treatments, apply compound benzoin tincture to the skin under the edge of the mask to reduce the risk of breakdown and necrosis. Check closely for air leaks around the mask near the eyes (an area difficult to seal); escaping air can dry the eyes, causing conjunctivitis or other problems.
• Check air intake ports (present on some CPAP devices) to detect obstructions.
• If the patient is using a nasal CPAP device for sleep apnea, observe for decreased snoring and mouth breathing during sleep, which indicates that nasal CPAP is effective. If these symptoms persist, notify the doctor; either the system is leaking or the pressure is inadequate.

Home care instructions
• If the patient is using CPAP for sleep apnea, explain the procedure to him and his caregiver, if appropriate. Ask his sleeping partner to monitor for symptoms. Ask the patient to demonstrate use of the system to make sure he can prevent excess leakage and maintain the prescribed pressures. Teach the patient how to clean the mask and change the air filter.
• Explain to the patient that he must use nasal CPAP every night even if he feels better after the initial treatments.
• Mention that apneic episodes will recur if he doesn't use CPAP as directed. However, if symptoms recur despite consistent use of CPAP, the patient should call his doctor.
• If the patient is obese, explain that losing weight may allow him to reduce the frequency of CPAP treatments.

COOLING TREATMENTS

Cooling treatments are fundamental procedures that, despite new high-tech medical therapies, are still commonly used. Cooling treatments include both moist and dry forms. Moist cold, which provides deeper penetration, includes tepid sponge baths, cold compresses for small areas, and cold packs for large areas. In severe hyperthermia, hypothermia blankets (which provide a type of dry cold) may be used. Other dry-cold methods include ice bags or collars, K pads, and chemical cold packs. Chilled enemas of 0.9% sodium chloride solution may control hyperthermia if other cooling treatments fail.

Purpose
• To lower body temperature, thereby preventing cellular death and organ damage by decreasing metabolic demands
• To relieve local pain by reducing nerve impulse conduction
• To prevent edema and relieve vascular congestion
• To slow or stop bleeding by constricting blood vessels.

Indications
Cooling treatments are used to lower body temperature in patients with hyperthermia. They are also useful in relieving acute pain and inflammation and are commonly used for initial treatment after eye injuries, strains, sprains, bruises, muscle spasms, and burns. Cooling therapy is also used to treat chronic pain and may be warranted for patients with bleeding episodes.

Cooling treatments should be used cautiously, if at all, in patients with impaired circulation, young children, and the elderly because of the risk of ischemic tissue damage.

Procedure
A properly prepared and covered ice bag, ice collar, K pad, or activated chemical cold pack is placed on the desired site for the required time. For hyperthermia, the cooling device will

be placed on the groin or axilla. The device is refilled or replaced, as necessary.

A cold compress or cold pack is wrung dry, covered with a waterproof cloth, then applied to the patient for the required time. The compress or pack is changed as needed to maintain the correct temperature.

A preset and covered hypothermia blanket is placed under the patient. The patient's head should not lie on the blanket's cold surface. The thermistor rectal probe is inserted and taped in place. The probe's other end is plugged into the blanket's control panel, which will indicate the patient's temperature. If necessary, a sheet or a second hypothermia blanket is placed over the patient to increase cold transfer.

A tepid sponge bath is administered by first sponging each extremity with moist, tepid washcloths for about 5 minutes. Then the patient's chest and abdomen is sponged for 5 minutes, followed by tepid sponging of the back and buttocks for 5 to 10 minutes. Throughout therapy, the patient is covered except for the area being sponged. A covered hot-water bottle is kept at the patient's feet to prevent chills and a covered ice bag is kept on his head to prevent headache and nasal congestion. Moist washcloths are placed on the axilla, groin, and popliteal areas.

Complications
In the hyperthermic patient, too-rapid cooling may cause a decrease in the patient's level of consciousness (LOC), pupillary response, and cardiac output. Chills may occur, which are detrimental because they increase metabolism, thereby raising body temperature.

Tissue damage, frostbite, or fat necrosis may also result from cooling procedures. Thrombi may result from hemoconcentration.

A hypothermia blanket can cause sudden changes in vital signs, increased intracranial pressure, respiratory distress or arrest, oliguria, and anuria.

Care considerations
Before therapy
• Explain the procedure to the patient. If the treatment is used to relieve pain, explain that the first few treatments may not be noticeably effective, but that significant analgesia (lasting from 15 minutes to several hours) can be achieved with repeated treatments.
• Obtain and prepare the necessary equipment. Select the correct size device, and check for leaks as well as frayed cords or broken plugs.
• If using an ice bag or collar, fill it halfway with crushed ice, which allows you to mold it to conform to the patient's body. Squeeze the bag to expel residual air, fasten the cap, and wipe any moisture from the outside cover.
• If using a K pad, fill the control unit two-thirds full with distilled water. Tilt the unit several times to clear air from the tubing. Then tighten the cap and check that the hoses between the control unit and pad are free of tangles. Place the unit on the bedside table, slightly above the patient so that gravity assists water flow. Set the temperature control to the lowest setting. Turn the unit on and allow it to cool for about 2 minutes.
• If using a chemical cold pack, follow the manufacturer's directions to activate the cold-producing chemicals.
• If using a cold compress or pack, cool a container of tap water by placing it in a basin of ice or by adding ice to the water. Chill the water to about 59° F (15° C) or as ordered, and immerse the compress or pack.
• If using a hypothermia blanket, after connecting the blanket to the control unit, specify the manual or automatic setting, as needed, and the desired temperature. Next, turn the unit on and add distilled water to the reservoir. Allow the blankets to cool, and place the control unit at the foot of the patient's bed.
• To give a tepid sponge bath, place a bath thermometer in a basin of warm water. Add cool water until the temperature reaches 93° F (34° C).
• To administer a chilled enema, place the solution container in a basin of ice water until it reaches the prescribed temperature.
• For all devices, make sure a protective covering is in place. Use a linen-saver pad if appropriate.
• Before proceeding with any cooling treatment, make sure the patient's room is warm and free of drafts. Obtain baseline vital signs and assess the patient's LOC.

During therapy
• When used for hyperthermia, monitor the patient's rectal temperature continuously (if he has a rectal probe in place) or every 10 minutes. Also monitor all other vital signs and the patient's LOC throughout therapy.
• Discontinue therapy and notify the doctor if the patient develops chills or signs of tissue intolerance – blanching, edema, mottling, graying cyanosis, maceration, and blisters – or if the patient reports new, intolerable, or unusual discomfort.
• If a hypothermia blanket is used, monitor for complications, such as altered vital signs and increased intracranial pressure, and institute emergency procedures if they occur.
• Stay with and carefully monitor patients at risk for tissue damage.
• Keep the patient's skin and bed linens free of moisture.
• Discontinue cooling treatment when the patient's temperature drops to 102° F (38.9° C), or as otherwise ordered. However, if administering a tepid sponge bath, discontinue therapy when the temperature decreases to 1° to 2° F (0.5° to 1° C) above the desired temperature because the temperature will decline naturally at that point. Report continued high fever to the doctor. If

using cold therapy to relieve pain, discontinue treatment as ordered. Continued application of cold to a small area may result in reflexive vasodilation.

After therapy

• Dry the patient's skin.
• Continue to monitor temperature and other vital signs for several days after cooling therapy.

Home care instructions

• Teach the patient how to perform the cooling treatment at home, if indicated.
• Tell the patient not to exceed the recommended duration of treatment because frostbite may result.
• Instruct the patient to report any change in symptoms or location of pain a well as any associated mottling, grayness, or blanching.
• Warn the patient not to put ice directly against his skin because the extreme cold can damage tissue.

CORDOTOMY

Cordotomy is the surgical destruction of sensory pathways that carry pain impulses to the brain. Unfortunately, this surgical procedure doesn't guarantee pain relief and its complications can be severe. Therefore, a cordotomy is rarely performed.

A cordotomy may be performed by one of two approaches: an open surgical procedure under general anesthesia or a percutaneous procedure under local anesthesia. An open cordotomy involves transection of the spinothalamic tract on the side opposite the pain. It provides pain relief below the level of transection. Percutaneous cordotomy, a closed technique, uses radio frequency coagulation to create a lesion on the anterolateral spinothalamic tract, thereby providing pain relief below the lesion.

The percutaneous approach is preferred; its results compare favorably with the open approach, and it's easier to perform, safer, and more precise. An open approach may be indicated in a patient unable to tolerate testing procedures while awake or one with anatomic changes, such as severe arthritis, in the cervical spine.

Purpose

• To relieve severe, intractable pain by preventing transmission of pain impulses to the brain.

Indications

Cordotomy is used for pain control, particularly in cancer patients experiencing unremitting pain in the thorax, abdomen, and lower extremities. It is most commonly performed on patients with extensive cancer of the pelvis. However, because a significant percentage of cordotomies lose their effectiveness in 1 to 5 years, this surgery is usually reserved for patients whose pain is unresponsive to more conservative treatments and whose life expectancy is under 2 years.

Procedure

For open cordotomy, the patient is given general anesthesia and is placed in a sitting or prone position, depending on the level of the procedure. The surgeon performs a laminectomy to expose the spinal cord, makes a small incision through the spinothalamic tract in the anterolateral quadrant of the cord, closes the dural flap with fine sutures, closes the laminectomy wound, and applies a pressure dressing.

During percutaneous cordotomy, the patient lies supine with his head immobilized by a head holder and with a pad placed beneath his shoulders to extend his neck. After administering a local anesthetic, the surgeon inserts a catheter into the patient's neck below and behind the mastoid process. He then injects radiopaque material and, guided by fluoroscopy, inserts an electrode through the catheter into the spinal cord.

To verify electrode placement, the surgeon stimulates the electrode, observing the patient's motor responses. Then he uses radio frequency currents to make a lesion at the desired spinal cord level. The patient should be warned when the electrode is being passed because the local anesthetic may not completely prevent pain.

After forming the lesion, the surgeon withdraws the electrode, sutures the incision, and applies a pressure dressing.

Complications

Cordotomy can cause severe complications, such as neurologic dysfunction, hemorrhage, respiratory distress, bladder dysfunction, and sexual impotence. It can also cause permanent loss of some sensations in the area of analgesia. Temporary paralysis or at least leg weakness and a loss of bowel or bladder control frequently follow a cordotomy; these result from edema of the spinal cord and will gradually disappear in 2 weeks.

Care considerations

Before surgery

• Reinforce the surgeon's explanation of the procedure, including benefits and risks. Explain that after surgery the patient won't feel pain, temperature, or other sensations within the area of analgesia. Inform the male patient that impotence commonly results from this surgery.

• Inform the patient who's undergoing a percutaneous cordotomy that muscle tests will be performed throughout the procedure. Tell the patient to immediately alert the surgeon to any sensations of pain, pressure, or weakness.

• Explain that after surgery the patient will lie flat in bed for 12 to 24 hours.

• Teach the patient the logrolling maneuver as well as coughing and deep-breathing techniques to help prevent respiratory complications. Make sure the patient or a responsible family member has signed a consent form.

• To serve as a baseline, take the patient's vital signs; evaluate the motion, strength, and sensation of each extremity; and obtain arterial blood gas (ABG) measurements, as ordered.

After surgery

• Keep the patient lying flat for the specified time. If the patient has had cervical incisions, keep the neck in a neutral position; don't elevate the head with pillows. The patient who has had a thoracic cordotomy may be turned to the prone position.

• Have the patient cough and deep-breathe every 2 hours. Observe for labored breathing, weakened voice, confusion, and drowsiness. Monitor the patient's ABG levels. Observe the patient's respiratory pattern during sleep. If periods of apnea or decreased respirations occur, wake the patient and have him breathe deeply. Report any signs of respiratory distress to the doctor. Be prepared to provide mechanical ventilation.

• Inspect the patient's dressing frequently for increased drainage, and report it promptly.

• Monitor the patient's vital signs, especially blood pressure. If the patient is severely hypotensive or symptomatic, notify the doctor immediately; if he remains hypotensive for more than 2 hours, again notify the doctor. Also monitor the patient's neurologic functioning. Report paresthesia and any decrease in movement, strength, or sensations.

• Check for urine retention, and notify the doctor if the patient hasn't voided in 8 hours. As ordered, instruct the patient to stand or sit to void, or institute intermittent catheterization.

• Turn the patient at least every 2 hours, and feel the skin regularly for temperature changes. Noticeably cool skin can indicate compromised circulation, which increases the risk of skin breakdown.

Home care instructions

• Explain that the patient may feel numbness or tingling in the area of analgesia.

• Remind the patient that the loss of sensation in areas affected by the cordotomy requires special safety precautions. Teach the patient to inspect his skin using a hand mirror to view hard-to-see areas because skin integrity may be compromised in areas of insensitivity. Also recommend protection against exposure to temperature and weather extremes; for example, suggest testing bath or shower water with a thermometer.

• Advise the patient to avoid constrictive clothing that may impair circulation in the area of analgesia.

• Inform the patient that temporary paresis is common and that weakness may persist on the affected side. Warn him to guard against falls caused by such weakness.

• Explain that most male patients experience some degree of impotence after cordotomy. Provide emotional support, and refer the patient to a specialist in sexual dysfunction.

• Reinforce the family's understanding that the analgesic effects of a cordotomy may diminish with time and that pain may recur. Explain that repeating cordotomy at another level is usually no more successful than the first procedure.

CORNEAL KERATOPLASTY

This procedure, commonly called a corneal transplant, replaces a damaged part of the recipient's cornea with healthy corneal tissue from a recently deceased human donor. A corneal transplant can take one of two forms: a full-thickness (penetrating) keratoplasty, involving excision and replacement of all corneal layers, or a partial-thickness (lamellar) keratoplasty, which removes and replaces only the outer layers of corneal tissue. The full-thickness procedure, by far the more common, produces a high degree of clarity and restores vision in 95% of patients. A lamellar transplant is performed rarely and selectively.

Because the cornea is avascular and doesn't recover as rapidly as other parts of the body, healing may take up to a year. Typically, sutures remain in place and vision isn't completely functional until healing occurs.

Purpose

• To replace damaged or opaque corneal tissue with a clear, healthy corneal graft.

Indications

Corneal transplants help restore corneal clarity lost through injury, inflammation, ulceration, or chemical burns. They may also correct corneal dystrophies as well as keratoconus, the abnormal thinning and bulging of the central portion of the cornea.

Procedure

A transplant is typically performed under local anesthesia and takes 1 to 2 hours. The patient must remain still until the surgery has been completed.

In a full-thickness or penetrating keratoplasty, the surgeon cuts a "button" from the recipient's diseased opaque cornea and replaces it with a precisely sized button obtained from healthy donor corneal tissue. The donor button is anchored in place with extremely fine sutures. To end the procedure, the surgeon patches the patient's eye and tapes a shield over it.

In a partial-thickness or lamellar keratoplasty, the surgeon excises only the superficial layers of corneal tissue in both the donor and recipient corneas. The donor graft is then sutured in place. As in the full-thickness procedure, the surgeon patches the eye and applies a rigid shield. (See *Comparing corneal transplants*.)

Comparing corneal transplants

A corneal transplant may involve replacement of the entire cornea or simply a thin layer of corneal tissue. In a full-thickness transplant, the surgeon removes the corneal disk, which measures 7 to 8 mm, and relaces it with a matching "button" from a donor. In a lamellar, or partial-thickness transplant, the surgeon removes superficial corneal tissue only and replaces it with donor tissue. By using this procedure, he spares the stroma and the entire endothelium.

Full-thickness transplant

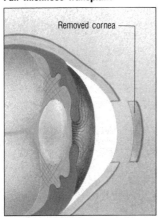

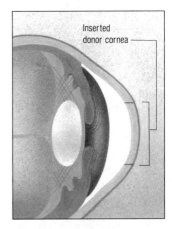

Lamellar transplant

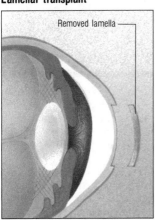

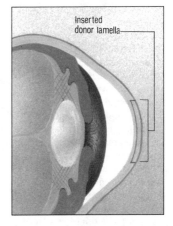

Complications

Graft rejection, which occurs in about 15% of patients, may happen at any time during the patient's life. Uncommon complications include wound leakage, loosening of the sutures, dehiscence, and infection.

Care considerations

Before surgery

• Explain the transplant procedure to the patient and answer any questions. Explain that healing will be slow and that vision may not be completely restored until the sutures are removed, which may be in about a year. Vision may then be improved further with a contact lens or glasses.

• Tell the patient that analgesics will be available after surgery because he may experience dull aching. Inform the patient that a bandage and protective shield will be placed over the eye.

• As ordered, administer a sedative or osmotic agent to reduce intraocular pressure.

• Assess the patient carefully. He should be free from respiratory or eye infections to promote postoperative healing.

• Ensure that the patient has signed a consent form.

After surgery

• After recovery from the anesthetic, assess for and immediately report sudden, sharp, or excessive pain; bloody, purulent, or clear viscous drainage; or fever. As ordered, instill corticosteroid eyedrops or topical antibiotics to prevent inflammation and graft rejection.

• To avoid increased intraocular pressure in the postoperative period, instruct the patient to lie on his back or on his unaffected side, with the bed flat or slightly elevated, as ordered. Tell the patient to avoid rapid head movements, hard coughing or sneezing, squinting or rubbing his eyes, bending over, and other activities that could increase intraocular pressure.

• Remind the patient to ask for help in standing or walking until he adjusts to vision changes. Make sure that all needed personal items are within the patient's field of vision.

Home care instructions

• Teach the patient and family to recognize the signs of graft rejection (cloudiness, drainage, and decreased vision). Instruct them to immediately notify the doctor if any of these signs occur. Emphasize that rejection can occur many years after surgery; stress the need for assessing the graft daily for the rest of the patient's life.

• Encourage the patient to keep regular appointments with his doctor.

• Tell the patient to avoid activities that increase intraocular pressure, including extreme exertion, sudden jerky movements, lifting or pushing heavy objects, or straining during defecation.

• Explain that photophobia, a common adverse effect, gradually decreases as healing progresses. Suggest wearing dark glasses in bright light.

• Teach the patient how to correctly instill prescribed eyedrops.

• Remind the patient to wear an eye shield when sleeping.

CORONARY ARTERY BYPASS GRAFTING

A surgical procedure, coronary artery bypass grafting (CABG) establishes a shunt to circumvent an occluded coronary artery. The number of obstructions bypassed varies from one to five or more.

The bypasses are made of autogenous grafts, usually from a segment of the saphenous vein or internal mammary artery, and permit blood flow from a major artery to the point past the coronary artery blockage, ultimately restoring blood flow to the myocardium. The internal mammary approach has recently become common.

CABG techniques vary according to the patient's condition and the number of arteries being bypassed. During the procedure, the patient must be placed on extracorporeal circulation (a heart-lung machine) because the heart must be immobilized for surgical manipulation. In patients with left main coronary artery stenosis exceeding 50% and those with three-vessel coronary artery disease and decreased left ventricular functions, CABG has been shown to provide symptomatic relief and longer survival than does medical therapy. Forthcoming comparisons of CABG and percutaneous transluminal coronary angioplasty may determine which method is best for multivessel disease.

Purpose

• To improve myocardial perfusion and relieve anginal pain.

Indications

Candidates for CABG include patients who have angiographic evidence of a diseased left main artery or significant triple vessel disease, multivessel coronary disease with left ventricular dysfunction, or vessel disease that includes proximal, severe left anterior descending artery stenosis and concomitant left ventricular dysfunction. Such patients may have experienced stable angina that is unresponsive to medical therapy for 5 months or more. Other appropriate candidates are patients with unstable angina unrelieved by medication and accompanied by electrocardiogram (ECG) changes. CABG benefits such patients by achieving revascularization before infarction occurs.

Patients at higher risk for morbidity after CABG include those with serious pulmonary problems, renal and metabolic dysfunction, and those with significant cerebrovascular atherosclerosis such as carotid artery stenosis, which increases the risk of perioperative cerebrovascular accident (CVA). Patients receiving anticoagulants must be identified before surgery. Those who are heavy smokers also have a greater risk of postoperative complications and death.

Procedure

Surgery begins with graft harvesting: The surgeon makes a series of incisions in the patient's thigh or calf, and removes a segment of saphenous vein for grafting. Most often, the surgeon uses a segment of the internal mammary artery.

When the grafts are obtained, the surgeon performs a median sternotomy, exposes the heart, and initiates cardiopulmonary bypass. This is accomplished by placing a catheter in the aorta and the right atrium or vena cavae. Cardiopulmonary bypass cools the body's temperature to 92° F (33° C). To further reduce myocardial oxygen demands during surgery and to protect the heart, the surgeon stops the electrical conductivity of the heart and induces cardiac hypothermia by injecting a cold cardioplegic solution (potassium-enriched 0.9% sodium chloride solution) into the aortic root and coronary arteries.

After the patient is fully prepared, the surgeon sutures one end of the venous graft to the ascending aorta and the other end to a patent coronary artery distal to the occlusion. (He sutures the graft in a reversed position to promote proper blood flow.) He repeats this procedure for each artery he bypasses. When the grafts are in place, the surgeon flushes the cardioplegic solution from the heart, discontinues cardiopulmonary bypass, implants epicardial pacing electrodes, inserts a chest tube, and closes the incision. A sterile dressing is applied.

Complications

CABG relieves pain in over 90% of patients, and its long-term effectiveness is well established. However, such problems as graft closure and development of atherosclerosis in other coronary arteries sometimes necessitate repeat surgery. Approximately 5% to 10% of patients develop graft closure within 1 year, and about 60% develop atherosclerotic disease of saphenous vein grafts within 10 years. Internal mammary bypass conduits remain patent much longer, sometimes indefinitely.

Potential intraoperative and postoperative complications include arrhythmias, hypertension or hypotension, cardiac tamponade, thromboembolism that may lead to a CVA, and myocardial infarction.

In the early postoperative period, postpericardiotomy syndrome and infection can occur. The patient may experience postoperative depression, but this may not develop until weeks after discharge.

Care considerations

Before surgery

• Reinforce the surgeon's explanation of the procedure. Explain the complex equipment and procedures used in the intensive care or postanesthesia unit. If possible and desired, arrange a tour of the unit for the patient and family before surgery.

• Tell the patient that he'll awaken from surgery with an endotracheal (ET) tube in place and will be connected to a mechanical ventilator. Warn the patient that he will be unable to speak while this tube is in place. He'll also be connected to a cardiac monitor and have in place a nasogastric tube, a chest tube, an indwelling urinary catheter, arterial lines, epicardial pacing wires and, possibly, a pulmonary artery catheter and an intra-aortic balloon pump (IABP). Reassure the patient that this equipment causes little discomfort and will be removed as soon as possible.

• Ensure that the patient or a responsible family member has signed a consent form.

• Explain that the evening before surgery, the patient will shower with an antiseptic soap and will be shaved from chin to toes.

• Restrict food and fluids after midnight and provide a sedative, if ordered. On the morning of surgery, also provide a sedative, as ordered, to help the patient relax.

• Before surgery, assist with pulmonary artery catheterization and insertion of arterial lines. Then begin cardiac monitoring.

After surgery

• Monitor for signs of hemodynamic compromise, such as severe hypotension, decreased cardiac output, and shock. Check and record vital signs every 15 minutes until the patient's condition stabilizes. Monitor the ECG for disturbances in heart rate and rhythm. Report serious abnormalities to the doctor, and be prepared to assist with epicardial pacing or, if necessary, cardioversion or defibrillation.

• Monitor core body temperature because the patient is at greatest risk for shock and arrhythmias during postoperative rewarming.

• To ensure adequate myocardial perfusion, maintain arterial pressure within the prescribed guidelines. Usually, mean arterial pressure below 70 mm Hg results in inadequate tissue perfusion; pressure above 110 mm Hg can cause hemorrhage and graft rupture. Also monitor pulmonary artery, central venous, and left atrial pressure, as ordered.

• Frequently evaluate the patient's peripheral pulses, capillary refill time, and skin temperature and color, and auscultate for heart sounds. Notify the doctor of any abnormalities. Also evaluate tissue oxygenation by assessing breath sounds, chest excursion, and symmetry of chest expansion.

• Check arterial blood gas (ABG) measurements every 2 to 4 hours, and adjust ventilator settings as needed to maintain ABG values within pre-scribed limits.

• Within 6 to 24 hours after CABG, all patients should begin a daily prophy-lactic dose of aspirin to reduce the in-cidence of saphenous vein graft throm-bosis.

• Monitor the patient's intake and out-put, and assess for electrolyte imbal-ance, especially hypokalemia, because this can lead to cardiac arrhythmias.

• Maintain chest tube drainage at the prescribed negative pressure (usually -10 to -40 cm H_2O). Verify the chest tube's patency according to the policy of the health care facility, checking regularly for hemorrhage, excessive drainage (greater than 200 ml/hour), and sudden decrease or cessation of drainage.

• As the patient's incisional pain in-creases, administer an analgesic, as or-dered.

• Throughout recovery, assess the pa-tient for signs and symptoms of CVA (altered level of consciousness, pupil-lary changes, weakness and loss of movement in extremities, ataxia, aphasia, dysphagia, sensory distur-bances), pulmonary embolism (chest pain, dyspnea, hemoptysis, pleural friction rub, cyanosis, hypoxemia), and impaired renal perfusion (decreased urine output and elevated blood urea nitrogen and serum creatinine levels).

• After weaning the patient from the ventilator and removing the ET tube, perform chest physiotherapy. Start in-centive spirometry, and encourage the patient to cough, turn frequently, and deep-breathe. Assist with range-of-motion exercises, as ordered, to en-hance peripheral circulation and pre-vent thrombus formation.

Home care instructions

• Instruct the patient to watch for and immediately notify the doctor of any signs of infection (fever; sore throat; or redness, swelling, or drainage from the leg or chest incisions) or possible arterial reocclusion (angina, dizziness, dyspnea, rapid or irregular pulse, or prolonged recovery time from exer-cise).

• Explain that postpericardiotomy syndrome often develops after open-heart surgery. Tell the patient to call his doctor if such symptoms as fever, muscle and joint pain, weakness, or chest discomfort occur.

• Prepare the patient for the possibility of postoperative depression, which may develop several weeks after discharge. Reassure the patient that this depres-sion is a normal reaction and should subside quickly.

• Make sure the patient understands the dosage, frequency of administra-tion, and possible adverse effects of all prescribed medications.

• Encourage the patient to follow the prescribed diet, especially noting any sodium and cholesterol restrictions. Explain that dietary compliance can help reduce the risk of recurrent ar-terial occlusion.

• Instruct the patient to maintain a bal-ance between activity and rest. He should try to sleep at least 8 hours a night, to schedule a short rest period for each afternoon, and to rest fre-quently during tiring physical activity. As appropriate, tell him he can climb stairs, engage in sexual activity, take baths and showers, and do light chores.

• Warn against lifting heavy objects (more than 20 lb [9 kg]), driving a car, or doing heavy work (such as mowing the lawn or vacuuming) until the doc-tor approves. Encourage the patient to follow a prescribed exercise program.

• Refer the patient to a local chapter of the Mended Hearts Club and the Amer-ican Heart Association for additional in-formation and support.

CORPUS CALLOSOTOMY

The corpus callosum is an area of transverse fibers connecting the two cerebral hemispheres. A corpus callosotomy is a surgical procedure in which the corpus callosum is divided by a fine suction aspirator. It is performed to reduce disabling seizure activity.

A corpus callosotomy is typically done in two stages. Initially, the anterior two-thirds of the corpus callosum is divided. If seizure activity is not reduced after several months, the final one-third is divided in a second operation. Corpus callosotomy is performed in two steps to prevent acute disconnection syndrome, which causes apraxia (loss of ability to carry out familiar movements), mutism, apathy, confusion, and infantile behavior.

Patients are discharged approximately 12 to 14 days after surgery. They may be discharged with some neurologic deficits and may require physical, occupational, or speech therapy. Rehabilitation may be completed as an outpatient. Severe neurologic deficits may require inpatient rehabilitation.

Corpus callosotomy is a palliative procedure. It is not expected to prevent all seizures. Because most patients who are eligible for a callosotomy have severely disabling seizures, the intention is to decrease the number and severity of the seizures.

Purpose

• To reduce the number of generalized seizures by interrupting the inter-hemispheric spread of epileptic discharges.

Indications

Corpus callosotomy is considered only after trials on all appropriate anticonvulsant drugs have failed to control seizure activity, if seizure activity is disruptive to daily life, and if the seizure activity does not arise from a single area of the brain.

If the diagnostic workup determines that the origin of the seizure activity is localized to a specific area of the brain, a cortical resection may be performed. (See *Cortical resection*.)

Patients who have generalized atonic, tonic, or tonic-clonic seizures and those who have seizures with a frontal focus are considered the best candidates for this surgery. EEG usually shows multifocal or bilaterally synchronous abnormalities.

Procedure

With the patient under general anesthesia, the neurosurgeon makes a vertex frontal craniotomy (opening of the scalp, skull, and dura) and divides the

---

Cortical resection

Cortical resection is a surgical procedure that removes epileptogenic tissue from the brain. Resection can remove any lobe but, most commonly, the temporal lobe is removed. Cortical mapping (electrocorticography) is used during surgery to identify and remove the smallest possible area of the brain while still excising all epileptogenic tissue.

Before surgery, an intracarotid amytal or Wada test is completed to identify the hemisphere that directs speech and memory. The results will indicate whether resection will affect speech and memory and will dictate the size and area of resection.

Healing may take up to a year, and the patient's seizure activity may continue during that time. Maintaining therapeutic blood levels of anticonvulsant drugs is important. If the patient is free of seizures for 2 years and the EEG shows no epileptic activity, anticonvulsant drugs may be gradually discontinued.

anterior two-thirds of the corpus callosum. If satisfactory seizure control has not been obtained after several months, a second craniotomy is performed and the final third of the corpus callosum is divided.

Complications

This surgical procedure has a low morbidity and mortality rate. Potential complications are those for any craniotomy: intracerebral hemorrhage, neurologic deficits, infection and, rarely, death. Mutism, lack of spontaneous speech, apathy, and infantile behavior have also been reported.

Care considerations

Before surgery

• Perform a neurologic evaluation to establish the patient's baseline status.
• Administer dexamethasone (Decadron), as ordered, to help control cerebral edema (swelling of the brain).
• Give the patient a povidone-iodine shampoo the night before surgery.
• The neurosurgeon shaves the patient's entire head before surgery.

After surgery

• Monitor vital signs for evidence of shock or increased intracranial pressure.
• Frequently monitor neurologic signs to detect evidence of increased cerebral edema.
• Monitor the patient for seizure activity.
• Administer dexamethasone, as prescribed, to control cerebral edema.
• Administer anticonvulsant drugs—for example, phenobarbital and phenytoin (Dilantin) I.V., as ordered.
• Monitor the patient's head dressing for excessive bleeding or cerebrospinal fluid leakage.
• After the dressing is removed, monitor the incision for infection.

Home care instructions

• Emphasize the importance of continuing anticonvulsant therapy, which will probably be needed indefinitely.
• Explain that because corpus callosotomy is a palliative procedure, the patient will continue to have some seizures. Typically, however, the seizures become less frequent and less severe. Emphasize that continued medical monitoring is required.
• Inform the patient that he can resume daily activities but should not plan to return to work for at least 6 months. Remind the patient to avoid activities that might cause head injuries.
• Teach the patient how to check the incision for signs of infection. Warn against rubbing the incision during bathing.

CORTICOSTEROIDS

Corticosteroids mimic the effects of natural hormones produced by the adrenal cortex. These drugs can be broadly classified as glucocorticoids or mineralocorticoids. The major glucortocoids include *hydrocortisone* and *cortisone* (short-acting corticosteroids) and *prednisone* and *prednisolone* (intermediate-acting); *desoxycorticosterone* and *fludrocortisone* represent the major mineralocorticoids. These drugs may be given alone or in combination, depending on the patient's condition, and may be administered orally, parenterally, or topically.

Purpose

• To reduce inflammation
• To produce immunosuppression
• To treat adrenocortical disorders.

Indications

Glucocorticoids have multiple clinical uses, such as the treatment of adrenal insufficiency; topical treatment of dermatologic and ocular inflammations; systemic or inhalation therapy for respiratory diseases such as status asthmaticus; relief of inflammation in conditions such as rheumatoid arthritis; suppression of inflammatory reaction in conditions such as asthma and food and drug allergies; emergency treatment of shock and anaphylactic reactions; immunosuppression and relief of inflammation to prevent rejection in organ and tissue transplants; adjunctive treatment of leukemias, lymphomas, myelomas, and spinal cord injury; and relief of cerebral edema.

Mineralocorticoids are used to treat salt-losing forms of adrenogenital syndrome (congenital adrenal hyperplasia) after electrolyte balance is restored. In combination with glucocorticoids, they are used to treat adrenal insufficiency (Addison's disease).

Because of their immunosuppressant effects, the corticosteroids are contraindicated in patients with systemic fungal infections. They should be administered cautiously to patients with GI ulcers, renal or hepatic disease, hypertension, congestive heart failure (CHF), osteoporosis, diabetes mellitus, hyperthyroidism or hypothyroidism, uncontrolled viral or bacterial infections, myasthenia gravis, tuberculosis, or AIDS. Because these drugs can precipitate depression or psychotic episodes, especially in high doses, they should be given judiciously to patients with a history of emotional instability or psychotic tendencies. Prolonged corticosteroid therapy requires careful monitoring of the patient's vital signs, fluid and electrolyte balance, mental status, and overall condition.

Adverse reactions

The chief adverse effects of corticosteroids depend on the duration of therapy and the dosage. Fluid and electrolyte disturbances can range from mild edema and sodium retention to CHF. Metabolic alkalosis, hypocalcemia, or hypokalemia may lead to arrhythmias, hypotension, or hypertension. Musculoskeletal effects may include muscle weakness or myopathy and weakening of the skeletal system, leading to pathologic fractures of the long bones or vertebral compression. GI disturbances may include nausea, vomiting, and peptic ulcers. Endocrine disturbances may include menstrual irregularities, growth suppression in children, cushingoid signs (moon face, buffalo hump, central obesity), or decreased carbohydrate tolerance. Other effects may include acne, hirsutism, impaired wound healing, emotional instability, and ophthalmic changes.

Abrupt withdrawal of corticosteroids after long-term, high-dose therapy can precipitate potentially fatal adrenal crisis. For this reason, the drug dosage should always be decreased gradually and discontinued under close supervision.

Care considerations

• Before beginning therapy, weigh the patient to establish a baseline. Weigh him regularly during therapy to detect any increases caused by corticosteroid-induced appetite stimulation and fluid retention.
• Check the patient for edema, thinning of the extremities, and elevated blood pressure. Notify the doctor if the patient gains weight rapidly or develops edema or hypertension.
• Because corticosteroids may cause GI upset when given orally, give the drug with milk or food.
• If the patient is receiving prolonged therapy, watch for cushingoid signs.
• Observe the patient on prolonged therapy for insomnia, emotional lability, and psychotic behavior – especially one with a history of instability. Report sudden mood swings to the doctor.
• If the patient has recently had surgery, monitor the wound for dehiscence and evisceration because corticosteroids may delay healing.

• Watch for such signs of infection as rhonchi and diminished breath sounds because corticosteroids may mask expected signs.

• Review the patient's medication regimen for possible drug interactions. Concurrent use of indomethacin or aspirin, for example, increases the risk of GI distress and bleeding. Barbiturates, phenytoin, and rifampin decrease corticosteroid effects.

• During withdrawal of corticosteroids, monitor the patient for symptoms of possible adrenal insufficiency: lethargy, weakness, dyspnea, orthostatic hypotension, syncope, fever, low blood sugar, diarrhea, arthralgia, and anorexia. Report any of these effects to the doctor immediately.

Home care instructions

• Instruct the patient to take a single daily dose in the morning to mimic the secretory pattern of endogenous corticosteroids, which peaks in the morning and reaches its nadir in the evening. If the patient is taking a divided dose, explain that the doctor has ordered the larger amount for the morning dose. Advise the patient to take divided doses at evenly spaced intervals throughout the day.

• Provide directions for missed doses. If the patient is on an alternate-day schedule, tell him to take the missed dose if he remembers later that morning; otherwise, he should take the dose the next morning and then omit the next day, resuming an alternate-day schedule. If the patient is on a daily schedule, tell him to take the missed dose as soon as he remembers, unless it's almost time for the next dose; warn the patient not to double-dose. If the patient is on a regimen with a divided dosage taken several times daily, tell him to take a missed dose as soon as he remembers and double-up if it's time for his next dose.

• Warn the patient against discontinuing the drug without the doctor's approval because sudden withdrawal can be fatal.

• To reduce GI upset, suggest taking the drug with food or milk. Advise the patient to avoid alcohol, which can increase the ulcerogenic effects of corticosteroids.

• Advise the patient to report minor stress or illness, such as a cold or a dental extraction, so that the doctor can increase the dosage. Explain that he'll require hospitalization and parenteral steroids if he suffers a major illness or requires an invasive procedure.

• Remind the patient who has primary adrenal insufficiency to maintain a liberal salt intake because his low aldosterone levels may cause sodium and fluid depletion. Advise him to be especially careful about salt intake during hot weather because perspiration increases sodium excretion.

• Explain that corticosteroids impair resistance to infection. As a result, the patient must avoid exposure to anyone with a known or suspected infection, and he must also avoid any vaccinations or immunizations during therapy and withdrawal.

• Instruct the patient to carry an identification card specifying the name and dosage of the prescribed drug.

• Warn the patient not to take any other drugs, including aspirin, without his doctor's approval.

COTREL-DUBOUSSET SPINAL INSTRUMENTATION

Cotrel-Dubousset spinal instrumentation was developed in France in 1984. This technique for treatment of spinal instability or deformity involves placing a series of rods and hooks to distract, compress, and derotate the spine. The cross-linking devices belonging to

Cotrel-Dubousset instrumentation

Cotrel-Dubousset instrumentation involves placing a series of rods and hooks to distract, compress, and derotate the spine. Cross-linking devices are added to provide further stability.

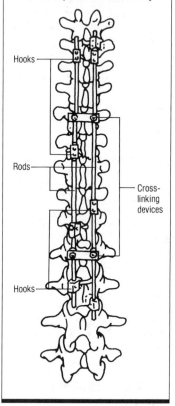

Hooks

Rods

Cross-linking devices

Hooks

this type of instrumentation serve to further stabilize the spine. Because the surgeon attaches this device to so many points of the spine, the patient may not need to wear a brace after the operation. Eliminating the need for a brace sets the Cotrel-Dubousset technique apart from other types of spinal instrumentation, such as the Harrington

rod and Zeike instrumentation. (See *Types of spinal instrumentation,* page 329.)

Purpose
• To provide stability of the spinal column during spinal fusion
• To correct spinal deformities.

Indications
Cotrel-Dubousset instrumentation is indicated when the spinal column is considered unstable secondary to tumor, infection, fracture, or increasing deformity. It provides segmental fixation for all problems of the thoracic, lumbar, and lumbosacral areas of the spine.

Cotrel-Dubousset instrumentation is contraindicated in patients who have significant osteoporosis.

Procedure
Cotrel-Dubousset spinal instrumentation is used by an experienced spinal surgeon and staff. Typically, a midline incision is made in the patient's back, and a spinal fusion (arthrodesis) is performed by stripping the paraspinal muscles from the area to be fused and by decorticating the bone. Then a bone graft is obtained – usually from the iliac crest – and placed along the area to be fused.

After the spine is prepared, multiple Cotrel-Dubousset hooks are placed at the previously determined levels and two Cotrel-Dubousset rods are placed into the hooks; then two cross-linking devices are added to provide greater stability (see *Cotrel-Dubousset instrumentation*). Any remaining bone graft is then placed along the length of the fusion and the back wound is closed according to the spinal surgeon's usual practice.

Complications
Pain, inflammatory reaction due to foreign body, local wound infection, and meningeal infection may complicate the patient's recovery. There is also the

risk that the instrumentation may loosen or break and require repair. Although the Cotrel-Dubousset instrumentation does not increase the incidence of complications, all spinal surgery carries a risk of neurologic deficit and paralysis.

Care considerations

Before surgery

• Perform a preoperative neurologic evaluation.
• Explain the surgery and postoperative course to the patient and his family. Include descriptions of postoperative assessment procedures.
• Demonstrate postoperative mobilization techniques, including logrolling, sitting, and standing.
• Ensure that laboratory values and preoperative X-rays are available to assess spinal and respiratory status.

After surgery

• Postoperatively, observe the patient in the intensive care unit for neurologic and hemodynamic changes.
• The patient should be transferred to the orthopedic unit for rehabilitation within 24 to 48 hours.
• Maintain accurate records of intake and output throughout the postoperative course. Monitor for fluid retention and hypovolemia.
• Institute the appropriate diet, observing for nausea and vomiting. Check bowel sounds for intestinal motility.
• Reinforce the dressing as needed. Document continuous or increased drainage, and notify the doctor.
• Instruct the patient on respiratory care, such as coughing and deep-breathing exercises and incentive spirometry. Continue intermittent positive-pressure breathing treatments.

Home care instructions

• Instruct the patient about gradual resumption of activity. The patient with fixation to the sacrum should avoid prolonged sitting.

• Advise the patient to avoid heavy lifting and strenuous activity and to avoid bending at the site.
• Discuss wound care as recommended by the doctor.
• Discuss pain management and the gradual withdrawal of narcotic analgesics and substitution of nonnarcotic medication.
• Emphasize the importance of a well-balanced diet to expedite bone growth, muscle strength, and return to normal bowel function. A high-fiber diet may be recommended because pain medication and iron can lead to constipation and the patient should avoid straining during elimination.
• Notify the doctor if the patient has a temperature over 101° F (38° C) for more than 24 hours, local redness, a swollen or inflamed wound, or any wound drainage.

CRANIOTOMY

A craniotomy is a surgical procedure that creates an opening in the skull, thereby exposing the brain for various treatments.

Craniotomy was previously the treatment of choice to remove brain tumors but has been replaced for this purpose by superior radiologic techniques that can localize intracranial lesions and enable neurosurgeons to use less invasive methods such as laser surgery or stereotaxic surgery, which involves guiding a probe into the brain to remove sharply circumscribed, deeply embedded tumors. The method used will depend on the patient's condition.

Purpose

• To expose the brain for surgical intervention.

Indications

Indications for craniotomy may include ventricular shunting, excision of a tumor or abscess, aspiration of a hematoma, or clipping of an aneurysm.

Procedure

Craniotomy is performed by a neurosurgeon using local or general anesthesia. Local anesthesia is used when the patient's response to manipulation of the brain must be assessed during surgery. Electrocortiography may also be performed to help assess these response areas of the brain. After making an incision through the scalp and stripping the muscle away from the scalp, the neurosurgeon drills several small burr holes into the skull and then cuts the bone between them with a pneumatic drill or a wire saw. The bone flap is turned down or completely removed. The surgeon then proceeds with the indicated surgery. After closing the incision, the surgeon covers the site with a sterile dressing.

Complications

Increased intracranial pressure (ICP) due to cerebral edema or bleeding is the major complication of intracranial surgery.

Cardiac and respiratory complications, such as cardiac or respiratory arrest, can occur from damage to the brain stem's vital centers. Potential postoperative complications include infection, hemorrhage, pneumonia, cardiac irregularities, renal and GI disorders, and meningitis.

Care considerations

Before surgery
• Perform a complete neurologic assessment. Carefully record your assessment data to use as a baseline for postoperative evaluation.
• The patient may receive anticonvulsant medication to reduce the risk of postoperative seizures.
• Steroids may be administered to prevent cerebral edema.
• Explain the procedure clearly, and provide thorough answers to questions.
• Try to relieve the patient's and family's anxiety. Although you can't guarantee a complete and uncomplicated recovery, you can help instill a sense of confidence in the surgeon and in a successful outcome.
• Wash the patient's hair with an antimicrobial shampoo on the night before surgery. Explain that his head may be partially or completely shaved, depending on the degree of surgery.
• Inform the patient that before surgery, his legs will be wrapped with elastic bandages to improve venous return (circulation) and reduce the risk of thrombophlebitis. An indwelling urinary catheter may be inserted.
• Explain to the patient that he will awaken from surgery with a large dressing on his head to protect the incision and possibly a surgical drain implanted in his skull for a few days, and that he will receive prophylactic antibiotics.
• Warn the patient to expect a headache and facial swelling for 2 to 3 days after surgery, and reassure him that medication will be given to reduce the pain. Explain that, if all goes well, he should be ambulatory within 2 to 3 days after surgery and the doctor will remove the sutures within 7 to 10 days.

After surgery
• Monitor vital signs and neurologic status.
• To help prevent increased ICP, elevate the head of the patient's bed 15 to 30 degrees to increase venous return and ease breathing.
• Turn the patient carefully every 2 hours.
• Observe the patient closely for signs of increased ICP. Immediately report worsening mental status, pupillary changes, or focal signs such as increasing weakness in an extremity.

• Closely observe respiratory status, noting rate and pattern. Immediately report any abnormalities. Encourage the patient to deep-breathe and cough, but not too strenuously.
• Carefully monitor fluid and electrolyte balance.
• Monitor and record intake and output, check urine specific gravity every 2 hours, and weigh the patient, as ordered.
• Check serum electrolyte levels every 24 hours and watch the patient for signs of imbalance. Low potassium levels may cause confusion and stupor; reduced sodium and chloride levels may produce weakness, lethargy, and even coma. Because fluid and electrolyte imbalance can precipitate seizures, report such signs immediately.
• Provide good wound care. Make sure the dressing stays dry and in place and that it's not too tight. Excessive tightness may indicate swelling—a sign of increased ICP. If the patient has a closed drainage system, periodically check drain patency and note and document the amount and characteristics of any discharge.
• Notify the doctor of excessive bloody drainage, which may indicate cerebral hemorrhage, or clear or yellow drainage or a halo shape on the dressing, which may indicate cerebrospinal fluid leakage.
• Monitor for signs of wound infection: fever, purulent drainage, or redness of the suture line.
• Provide supportive care. Ensure a quiet, calm environment to minimize anxiety and agitation and help lower ICP.
• Administer anticonvulsants, as prescribed, as well as other medications: corticosteroids to prevent or reduce cerebral edema, stool softeners to prevent increased ICP caused by straining, analgesics to relieve pain, and antibiotics to decrease the risk of infection.

Home care instructions

• Make sure the patient knows proper wound care. He can allow shower water to run over the incision and wash it gently with soap but not scrub. Otherwise, tell him to keep the suture line dry.
• Tell the patient to evaluate the incision regularly for redness, warmth, or tenderness and to report such findings to the doctor.
• If the patient is self-conscious about his appearance, suggest wearing a wig, hat, or scarf until his hair grows back. As the hair begins to grow back, tell him to apply a lanolin-based lotion to the scalp—except for the suture line—to keep it supple and decrease itching.
• Remind the patient to continue taking prescribed anticonvulsants to minimize the risk of seizures. Depending on the type of surgery, the patient may need to continue anticonvulsant therapy for up to 12 months after surgery.
• Tell the patient to report any drug reactions, such as excessive drowsiness or confusion, and increased headache, photophobia, or neck stiffness, which might indicate meningitis.

CRYOSURGERY

Cryosurgery is the destruction of tissue by the application of extreme cold. This procedure is often performed in the doctor's office. It can be performed simply, with a cotton-tipped applicator dipped into liquid nitrogen and applied to the lesion, or it may involve a complex cryosurgical unit (CSU).

The success of cryosurgery depends on the type of lesion, the extent and depth of the freeze applied, and the duration between freezing and thawing. A slow thaw destroys lesions most effectively. Liquid nitrogen and nitrous oxide are the most commonly used cryogens, but some CSUs employ carbon dioxide or Freon. Liquid nitrogen is by far the most powerful cryogen and is especially useful for treating cancerous lesions, which resist cold because of their vascularity. Nitrous oxide is often favored for less extensive procedures because the surgeon can more easily control its effects.

Purpose
• To destroy diseased tissue by the application of extreme cold
• To create a chorioretinal scar to seal retinal tears or holes.

Indications
Cryosurgery is used to treat actinic and seborrheic keratoses, leukoplakia, molluscum contagiosum, verrucae, and sometimes early basal cell epitheliomas and squamous cell carcinomas. Cryosurgery may also be indicated for various gynecologic conditions, including cervicitis, chronic cervical erosion, cervical polyps, and condyloma accuminata, and for cataract removal or treatment of retinal pathology, such as tears or holes in the anterior or peripheral retina. Retinopathy of prematurity may also be treated by cryosurgery.

Contraindications to cryosurgery include an underlying cryoglobulinemia, cryofibrinogenemia, cold intolerance, Raynaud's disease, cold urticaria, pyoderma gangrenosum, collagen and autoimmune disease, concurrent dialysis or immunosuppressant drug therapy, platelet deficiency, blood dyscrasias, multiple myeloma, and agammaglobulinemia.

Procedure
For dermatologic cryosurgery, the surgeon may give a local anesthetic, depending on the type of procedure. When freezing superficial lesions, the surgeon can often determine the correct temperature and depth of freezing simply by palpating and observing the lesion. When treating skin cancers, however, he uses thermocouple needles (inserted and secured into the base

of the tumor) and a tissue temperature monitor (pyrometer) to ensure that the tissue at the deepest part of the lesion has been adequately frozen. In such cases, a nurse is often responsible for operating the needles and pyrometer. (See *Positioning thermocouple needles.*)

The surgeon uses the cotton-tipped applicator or the CSU to freeze the lesion and may refreeze a tumor several times to ensure its destruction.

If cryosurgery is used to treat retinal pathology, the patient receives topical anesthetic eyedrops, and the pupils are well dilated. A cryoprobe is then used to freeze affected tissue. The affected eye is patched until anesthesia has worn off.

However, if cryosurgery is used to treat posterior retinal pathology, the conjunctiva is incised to enable eye rotation with scleral exposure. This procedure then will require strict sterile technique.

Cryosurgery to treat a gynecologic disorder is usually performed 1 week after a woman's menstrual period. The procedure is performed with a vaginal speculum in place.

Complications
Complications of cryosurgery are usually minor and may include hypopigmentation (from destruction of melanocytes) and secondary infection. Rarely, the procedure may damage blood vessels, nerves, and tear ducts. After gynecologic cryosurgery, cervical stenosis may result if too large an area of the cervix is frozen at one time. Any procedure requiring cryosurgery carries a risk of infection.

Care considerations
Before the procedure
• Explain the procedure to the patient. Clarify that an incision is not made (unless treating posterior retina).
• Tell the patient to expect to initially feel cold, followed by burning, during the procedure. Warn him to remain as

Positioning thermocouple needles

During cryosurgery, you may be responsible for positioning thermocouple needles. These needles measure the temperature of the tissue and help the doctor gauge the depth of freezing—a vital factor when destroying cancerous lesions.

The needle may be placed in any of several positions. The illustration at the right shows the needle inserted at an angle so that the tip rests about 5 mm below the base of the tumor to give a direct reading of tissue temperature. When used in this fashion, the temperature reading may be affected by chilling of the shaft within the frozen tissue, but the error isn't likely to be significant. The bottom illustration shows a needle inserted perpendicularly about 5 mm to one side of the frozen tissue at a depth of about 3 mm. In this position, it will register the same temperature as the probe at the left because both tips are about the same distance from the frozen tissue.

Precise temperature measurement can be difficult because a variation of only 1 mm in the probe's position can translate into a difference of 10° to 15° C (18° to 27° F). For that reason, you'll usually place two or more probes in different areas to increase the accuracy of the reading.

Needle at an angle

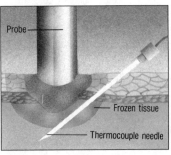

Probe

Frozen tissue

Thermocouple needle

Needle perpendicular

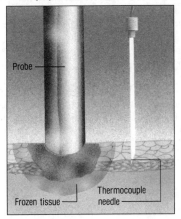

Probe

Frozen tissue

Thermocouple needle

still as possible during the procedure to prevent inadvertent freezing of normal tissue.
• If appropriate, gather the necessary equipment. If thermocouple needles and a pyrometer will be used, make certain that they are sterile and in good working order.
• Ensure that the patient has signed a consent form.

• If assisting with the procedure, position the patient comfortably and as required by the site of treatment.
• If necessary, shield the patient's eyes or ears to prevent damage.

During the procedure
• Assist the surgeon as appropriate. You may be responsible for positioning thermocouple needles.
• Provide reassurance and psychological support. Tell the patient what to

do to help the procedure proceed quickly and smoothly. Suggest that the patient breathe slowly and deeply to manage discomfort.

• During gynecologic cryosurgery, anticipate that the patient may experience headaches, dizziness, flushing, or cramping.

After the procedure

• After dermatologic cryosurgery, clean the area gently with a cotton-tipped applicator soaked in hydrogen peroxide. Because cryosurgery doesn't cause bleeding, don't apply a bandage. In fact, occlusive dressings are contraindicated.

• If necessary, apply an ice bag to relieve swelling and give analgesics to relieve pain, as ordered. Cryosurgery may cause considerable pain, especially if it was performed on or near the lips, eyes, eyelids, tongue, or plantar surfaces of the feet.

Home care instructions

• Tell the patient to expect pain and to manage it with the prescribed analgesic.

• Tell the dermatologic patient to expect redness and swelling and the formation of a blister. Tell him not to touch the blister. It will slough off in 2 to 3 weeks. If it becomes extremely uncomfortable or interferes with daily activities, the patient can ask the doctor to decompress it.

• Tell the patient to immediately report new, intense pain; fever; or purulent drainage to the doctor.

• Tell the dermatologic patient to clean the area gently with soap and water, alcohol, or a cotton-tipped applicator soaked in hydrogen peroxide. To prevent hypopigmentation, instruct him to cover the wound with a loose dressing when he's outdoors. After the wound heals, he should apply a sunscreen over the area. If the patient has had a malignant lesion destroyed, urge him to have regular checkups because skin cancers may recur.

• Instruct the gynecologic patient to avoid intercourse for 2 weeks and to return for regularly scheduled physical examinations.

CYSTOSTOMY

Cystostomy is a type of urinary diversion. It involves transcutaneous insertion of a catheter through the suprapubic area into the bladder, with connection of the device to a closed drainage system.

Purpose

• To provide temporary urinary diversion when urethral catheterization is contraindicated or not possible.

Indications

Typically, cystostomy provides temporary urinary diversion after certain gynecologic procedures, bladder surgery, or prostatectomy and relieves urinary obstruction resulting from severe urethral strictures or pelvic trauma. Rarely, it may be used to create a permanent urinary diversion to relieve urinary obstruction by an inoperable tumor or other lesions.

It's often useful in infants and young children, whose narrow urethras may hinder insertion of an indwelling urinary catheter.

Procedure

Cystostomy may be performed during other surgery while the patient is under general anesthesia. It may also be performed under local anesthesia at the patient's bedside. The procedure causes little or no discomfort and takes 5 to 10 minutes.

To perform a percutaneous cystostomy, the surgeon makes a stab wound in the area above the symphysis pubis, inserts a trocar and catheter, and advances them into the bladder until he detects urine return. Next, he stabilizes the catheter while the trocar is removed and then secures the catheter to the skin with sutures and tape. Percutaneous cystostomy requires a distended bladder and the absence of suprapubic or groin surgery (or scarring). If bladder distention is doubtful—for example, in an obese patient—it may be verified by ultrasonography.

To perform an open suprapubic cystostomy, the surgeon makes a short 2" to 3" (5- to 7.6-cm) transverse incision two finger-breadths above the symphysis pubis. He divides the anterior fascia and separates the rectus muscles to expose the anterior bladder wall. Next, he introduces a Malecot catheter into the bladder and brings the catheter out to the skin surface through the stab incision, or, more commonly, through a stab wound above the incision. After closing the incision, he sutures the catheter in place and secures it with tape.

With either approach, the cystostomy tube is connected to a closed drainage system. After removal of the cystostomy tube, the doctor will place sterile dressings over the site. Rapid healing generally occurs, sealing over the insertion site. However, if a catheter with a larger bore is inserted, healing may be delayed.

Complications

Cystostomy can lead to urine retention from catheter obstruction, evidenced by leaking around the catheter; bladder infection; hematuria; and skin breakdown.

Care considerations
Before the procedure
• Explain the procedure and postoperative care to the patient or family.
• Ensure that the patient or a responsible family member has signed a consent form.

During the procedure
• As appropriate, assist the surgeon and provide emotional support and reassurance to the patient.
After the procedure
• Provide routine postoperative care: monitor vital signs, intake and output, and fluid status, and encourage coughing, deep-breathing, and early ambulation. In addition, focus on providing tube care and assessing for possible complications.
• To ensure adequate drainage and tube patency, check the cystostomy tube at least hourly for the first 24 hours after insertion. Carefully document the color and amount of drainage from the tube; note particularly any color changes.
• Make sure that the catheter and the drainage tube are kink-free and that the collection bag is below bladder level to enhance drainage and prevent backflow, which can lead to infection.
• Irrigate the cystostomy tube as ordered, using the same technique as for irrigating an indwelling urinary catheter. Check the tube frequently for kinks or obstruction. A decrease in urine output and a distended, tender bladder indicate obstruction. If a blood clot or mucus blocks the tube and you can't clear the obstruction promptly, notify the doctor.
• To prevent kinks in the tube, curve it gently but don't bend it. Tape the tube securely in place on the abdomen to reduce tension and prevent dislodgment. However, if the tube does become dislodged, immediately notify the doctor; he may be able to reinsert it through the original tract. Remember that the longer the interval between catheter dislodgment and replacement, the less likely is successful catheter reinsertion.
• If ordered, perform a voiding trial: Instill fluid through the catheter to the point of bladder discomfort; then clamp the catheter and tell the patient to void as he would normally. Observe and re-

cord the instilled and voided urine volumes.

• Check the dressing often, and change it at least once a day or as ordered. Anticipate wet dressings for the first few days after removal of the cystostomy tube; change these dressings frequently, as needed.

• Observe the skin around the insertion site for encrustation and signs of infection.

Home care instructions

• Teach the patient or parents how to change the dressing and, if the cystostomy tube is still in place, how to empty and reattach the collection bag.

• Advise the patient to see the doctor or return to the hospital if the catheter becomes completely dislodged. Remind the patient that excessive urine leakage around the catheter may indicate partial dislodgment, requiring catheter replacement.

• Tell the patient or family caregiver to promptly notify the doctor of signs of infection, such as discolored or foul-smelling discharge; impaired drainage; swelling, redness, or tenderness at the tube insertion site; and decreased urine output.

• Encourage the patient to drink plenty of fluids to reduce the risk of complications.

• Emphasize the importance of regular follow-up examinations to allow early detection of complications.

DEBRIDEMENT

Debridement is the mechanical, chemical, or surgical removal of necrotic tissue from a wound. This procedure can be extremely painful, but it is necessary to promote healing and prevent infection of burns, pressure ulcers, and nonhealing surgical or traumatic wounds.

Mechanical debridement includes application of wet-to-dry dressings, irrigation, hydrotherapy, and bedside debridement. *Chemical debridement* uses enzymes that selectively digest necrotic material. These agents also absorb bacteria and thus reduce the risk of infection. *Surgical debridement*, performed under general or regional anesthesia, affords the fastest and most complete debridement. The method selected depends on the type and extent of injury and the patient's overall condition.

Caution should be used when applying wet-to-dry dressings because they can have a deleterious effect on healing tissues. Enzyme debridement should not be used on wounds with exposed bone.

Purpose
• To promote wound healing
• To prepare the wounded skin area for grafting
• To prevent secondary infection.

Indications
The use of mechanical, chemical, or surgical debridement depends on the size and extent of the patient's wound and the patient's overall condition. The simplest type of mechanical debridement, wet-to-dry dressings are appropriately applied to partially healed wounds with only slight amounts of necrotic tissue and minimal drainage; they're most commonly used to treat pressure ulcers rather than burns. Irrigation and wound packing are indicated for deeper wounds to allow proper healing from the inside outward to the skin surface and to prevent abscess formation. Hydrotherapy, another type of mechanical debridement, is usually performed on burned patients. It allows relatively nontraumatic wound debridement, dressing changes, removal of previously applied topical agents, and general body cleaning. A third type of mechanical debridement, so-called bedside debridement (not always done at the bedside), can be used in the treatment of burns, pressure ulcers, and nonhealing surgical or traumatic wounds.

Chemical debridement is most often used for pressure or stasis ulcers, traumatic infected surgical wounds, and sickle cell ulcers. Sometimes chemical and mechanical debridement are combined by applying bandages saturated with various medications.

Surgical debridement is usually reserved for burns or extremely deep or large ulcers. It is typically performed along with skin grafting.

Procedure
Wet-to-dry dressings are placed in contact with the wound and covered with an outer layer of bandages. As the dressing dries, it sticks to the wound and, when the dry dressing is removed,

the attached necrotic tissue comes off with it.

When irrigating a wound, the prescribed solution is instilled with an irrigation syringe. The solution should flow from the cleanest part of the wound to the dirtiest to prevent cross-contamination. The irrigation is repeated until the prescribed amount of solution has been used or until the return is clear. After irrigation, a wound is usually packed with dressings to absorb additional drainage.

Usually performed by a nurse assisted by a physical therapist, hydrotherapy—also called "tubbing" or "tanking"—involves immersion of the patient in a tank of warm, chemically treated water that is intermittently agitated. The patient soaks for a predetermined time to loosen the old dressings (gentle agitation may be needed), and the burned areas are gently scrubbed to remove topical agents, exudates, necrotic tissue, and debris. Debridement is then performed as necessary, usually by a doctor, and the areas are re-dressed with sterile dressings. (Also see the entry "Hydrotherapy.")

Bedside debridement of a wound involves careful prying and cutting of loosened eschar (burned tissue) or necrotic tissue with forceps and scissors to separate it from the viable tissue beneath. Depending on the size and severity of the burn, bedside debridement may be performed during hydrotherapy or afterward in the procedure room. One of the most painful types of debridement, it may be the only way to remove necrotic tissue from a severely burned patient. Bedside debridement of pressure ulcers can be performed by specially skilled nurses. If the patient is at home, it can be performed there.

Chemical debridement is performed by a nurse and is accomplished by first gently irrigating the wound with 0.9% sodium chloride solution to remove the previous application and any exudate

and necrotic tissue. The topical debriding agent is then applied to the necrotic area, and the wound is covered with a sterile dressing. Surrounding healthy tissue may require protection from the debriding agent with a skin-toughening agent such as Skinprep.

Surgical debridement is performed by the doctor in the operating room using one of two procedures, depending on the depth and extent of the wound. In the first, tangential excision, he uses a dermatome or knife to remove sequential layers of dead tissue until viable tissue is reached. In the second, fascial excision, the surgeon removes all injured tissue and underlying fat down to the fascia by using avulsion, a scalpel, or a laser.

Complications

In any type of debridement, there is a risk of infection. Surgical debridement may cause sepsis, if the wound is grossly infected at the time of excision, as well as hemorrhage and the usual risks of surgery.

In debridement of extensive wounds, fluid and electrolyte imbalance may occur. Also, application of wet-to-dry dressings may lead to destruction of newly healed skin.

Care considerations
Before the procedure
• Explain the type of debridement that will be used.
• Teach relaxation techniques.
• When applicable, administer analgesics, as ordered, 20 minutes before the procedure.
• Position the patient comfortably and provide maximum access to the site.
During the procedure
• Provide emotional support.
• Perform the procedure as gently as possible.
• Note the amount of granulation tissue, necrotic debris, and drainage.

• Be alert for signs of wound infection. Report such signs immediately because infection in compromised patients can quickly grow to life-threatening severity.

After the procedure
• Assess the patient's pain level, both from his own reports and from such signs as restlessness, increased muscle tension, and rapid respirations.
• Provide additional analgesics as appropriate.
• Assess fluid and electrolyte status, especially if the patient has burns. Weigh the patient daily, maintain accurate intake and output records, and closely monitor laboratory test results.
• Watch for and report signs of electrolyte imbalance: poor skin turgor, cardiac disturbances, tremors, weakness or spasms, or confusion.
• If a limb was debrided, keep it elevated to promote venous return — especially for stasis ulcers.
• Watch for excessive bleeding after bedside and surgical debridement.
• Assess for signs of infection.

Home care instructions
• Pressure or stasis ulcers and other nonhealing wounds are often managed at home by a home care nurse, the patient, or caregiver.
• Instruct the patient on the signs and symptoms of infection and when to notify the home care nurse or doctor.
• If the patient will be performing dressing changes, provide instructions on aseptic technique.

DECONGESTANTS AND ANTIHISTAMINES

Antihistamines relieve allergic symptoms by competing with histamine for receptor sites on effector cells. They include such drugs as *azatadine, astemizole, brompheniramine, carbinoxamine, chlorpheniramine, clemastine, cyproheptadine,* *diphenhydramine, methdilazine, promethazine, terfenadine, trimeprazine, tripelennamine,* and *triprolidine.*

Most antihistamines are given orally; some, including brompheniramine, diphenhydramine, chlorpheniramine, and promethazine, can also be given by deep I.M. injection. Such injection brings rapid relief of allergic symptoms but may cause local stinging and burning, sweating, and transient hypotension.

Decongestants, including *ephedrine, pseudoephedrine,* and *phenylpropanolamine,* relieve nasal stuffiness by acting on the respiratory tract's alpha-adrenergic receptors to produce vasoconstriction. They're available for oral use in tablets, extended-release capsules, and liquid.

Antihistamines and decongestants are often combined in cold and allergy medications to relieve a wide range of symptoms. For example, chlorpheniramine and phenylpropanolamine are combined to relieve rhinorrhea and nasal stuffiness.

Purpose
• To decrease allergic reactions and decrease allergy symptoms (antihistamines)
• To decrease nasal stuffiness (decongestants).

Indications
Decongestants and antihistamines relieve sneezing, rhinorrhea, and nasal congestion associated with colds and allergies. Antihistamines are also used to prevent or treat allergic reactions ranging from the symptoms of hay fever or insect bites to anaphylaxis.

Antihistamines should be avoided in patients with acute asthma because they increase the viscosity of tracheobronchial secretions. They should also be avoided in patients with urine retention or prostatic hyperplasia because they may worsen urine retention. Decongestants should be avoided in patients with hypertension because these agents, which cause vasoconstriction of the blood vessels, may further elevate blood pressure.

Adverse reactions

Antihistamines and decongestants are typically well tolerated but can produce many systemic effects. Most antihistamines (except astemizole and terfenadine) cause drowsiness, fatigue, and some confusion. They may also cause epigastric distress, postural hypotension, dry mouth, nausea, and vomiting.

The nonsedating antihistamines astemizole and terfenadine cause different reactions. Terfenadine is associated with alopecia, visual disturbances, cough, rash, and itching; astemizole, with headache, increased appetite, weight gain, abdominal pain, and dry mouth. High doses can cause cardiac rhythm disturbances.

Decongestants, which affect the same systems, may cause restlessness, irritability, insomnia, and palpitations. Neither is recommended for use in neonates, premature infants, or elderly patients.

Care considerations

• Before giving an antihistamine or a decongestant, check the patient's drug regimen for possible interactions. For instance, concurrent use of antihistamines with central nervous system (CNS) depressants may cause increased sedation. Use of decongestants with monoamine oxidase inhibitors can cause life-threatening hypertensive crisis. Use of terfenadine with ketoconazole or erythromycin and its derivatives can cause cardiac rhythm disturbances.
• If administering antihistamines by deep I.M. injection, monitor the patient's vital signs, noting hypotension, irregular pulse, or other untoward reactions. Be alert for signs of overdose: hypotension, seizures, flushing, palpitations, restlessness, and chest tightness.
• Watch for changes in mental status. If the patient is taking an antihistamine and experiences drowsiness, raise the side rails of the bed and assist with ambulation, if necessary. If the patient is taking a decongestant, watch for increased restlessness and insomnia. Give the last dose 2 to 3 hours before bedtime. Warn the patient not to crush or chew the extended-release tablets or capsules.

Home care instructions

• Tell the patient to take the drug exactly as directed. Explain that a tolerance to it may develop; however, he shouldn't increase the dosage on his own, but should contact the doctor.
• Instruct the patient to take a missed dose as soon as possible, unless it's within 2 hours of his next dose (or within 12 hours if taking an extended-release product). Warn him not to double-dose.
• If the patient is taking an antihistamine, explain that drowsiness is common. Instruct him to avoid hazardous tasks that require alertness until CNS response is clearly established. Suggest that caffeinated beverages may combat drowsiness, and warn against drinking alcohol or taking sedatives unless directed otherwise by the doctor. Suggest relieving dry mouth with ice chips, sugarless gum, or hard candy. If GI irritation develops, advise taking the drug with soup or milk.
• Tell the patient who is taking a decongestant to avoid excessive intake of caffeinated beverages because these increase CNS stimulation. Instruct him to notify the doctor if his symptoms don't improve in a week or if fever persists.

Defibrillation

Defibrillation is delivery of a brief electric shock to the heart during a life-threatening arrhythmia. This burst of electric current completely depolarizes the myocardium, allowing the heart's natural pacemaker (the sino-atrial [SA] node) to regain control of cardiac rhythm.

Life-threatening arrhythmias, such as ventricular fibrillation or pulseless ventricular tachycardia, cause cardiac output to drop to zero. If zero output persists for more than 4 to 6 minutes, irreparable brain damage results from lack of oxygenated blood. Once the emergency situation is identified, defibrillation must be performed immediately. According to recent literature, when advanced cardiac life support (including defibrillation) is given to a person in ventricular fibrillation within 5 minutes, about 40% of victims are successfully resuscitated.

The patient receiving defibrillation must be pulseless and unresponsive. No matter what the electrocardiogram (ECG) indicates, *never defibrillate a patient who's alert or has a pulse.* Defibrillating an alert patient could trigger lethal arrhythmias and cardiac standstill. The patient who has an abnormal cardiac rhythm with a pulse may be a candidate for synchronized cardioversion instead. (See the entry "Cardioversion, Synchronized.")

Purpose

• To correct pulseless ventricular tachycardia or fibrillation and allow the SA node to resume initiation of the heartbeat.

Indications

Defibrillation is the treatment of choice for ventricular fibrillation and pulseless ventricular tachycardia.

Procedure

Defibrillation is performed by a health professional specially skilled in advanced cardiac life support. It is administered with other resuscitation measures, such as mechanical ventilation, cardiopulmonary resuscitation (CPR), and emergency medications. As soon as pulseless ventricular tachycardia or ventricular fibrillation has been confirmed on the monitor, the defibrillator is brought to the patient's bedside. The defibrillator paddles are coated with conductive gel or paste and are positioned on the patient's chest. Standard placement requires one paddle positioned to the right of the upper sternum and below the clavicle; the other paddle is positioned to the left of the apex in the midaxillary line. (Alternate positioning, using anterior-posterior [A-P] paddles, places the anterior paddle over the left precordial area and the posterior paddle behind the heart just below the left scapula.) The machine is charged. Immediately before delivering the shock, the health care worker holding the paddles must notify the rest of the emergency team to stand clear of the bed and the patient. Then, the electric shock is delivered. The American Heart Association recommends a charge of 200 joules for the first attempt, 200 to 300 joules for the second attempt, and 360 joules for subsequent attempts.

An alternative type of external defibrillator uses pre-gelled, self-adhesive, conductive, disposable defibrillator pads. These pads can remain on the patient's chest; if a lethal arrhythmia develops, defibrillation can be performed without the need to reapply gel or reposition the paddles. This is especially useful for patients with recurrent ventricular tachycardia.

Defibrillation and other resuscitation measures continue until the patient's cardiac condition stabilizes or the doctor orders discontinuation.

Complications

The most common complication from defibrillation is skin burn from the defibrillator paddles.

Other complications include myocardial injury, postconversion tachyarrhythmias, and embolization. Safety precautions must be taken to avoid delivering electric shocks to the emergency health care team.

Care considerations

Before the procedure

• Maintenance of defibrillation equipment is of vital importance. It should be checked according to the facility's policy to ensure that the defibrillator charges and releases the electric currents appropriately.

• When a cardiac emergency situation arises, promptly call for help (health care facilities ordinarily have an intercom system to summon the emergency team) and begin CPR.

• When the defibrillator arrives, continue CPR during preparation of the equipment.

• Set up the defibrillator and attach ECG leads to the patient.

• Make sure the synchronizer control is turned off; if it's set on the synchronous mode, it won't discharge during ventricular fibrillation or ventricular tachycardia.

• Apply conductive gel or paste to the paddles or place two gel pads on the patient's bare chest in the appropriate position. If using gel or paste, coat the entire surface of the paddles by rubbing them together. Be sure to remove any gel from your hands and the sides of the paddles because excessive conductive gel will provide a pathway for the electric current and cause burns.

• Verify pulselessness by checking for a carotid pulse and verify ventricular fibrillation, ventricular tachycardia, or asystole on the monitor.

• Select the charge and place the prepared paddles on the patient. Avoid placing them over a permanent pacemaker or on a woman's breast.

• Instruct all caregivers to stand clear before discharging the defibrillator. Make sure there is no water on the floor because it can transmit an electric charge.

During the procedure

• Continue to monitor for pulse and cardiac rhythm.

• Administer medications, as ordered, to treat possible causes of fibrillation, such as hypoxia, hypokalemia, and acidosis.

After the procedure

• Continue to monitor cardiac and respiratory status as well as vital signs until the patient is stable.

• Obtain a 12-lead ECG and chest X-ray.

• Clean the patient's skin and the defibrillator paddles to remove conductive gel or paste.

• Evaluate the skin for burns and apply prescribed ointment.

• Maintain patent I.V. access and continue to monitor for precipitating causes of ventricular tachycardia or fibrillation.

• Document the date and time arrhythmia occurred, the therapy initiated, and the patient's status before and after arrhythmia and defibrillation.

Home care instructions

• Instruct the patient to take his pulse for a full minute before taking prescribed medication and to notify the doctor of palpitations, dizziness, faintness, or alteration of rate and rhythm from what is typical for him.

• Emphasize the need to continue regular medical follow-up appointments for routine ECGs and evaluation of the patient's response to medication.

• If your patient will have an implantable cardiac defibrillator, outline the special precautions he'll have to take (see the entry "Implantable Cardioverter Defibrillator").

DERMABRASION

Dermabrasion is the surgical removal of the surface layer of the skin by high-speed sanding to improve many superficial skin problems. Dermabrasion removes the epidermis and some superficial dermis, while preserving enough skin for reepithelialization (regrowth). In some cases, patients require two to three dermabrasion procedures for optimal results.

Careful patient selection is essential. Patients who have unrealistic expectations are not appropriate candidates. The candidate for dermabrasion must understand the limitations of this procedure and be able to accept the fact that some skin defects will remain after the procedure.

Pigmentary changes following a dermabrasion procedure may occur in individuals with pigmented skin such as brunettes, Asians, and light-skinned Blacks.

Purpose

• To remove minor imperfections from the surface of the skin
• To improve the patient's appearance and thereby boost self-esteem
• To reconstruct a skin area after surgery.

Indications

The most frequent indication for dermabrasion is postacne scarring. It has also been useful for removing superficial scars after traumatic injury or surgery. Other indications for dermabrasion include smallpox scars, removal of decorative or traumatic tattoos, solar elastosis (sun damage), actinic keratoses, and seborrheic keratoses.

Dermabrasion is contraindicated in patients who have undergone radiation therapy that has weakened underlying skin structure, and in those with uncontrolled diabetes mellitus or severe cardiovascular disease. It should not be used for at least 6 to 12 months after a course of isotretinoin (Accutane) or in a patient with a positive blood test for the human immunodeficiency virus.

Procedure

Dermabrasion may be performed by a dermatologic surgeon, a plastic surgeon, or a cosmetic surgeon. The dermabrasion may take place in an office, an outpatient clinic, or a hospital operating room.

A sedative is administered either orally or by injection. After the skin is cleaned with an antimicrobial soap, gentian violet is painted on the areas to be planed. This fills and identifies the deepest pits for abrasions. The patient is asked to hold a cold pack on the area to be planed to lower the temperature of the skin.

A local anesthetic is administered to provide regional anesthesia. A refrigerant spray may be used to freeze the skin and to harden the surface for improved abrasion. The surgeon then removes the area that is to be abraded with a high-speed diamond fraise or a wire brush. A thick, nonadherent pad is then applied directly to the abraded area to absorb the drainage.

Deep scars that cannot be dermabraded can be excised and sutured closed or later filled with collagen.

Complications

Hypopigmentation and hyperpigmentation may follow dermabrasion. Hypopigmentation occurs in about 50% of all dermabrasions. Other rare complications include infection, scarring, or keloid formation. In a patient with a history of herpes simplex, dermabrasion may reactivate the virus. Because the results of dermabrasion are never perfect, patients who are unable to accept the remaining defects may develop emotional problems.

Care considerations

Before therapy

• Assure proper patient selection. Interview the patient for medical history, level of knowledge about the procedure, and expected outcome.

• Inform the patient about the procedure, risks, complications, and possible outcomes.

• The patient's skin must be free of cosmetics and washed with soap and water or an antimicrobial soap. The area to be abraded must be clean-shaven.

• The patient should bring someone along to provide transportation home.

• Make sure the patient signs a consent form.

After therapy

• Monitor vital signs.

• Demonstrate wound care to the patient or caregiver and make sure they can identify signs of infection, such as fever or purulent drainage.

Home care instructions

• Inform the patient that he will experience edema, erythema, crust formation, and some discomfort and itching after the procedure.

• Advise the patient to remove the dressing the next day and to clean the skin with soap and water. The skin should be patted dry, not rubbed, then covered with an antibacterial ointment.

• Emphasize the importance of keeping follow-up appointments to treat problem areas.

• Tell the patient to avoid sun exposure for 3 to 6 months and, afterward, to use a sunscreen with a skin protection factor of at least 15 when outdoors.

• Advise patients who received dermabrasion for sun-damaged skin to alter their outdoor activities to prevent further damage.

DETOXIFICATION

Detoxification refers to withdrawal from the effects of prolonged dependence on alcohol or other drugs. Detoxification programs are designed to help the patient maintain abstinence and to provide a relatively safe alternative to self-withdrawal, which is difficult and often dangerous. Provided in outpatient centers or in special hospital units, detoxification programs offer treatment of symptoms as well as counseling or psychotherapy for an individual, group, or family.

Treating patients during detoxification requires skill, compassion, and commitment. Because substance abusers have low self-esteem and commonly try to manipulate others, health care workers who manage their care need to recognize attempts at manipulation and to control natural feelings of anger and frustration.

Detoxification programs are only one part of the total treatment plan for a drug- or alcohol-dependent patient; they are used with psychotherapy, counseling and, ultimately, rehabilitation.

Purpose

• To help the patient achieve abstinence from alcohol or drugs while providing supportive and symptomatic care.

Indications

Detoxification programs are the treatment of choice for alcohol and drug dependence.

Procedure

Alcohol withdrawal requires total abstinence and usually proves more severe and hazardous than drug withdrawal. The procedure for alcohol detoxification involves providing a safe, softly lit environment to avoid overstimulation and agitation, which can cause tremors, and removing any potentially harmful objects from the patient's room. The patient is usually treated symptomatically with antianxiety agents, anticonvulsants, antiemetics, and antidiarrheals, as needed.

The patient who experiences hallucinations may need frequent orientation to reality (time, place, and person) and may require short-term use of restraints for combative behavior. Seizure and suicide precautions are recommended.

Detoxification from opioids, benzodiazepines, depressants, or other drugs is achieved by gradually lowering the dosage of the abused drug or by substituting a drug with similar action; for example, methadone may be substituted for heroin; cocaine addiction may be treated with bromocriptine or naltrexone. The patient may be taught relaxation techniques, encouraged to perform mild exercise, and provided with nutritional support.

Some drug abusers who enter detoxification programs require emergency treatment, typically for an overdose of opioids (narcotics), barbiturates, cocaine, or amphetamines. (See *Treating drug intoxication*, page 226.) This treatment is aimed at preventing shock and maintaining respirations. Gastric lavage or induction of vomiting may be used if the drug was ingested within 4 hours of treatment. Dialysis, cardiopulmonary resuscitation, and defibrillation may also be required.

Complications

During withdrawal from prolonged abuse of alcohol, autonomic hyperactivity results in tachycardia, hypertension, fever, flushing, and diaphoresis. Central nervous system symptoms include anxiety, tremors, and irritability, which may progress to seizure activity. Anorexia, nausea, vomiting, and diarrhea are also seen. Alcohol withdrawal syndrome, an acute toxic state characterized by agitation, confusion, delusions, hallucinations, and tonic-clonic seizures, is a life-threatening response to withdrawal.

Care considerations
Before therapy
• Reassure the patient in acute distress, along with his family, that he'll receive immediate treatment.
• If the patient is not in acute distress, perform a psychosocial evaluation to assess family and social life.
• Take a medical history, noting especially any history of psychiatric disorder, seizures, and specific substance dependence.
• Perform a complete neurologic assessment.
• Obtain blood samples and urine specimens for alcohol and drug screening.
During therapy
• Be alert for any continued substance abuse after admission to the detoxification program.
• Administer prescribed medications carefully to prevent hoarding by the patient.
• Closely monitor visitors, who might supply drugs or alcohol from the outside.
• If you suspect continued abuse, obtain a blood sample and urine specimen for screening and report any positive findings to the doctor. This procedure may depend upon the facility's policy.
• Because immunity can be lowered in drug or alcohol abuse, observe the patient for signs of infection.
• Provide adequate nutrition and assess for signs of vitamin deficiency and malnutrition.
• If the patient shows impaired mobility, assist with ambulation as necessary and encourage bed rest until he regains stability.
After therapy
• Encourage participation in rehabilitation programs and self-help groups.

Treating drug intoxication

Sometimes drug abusers enter detoxification programs requiring emergency treatment, typically for an overdose of opioids (narcotics), barbiturates, cocaine, amphetamines, or benzodiazepines.

Opioid overdose
The immediate goal is to prevent shock and maintain respirations. Intubate the patient and give oxygen, I.V. fluids, and plasma expanders. Also give naloxone (Narcan), a specific opioid antagonist, to reverse central nervous system (CNS) depression.

Barbiturate overdose
Like treatment of opioid overdose, treatment of barbiturate overdose aims to prevent shock and maintain respirations. It may also include gastric lavage or induced vomiting if the patient ingested the drug within the previous 4 hours. Or it may include administration of activated charcoal, followed by a cathartic, to eliminate the toxic drug. Extreme intoxication requires dialysis.

Cocaine intoxication
Because cocaine is cardiogenic, monitor the patient's heart rate and rhythm. If ventricular fibrillation or asystole occurs, institute cardiopulmonary resuscitation and defibrillation. Provide supportive care—for example, administer an antipyretic to reduce fever, an anticonvulsant to prevent seizures, and propranolol to treat tachycardia.

Amphetamine overdose
If the drug was taken orally, induce vomiting or perform gastric lavage. Give a sodium or magnesium sulfate cathartic to hasten evacuation, mannitol to induce diuresis, pentobarbital or chlorpromazine to treat agitation and CNS stimulation and to prevent or control seizures, and phentolamine to lower blood pressure. To increase amphetamine excretion, acidify the patient's urine by giving ammonium chloride or ascorbic acid I.V.

Benzodiazepine overdose
If the drug was taken orally, induce vomiting when ingestion is recent and the patient is fully conscious. If the patient is lethargic or comatose, gastric lavage may be performed after the airway is protected through endotracheal intubation. Follow induction of vomiting with activated charcoal and a cathartic of 0.9% sodium chloride solution to remove residual drug from the GI tract. Give flumazenil (Mazicon), a specific benzodiazpine antagonist, to reverse CNS depression.

Home care instructions
• Patients who return to a social setting where substance abuse is common are likely to have a relapse. As a result, encourage continuing professional support for the patient and his family after the detoxification program ends.
• Emphasize the need to join an appropriate self-help group, such as Alcoholics Anonymous or Narcotics Anonymous, for continued support and encouragement. Recommend that the patient's spouse or mature children accompany the patient to group meetings. Also refer the patient's family to a support group if necessary.
• Emphasize to the patient that he ultimately must accept responsibility for avoiding abused substances.

DIET, CALORIE-MODIFIED

Say the word "diet" to most patients and they'll think of a calorie-modified diet—specifically, a low-calorie diet. These diets are among the most popular—and most abused—forms of self-treatment. In the United States, 25% to 50% of all adults are obese.

High-calorie diets are another type of calorie-modified diet. High-calorie diets are typically used to rehabilitate people who are malnourished or underweight and to prevent malnourishment in conditions of increased energy needs.

Compliance is the major obstacle to the success of a calorie-modified diet. That's obvious for patients requiring a low-calorie diet, but those who need a high-calorie diet may also find compliance difficult. In the hospital setting, the latter group of patients poses the greatest challenge. Both types of calorie-modified diets may require ingenuity and creativity to help the patient comply.

Purpose
• To help correct weight imbalances through balanced nutritional practices.

Indications
Low-calorie modified diets are typically used for weight reduction and maintenance. They are indicated for patients who are overweight or have mild, moderate, or morbid obesity.

A high-calorie modified diet is typically used in conditions that produce greatly increased food energy needs, such as cancer, hyperthyroidism, cachexia, cystic fibrosis, chronic lung disease, acquired immunodeficiency syndrome, severe stress, and trauma, and when the patient is involved in excessive activity, such as athletic training. Treatment of anorexia nervosa also includes a high-calorie diet.

Procedure
Calorie-modified diets should be planned by a registered dietitian. In many cases, the U.S. food exchange system lists are used in formulating realistic calorie-modified diets. These lists are helpful in controlling calories and energy nutrients. Exchange lists consider proportions and portion sizes, which may be easier for a person than counting calories.

For a low-calorie diet
A low-calorie diet should provide sufficient calories to meet the patient's metabolic needs and activity level, can be followed realistically, and will promote weight loss of about 1 to 2 lb (0.5 to 1 kg)/week. The low-calorie diet includes foods from all four food groups but limits carbohydrates and restricts fats and alcohol. It also includes fiber to reduce caloric density and slow digestion. The overall treatment plan for weight reduction should include diet, exercise, and behavior modification.

Depending on the patient's sex, weight, and activity level, a low-calorie diet may provide 1,000 to 1,800 calories/day, with about 20% of calories obtained from protein. For morbid obesity, the doctor may recommend an extreme low-calorie diet—providing only 300 to 700 calories/day—that includes high-quality protein and few carbohydrates.

For a high-calorie diet
A high calorie diet should have a high-protein content and provide 500 to 1,000 additional calories with a goal for weight gain of about 1 lb/week for most patients. Fat intake should remain within normal limits to prevent anorexia (appetite loss) and nausea.

High-calorie diets are commonly planned to provide as many calories in as small a volume as possible. Between-meal snacking is often encouraged as an effective strategy for weight gain. Milk shakes, cream soups, peanut butter, and commercially prepared liquid supplements or powdered breakfast drinks are commonly used to increase caloric intake.

Typically, these diets increase caloric intake gradually so that the patient can adjust to the added food amounts. Use extra helpings, snacks, and concentrated supplements to increase caloric intake.

Complications

Severely restricted low-calorie diets can be complicated by weakness, apathy, fatigue, and dehydration. If the calories and nutrients are inadequate for prolonged periods, protein-calorie malnutrition may result.

High-calorie diets can result in hyperlipemia if the patient eats too many fatty foods.

Care considerations

• Ensure that a thorough medical examination is performed before a calorie-modified diet is begun.
• Take a complete dietary history. Ask what kinds of food the patient likes and dislikes and how they're prepared. Discuss eating habits; find out if the patient eats regular meals, skips some meals, or snacks between meals. Explore food-related behavior. For example, ask the patient whether he sits down at a table to eat or if he eats while standing, driving, or watching TV. Ask about smoking and whether he's trying to quit; a patient who's trying to quit smoking commonly has difficulty following a diet.
• With an obese patient, discuss the benefits of exercise and the role of behavior modification, psychotherapy, and prescribed drugs in weight loss. Encourage participation in a weight-loss support group. Help the patient set reasonable weight-loss goals, and emphasize that slow, gradual reduction helps keep weight from returning.
• With an underweight patient, set a realistic goal for weight gain (typically about 1 lb/week). Recommend a hearty meal at breakfast and regular meals.
• Weigh the patient before the diet begins and once weekly afterward to chart his progress. Tell the patient that daily weighings are not necessary. Explain that daily weight fluctuations, usually due to fluid retention, can be misleading.
• Encourage the patient to keep a food diary, which he should bring to follow-up office visits. At that time, review the patient's food diary with him, and make suggestions, as appropriate, that will help improve his diet. Check the diary for adequate fluid intake.
• Monitor blood urea nitrogen levels in the overweight patient who is on a severely restricted diet that provides less than 800 calories a day.

Home care instructions

• Enlist the support of the patient's family. Their encouragement and cooperation are vital to the patient's success with the diet.
• Suggest planning menus and shopping lists for the week to prevent impulse buying and eating. Encourage eating fish and poultry instead of red meat, substituting polyunsaturated fats for saturated ones, and eating vegetables and fruits instead of sweets.
• For the underweight patient, suggest dried fruits and nuts for between-meal snacks because they're high in calories and nutritious. Recommend bananas with breakfast and potatoes, pasta, noodles, or rice at least twice a day.
• Arrange a consultation with a dietitian for the patient with a severe weight imbalance. A team effort — with doctor, nurse, dietitian, and therapist participating — may be necessary to help the patient.
• Encourage the patient not to abandon his diet simply because he sometimes cheats: Explain that occasional noncompliance matters little to long-term success. Help him use behavior modification techniques to reduce noncompliance; for example, set a goal of slowly reducing the number of cheating episodes per week.

• Explain the need for the underweight patient to regulate his energy expenditures. Such a patient may need to reduce his activities.
• Warn against fad and gimmick diets. These diets commonly severely restrict one or more food groups and may cause dangerous adverse effects.

DIET, DIABETIC

Diet management is a cornerstone of diabetes treatment. A diabetic diet requires the development of an individual meal plan that allows the patient to maintain a normal life-style while keeping blood glucose and weight at appropriate levels.

The patient with Type I (insulin-dependent) diabetes is unable to produce insulin. Thus, he must administer insulin, schedule meals and snacks to offset peak insulin action, and follow a prescribed diet to avoid hypoglycemia and hyperglycemia. He also needs to follow an exchange system to balance dietary protein, carbohydrate, and fat.

The patient with Type II (non-insulin-dependent) diabetes produces some insulin but also has insulin resistance (the inability of the cells in the body to effectively use the insulin). Insulin resistance is intensified if the patient has excess body fat; therefore, diet therapy in Type II diabetes focuses on weight loss to reduce insulin resistance; a balance of dietary protein, carbohydrate, and fat; and avoidance of hypoglycemia and hyperglycemia.

Purpose
• To provide a meal plan for the patient with diabetes that meets that patient's nutritional requirements, weight goals, life-style needs, and activity level.

Indications
This diet is indicated for all patients with diabetes mellitus.

Procedure
The patient's doctor commonly prescribes a caloric level, which is adjusted as necessary to maintain stable weight control. A dietitian or nurse then develops an individual meal plan, often using an exchange list. The exchange lists that are currently used were developed by a committee of the American Diabetes Association and American Dietetic Association primarily to meet the needs of diabetic patients and others who must follow special diets. The exchange lists are based on universal principles of good nutrition, and they divide foods into equivalent groups (exchanges) according to calorie and nutritional content. In the diabetic patient's diet, carbohydrates contribute 50% to 60% of his total daily calories; proteins contribute 12% to 20%; and fat should contribute no more than 30% of total calories.

For the individual taking insulin, a bedtime snack may be necessary to prevent hypoglycemia during sleep. The scheduled times for other snacks depend on the patient's activity level, meal times, and the type of insulin or oral antidiabetic agents used.

Complications
Hypoglycemia and hyperglycemia are the primary complications of a diabetic diet. They may occur if the patient does not follow the prescribed diet, if his activity level or life-style changes, or if his insulin dosage or the dosage of antidiabetic agents is altered without compensatory diet changes.

Care considerations
• Before beginning the diet, assess the patient's prior knowledge of nutrition and teach about nutritional requirements as appropriate.
• Take a thorough dietary history, keeping in mind that noncompliance with the diabetic diet may result from unnecessary restriction of preferred foods and habits. Consider not only *what* the pa-

tient eats, but also *when* he eats, which will help you set up meal and snack times.
• Explain that the patient will require a prescribed diet and that the diet is based on the patient's individual needs. Tell him that he'll need to keep track of all the foods he eats and that he may need to categorize them according to food exchanges if he's using that system. Mention that no foods are exempt—even so-called dietetic foods.
• Monitor the patient for signs of hypoglycemia: nervousness, faintness, dizziness, diaphoresis, hunger, shakiness, possible seizures, and coma; and for signs of hyperglycemia: polyuria, polydypsia, polyphagia, weight loss, and dehydration.

Home care instructions

• Work closely with the patient and, as necessary, his family to reinforce prescribed diet therapy. If needed, review food exchange lists carefully. (Teaching materials are available from the American Diabetes Association.)
• Teach the patient and family members the signs of hypoglycemia and hyperglycemia.
• Show the patient how to keep a food diary. Show how and where his current eating habits deviate from his prescribed diet. (For example, the patient may have been eating 2,400 calories/day rather than the 2,000 he needs, or he may have been getting 50% of his calories from fat rather than the recommended 30%.) Explain that his food diary can be used to make necessary diet adjustments. If appropriate, show the patient how to use the exchange lists to work out a meal plan that incorporates some of the same foods but falls within the recommended guidelines. Then, if appropriate, have him develop a meal plan using the exchange lists. (Working with exchange lists can be extremely confusing at first, so allow the patient to work at his own pace.) The more practice the patient has in planning enjoyable meals, the more likely he is to com-

ply with his diet. Suggest planning meals a few days in advance to have correct ingredients on hand and to avoid inappropriate substitutions.
• Provide reassurance and support as the patient adjusts to the diet, and offer referral to local support groups such as the American Diabetes Association.
• If the patient habitually consumes alcohol, explain that certain restrictions are necessary to avoid complications. The American Diabetes Association recommends limiting alcohol consumption to two exchanges of an alcoholic beverage once or twice a week. One alcohol exchange is 1½ oz of whiskey, 4 oz of wine, or 12 oz of beer. If the patient uses insulin, the alcohol exchanges can be used in addition to the usual meal plan. If he does not require insulin, alcohol should be substituted for fat exchanges; one alcohol exchange is equal to two fat exchanges. Explain that hypoglycemia is the major concern when alcohol is taken without food.
• Encourage the patient to eat foods that contain unrefined carbohydrates and are high in fiber. Daily intake of 25 to 30 g of fiber delays gastric emptying and slows carbohydrate absorption, which can lower blood glucose levels and reduce insulin requirements.
• If the patient is insulin-dependent or taking oral antdiabetic agents, stress the importance of eating on a regular, consistent schedule, even during an illness, to balance insulin therapy. Explain that hypoglycemia can result from lack of food, vomiting, diarrhea, or too much exercise.
• Tell the patient that if he is able to eat regular meals during an illness, he should also increase his fluid intake to three times his typical daily intake or 12 oz (360 ml)/hour for the average adult patient. (Be sure to inform the parents or caregivers of young patients about this increased fluid requirement.) If vomiting occurs, the patient

should try to drink liquids containing glucose and electrolytes (regular soda, fruit juices, fluid electrolyte replacement [such as Gatorade], or ice pops containing 15 g of carbohydrate) every 30 minutes.

• Explain that the patient should continue to take prescribed insulin and oral antidiabetic agents during stress or illness unless told to stop by his doctor. Advise the patient to notify the doctor about any illness because stress and illness often cause blood glucose levels to rise.

• Encourage the patient to carry a form of simple carbohydrate, such as hard candy or a fruit juice, to prevent hypoglycemia when away from home or if a meal may be delayed.

DIET, FIBER-MODIFIED

Fiber makes up a crucial part of the diet and yet, paradoxically, it's not completely digestible. The benefits of fiber are primarily mechanical: It promotes peristalsis, reduces intestinal transit time, and increases stool volume and weight.

Essentially, a high-fiber diet is a normal diet that substitutes high-fiber foods for low-fiber foods. A low-fiber diet, also called a low-residue diet, restricts dietary fiber and residue to eliminate or reduce mechanical stimulation of the GI tract. Low-residue dietary restrictions range from mild to severe. Because low-fiber diets lack sufficient vitamins and minerals, they can be used for only a limited time.

Purpose
For a high-fiber diet
• To increase fecal bulk
• To increase GI motility
• To decrease pressure within the bowel.

For a low-fiber diet
• To reduce stool bulk
• To slow transit time through the bowel
• To limit gastric secretion.

Indications
High-fiber diets are indicated for prevention and treatment of constipation, irritable bowel syndrome, Crohn's disease, and diverticulosis and to help lower cholesterol levels in patients with hypercholesterolemia. Adding high-fiber foods to the diet is also often indicated for weight loss in obesity, in diabetes mellitus to improve glucose tolerance, and in coronary artery disease. Researchers believe that a high-fiber diet may reduce the risk of bowel cancer by reducing the number of carcinogens in fecal matter.

Low-fiber diets are generally indicated for patients with indigestion, nausea, esophageal varices, gastritis, diarrhea, bowel inflammation (as seen in the acute stages of diverticulosis, ulcerative colitis, and regional enteritis), myocardial infarction, and congestive heart failure, and during preparation for bowel procedures.

Procedure
The registered dietitian frequently explains and reviews the prescribed diet with the patient and, if appropriate, with the family. The nurse commonly reinforces these diet instructions with the patient and family.

Extra fiber should be introduced gradually. If large amounts of fiber are introduced all at once, complications are more likely. Diabetic patients on a high-fiber diet should consume 30 to 50 g/day of fiber; for other patients, the diet is more flexible and should simply include as much fiber as is practical.

A high-fiber diet should include breads and other baked goods made from whole grains, especially bran. Coarsely ground bran can be added to cereals, muffins, or bread as an additional fiber supplement. Vegetables should be eaten raw or cooked with minimal preparation. Those most helpful include carrots, peas, broccoli, corn, lettuce, dried peas, and beans. Fresh fruits should be eaten unpeeled (especially apples and pears). Other high-fiber fruits include berries, oranges, and stewed and dried fruits. Nuts and seeds are also considered high in fiber.

A low-fiber diet consists of soft, mild food. It excludes raw vegetables and fruits, nuts, seeds, coarse breads, and strong seasonings and limits fried foods and fats because they can increase gastric reflux.

The low-fiber diet includes ground or well-cooked tender meat, fish, and poultry as well as eggs and up to 16 oz of milk per day and mild cheese. It may also include strained fruit juices, except prune juice; cooked or canned apples, apricots, white cherries, peaches, pears and ripe bananas; strained vegetable juices; canned, cooked, or strained asparagus, beets, green beans, pumpkin, acorn squash, and spinach; white bread, toast, crackers, bagels, melba toast, and waffles; and refined cereals, such as cream of wheat, cream of rice, and puffed rice. Other foods that are permitted on the low-fiber diet include plain desserts made with soft, seedless foods; gelatin; candy, such as butterscotch, jelly beans, marshmallows, and plain hard candy; and honey, molasses, and sugar.

Complications

Patients can show intolerance to a high-fiber diet, exhibiting such symptoms as flatulence, abdominal distention, cramping, and diarrhea.

Nutrient deficiencies, for example iron deficiency or calcium deficiency, may occur in patients on high- or low-fiber diets. Constipation can also occur because the low-fiber diet decreases stool bulk and slows transit time through the bowel. Low-fiber diets may be calorically inadequate if used for extended periods.

Care considerations

• Explain the diet to the patient. Reinforce the dietitian's explanation as necessary.
• Explain to any patient on a fiber-modified diet that mineral and vitamin deficiencies may occur. Mention that he should eat a variety of foods and may have to take vitamin and mineral supplements.
• Monitor laboratory test results for signs of calcium, zinc, or iron deficiency. If the patient is on a high-fiber diet, explain that these minerals may be eliminated in feces because of the increased intestinal transit time. If the patient is on a low-fiber diet, explain that restriction of milk and other dairy products may cause calcium deficiency and that restriction of sources of iron, such as dried fruit and iron-fortified cereal, can cause iron deficiency.

For a high-fiber diet

• Review the patient's dietary intake and explain the benefits that the diet offers.
• Explain that fiber is a component of plants and is therefore abundant in fruits, vegetables, and grains. Also tell this patient that signs of intolerance, such as a bloated feeling and diarrhea, can be minimized by increasing fiber content gradually.
• Encourage the patient to drink at least six to eight 8-oz glasses of water daily. If he doesn't have at least one soft stool per day, tell him to add a bran supplement to his diet.

For a low-fiber diet

• Explain the rationale for prescribing a low-fiber diet: reducing fiber intake will slow the passage of food through the bowel.
• Monitor for inadequate calorie intake, especially important because of the diet's restrictions.
• Monitor for constipation. Explain that the diet causes a decrease in stool bulk and slows intestinal transit time.

Home care instructions

• Tell the female patient on a high-fiber diet to increase calcium intake to prevent osteoporosis. Tell her to drink at least two 8-oz glasses of milk a day and to eat cheese and yogurt. If she's trying to lose weight or has diabetes, recommend skim milk and low-fat cheese.

• Tell the patient on a high-fiber diet to eat iron-rich foods, such as liver. To increase his intake of zinc, recommend meat, nuts, beans, wheat germ, and cheese.

• Suggest taking a list of high-fiber foods with him when grocery shopping.

• Emphasize the need to schedule medical follow-up for evaluation of progress and assessment of nutritional status.

• Advise the patient to take prescribed vitamin and mineral supplements.

DIET, GLUTEN-FREE

A gluten-free diet helps prevent the bloating, projectile vomiting, diarrhea, weight loss, malnutrition, and poor growth patterns associated with celiac disease. In this disorder, which is usually first diagnosed in infancy or early childhood, the intestinal lining is damaged by the glutamine-bound fraction of protein (gliadin) in many grain products. Researchers aren't sure why celiac disease occurs: It may result from an abnormal enzyme in the mucosal cell that doesn't digest a toxic peptide in gluten or from an immune reaction within the mucosal cell membrane. According to the latter theory, which is gaining increased support, gliadin acts as an antigen that causes a damaging immune response.

A gluten-free diet can't reverse the intestinal damage of celiac disease, but it can usually prevent further damage, relieve symptoms, and correct malab-sorption of nutrients. Children may show improvement after 2 weeks on a gluten-free diet; in adults, results take a little longer – typically a month or two.

Initially, the patient's diet excludes sources of gluten but may include supplementary protein, calories, vitamins, and minerals to correct previous dietary deficiencies. After such deficiencies are corrected, the patient follows a diet that's normal except for its gluten content. The patient must follow this diet scrupulously for the rest of his life; ingesting even small amounts may prevent remission or induce relapse. Patients who repeatedly go on and off the gluten-free diet may eventually fail to respond to it.

Purpose

• To prevent complications of celiac disease.

Indications

This diet is used as part of the treatment for celiac disease.

Procedure

The doctor commonly prescribes a gluten-free diet that must be adhered to for life. The dietitian outlines any specific restrictions of the diet and then assists the family with continued dietary management. The nurse commonly reinforces these instructions with the patient and, if applicable, the family.

A gluten-free diet eliminates all products containing wheat, rye, oats, barley, and malt. In their place, the patient may eat cereals and breads made from rice, corn, soy, and potatoes. Initially, milk and milk products are also withheld because intestinal damage often causes an intolerance to lactose. (See *Gluten-free diet guidelines*, page 234.) As the patient's symptoms improve, these dairy products can be gradually reintroduced.

Gluten-free diet guidelines

Patients who follow a gluten-free diet must do so for life. Review this list with the patient and his family or caregivers, and answer their questions about permitted and forbidden foods in a gluten-free diet.

Meat and meat alternatives
Any allowed except those that are breaded, prepared with bread crumbs, or creamed. Avoid sausage, hot dogs, and turkey injected with hydrolyzed vegetable protein.

Milk and milk products
Any allowed except milk mixed with Ovaltine, commercial chocolate milk with a cereal additive, pudding thickened with wheat flour, or ice cream or sherbet containing gluten stabilizers.

Fruits and vegetables
Any allowed except those that are breaded, prepared with bread crumbs, or creamed.

Grains
Allowed: Bread, cereal, or dessert products made from arrowroot, soybean flour, rice flour, potato flour, or gluten-free starch; gluten-free macaroni or porridge; tapioca; cornmeal, cornflakes, popcorn, hominy; rice, cream of rice, puffed rice, rice flakes; buckwheat products; and potato chips.
Not allowed: Bread, cereal, or dessert products made from wheat, rye, oats, or barley; commercially prepared mixes for biscuits, cornbread, muffins, pancakes, cakes, cookies, and waffles; bran, pasta, macaroni, and noodles; malt; pretzels; wheat germ; doughnuts; or ice cream cones.

Miscellaneous
Not allowed: Beer; ale; certain whiskeys (Canadian rye); cereal, beverages such as Postum; root beer; commercial salad dressings that contain gluten stabilizers; soups containing any ingredient not allowed (such as barley).

Complications

Noncompliance with the gluten-free diet causes the complications of celiac disease: projectile vomiting, chronic diarrhea, and poor growth patterns.

Care considerations

• Carefully explain the role of gluten in celiac disease and then explain the gluten-free diet to the family and, as appropriate, to the child. Have the dietitian visit the family to ensure that they fully understand the diet.
• Explain that the gluten-free diet is difficult to follow because gluten is hidden in many foods—for example, in chocolate syrup (where it's used as a stabilizing and thickening agent); in sausages, hot dogs, and turkey injected

with hydrolyzed vegetable protein; and in distilled white vinegar and whiskeys.
• Be sure that the family and, as appropriate, the child understand that this is a lifelong diet.
• The patient may initially require hospitalization to stabilize his condition and provide nutritional supplementation. While he's in the hospital, monitor hemoglobin and hematocrit levels for signs of anemia and administer iron, folate, or vitamin B_{12}, as prescribed. Monitor prothrombin time to detect bleeding as a result of vitamin K deficiency, and observe for signs or symptoms of osteomalacia (rheumatic pain in pelvis and limbs). Osteomalacia may

result from vitamin D and calcium deficiencies.

• Tell parents to observe the child closely for improvement once the diet begins. Explain that dramatic improvement is common within the first few days and that the child will continue to improve as long as he follows the diet.

Home care instructions

• Tell the patient and family that special foods are commercially available for persons with celiac disease. Have the dietitian recommend brands.

• Suggest the use of rice and rice flour, often available in Asian food stores. Health food stores also carry many of the appropriate foods.

• Teach the patient and family how to read food labels for gluten content. Many foods contain hidden gluten. Be sure the family knows that products that contain "hydrolyzed vegetable protein" or that have "vegetable protein added" must be avoided.

• Suggest broiled or boiled meat or fish and the avoidance of sauces, gravies, and breaded foods when eating out in restaurants.

• Explain that foods made with gluten-free flours may be less grainy if the flour is mixed with a liquid in a recipe. Tell the parents to boil the flour with the liquid and to cool this mixture.

• Emphasize the need for frequent medical checkups to evaluate nutritional status.

• Tell the parents to notify the doctor if the child ingests foods containing gluten.

DIET, LACTOSE-REDUCED

A lactose-reduced diet is the only treatment for lactose intolerance (lactase deficiency), a common disorder that causes difficulty in digesting dairy products. (See *What happens in lactose intolerance,* page 236.)

Beginning after age 4, nearly 70% of people develop some degree of lactose intolerance. The incidence of this disorder increases with age, perhaps because lactase activity decreases as a person grows older. Lactase activity is at its peak during infancy. For reasons not entirely understood, lactose intolerance is usually more pronounced among Blacks, Jews, Native Americans, and Asians. Rarely, complete lactose intolerance is present from birth. Secondary lactose intolerance may occur in patients with disorders such as celiac disease, sprue, colitis, enteritis, cystic fibrosis, or malnutrition and in patients who have undergone a gastrectomy or small-bowel resection.

Few patients require a diet that's totally free of lactose; this depends on whether or not the patient has a complete or partial lactase deficiency. Most people can tolerate some milk if it's carefully spaced throughout the day, and many can tolerate cheese or yogurt (in which lactose is broken down by the active cultures) as well as sweet acidophilus milk (which contains an enzyme that hydrolyzes lactose). Some patients benefit from lactose enzyme tablets, an over-the-counter product, which permit digestion of lactose-containing foods.

Because the lactose-reduced diet is somewhat flexible, it's easy to follow, and, unlike many other diets, it need not be permanent. Many patients can gradually add dairy products without suffering ill effects.

Purpose

• To reduce dietary lactose and thereby alleviate GI symptoms, such as abdominal cramps, distention, and diarrhea.

Indications

The lactose-reduced diet is indicated for patients with GI symptoms resulting from lactose intolerance.

What happens in lactose intolerance

Normal digestion

Carbohydrates typically reach the small intestine in disaccharide form. In normal digestion, lactose, one of these disaccharides, is hydrolyzed by lactase—an enzyme located in the intestinal mucosa—before absorption takes place.

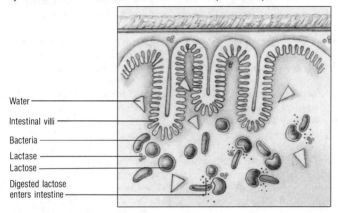

Water

Intestinal villi

Bacteria

Lactase

Lactose

Digested lactose enters intestine

Digestion in lactose intolerance

In lactose intolerance, the classic signs—bloating, flatulence, diarrhea, and malabsorption—result from undigested lactose in the small intestine (the undigested lactose is caused by a lactase deficiency). In the intestine, this lactose is attacked by bacteria giving off hydrogen as it's broken down. Lactose also draws water into the intestine by osmosis. The gas and increased fluid load trigger hyperperistalsis, which in turn inhibits absorption of other nutrients.

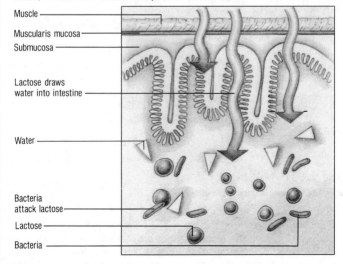

Muscle

Muscularis mucosa

Submucosa

Lactose draws water into intestine

Water

Bacteria attack lactose

Lactose

Bacteria

Procedure

Before prescribing this diet, the doctor will measure the patient's ability to digest lactose by performing either of two tests: the lactose tolerance test or the lactose malabsorption test.

After evaluating the patient's ability to digest lactose, the doctor may recommend that the patient limit or eliminate consumption of milk and milk products, or use lactose enzyme tablets.

After the doctor makes this recommendation, the health care team—including the registered dietitian and nurse—teaches the patient the sources of lactose and works with him to establish his level of tolerance.

Complications

Calcium deficiency can complicate the lactose-reduced diet as a result of reduced intake of milk and milk products.

Care considerations

• Explain to the patient why he has trouble digesting dairy products: undigested lactose is fermented by intestinal bacteria and it draws water into the intestine; the acids and gases formed by fermentation then combine with the excess water to cause bloating, cramping, and diarrhea. Because milk and milk products are the only sources of lactose, eliminating or limiting them can prevent GI distress.

• Teach the patient how to identify lactose-containing foods that produce GI complications so that he can eliminate them as necessary.

• Suggest limiting or eliminating consumption of ordinary milk and milk products. For example, suggest drinking no more than half a cup of ordinary milk per day. Also recommend substituting sweet acidophilus milk, eating small quantities of cheese or yogurt, and drinking small amounts of buttermilk because doing so will break down or hydrolyze lactose. The patient should avoid baked goods made with milk, sausages that contain milk solids, creamy sauces and gravies, and processed foods that contain other less obvious sources of lactose (chocolate, caramel, cocoa mixes, certain nondairy creamers, vitamins, instant potatoes, and frozen french fries).

• While the patient is on a lactose-reduced diet, monitor his intake of calcium and riboflavin, which are usually supplied by milk. Provide dietary supplements, if ordered. Also evaluate the patient's diet for sufficient intake of protein and calories.

• Observe the patient for signs and symptoms of lactose intolerance, including cramping, bloating, distention and diarrhea. These are most likely to occur when the patient is establishing his level of tolerance, or when lactose-containing foods are gradually being reintroduced into his diet.

Home care instructions

• Advise the patient to read food labels carefully to detect the presence of milk, milk solids, whey, lactose, or casein.

• Suggest substitution of water or fruit juices for milk in recipes, and, when eating in restaurants, avoidance of foods prepared with sauces, gravies, or bread.

• If the patient's symptoms improve, he can try adding small amounts of dairy products at one meal; if he tolerates them well, he may gradually increase his intake. Tell the patient that sometimes chocolate milk is tolerated better than regular milk. If he wants to try adding cottage cheese to his diet, tell him to try different brands, since the amount of lactose they contain varies widely.

• Suggest adding an enzyme preparation (such as Lact-Aid) to milk before drinking. The enzyme breaks down much of the lactose in milk.

• Suggest using calcium-fortified soy milk as a milk substitute.

• Explain that other calcium-rich foods (such as dark green leafy vegetables, and grains) may provide small amounts of available calcium, but that calcium from these sources is largely unavailable for absorption.

DIET, LOW-CHOLESTEROL

Dietary therapy is the primary defense against high serum cholesterol levels and their cardiovascular complications. It's an important part of an overall campaign against risk factors for heart disease. The patient must also be encouraged, if necessary, to stop smoking, lose weight, and exercise more, and he may require drug therapy for hereditary hypercholesterolemia.

A low-cholesterol diet isn't curative, so most patients must remain on it permanently. Typically, results don't become apparent for at least 3 months.

Because serum cholesterol levels reflect overall fat intake, a low-cholesterol diet has much in common with a low-fat diet. But there are some differences because of the role that certain foods play in hypercholesterolemia. For example, research has shown that serum cholesterol levels can be significantly reduced by substituting monounsaturated and polyunsaturated fats (such as olive oil, safflower oil, and corn oil) for saturated fats. Dietary fiber also lowers serum cholesterol levels, and some research suggests that leafy and root vegetables do so as well.

Purpose

• To lower serum cholesterol levels and reduce the risk of heart disease.

Indications

Low-cholesterol diets are generally indicated for use in treatment of atherosclerosis, diabetes mellitus, hypercholesterolemia, hypertension, and myocardial infarction.

Procedure

A low-cholesterol diet is generally prescribed by the doctor. A registered dietician may be consulted to assist in menu planning.

Usually, the patient is advised to follow one of three diets recommended by the American Heart Association (see *Three ways to combat cholesterol*). Each of these diets provides adequate nutrition. If necessary, caloric intake can be reduced to help the patient lose weight, and salt may be restricted to curb hypertension. The low-cholesterol diet is phased in gradually, both to improve compliance and to permit assessment of the patient's response, which can vary greatly.

Complications

The low-cholesterol diet doesn't typically produce complications.

Care considerations

• Before the patient's diet begins, take a careful dietary history. Ask the patient if he cooks in animal fats, uses butter or margarine, and if he typically bakes, broils, or fries his food. Also find out how many eggs he eats every week.

• Explain to the patient and family how high cholesterol levels increase the risk of cardiovascular disease and how dietary control can reduce this risk.

• Explain that not all fats are the same; saturated fats (which are often solid, such as butter or animal fat) contain cholesterol. Encourage the patient to try to maintain a diet in which the ratio of polyunsatured to saturated fats is about 2:1 (in the typical American diet, this ratio is about 1:3).

• Explain the role of low-density lipoprotein (LDL) in cardiovascular disease. Tell the patient that LDL carries cholesterol to the cells and that high LDL levels can therefore promote the

Three ways to combat cholesterol

The American Heart Association recommends three diets for combating elevated serum cholesterol levels. These diets range from a slightly restrictive one, which aims to prevent excessive cholesterol intake, to a severely restricted one.

Accent on prevention
In the preventive diet, suitable for most people, about one-third of the calories are evenly divided among the saturated, monounsaturated, and polyunsaturated fats. Carbohydrates — ideally, complex ones — make up half the calories, with protein making up the remainder. Total cholesterol intake doesn't exceed 300 mg/day.

This diet limits egg yolks to two weekly. Most organ meats are omitted. Soft margarine, vegetable oils and shortening, skim milk, and egg whites replace butter, lard, whole milk, and whole eggs. Beef may be eaten three times weekly.

Strictly lean
The American Heart Association's "phase 2" diet aims to correct mild hypercholesterolemia. It contains the same distribution of fats, carbohydrates, and protein as the preventive diet but restricts cholesterol to 200 mg/day. It also limits the intake of milk, poultry, and seafood to 6 oz a day, while emphasizing legumes, grains, fruits, and vegetables. Only extremely lean cuts of meats and skim-milk cheeses are permitted.

Lean and mean
The most restrictive diet is used for severe hypercholesterolemia. Fats account for more than 25% of the calories consumed (again, equally distributed among saturated, monounsaturated, and polyunsaturated fats). Between 55% and 60% of calories come from carbohydrates. Meat, shellfish, and poultry servings are limited to 3 oz daily.

accumulation of cholesterol in arterial walls. Explain that high-density lipoprotein (HDL) is desirable because it helps to remove cholesterol from the blood and transport it to the liver for elimination.

• Inform the patient that new, tasty foods can be exchanged for foods that are high in saturated fats. For example, suggest beans as an alternative source of protein and whole grain cereal and bread, fruits, and raw vegetables to increase fiber content. Oat cereals and apples also help reduce cholesterol levels.

• Arrange for a consultation with a dietitian to help the patient plan a low-cholesterol diet and to provide additional support and reinforcement of dietary measures.

• During the diet, provide mineral supplements as necessary. Explain that these may be necessary because high intake of dietary fiber may interfere with absorption of calcium, iron, and zinc.

• Monitor serum cholesterol levels and HDL, LDL, and very-low-density lipoprotein (VLDL) reactions to evaluate the effectiveness of treatment. Advise the patient to keep a chart of these values to provide positive reinforcement of the diet.

Home care instructions

• Review low-cholesterol food choices with the patient.

• Explain that adapting to new eating patterns may take several months. To promote compliance, encourage the patient to master one part of the diet at a time: for example, to limit consumption of red meat before reducing the number of eggs that he eats.

• When eating out, the patient should select salads and vegetables, choose poultry over red meat, avoid fried food, and choose simply prepared dishes instead of those with rich sauces or dressings. Vegetarian Chinese food and pasta are often good choices, except for pasta with large amounts of whole-milk cheeses.

• Be sure the patient understands the need to consume enough dairy products to make up for impaired calcium absorption and to eat beans and leafy vegetables to obtain iron and zinc.

• Recommend a cooking spray for frying and baking and tub margarine of a type that's high in polyunsaturated or monounsaturated fat. Recommend using a brand that shows vegetable oils first in the list of ingredients. Hydrogenated vegetable oils have more saturated fat than nonhydrogenated oils.

• Suggest making soups or stews a day ahead and refrigerating them; the patient should then skim off the hardened fat before reheating.

• Recommend using low-cholesterol substitutes for mayonnaise, salad dressings, hot dogs, egg noodles, ice cream, and many other foods.

• Tell the patient that the American Heart Association publishes and distributes pamphlets and recipe books for the low-cholesterol diet.

DIET, LOW-FAT

Fat is a vital nutrient that supplies energy and fat-soluble vitamins, but most Americans eat too much of it—about 160 g/day, on average, accounting for some 40% of their caloric intake. In fact, excessive dietary fat has been linked not only to obesity but also to cardiovascular disease and to colon, prostate, and breast cancer.

Nutrition experts recommend that fat intake be limited to no more than 30% of total caloric intake—that is,

about 120 g/day—including 10% from unsaturated fats and 8% from saturated fat. Patients with certain disorders may require even lower fat intake. A low-fat diet limits the daily amount to 50 g/day; an extremely low-fat diet limits intake to only 25 to 30 g/day.

Compliance is a major problem with a low-fat diet. Simply reducing fat intake to 30% of ingested calories, for example, limits the patient to three eggs a week and requires substitution of skim milk, margarine, and vegetable oils for whole milk, butter, and lard. More stringent diets, of course, are even more restrictive.

Purpose

• To prevent problems associated with the malabsorption of fat by reducing dietary fat

• To prevent or reduce elevated lipid levels in the blood, lymph system, gallbladder, and other tissue by reducing dietary fat.

Indications

Low-fat diets are indicated for use in the treatment of acquired immunodeficiency syndrome, blind-loop syndrome (depletion of B_{12} and fat malabsorption that results from bypassed intestinal segments), steatorrhea, gallbladder disease, inflammatory bowel disease, liver disease, pancreatitis, short-bowel syndrome, celiac disease, topical sprue, radiation enteritis, and reflux esophagitis. In patients with gout, a low-fat diet can help prevent uric acid retention. In hyperlipoproteinemia, a low-fat diet can sometimes reduce the serum levels of lipoproteins. If started early in life, it can help prevent atherosclerosis in patients with hereditary hyperproteinemia.

Procedure

A low-fat diet is typically prescribed by the doctor. A registered dietitian commonly reviews the diet with the patient. The nurse can also help the patient understand the diet and answer questions that he might have after he begins the diet.

The restriction of fat intake depends on the grams of fat permitted per day. Most low-fat diets eliminate whole milk and whole-milk cheeses; pastries, cake, and pies made with fat; and desserts and soups made from cream, chocolate, or nuts (see *Foods not permitted on a low-fat diet*). The patient is encouraged to substitute vegetables, fruits, bread and cereals without added fats, rice, and pasta for high-fat foods (see *Foods with little or no fat*, page 242). The patient is also limited to 6 oz of lean meat per day. Meat substitutes (such as eggs) are also limited because two medium eggs provide 10 grams of fat. Intake of butter, margarine, oils, salad dressings, cream, and nuts is also very limited.

A diet allowing 30 to 40 g/day of fat excludes whole milk and its products and limits eggs to three per week. However, the patient may use skim milk and products made from it and can have 1 tbs of oil, lard, butter, or mayonnaise and 4 oz of lean meat daily. The patient should avoid such high-fat snacks as chocolate, nuts, cheese crackers, and potato chips.

Complications

Vitamin deficiencies can occur if the patient does not take vitamin supplements, and sometimes adequate calorie ingestion is difficult. Noncompliance is a major problem.

Care considerations

• Discuss the low-fat diet with the patient and his family members. Reinforce the dietitian's explanations as necessary, and answer the patient's questions.
• Explain the importance of the low-fat diet in the patient's condition. Emphasize that the diet won't cure the underlying condition but can relieve symptoms and prevent complications.

Foods not permitted on a low-fat diet

Meats
• Sausage
• Lunch meat
• Spareribs
• Hot dogs
• Bacon
• Tuna packed in oil
• Salmon packed in oil

Dairy products
• Whole milk
• Whole-milk cheeses
• Yogurt (low-fat or nonfat is permitted)
• Ice cream

Fruits and vegetables
• Buttered or au gratin, creamed or fried vegetables

Breads and cereals
• Products made with added fat: biscuits, muffins, pancakes, doughnuts, waffles, and sweet rolls
• Breads made with eggs, cheese, or added fat

Miscellaneous
• Gravy
• Peanut butter
• Desserts
• Candy
• Any food containing chocolate or nuts

• Take a dietary history focusing on the patient's food preferences. Ask how often he eats out in restaurants, especially the fast-food type.
• Help the patient identify sources of dietary fat. Point out that fat is often invisible—for example, when it's in milk, eggs, or some meats.
• Discuss methods of food preparation. Tell the patient to use fish, poultry, and veal, and lean cuts of beef and pork as allowed. Tell him to remove visible fat and skin from meat and to broil, bake, or steam foods instead of frying them.

Foods with little or no fat

- Coffee
- Tea (regular and herbal)
- Pasta
- French bread
- Rice
- Fruit juices
- All fruit except coconuts and avocados
- All vegetables
- Hot cereals
- Most cold cereals (check food labels for additives)
- All legumes (dry beans and peas)
- Air-popped corn
- Baked potatoes

• Explain that vitamin supplements are necessary because a low-fat diet reduces intake of fat-soluble vitamins.
• Monitor nutritional status—for example, by weighing the patient on a regular basis. (A low-fat diet tends to be low in calories and, in some cases, weight loss may be excessive.) Also monitor for electrolyte imbalances.

Home care instructions

• Teach the patient how to shop for low-fat foods. For example, tell him to look for dairy products made with skim milk and for pasta that doesn't contain eggs. Suggest that the patient explore certain ethnic foods. Italian, Japanese, and Chinese foods are often low in fat and offer helpful variety to the diet. Warn against Italian foods that contain cheese.
• Explain that foods must be properly prepared to reduce dietary fat. For example, tell the patient to put baked meats or poultry on a rack away from the drippings and to remove skin and fat from foods before cooking them.
• Recommend using egg whites for cooking.
• Counsel the patient about eating out. Suggest that he order juice for an appetizer and use lemon juice or vinegar on salads. Remind him that he must limit portions of meat; order foods that are broiled, baked, or poached; omit sauces and gravies; and select ices or fruit for dessert.

• Suggest low-calorie cookbooks, which feature appealing low-fat recipes.
• Substitute reduced-calorie, reduced-fat, and no-fat items for regular margarines, salad dressings, and mayonnaise.
• Check with the doctor to find out if the patient's diet can include medium-chain triglycerides. These synthetic substances, which are absorbed directly into the portal vein, may be used in place of cooking oil. They're expensive, but they can improve the patient's compliance with fat restrictions and increase caloric intake.

DIET, LOW-PHENYLALANINE

The low-phenylalanine diet, if begun shortly after birth and scrupulously followed, prevents mental retardation and neurologic damage in children with phenylketonuria (PKU), a congenital deficiency of the liver enzyme phenylalanine hydroxylase. (Most infants in the United States are screened for the disorder soon after birth.) The low-phenylalanine diet effectively maintains low serum phenylalanine levels to prevent clinical symptoms. The low-phenylalanine diet is difficult to follow. Nevertheless, the child with PKU must begin to take responsibility for the diet at an early age and may not understand the consequences of noncompliance.

Outside the home, the child may find that the diet sets him apart from his friends.

Unfortunately, there is no safe age at which to discontinue the diet. Young women with PKU who are pregnant must not deviate from the diet because excess phenylalanine can be transmitted to the fetus and cause congenital defects.

Purpose
• To reduce phenylalanine intake and prevent accumulation of excessive phenylalanine levels in the blood, while providing sufficient amino acids and nutrients for normal growth and development.

Indications
The low-phenylalanine diet is indicated for all patients with PKU.

Procedure
When the patient's blood level of phenylalanine is determined, the nutritionist establishes a diet that permits the patient to maintain a tolerable blood phenylalanine level. The diet consists of two parts: milk substitutes for the infant's first food and guidelines for adding solid foods. The diet is continuously monitored and adjusted by the nutritionist according to the patient's blood phenylalanine level, age, and weight.

To eliminate milk, which has a high phenylalanine content, the infant is fed a special formula containing casein hydrolysate products or elemental crystalline amino acids. Such formulas contain a limited amount of phenylalanine or are phenylalanine-free; all are balanced with fats, carbohydrates, vitamins, and minerals. A small amount of milk or regular infant formula can be added to the special formula to adjust the phenylalanine content and maintain an appropriate blood level.

As the infant grows, solid foods selected from a list of phenylalanine food exchange groups or equivalents are added according to their phenylalanine content. Specially prepared beverages and other phenylalanine-free products are also used for growing children.

Complications
The low-phenylalanine diet can cause stunted growth if the diet is not properly regulated and phenylalanine is eliminated totally from the diet.

Care considerations
• Explain the diet thoroughly to the parents.
• Explain how excess phenylalanine affects the developing nervous system. Emphasize that their child can develop normally – physically and psychologically – *only* if the diet is followed scrupulously. Offer suggestions early in treatment to limit psychosocial problems. For example, warn the parents against overemphasizing food intake or overprotecting their child; advise them to treat him as normally as possible. Suggest family counseling to aid adjustment to the child's dietary regimen.
• Check serum phenylalanine levels once weekly in early infancy and then monthly as the child matures to determine response to diet therapy. Serum phenylalanine levels should be kept between 2 and 10 mg/dl.
• Regularly assess the child's height, weight, and head circumference to ensure that the diet provides adequate nutrition for normal growth. Monitor hemoglobin levels because this diet is low in protein, magnesium, and zinc. If deficiencies of these elements develop, vitamin and mineral supplements may be required.
• Inadequate phenylalanine intake may result in phenylalanine deficiency. Watch for signs of phenylalanine deficiency: listlessness, anorexia, or stunted growth.
• Emphasize the importance of dietary compliance for the woman with PKU

who is pregnant or plans to get pregnant. Explain that congenital malformations and mental and physical retardation are likely when the fetus is exposed to high phenylalanine levels.

Home care instructions

• Instruct the parents to keep a daily food diary, which should be reviewed during follow-up visits, to assess phenylalanine intake and overall nutrition.

• Explain that tissue breakdown during illness can cause an accumulation of phenylalanine in the blood; therefore, the child may be restricted to clear liquids during illness. Tell parents to reintroduce the formula or diet as soon as possible after the child recovers.

• Parents need additional support and guidance as they introduce new foods to an infant. Have them demonstrate their ability to weigh and measure food properly and to make appropriate choices from the exchange lists.

• Emphasize to the parents that the child must learn to become responsible for his own diet. Help them develop this responsibility early. For example, explain that by age 3 or 4, children can learn that some foods are "no" foods and others are "yes" foods. Children can be taught to count out how many crackers they're allowed to eat.

• Help the parents find sources of low-protein foods, such as specialty shops and mail-order firms, and suggest that they use cookbooks designed for a low-phenylalanine diet and vegetarian cookbooks that include dairy products.

DIET, LOW-PURINE

This diet restricts foods—for example, liver, eggs, and sardines—that contain preformed purines, which the body breaks down into uric acid. This diet was commonly prescribed to control gout and prevent renal calculi, but its use has recently become controversial. Because the body is now known to synthesize purines, dietary measures alone will not control the uric acid level. The low-purine diet is now prescribed with a weight-control and exercise program to supplement therapy with uricosuric drugs, such as allopurinol and probenecid.

Purpose

• To lower serum uric acid levels while supplying adequate nutrients.

Indications

The diet may be used as part of the treatment of gout and renal calculi and in the treatment of patients with increased uric acid levels secondary to obesity, hypertension, hypertriglyceridemia, alcoholism, lead toxicity, pregnancy-induced hypertension, leukemia, polycythemia, psoriasis, or diuretic therapy.

Procedure

This diet is prescribed by the doctor as part of the patient's treatment. Typically, the dietitian explains the diet to the patient.

The low-purine diet contains limited amounts of fats, moderate amounts of protein, and plentiful amounts of complex carbohydrates. It also includes about 2 qt (2,000 ml)/day of water and fruit juice to help promote uric acid excretion, decrease the risk of renal calculi, and prevent the dehydration associated with antigout medications. This diet also includes fruits and vegetables to increase the alkalinity of the urine and thereby increase the solubility of uric acid.

The diet permits limited amounts of foods containing moderate amounts of purines, such as meats and dairy products and any food containing less than 150 mg of purines per 100 g.

Foods that are excluded include organ meats, such as liver, kidney, sweetbreads, brains, and heart; certain types of fish, including mussels, anchovies, sardines, fish roe, herring, shrimp, and mackerel; and certain other foods, such as mincemeat and yeast.

Complications

The low-purine diet doesn't typically cause complications.

Care considerations

• Review the patient's dietary and medication history. Ask about alcohol consumption, which can aggravate gout. Review the patient's use of medications because hydrochlorothiazide, pyrazinamide, and other drugs can cause accumulation of uric acid in body tissues.
• Emphasize that the low-purine diet is only part of a comprehensive regimen.
• Closely monitor serum uric acid levels. Notify the doctor if levels begin to rise sharply.
• Regularly assess for diffuse swelling in the joints and for nodular deposits of sodium urate crystals. Closely monitor intake and output, and encourage intake of fluids.
• Check urine pH. If ordered, administer sodium bicarbonate or potassium carbonate to increase urine alkalinity.
• Monitor laboratory studies for deficiencies of sodium, potassium, carotene, riboflavin, and vitamin B_{12} because antigout drugs can decrease absorption of these substances. If ordered, administer vitamin and mineral supplements.

Home care instructions

• Advise the patient to keep a food diary and review it at follow-up visits.
• Discourage fasting, low-carbohydrate diets, and rapid weight loss; all favor the formation of ketones, which inhibit the excretion of uric acid. The patient who wishes to lose weight should do so gradually.
• Suggest ways to increase fluid intake—for example, by having soup or drinking a glass of water before each meal and at bedtime.

• Help the patient develop an exercise and weight-control program.
• Discourage the consumption of alcoholic beverages, which can aggravate gout.
• Mention that avoiding coffee, tea, and cocoa is no longer considered necessary.
• Tell the patient to avoid aspirin and other salicylates; they can interact with certain antigout drugs to prevent uric acid excretion.
• Emphasize the need for regular follow-up visits to monitor progress and detect dietary deficiencies.

DIET, LOW-SODIUM

The low-sodium diet is one that patients find difficult, often describing it as tasteless and bland. Most Americans typically consume over 5,000 mg of sodium daily. A low-sodium diet may restrict sodium to as little as 250 mg daily.

Purpose

• To restrict dietary sodium, thereby preventing or correcting water retention associated with increased cardiac work load and edema or ascites.

Indications

Low-sodium diets are recommended for a variety of disorders, including hypertension, congestive heart failure, some renal diseases characterized by edema and hypertension, liver diseases characterized by edema and ascites, and myocardial infarction. Low-sodium diets may also be indicated in diabetes, coronary artery disease, and in conjunction with corticosteroid treatment.

This diet is contraindicated in patients with sodium-wasting renal diseases, such as pyelonephritis, polycystic renal disease, and bilateral hydronephrosis; in pregnancy; in myxedema; and in patients with ileostomies.

Procedure

A doctor usually prescribes the diet, and a dietitian assists in planning food choices. Depending on the patient's condition, the prescribed restriction of sodium can be mild or strict. (See *Meal planning for a low-sodium diet*.) Sodium diets that limit intake to 250 mg or 500 mg/day should be used only briefly – for example, in preparation for diagnostic testing. If sodium intake is limited to 250 mg/day, the patient must use distilled water for drinking and for making coffee, tea, and other beverages. All other diets allow 100 mg of sodium for 1,000 ml (1 qt) of tap water.

Complications

Patients restricted to 500 mg/day or less of sodium may develop hyponatremia, hypochloremia, and sodium depletion azotemia.

Care considerations

• Take a diet history to estimate the sodium content of the person's typical food choices as well as the amount of salt added at the table. Note any specific cultural or ethnic influences on diet. Also determine how often the patient eats out in order to plan a realistic allowance of sodium and predict how the patient will adjust to it.
• To encourage compliance, explain the role of sodium in water retention. Describe how water retention contributes to edema, ascites, and hypertension.
• Help the patient identify dietary sources of sodium. Typically, the patient can easily recognize salt (sodium chloride) because of its distinctive taste. But remember that he may equate sodium solely with table salt (which is 46% sodium). Make sure the patient realizes that sodium is a natural component in many foods; generally, meat, fish, milk, and eggs contain more sodium than do whole grain cereals, fruits, and vegetables.
• Explain that food additives – such as monosodium glutamate (MSG), found in many prepared foods; sodium alginate, which is added to chocolate and ice cream; and baking soda (soda bicarbonate) – can significantly increase the sodium content of the diet. When teaching about these sodium sources, point out that many food additives that add sodium do not give the food a salty taste.
• Monitor the patient restricted to 500 mg or less of sodium for hyponatremia, hypochloremia, and sodium depletion azotemia. Observe for weakness, lassitude, anorexia, abdominal cramps, confusion, and aching skeletal muscles. To detect fluid retention, weigh the patient daily. Also watch for diminished urine output, which may signal renal failure. Patients who are restricted to 500 mg/day or less of sodium are usually hospitalized.
• Check the hospitalized patient's food before he eats to be sure that salt hasn't been added accidentally.

Home care instructions

• Teach the patient how to read food labels to determine sodium content. The sodium content is noted on the label (200 mg of salt equals 80 mg of sodium). Also inform the patient that additives are listed in order of greatest quantity. Tell him to avoid a product if one of the following additives is among the first five listed: salt, sodium benzoate, sodium nitrate, or MSG.
• Warn that many over-the-counter medications contain sodium. Some examples include Alka-Seltzer, Di-Gel, Maalox Plus, Metamucil, Rolaids, and Vicks Formula 44 Cough Mixture. The patient should consult his doctor or pharmacist about the sodium content of any unprescribed medicine that he wishes to take.
• To help make the sodium-restricted diet more palatable, suggest seasoning foods with herbs and spices instead of salt. Tell the patient to avoid salt substitutes, unless his doctor approves. Explain that some products advertised

Meal planning for a low-sodium diet

The patient whose sodium intake is restricted needs guidance to plan meals appropriately.

Mild restrictions
Sodium restricted to 4,000 to 5,000 mg/day
- Cook with a minimum of salt (up to ½ tsp/day).
- Use regular milk—limit buttermilk to once a week.
- Use fresh or frozen vegetables and low-sodium vegetable juices. Avoid sauerkraut and other pickled vegetables prepared in brine.
- Eat fruits as desired.
- Beverages, sweets, and desserts may be taken as desired.
- Use regular bread, but avoid breads with salted tops.
- Use limited amounts of canned and dehydrated soups.
- Avoid any meat, fish, or poultry that is smoked, cured, or salted. Avoid lunch meat, hot dogs, sausages, sardines, anchovies, marinated herring, pickled meats and eggs, and processed cheese.
- Avoid salad dressing containing bacon fat, bacon bits, and salt pork.
- Avoid all seasonings or herbs labeled with the word SALT (garlic salt, celery salt, onion salt, and seasoned salt).
- Avoid commercially prepared potato, stuffing, and rice mixes.
- Avoid obviously salty foods, such as pickles and salted snacks.

Sodium restricted to 2,000 to 3,000 mg/day
- Cook food with a minimum of salt (up to ½ tsp/day) and don't use salt at the table.
- Avoid obviously salty foods, such as potato chips, pretzels, and snack crackers, and other high-sodium foods, such as canned soups and vegetables, prepared foods (such as TV dinners and frozen entrees), lunch meats, cheeses, or pickles, and any other foods preserved in brine. (Low-sodium canned products may be included.)
- Avoid using canned tomatoes and tomato products, unless they are low-sodium products.
- Avoid salted sauces or seasonings, such as chili sauce, mustard, catsup, and relish.
- Use unsalted meat, broth, soups, and butter.

Severe restrictions
Have the patient follow these same guidelines for all other levels of sodium restriction, but tell him to cook his food without salt. Then suggest the daily meal plan below, as appropriate.

Sodium restricted to 1,000 mg/day
- Regular milk, 1 pt
- Unsalted eggs
- Unsalted meat, 6 oz, cooked
- Unsalted vegetables, three servings
- Citrus fruit, as desired
- Unsalted bread and its exchanges, as desired
- Regular bread, four slices
- Fats, sugars, and jellies without sodium preservatives

(continued)

Meal planning for a low-sodium diet *(continued)*

Severe restrictions *(continued)*

Sodium restricted to 800 mg/day
• Regular milk, 1 pt
• Unsalted eggs
• Unsalted vegetables, three servings
• Citrus fruit, as desired
• Unsalted bread and its exchanges, as desired
• Regular bread, one slice
• Unsalted butter, sugars, and jellies without sodium preservatives

Sodium restricted to 500 mg/day
• Regular milk, ½ pt
• Low-sodium milk, ½ pt
• Unsalted egg, one (in place of 1 oz of meat)
• Unsalted meat, 6 oz, cooked
• Unsalted vegetables, three servings, but exclude beets, beet greens, carrots, kale, spinach, celery, white turnips, rutabagas, mustard greens, chard, and dandelion greens
• Citrus fruit, one serving
• Unsalted bread and its exchanges, as desired
• Fats, sugar, and jellies without sodium preservatives (no sherbet or gelatin)

Sodium restricted to 250 mg/day
• Low-sodium milk, 1 pt
• Unsalted meat, 5 oz, cooked (one unsalted egg can be substituted for 3 oz meat)
• Unsalted vegetables, three servings (omit the same vegetables as those listed in the 500-mg diet)
• Citrus fruit, three servings
• Unsalted bread and its exchanges, six servings
• Fats, sugar, and jellies without sodium preservatives

---

as low-sodium salt substitutes contain sodium chloride and may contain potassium or ammonium salts, which could be harmful if the patient has kidney or liver disease. Other products, classified as vegetized salts, use powdered dehydrated vegetables as a base and may contain considerable amounts of sodium.
• Advise the patient when eating out to order baked, broiled, or roasted foods and to avoid gravies, soups, and cheesy dressings.
• Teach the patient how to modify ethnic food practices, as necessary. For example, advise the patient who likes southern cuisine to avoid cooking with bacon or salt pork.

• Help the Jewish patient who wishes to follow orthodox dietary laws regarding meat and poultry. To be kosher, ritually slaughtered meat and poultry must be salted for 1 hour to remove the blood. Although the meat or poultry is thoroughly washed before cooking, some sodium is retained, increasing its sodium content by as much as 400%. Suggest using ammonium chloride instead of sodium chloride for drawing out the blood. Or suggest boiling the meat and discarding the broth before serving.
• Advise patients to use fresh tomatoes for soups and sauces; to use unsalted canned tomatoes, tomato paste, or tomato juice; and to avoid or restrict in-

take of olives, Italian cheeses, and Italian bread.

• Warn patients to avoid seasoning food with MSG or soy sauce. A low-salt soy sauce is available but should be used carefully because it contains a considerable amount of sodium.

• Inform the patient about the availability of specially prepared low-sodium products, such as low-sodium milk, unsalted canned vegetables, unsalted butter and margarine, low-sodium soups, and low-sodium baking powder.

• Collaborate with the dietitian to help the patient plan low-sodium menus and appropriate methods of preparing foods at home. Dietitians use a system similar to counting calories for counting the milligrams of sodium. The patient can eat small portions of sodium-containing food as part of the daily sodium allotment. Suggest sources of low-sodium recipes to keep his diet varied and enjoyable.

• Explain that bottled soft drinks may be high in sodium, depending on the sodium content of the water where they're manufactured.

• Eliminating dietary salt may place the patient at risk for iodine deficiency if iodine intake depends mainly on iodized salt. Encourage the use of other dietary sources of iodine, such as seafood and vegetables grown in iodine-rich soil. Explain that he can have the iodine content of his garden soil analyzed. Advise the patient to take supplemental iodine tablets, as ordered, if the iodine content of his diet and local drinking water is inadequate. Tell him to contact the local water authority or have his well water tested to establish iodine content.

• Refer the patient to the American Heart Association for additional information about sodium-restricted diets.

DIET, PROTEIN-MODIFIED

A high-protein diet can benefit patients with increased tissue breakdown, nitrogen depletion caused by stress or increased secretions of thyroid or glucocorticoid hormones, or protein loss. Contrary to popular belief, the protein recommendation for athletes is the same as that for the general population; athletes require more food due to increased energy expenditure, but a balanced diet provides sufficient protein.

When a high-protein diet is necessary, its beneficial effects can be striking. In just a few weeks, the patient's general health and well-being begin to improve. He gains weight and feels stronger; his resistance to infection increases, and wounds heal faster.

Some patients require a low-protein regimen. Protein restrictions may be necessary to keep a particular balance or to prevent the harmful accumulation of ammonia, urea, and other by-products of protein catabolism. Typically, such patients have illnesses that impair the body's ability to eliminate the by-products of protein catabolism — for example, end-stage renal disease or severe hepatic disease.

Purpose

• To meet the body's increased or decreased requirements for protein.

Indications

High-protein diets are generally indicated for patients with protein-calorie malnutrition, severe stress, and hypermetabolism resulting from conditions such as burns, cancer, acquired immunodeficiency syndrome, or damaged kidneys that lose large amounts of protein. High-protein diets may also be used in malabsorption syndromes, including protein-wasting enteropathy, short-bowel syndrome, inflammatory bowel diseases, and celiac disease.

Low-protein diets are indicated in the anuric phase of acute renal disease, chronic renal disease not treated with dialysis, cirrhosis, and hepatic coma. Some diseases—for example, alcoholism—require different modification of protein at different stages.

Procedure

Protein-modified diets are typically prescribed by the doctor according to the patient's condition. A registered dietitian frequently calculates allowed protein intake and reviews it with the patient. A nurse reinforces and works with the patient, family, and support team to promote the individualized plan.

The goal of a high-protein diet is to provide approximately 1.5 g of protein per kilogram of body weight and approximately 2,500 calories each day. One-half to two-thirds of the day's protein allowance should be selected from complete proteins, such as milk and meats (vegetables, bread and cereals contain incomplete protein), and the protein allowance should be divided as evenly as possible among the meals of the day. Nonfat dry milk may be added to regular milk and to casseroles to increase their protein content.

A low-protein diet should provide 75% of the dietary allowance in the form of high-value protein, such as that found in eggs. A low-protein diet excludes meats and dairy products, which are high in protein. It includes beverages, such as carbonated soft drinks, fruit drinks and punches, lemonade, and limeade; candies, such as candy corn, fondant (made with egg white only), hard candies, gum, gumdrops, jelly beans, lollipops, marshmallows, and mints; flour products, such as arrowroot, cornstarch, rice starch, tapioca, and wheat starch; certain sweeteners, such as corn syrup, honey, jams, jellies, maple syrup, and confectioner's

sugar; and most varieties of fruits and vegetables. Allowed fats include butter and margarine (unsalted), mayonnaise (without eggs), oils, and shortening. The protein allowance should be divided as evenly as possible among meals. Each patient's diet should contain enough calories to meet energy requirements; it may include supplements to prevent amino acid deficiencies.

Complications

A low-protein diet can lead to malnourishment if the patient does not receive adequate calories and nutrients. Amino acid deficiency can also occur.

Care considerations

• Explain the rationale for increasing or decreasing protein intake.
• Review the patient's diet history, considering sources of complete and incomplete protein. If the patient requires a high-protein diet, explain the need to eat plenty of carbohydrates; otherwise, the body simply burns protein as fuel.
• If the patient requires a low-protein diet, work with the dietitian to develop an individualized plan. Emphasize that the patient will need to limit the size of portions as well as the types of foods. Using the food on a hospital tray or plastic models, show the correct portion size for various foods; also show the patient how to use a food scale and have him give a return demonstration. Include the patient's family—especially the primary food preparer—in such discussions. Be sensitive to ethnic and cultural influences; most Americans consume large amounts of protein.
• Weigh the hospitalized patient on a high-protein diet daily; weigh an outpatient weekly. Expect a weight gain of 1 to 2 lb (0.5 to 1 kg)/week. Monitor for signs of protein deficiency, such as weakness, decreased resistance to infection, and low hemoglobin levels. In severe protein deficiency, monitor

serum albumin levels. Also check for edema, a sign of albumin deficiency.

• If the patient on a low-protein diet has end-stage renal disease, monitor blood urea nitrogen and serum creatinine levels, which reflect the clearance of the end products of protein metabolism. Also monitor the glomerular filtration rate (GFR); it can guide the degree of protein restriction. For example, a patient with a GFR of 10 to 15 ml/minute should restrict protein intake to 0.7 g/kg of body weight, but not less than 35 to 40 grams daily. Similarly, monitor urine flow to determine appropriate fluid intake; daily fluid intake should be 500 to 600 ml more than urine output.

• If the patient is receiving a low-protein diet because of liver disease, monitor serum ammonia levels daily and watch for signs of ammonia intoxication, such as flapping hand motions or tremors. Elevated ammonia levels will require further dietary restrictions.

Home care instructions

• Reinforce diet guidelines, and, if necessary, arrange a referral to a nutritionist or dietitian.

• Encourage the patient to return for frequent checkups.

• Remind the patient on a high-protein diet to increase protein and calorie consumption gradually.

• Inform the patient on a low-protein diet that specialized low-protein breads and other low-protein foods are commercially available. Provide the titles of appropriate cookbooks, particularly vegetarian cookbooks.

• Emphasize the importance of continuing to take prescribed vitamin and mineral supplements at home.

DIGITALIS GLYCOSIDES

The digitalis glycosides include digitoxin, derived from the dried leaves of the plant *Digitalis purpurea*, and digoxin and deslanoside, derived from *Digitalis lanata*.

All the digitalis glycosides produce similar cardiovascular effects; however, they differ in rates of absorption, metabolism, and excretion. The choice of drug and method of administration depend on the disorder and the desired onset of activity. For example, digoxin, the most commonly prescribed digitalis glycoside, requires several I.V. loading doses over a 24- to 48-hour period to reach therapeutic serum levels for congestive heart failure (CHF) maintenance.

Purpose

• To increase cardiac output
• To control atrial flutter or fibrillation.

Indications

Digitalis glycosides are used to increase cardiac output in acute or chronic CHF. They control the rate of ventricular contraction in atrial flutter or fibrillation, and they are also used to prevent or treat paroxysmal atrial tachycardia and angina associated with CHF. Digoxin is the drug of choice for maintenance therapy in CHF. Deslanoside has only one use: loading dosage in adults who require rapid digitalization.

Contraindications include ventricular tachycardia and fibrillation and hypersensitivity reactions. Digitalis glycosides should be used cautiously in elderly patients and in those with renal or hepatic insufficiency, hypothyroidism, severe pulmonary disease, acute myocardial infarction (MI), atrioventricular block, constrictive pericarditis, or idiopathic hypertrophic subaortic stenosis.

Adverse reactions

The digitalis glycosides have a narrow range between therapeutic and toxic blood levels and therefore carry a high

Recognizing digitalis toxicity

Digoxin and digitoxin, two commonly prescribed digitalis glycosides, have a narrow therapeutic range. As a result, toxicity is a common problem. In infants and young children, the first symptoms are usually arrhythmias; in older children and adults, GI symptoms usually herald toxicity.

Detecting toxicity
To detect toxicity, watch for extracardiac symptoms: anorexia, nausea, vomiting, abdominal pain, diarrhea, headache, fatigue, and weakness. The patient may also experience visual disturbances, such as blurring, halos around lights, or diplopia.

Be alert for signs of heart failure, and check the pulse for bradycardia or tachycardia. Monitor the electrocardiogram for premature ventricular contractions, atrial fibrillation, accelerated junctional nodal rhythm, atrioventricular dissociation, or heart block.

Confirming toxicity
Draw serum samples for measuring drug levels at least 6 hours after an oral dose, the duration necessary for the serum and tissues to reach equilibrium levels. The therapeutic level for digoxin ranges from 0.5 to 2 ng/ml; levels greater than 2.5 ng/ml cause toxicity. The therapeutic level for digitoxin ranges from 14 to 26 ng/ml; serum levels over 35 ng/ml cause toxicity.

risk of toxicity. Nearly one-third of patients treated with these agents develop toxic reactions, which may include life-threatening arrhythmias, hypotension, or severe CHF. Toxic effects may result from overdosage or altered absorption, changes in serum electrolyte levels (especially hypokalemia), renal or hepatic dysfunction, drug interactions, or other factors. In a patient with sensitivity to digitalis glycosides, toxicity can develop even with normally therapeutic doses. (See *Recognizing digitalis toxicity*.)

Care considerations
• Before administering the first dose of a digitalis glycoside, obtain baseline heart rate and rhythm, blood pressure, and serum electrolyte levels; before each subsequent dose, monitor the patient's apical-radial pulse for 1 minute. If any sudden increase or decrease in rate or new irregularities are noted, withhold the drug and inform the doctor.
• Monitor serum potassium levels carefully, and notify the doctor of falling levels, which require corrective action to prevent hypokalemia.
• Throughout therapy, carefully monitor for symptoms of toxicity.
• Notify the doctor immediately of any early symptoms; they require prompt measurement of serum electrolyte and drug levels.
• To prevent toxicity from drug interactions, closely review the patient's drug regimen. Agents such as beta-adrenergic blockers, thiazide-like and loop diuretics, calcium channel blockers, quinidine, and cimetidine may raise serum levels of digitalis glycosides. Antacids, kaolin-pectin, colestipol, cholestyramine, and metoclopramide may decrease absorption of digitalis glycosides and should be given as far apart from them as possible. Amphotericin B, carbenicillin, ticarcillin, corticosteroids, and diuretics can cause hypokalemia, and parenteral calcium and thiazides can produce hypercalcemia and hypomagnesemia. Remember that such electrolyte imbalances can increase the risk of digitalis toxicity.

• Check the patient's regimen for concurrent use of phenylbutazone, phenytoin, phenobarbital, and rifampin, which can speed hepatic metabolism of digitalis glycosides and shorten their therapeutic duration. Similarly, check for propranolol, reserpine, succinylcholine, epinephrine, and isoproterenol, which may increase the risk of arrhythmias.

Home care instructions

• Instruct the patient to take this medication at the same time each day. Or tell parents to give the drug to an infant or young child in divided doses, as ordered.
• Tell the patient or caregiver to count the pulse for 1 minute before each dose. Emphasize the importance of notifying the doctor if the rate is below 60 beats/minute or over 100 beats/minute or if skipped beats or new irregularities are detected.
• Instruct the patient or caregiver to watch for and immediately report early symptoms of toxicity, such as anorexia, nausea, diarrhea, or a bloated feeling. Other symptoms include weakness, blurred vision, and halos around lights.
• Also emphasize the importance of informing the doctor about signs of fluid retention, such as lung congestion, shortness of breath, or swelling.
• Tell the adult patient to weigh himself once a week on the same scale, at the same time of day, and wearing similar amounts of clothing, and to notify the doctor if he gains 3 lb (1.4 kg) or more.
• If the doctor also has prescribed a loop or thiazide diuretic, instruct the patient to take a potassium supplement or to eat foods high in potassium, as recommended.
• Tell the patient to avoid over-the-counter products such as cough and cold medicines, antacids, and diet medicine unless the doctor has recommended their use.
• If appropriate, tell the patient to follow a low-salt diet.

DILATATION AND CURETTAGE OR EVACUATION

Dilatation and curettage (D and C) is a gynecologic procedure that involves widening the cervical canal with a dilator and scraping the uterine cavity with a curette. Dilatation and evacuation (D and E) involves widening the cervical canal with a dilator and then evacuating the contents of a pregnant uterus with a curette or a curette with suction attached.

Purpose
For a D and C
• To remove tissue after an incomplete, early abortion
• To control and diagnose the cause of abnormal uterine bleeding
• To explore the uterus
• To obtain endocervical and endometrial tissue for cytologic study.
For a D and E
• To perform a therapeutic abortion
• To treat an incomplete abortion occurring in the late first trimester or in the early second trimester.

Indications

D and C provides treatment for an incomplete abortion, controls abnormal uterine bleeding, and can secure an endometrial or endocervical tissue sample for cytologic study. D and E can also be used for an incomplete or a therapeutic abortion, usually up to 12 weeks of gestation but occasionally as late as 16 weeks. The procedure may be done as late as 20 weeks but is associated with increased risks in advanced pregnancy.

Procedure

These procedures are performed by the doctor in the operating room or short procedure unit. They require anesthesia (general, paracervical block, or local, supplemented with diazepam or meperidine) and asepsis. After receiving an anesthetic, the patient is placed in the dorsal lithotomy position; the doctor performs a pelvic examination, dilates the cervix with an instrument called a dilator, and then removes the superficial layer of the endometrium with a curette. Biopsy specimens can also be taken if warranted.

If a D and C is used to treat an incomplete abortion, the doctor also removes the remaining products of conception.

In a D and E, the surgeon dilates the cervical canal with a dilator. In a therapeutic abortion, he may use a synthetic dilator (Dilipan) or laminaria wedges (seaweed wedges that swell) that are inserted the evening before surgery. He then uses either a sharp curette or a suction curette to extract the contents of the uterus. He then explores the uterine cavity to ensure complete removal of the products of conception.

Complications

Potential complications of D and C include uterine perforation, hemorrhage, and infection. Second-trimester D and E may cause cervical trauma and may affect subsequent pregnancies; it can lead to spontaneous abortion, cervical incompetence, or premature birth.

Care considerations

Before the procedure

• Review the procedure with the patient and answer her questions.
• Inform the patient that after the procedure she will have some vaginal drainage and a perineal pad in place.
• Explain that temporary abdominal cramping and pelvic and low-back pain are normal symptoms after this procedure.
• Ensure that preliminary studies have been completed.

• Be sure that the patient has followed preoperative directions for fasting before admission.
• Inform the patient that she'll be groggy after the procedure and won't be able to drive.
• Make sure the patient has signed a consent form.
• Ask the patient to void before you administer any preoperative medications.

After the procedure

• Administer analgesics, as ordered. Expect the patient to have moderate cramping and pelvic and low-back pain, but be sure to report any continuous, sharp abdominal pain that doesn't respond to analgesics; this may indicate perforation of the uterus.
• Monitor the patient's vital signs and assess for possible hemorrhage and signs of infection, such as purulent, foul-smelling vaginal drainage.
• Administer fluids, as tolerated, and allow food if the patient requests it. Keep the bed's side rails raised, and help the patient walk to the bathroom, if appropriate.

Home care instructions

• Instruct the patient to report any signs of infection.
• Tell the patient to use analgesics to control pain but to report any unrelenting sharp pain.
• Inform the patient that spotting and discharge may last a week or longer, but that she should report any bright red blood.
• Instruct the patient to schedule a follow-up appointment with the doctor.
• Tell the patient to resume activity as tolerated, but remind her to follow her doctor's instructions for vigorous exercise and sexual intercourse. This usually includes maintaining pelvic rest (no sexual intercourse, tampons, or douching) for 10 days after the procedure.

• Advise the patient to seek birth control counseling, if needed, and refer her to an appropriate center.

DIURETICS

Diuretics satisfactorily control mild hypertension in about one-third of all patients. Because of their safety, effectiveness, and reasonable cost, they're often the first choice for treating hypertension and congestive heart failure (CHF). They are also used to reduce intraocular pressure in acute angle-closure glaucoma. (See *Osmotic drugs: Emergency prevention of blindness*.)

The four types of diuretics — thiazide, thiazide-like, potassium-sparing, and loop — possess somewhat different mechanisms of action. (See *Comparing diuretics*, pages 256 to 258.)

Purpose
• To control hypertension
• To reduce fluid volume.

Indications
Diuretics represent the mainstay in pharmacologic management of hypertension. Diuretics also prove valuable in managing fluid overload, especially in pulmonary edema, ascites, cirrhosis, peripheral edema, or anasarca.

Typically, diuretics are contraindicated in patients with anuria, hepatic coma, severe fluid and electrolyte depletion, and hypersensitivity to another diuretic. They should be used cautiously in patients with renal or hepatic failure, in pregnant patients, and in children. They should also be used cautiously in elderly patients, who are most likely to experience adverse reactions and fluid and electrolyte imbalances.

(Text continues on page 258.)

Osmotic drugs: Emergency prevention of blindness

In acute angle-closure glaucoma, hyperosmotic solutions, such as *glycerin, isosorbide, urea,* and *mannitol,* effectively control sharply rising intraocular pressure. Without prompt treatment, this ophthalmic emergency could result in blindness.

How osmotics work
Hyperosmotic solutions rapidly reduce intraocular pressure and vitreous volume while the patient is prepared for surgery or laser treatment. These drugs draw fluid from the eyeball by osmosis to increase blood osmolarity; at the same time, they decrease corneal edema. Their effectiveness hinges on an intact blood-aqueous vascular system and on the absence of inflammatory disease.

Comparing osmotics
In an emergency, mannitol and urea are equally effective in reducing intraocular pressure and vitreous volume. They reduce intraocular pressure in 30 to 60 minutes and remain effective for 6 to 8 hours. Both are given I.V., but mannitol is more convenient to administer and less toxic. Urea irritates the tissues, causing pain at the infusion site. And if this drug is infused into a leg vein, it can also precipitate thrombosis.

In contrast, glycerin and isosorbide are given orally. They work more slowly than the other osmotics, but they're safer and more convenient to use. Glycerin reduces intraocular pressure in about 1 hour and its effects subside after 5 hours. Isosorbide has a similar duration of action. However, it's preferred over glycerin in diabetic patients because it doesn't alter their blood glucose levels.

Comparing diuretics

DRUG AND MECHANISM OF ACTION	INDICATIONS	SPECIAL CONSIDERATIONS
Loop diuretics		
furosemide Inhibits the absorption of sodium, chloride, and water in the ascending loop of Henle, promoting the excretion of sodium, water, chloride, and potassium.	Used to treat edema associated with congestive heart failure (CHF), cirrhosis, and renal disease; less ototoxic than ethacrynic acid.	• Advise the patient to increase intake of potassium-rich foods to avoid hypokalemia. • Tell the patient to avoid eating natural black licorice; the glycyrrhizic acid it contains can cause hypokalemia. • Watch for swelling or pain in the joints, which may indicate gout. Monitor uric acid levels. • Tell the patient to report ototoxic signs: vertigo, tinnitus, or hearing loss.
ethacrynic acid Inhibits sodium and chloride reabsorption in the proximal tubule and loop of Henle, promoting potassium and hydrogen ion excretion. Hypotensive effects result from hypovolemia and decreased vascular resistance.	Used to treat severe edema associated with CHF, cirrhosis, and renal disease. Because of severe side effects, typically used after furosemide for these applications.	• Same special considerations as for furosemide. • Immediately report profuse, watery diarrhea to doctor.
bumetanide Inhibits reabsorption of sodium and chloride in the ascending loop of Henle; may have additional activity in the proximal tubule to promote phosphate excretion.	Used to treat edema associated with CHF, cirrhosis, and renal disease; may be less ototoxic than furosemide; can be safely prescribed for patients allergic to furosemide.	• Same special considerations as for furosemide. • Use with antimuscarinics can increase GI irritability. • Use with corticotropin or with sodium bicarbonate or insulin infusion can decrease serum potassium levels.

Comparing diuretics *(continued)*

DRUG AND MECHANISM OF ACTION	INDICATIONS	SPECIAL CONSIDERATIONS
Thiazide diuretics		
chlorothiazide and hydrochlorothiazide Reduce sodium reabsorption and increase potassium secretion in the distal tubule; promote sodium, bicarbonate, and potassium excretion and retention of calcium and uric acid.	Used alone or with other drugs in step 1 treatment of hypertension. Also used to treat edema associated with CHF, cirrhosis, renal disease, and corticosteroid therapy.	• Advise the patient to increase intake of potassium-rich foods to avoid hypokalemia and to avoid natural black licorice. • Monitor calcium and uric acid levels. • Can cause photosensitivity; avoid excessive sun exposure.
Thiazide-like diuretics		
chlorthalidone Structurally related to thiazides, with a similar mechanism of action.	Used alone or with other drugs to treat essential hypertension. Also used to treat edema associated with CHF.	• Same special considerations as for thiazide diuretics.
metolazone Structurally related to thiazides, with a similar mechanism of action.	Used in severe hypertension; more effective than thiazides in severe renal failure.	• Same special considerations as for thiazide diuretics.
Potassium-sparing diuretics		
amiloride Inhibits sodium reabsorption and potassium excretion by direct action on the distal tubule.	Used for adjunctive treatment of hypertension when a potassium-sparing diuretic is needed.	• Watch for signs of hyperkalemia, such as weakness, confusion, and paresthesia of or heaviness in the legs. • Don't use in patients whose serum potassium levels exceed 5.5 mEq/L. • Tell the patient to limit potassium intake. • Can cause central nervous system disturbances. Advise the patient to use caution when driving a car or operating machinery.

(continued)

Comparing diuretics *(continued)*

DRUG AND MECHANISM OF ACTION	INDICATIONS	SPECIAL CONSIDERATIONS
Potassium-sparing diuretics *(continued)*		
spironolactone Competes with aldosterone for cellular receptor sites in the distal tubule; promotes sodium, chloride, and water excretion without potassium loss.	Moderate diuretic action (less than that of thiazides); used to potentiate actions of other diuretics and to spare potassium.	• Same special considerations as for amiloride (first three bullets). • Can cause breast swelling and tenderness as well as menstrual abnormalities.
triamterene Promotes excretion of sodium and carbonate, with little or no excretion of potassium; blocks potassium excretion by direct action on the distal tubule.	Weak diuretic action; used with other diuretics because of potassium-sparing ability.	• Same special considerations as for amiloride (first three bullets). • Can cause gout. Check for swollen or painful joints. Monitor uric acid levels. • Withdraw drug over several days to avoid excessive rebound potassium excretion.

Adverse reactions

The most common adverse reaction to thiazide and loop diuretics is potassium depletion. Hypokalemia may be associated with hypochloremic alkalosis, especially in patients with other losses of chloride and potassium, such as vomiting and diarrhea. Dilutional hyponatremia may occur. Hyperuricemia may occur but is usually asymptomatic, except in patients predisposed to gout or chronic renal failure.

Thiazides and thiazide-like diuretics can produce hyperglycemia, glycosuria, and elevated triglyceride and cholesterol levels. GI reactions include anorexia, nausea, and pancreatitis. Cardiovascular reactions can include orthostatic hypotension and volume depletion; electrolyte disturbances can include dehydration, hypocalcemia, and hypomagnesemia. Rarely, agranulocytosis, leukopenia, and thrombo-

cytopenia may occur. When given I.V. rapidly or in high doses, the loop diuretics have been associated with ototoxicity.

Potassium-sparing diuretics may cause hyperkalemia. Nausea, vomiting, anorexia, headache, and dizziness occur less frequently. Amiloride may cause impotence; spironolactone may cause gynecomastia in men and breast soreness in women; triamterene has caused anaphylaxis, photosensitivity, and megaloblastic anemia.

I.V. doses of diuretics should be given slowly over several minutes. Rapid or excessive diuresis can cause hypovolemia, hypotension, and vascular collapse.

Care considerations

• During therapy, regularly assess the patient's vital signs, intake and output, and weight. If administering a diuretic

I.V., check blood pressure frequently and be alert for pain and irritation at the insertion site, possibly indicating drug extravasation. If you detect severe hypotension, hematuria, diarrhea, or hypovolemia, discontinue the drug and notify the doctor.

• Throughout diuretic therapy, monitor levels of serum electrolytes, serum creatinine, and blood urea nitrogen (BUN). Diuretics can alter levels of serum electrolytes, especially potassium. Elevated levels of serum creatinine and BUN may indicate renal damage and can decrease the effectiveness of diuretics.

• If the patient has a history of gout, watch for elevated serum uric acid.

• If the patient has diabetes, carefully monitor blood and urine glucose levels; thiazide-induced glucose intolerance may require an adjustment of therapeutic regimen when hypoglycemic effects are decreased. The patient may need increased dosage of insulin.

• Check the patient's drug regimen for possible interactions. Potassium depletion is an important consideration in patients receiving digitalis glycosides because a low potassium level increases the cardiotoxicity of these agents. If you're giving the two drugs concurrently, monitor for signs of toxicity: fatigue, weakness, arrhythmias, blurred vision, anorexia, and nausea. Diuretics may increase the therapeutic and toxic effects of lithium by decreasing its renal excretion. Lithium levels must be monitored and dosage lowered as necessary.

Home care instructions

• Tell the patient to notify his doctor about adverse reactions, especially if he's taking furosemide. GI adverse reactions commonly develop after 1 or 2 months of treatment.

• Tell the patient to expect increased frequency and amount of urination.

• Recommend taking the drug in the morning or afternoon to avoid nocturia and taking it with meals or a snack to reduce GI upset.

• Teach the patient how to recognize symptoms of hypokalemia or hyperkalemia (depending on the type of diuretic he's taking). Instruct him to report any of these symptoms to his doctor. Emphasize the importance of keeping appointments for serum potassium determinations.

• Tell the patient to weigh himself every week at the same time of day, on the same scale, and wearing similar clothing, and to notify the doctor of any weight loss or gain exceeding 3 lb (1.4 kg).

DOUCHING

Douching, or vaginal irrigation, is the instillation of fluid with or without medication into the vagina. It may be performed in the hospital by a nurse either preoperatively or postoperatively, or to treat a specific condition, but it is often performed at home by the patient for cleanliness or to treat infection and inflammation.

Commonly used solutions include sterile water, 0.9% sodium chloride solution, and antiseptic solutions such as povidone-iodine. Various disposable douches are commercially available for the treatment of vaginal inflammation. When performed after surgery, douching requires aseptic technique.

Douching for treatment of infection or infertility is usually done by the patient in her own home. Frequent douching (more than twice a month) is not recommended unless prescribed because it can irritate the vaginal mucosa and increase the risk of infection by disrupting the vagina's normal protective mechanism. Self-prescribed treatment for vaginal irritation or infections is strongly discouraged by most health care providers.

Purpose

- To clean and disinfect the vagina
- To relieve pain and inflammation
- To instill medication into the vagina
- To alter vaginal pH.

Indications

Douching is commonly used in the treatment of gynecologic disorders, such as vaginal infection and inflammation; it is also used preoperatively and postoperatively. For example, vaginal douching with a povidone-iodine-and-water solution is frequently performed before a hysterectomy to prevent the transmission of microorganisms from the vagina into the operative area.

Solutions that contain vinegar or sodium bicarbonate and water, which alter vaginal pH and thereby create a compatible environment for sperm, are commonly used in the treatment of infertility. Many women douche with commercial solutions for personal hygiene after intercourse or at the end of the menstrual cycle to remove blood and tissue.

Vaginal douching is contraindicated in untreated sexually transmitted disease and during pregnancy because it may cause an air embolism and death. It is also contraindicated for 4 to 6 weeks after miscarriage or childbirth because it may increase the risk of infection.

Procedure

Preoperative douching is usually performed by the nurse and given with the patient in bed on a bedpan to ensure maximum cleaning. The patient may also douche in the bathtub or while sitting on the toilet.

One tablespoon of povidone-iodine solution is mixed with approximately 1,000 ml (about 1 qt) of warm tap water.

Water temperature should be between 100° and 110° F (37.7° and 38.3° C).

Douching for the purpose of altering pH for infertility is usually done by the patient at home and should be performed about 30 minutes before intercourse. Vinegar-and-water solutions are prepared with 1 tbs of white vinegar in about 16 oz (500 ml) of warm tap water; sodium bicarbonate douches require 1 tbs of baking soda in 1 qt of warm tap water.

The patient should empty her bladder before the procedure. After mixing the douche solution, the irrigating receptacle is hung at a level just above the patient's hips to allow the solution to flow freely and gently. The nozzle is lubricated and inserted about 2″ (5 cm) into the vagina in a downward and backward direction. Then, the solution is allowed to flow until the container is empty. The nozzle can be gently rotated during the instillation. If the patient is using a prefilled container, the nozzle is usually prelubricated. The nozzle is inserted in the same way; then the container is gently squeezed to instill the premeasured solution.

Complications

Complications are rare, but routine, frequent douching may eliminate normal vaginal flora. This can lead to an alteration in vaginal pH and subsequent vaginal dryness, irritation and, possibly, infection.

Care considerations

Before the procedure

- Explain the procedure to the patient and provide privacy.
- Check to make sure the patient has no allergies to the medications to be used.
- Ensure the proper amount and temperature of the irrigating solution.
- Make sure the patient empties her bladder.
- The patient should wash her hands before self-administering the douche.

During the procedure
• Monitor for any irritation caused by the douching.
• Insert the douche nozzle gently and for the correct distance of 2" to prevent injury to the vaginal mucosa.
• Ensure the correct level for the douche bag of no more than 2' (0.6 m) above the level of the patient's hips.
• When administering a douche post-operatively, use aseptic technique.

After the procedure
• Encourage the patient to lie recumbent for 1 hour after the povidone-iodine douche to obtain maximum therapeutic benefit.
• Dispose of all equipment used in the hospital setting to prevent cross-contamination.

Home care instructions
• Provide an adequate explanation and written instructions for the patient performing the procedure at home.
• Tell the patient to report vaginal discharge, itching, odor, or irritation to her health care provider immediately.
• Teach the importance of following the written instructions. Allow time for the patient to ask questions.
• Advise the patient against frequent douching unless recommended by her doctor.

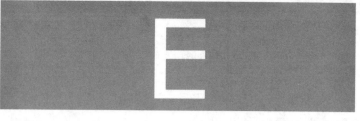

EAR IRRIGATION

Ear irrigation involves washing the external auditory canal with a stream of solution (usually water) to clean the canal of debris, remove impacted cerumen, or dislodge a foreign body. If a fungal (mycotic) infection is present, alcohol may be used as the irrigant to facilitate evaporation of moisture. Because ear irrigation may contaminate the middle ear if the tympanic membrane is ruptured, an otoscopic examination always precedes ear irrigation.

Purpose
• To remove impacted cerumen from the external auditory canal
• To clean the external auditory canal of discharges or debris
• To dislodge a foreign body from the external auditory canal
• To eliminate moisture from the external auditory canal.

Indications
Ear irrigation is indicated when otoscopic examination reveals the need to remove impacted cerumen, debris, or a foreign body from the external auditory canal. Alcohol irrigation may be indicated to treat a fungal infection.

Ear irrigation is contraindicated when a vegetable foreign body (such as a pea, bean, or corn kernel) obstructs the auditory canal. A vegetable foreign body attracts and absorbs moisture. In contact with an irrigant, it swells, causing intense pain and complicating removal of the object. Ear irrigation is also contraindicated if the patient has a cold, fever, nonmycotic ear infection, or an injured or ruptured tympanic membrane.

Procedure
Ear irrigation may be performed by a doctor or specially trained nurse. For an adult, the pinna is gently pulled up and back; for a child, the pinna is pulled down and back. This straightens the auditory canal, thus allowing the solution to flow through the entire length of the canal.

The syringe is filled with tepid water because too cold or too hot water will affect inner ear fluids and induce vertigo and nausea. The tip of the syringe is inserted approximately one-third of the way into the external auditory canal and is pointed upward and toward the posterior auditory canal to prevent damage to the tympanic membrane. A steady stream of irrigant is directed against the side of the canal.

An initial return of discolored water and debris is expected. The syringe is refilled and irrigation continued until return flow is clear and otoscopic examination reveals a clean auditory canal. However, ear irrigation should not use more than 500 ml (about 18 oz) of irrigant.

Complications
Perforation of the tympanic membrane and laceration of the external auditory canal can occur but rarely do so when ear irrigation is performed by

an experienced person. Other complications include vertigo, nausea, otitis externa, and otitis media (if the patient has a ruptured tympanic membrane).

Care considerations
Before the procedure
• Before irrigating, ask if the patient has had previous ear surgery, a history of a perforated tympanic membrane, or repeated episodes of middle ear infection. If the patient has a history of ear problems, the irrigation should be performed by an ear specialist (otolaryngologist).
• A ceruminolytic agent containing peroxide and a lubricant may be instilled several times a day for 4 to 7 days before irrigation. This procedure, which softens the earwax, is especially important in elderly patients because their cerumen contains a high content of keratin, which is not easily removed by ordinary irrigation.
• Before irrigation, explain the procedure to the patient and position him seated with his head tilted slightly forward and toward the affected ear. If the patient cannot sit, he should lie on his back with his head tilted slightly forward and toward the affected ear. Have him hold an emesis basin close to his head under the affected ear.
During the procedure
• Watch for and ask the patient to report any pain or dizziness. If either occurs, the procedure should be discontinued.
After the procedure
• Dry the patient's pinna and neck.
• If the patient has an external mycotic infection, topical antifungal therapy is needed after cleaning.

Home care instructions
• Advise the patient to contact his doctor if he has any pain or excessive drainage.

ELECTROCONVULSIVE THERAPY

Electroconvulsive therapy (ECT), also referred to as electroshock therapy, was first used in 1937 as a somatic treatment for various emotional disorders. During ECT, an electric current travels through electrodes placed on the temples, causing a generalized tonic-clonic seizure. Exactly how ECT works remains unclear, but it seems to produce biochemical changes in the brain that increase levels of norepinephrine and serotonin.

Despite its controversial history, ECT is now considered a relatively simple procedure. Decisions regarding its use are based on the risks and benefits of all available treatments.

Purpose
• To relieve major depression or other severe mental disorders.

Indications
ECT is primarily used to treat major depression in patients who do not respond to or cannot tolerate drug therapy or its adverse effects. It is also indicated for actively suicidal patients who could die while waiting for antidepressant medication to become effective.

When standard therapies produce inadequate results, ECT also may be used to treat other mental disorders, organic mental syndrome, reduced pituitary hormone levels, seizure disorders, and Parkinson's disease. Other candidates for ECT may include patients with manic disorders, schizophrenia, or catatonic syndromes.

ECT is contraindicated in patients who cannot tolerate the increase in either intracranial pressure (ICP) or myocardial oxygen consumption. It should not be used in patients who have increased ICP or an intracranial mass or in patients who have an unstable vascular anomaly such as an aortic or intracranial aneurysm, or who have had a recent cerebrovascular accident, myocardial infarction, or decompensated congestive heart failure. Such patients are at higher risk for complications from the ECT-induced seizure and the anesthesia. ECT should be used cautiously during pregnancy and in elderly patients.

Procedure

The patient, accompanied by staff, is taken to a treatment room equipped with specialized ECT and emergency resuscitation equipment. The patient is placed on a padded bed and may be gently restrained. An I.V. line is started to deliver medication as needed. An oxygen mask is used for respiratory support. An oral airway is inserted to prevent airway obstruction and biting of the tongue. Electrocardiogram (ECG) electrodes are applied to monitor cardiac function. EEG electrodes are applied to monitor brain electrical activity. Usually the ECT electrodes are placed on each temple, although some psychiatrists prefer to place both electrodes on the nondominant side because it produces less memory disturbance. An alternating current of 400 milliamperes and 70 to 120 volts is passed between the ECT electrodes for 0.1 to 0.5 second.

A psychiatrist administers the ECT and is supported by a specially trained anesthesia and nursing staff. Usually a short-acting general anesthetic and a muscle relaxant are administered. Treatments vary depending on the severity of symptoms and the patient's responsiveness to treatment. Usually ECT treatments are given on alternate days, 3 to 4 times a week. An average of 6 to 10 treatments are given for depression; 20 to 30 treatments may be given for schizophrenia.

ECT is not used indiscriminately or for a long time. Psychotropic drugs and psychotherapy may be used as adjunctive therapy with ECT.

Complications

The two most common adverse reactions to ECT are temporary memory loss and confusion. These reactions are transient and are related to the number of treatments, the technique of electrode placement, the voltage used, and the age and mental status of the patient before therapy. Memory and cognitive function routinely return to normal 1 to 6 months after treatment.

Cardiac complications include bradycardia, tachycardia, and blood pressure changes, which are related to the use of muscle relaxants, anesthesia, and the induced tonic-clonic seizure.

Historically, fractured bones and strained muscles of the neck, back, and extremities were common with the use of ECT. The use of muscle relaxants and anesthesia has virtually eliminated these problems. Some clinicians report that patients who have received ECT have suffered social stigmatization because of others' negative perceptions of them.

Care considerations

Before therapy

• Explain the procedure to the patient and family, correct any misconceptions, and answer their questions. Provide emotional support.

• Obtain the patient's or caregiver's informed consent before ECT is administered.

• A thorough medical evaluation before treatment should include a physical examination, standard laboratory tests, ECG, EEG, and X-rays.

• Because depressed patients may experience sleeping and eating disturbances, assist them in maintaining adequate nutrition, proper elimination, and effective sleeping patterns.

• The patient should have nothing to eat or drink for at least 4 hours before treatment and should wear loose-fitting clothes and remove contact lenses and jewelry.

• Psychotropic drugs should be discontinued the day before ECT to prevent any interactions.

• Ask the patient to void just before the procedure to prevent incontinence during the induced seizure.

• Ask the patient who wears dentures to remove them to prevent airway obstruction.

• Make sure emergency resuscitation equipment is available.

• A premedication may be administered 30 minutes before the treatment to assist with anesthesia and provide sedation.

After therapy

• Posttreatment care includes continued respiratory support until the patient can breathe unassisted. Monitor vital signs and neurologic status every 5 minutes until the patient is awake and then every 15 minutes until the patient is alert. Continue to orient the patient and provide emotional support as needed.

• To prevent injury, keep the bed's side rails raised until the patient becomes oriented.

• Administer posttreatment analgesics and antiemetics as necessary to relieve headache or nausea.

• Discharge the patient from the recovery room when stable.

Home care instructions

• If the patient receives ECT as an outpatient, make sure a family member or caregiver is available to provide transportation home. Warn the patient against driving and other hazardous tasks until confusion and drowsiness completely subside. The patient may resume his daily activities only when he feels physically able.

• Remind the patient's family or caregiver that temporary amnesia and mild confusion can occur after ECT, but that these symptoms usually diminish or disappear.

• Encourage the patient's family to support the patient once he's home. Allay their fears and encourage them to make sure the patient follows the doctor's recommendations and keeps follow-up appointments.

• The patient may need to continue taking antidepressant medication after ECT. Encourage compliance.

EMBOLIZATION OF ARTERIOVENOUS MALFORMATION

Arteriovenous malformations (AVMs) are developmental anomalies in which the normal communication between the arterial and venous systems is absent; arterial blood is shunted directly from feeder arteries to draining veins without perfusion of underlying tissue. Ischemia or infarction of underlying and surrounding tissue may occur even without rupture, although the severity of these complications is increased with rupture. The size of an AVM varies from a small malformation of a few millimeters to a large tangled mass of arteries and veins.

Surgical excision is commonly the treatment for an AVM but may not be an option for some patients. An alternative treatment, embolization, also known as transcatheter arterial embolization therapy, is now being used more often for cranial AVMs. Embolization therapy aims to occlude the abnormal vessels and obliterate or at least decrease the size of the AVM. To do this, an embolizing substance is introduced into the nidus (point of vessel entry) of the feeder vessel (see *Describing AVM embolization*, page 266). This procedure may stabilize or reverse neurologic deficits.

The success of the procedure depends on the AVM's vascularity and its size as well as the patient's overall health status. Recent improvements in mate-

Describing AVM embolization

This illustration shows the feeder artery of an arteriovenous malformation (AVM). For AVM embolization, the surgeon injects small Silastic beads through a catheter placed in the malformation's feeder artery. These beads lodge in the artery, forming an embolus that occludes blood flow to the malformation.

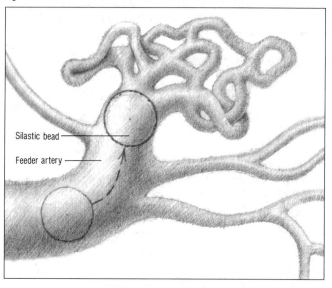

Silastic bead

Feeder artery

rial and methods have made this procedure much safer. However, significant risks still exist.

Purpose

• To occlude blood flow to an AVM, destroying it or decreasing its size.

Indications

Embolization therapy may be indicated when surgical removal of the AVM is contraindicated in a patient at high risk or when the location of the AVM makes surgery impossible. The procedure may also be used to decrease the size of large AVMs before attempting surgical resection. This helps to reduce risks, especially bleeding, associated with subsequent surgery.

Procedure

The doctor, using angiography, performs embolization therapy. A temporary or permanent substance may be used to occlude the AVM. Temporary materials, such as absorbable gelatin sponge (Gelfoam) or autologous blood clots, are typically used when surgical resection is planned. Permanent materials, such as silicone liquid, Silastic beads, polyvinyl alcohol, bukrylate, or stainless steel or platinum coils, are used to provide longer stability.

The procedure is usually performed under local anesthesia. Most commonly, a femoral artery approach is used for catheter insertion. The flexible catheter is threaded to the AVM site and the tip is positioned as close as possible to the vessel nidus. The selected embolizing substance (for example, small Silastic beads) is injected and carried by blood flow to occlude the AVM. A calibrated-leak balloon may be used instead to release embolizing material.

Two or more embolizing procedures may be required to provide adequate occlusion of the AVM. Using several procedures instead of attempting to embolize a large AVM in a single procedure decreases the incidence of associated complications. A second embolization is typically performed several weeks after the first.

Complications

The major complication of embolization is neurologic deficit related to occlusion of normal vessels by the substance used for AVM embolization. If the substance passes into the systemic circulation, a pulmonary embolus may occur. Other complications include intracranial hemorrhage, postembolytic inflammatory reaction, sepsis, and complications related to angiography (such as allergic reaction, femoral artery thrombosis, and hemorrhage at the catheter insertion site).

Care considerations

Before the procedure

• Reinforce the doctor's explanation of the procedure. Tell the patient what to expect before, during, and after the procedure.
• Ensure that the patient has fasted for 6 to 8 hours before the procedure.
• Obtain baseline vital signs and a neurologic assessment. Obtain and mark pedal pulses.
• Initiate I.V. fluid therapy, as ordered.
• Check the patient's history for hypersensitivity to iodine, iodine-containing foods (such as shellfish), or other radiographic contrast media. Notify the doctor of any such hypersensitivities; they may require prophylactic medications or cancellation of the procedure.

• Prepare the catheter insertion site. As ordered, shave the area and clean it with an antiseptic solution.
• Ask the patient to void just before the procedure.
• Administer ordered preoperative medications.
• Ensure that the patient or a responsible family member has signed a consent form.

During the procedure

• Monitor for signs of hypersensitivity, and report them immediately. Keep emergency resuscitation equipment available.
• Support the patient.
• Monitor for signs of neurologic deficits, and report them immediately.

After the procedure

• Enforce bed rest for 24 hours.
• Monitor the patient's vital signs and check all pulses distal to the insertion site. Assess the affected leg's temperature, color, and sensation.
• Assess the groin site for bleeding or hematoma. Apply an ice bag to relieve pain and reduce swelling. Control bleeding with firm pressure.
• Keep the affected leg extended and immobilized for 12 hours after the procedure.
• Assess neurologic status, including level of consciousness (LOC), pupil size and reactions, motor function, and speech. Report signs of neurologic deterioration immediately.
• Check that the patient has voided within 8 hours after the procedure. Intermittent urinary catheterization may be ordered if the patient has not voided.
• To help reduce the risk of AVM bleeding after embolization, provide a quiet, softly lit environment and limit visitors. Administer analgesics and sedatives, as ordered, and provide a soft, high-fiber diet with stool softeners, as needed.

Home care instructions

• Instruct the patient and family to immediately report any abnormal symp-

toms, such as severe headache, weakness in the extremities, or deteriorating LOC. Explain that such symptoms, which may indicate that the AVM is bleeding or increasing in size, require immediate medical evaluation.
• Instruct the patient to keep follow-up appointments.

ENDOCARDIAL RESECTION

Endocardial resection is an open-heart surgical procedure in which scar tissue from the inner lining of the left ventricle (endocardium) is removed to permanently cure the patient with recurrent sustained ventricular tachycardia (VT). Besides this direct surgical intervention for recurrent sustained VT, other interventions include encircling endocardial ventriculotomy, cryosurgery, laser therapy, and heart transplantation.

Endocardial resection is often combined with mapping to define the site of origin of the arrhythmia and with aneurysmectomy (removal of a left ventricular aneurysm) and cryoablation (freezing) of endocardial tissue. Such techniques improve the chance of destroying the arrhythmia focus.

Purpose
• To remove or destroy diseased endocardial tissue that provides the site of origin for sustained malignant ventricular arrhythmias.

Indications
Endocardial resection is indicated for patients with recurrent sustained ventricular arrhythmias that do not respond to conventional therapies. It is most successful in those patients with tachycardia that can be localized by mapping to a discrete left ventricular aneurysm.

Mapping involves sampling electrograms from strategically selected sites of the heart. Preoperative electrophysiologic testing and mapping for evaluation of tachycardia contribute to operative success and should be done in patients clinically able to tolerate repeated inductions of VT, especially since the arrhythmia may not be induced under general anesthesia. The type of VT most amenable to endocardial resection is uniform in morphology and tolerated well enough hemodynamically to allow for extensive left ventricular mapping. Resection can be performed for more rapid tachycardia even if mapping is not performed in the operating room.

Procedure
Under general anesthesia, a midsternal incision is made to visualize the heart. VT is induced repeatedly by either pacing protocols or I.V. isoproterenol. Localization of the site of origin of the arrhythmia is done through epicardial mapping and, after the aneurysm is opened, by endocardial mapping.

After the arrhythmia focus is identified, a 2- to 3-mm thickness of subendocardial (beneath the lining membrane on the inner surface of the heart) scar tissue is dissected away from healthy myocardium. This resection usually includes the full extent of visible scar tissue. Border zones of diseased endocardium may be treated by cryoablation, in which a special probe is used to freeze tissue surrounding the resection site. This further aids in interrupting the VT circuit without producing structural damage to the myocardium. Endocardial resections may be performed with left ventricular aneurysmectomy or coronary artery bypass surgery in patients who require such intervention.

Complications
Associated morbidity and mortality vary greatly, depending on the patient's underlying cardiac function.

Patients with a preoperative left ventricular ejection fraction below 25% have a higher risk of cardiogenic shock after such extensive surgery. Patients who have multiple VT morphologies or rapid, poorly tolerated VT that is difficult to map have a higher rate of postoperative recurrence. Because this procedure requires an incision into the left ventricle to open the aneurysm, there is a risk of postoperative cardiac tamponade. Also, because endocardial resection requires open-heart surgery, the patient is at risk for the complications associated with bypass surgery: hemorrhage, infection, cerebrovascular accident, and shock.

Care considerations
Before surgery
• Explain the surgical procedure to the patient and family.
• Prepare the patient and family for the postoperative course.
• Perform a baseline evaluation of patient's neurologic, physical, and emotional status.
• Make sure that preoperative testing is complete and that an informed consent form has been signed.
After surgery
• Postoperatively, the patient is sent to the intensive care unit.
• Monitor the patient with continuous telemetry for recurrence of VT, and observe for cardiac tamponade or cardiogenic shock.
• Monitor neurologic status.
• Maintain aseptic technique with wound care.
• Provide aggressive pulmonary care.
• Before hospital discharge, electrophysiologic testing should be repeated to evaluate the effect of surgery. If VT remains inducible, appropriate drug or device (implantable cardioverter-defibrillator) therapy must be identified and initiated.

Home care instructions
• Give the patient routine postoperative open-heart home care instructions.
• Provide teaching about drug or device therapy as appropriate.

ENDOSCOPIC RETROGRADE SPHINCTEROTOMY

Endoscopic retrograde sphincterotomy (ERS) is a procedure that widens the biliary sphincter to aid in removal of retained gallstones after cholecystectomy or to insert biliary stents for drainage. ERS allows treatment without general anesthesia or a surgical incision, assuring a quicker, safer recovery. And because it may be performed on an outpatient basis for some patients, it is a cost-effective alternative to surgery.

Purpose
• To relieve obstruction of biliary drainage.

Indications
Originally developed to remove retained gallstones from the common bile duct after cholecystectomy, ERS is now also used to treat high-risk patients with biliary dyskinesia and to insert biliary stents for drainage of malignant or benign strictures in the common bile duct.

Procedure
After anesthetizing the patient's throat, the doctor advances a fiber-optic endoscope through the stomach and duodenum to the ampulla of Vater. Then the doctor passes a cutting wire, known as a sphincterotome or papillotome, through the endoscope and, under fluoroscopic guidance, makes a small incision to widen the biliary sphincter. The stone may then drop out into the duo-

denum; if not, the doctor may need to introduce (through the endoscope) a Dormia basket, a balloon to remove the stone, or a lithotriptor to crush the stone. Cholangiography confirms passage or removal of the stone. Alternatively, the doctor may introduce an endobiliary prosthesis, or stent, through the endoscope to bypass a bile duct obstruction and restore normal biliary drainage. After sphincterotomy, the doctor may insert a nasobiliary catheter to drain bile and temporarily decompress the biliary tree.

Complications

Complications of ERS include hemorrhage, transient pancreatitis, cholangitis, and sepsis.

Care considerations
Before the procedure
• Explain the treatment, and answer any questions. Reassure the patient that the sphincterotomy should cause little or no discomfort.
• Position the patient on the fluoroscopy table in a left side-lying position, with the left arm behind him. Encourage him to relax, and, if ordered, administer a sedative.
After the procedure
• Keep in mind that the anesthetic's effects may hinder expectoration and swallowing. Withhold food and fluids until the anesthetic wears off and the patient's gag reflex returns.
• Check the patient's vital signs frequently and monitor carefully for signs of hemorrhage: hematemesis, melena, tachycardia, and hypotension. Report any of these signs immediately.
• Also observe for signs and symptoms of other complications. Cholangitis, for instance, produces hyperbilirubinemia, high fever and chills, abdominal pain, jaundice, and hypotension. Pancreatitis may be marked by abdominal pain and rigidity, vomiting, low-grade fever, tachycardia, diaphoresis, and elevated serum amylase levels (al-

though elevated serum amylase by itself doesn't confirm pancreatitis). Report any complications promptly, and prepare to obtain serum samples for culture and sensitivity studies and to administer prescribed antibiotics.

Home care instructions
• Instruct the patient about signs and symptoms of complications, and tell him to report them to the doctor immediately.
• Advise the patient to report any recurrence of jaundice or pain of biliary obstruction. He may need repeat ERS to remove new stones or replace a malfunctioning biliary stent.
• Advise the patient to keep follow-up appointments with the doctor.

ENEMAS

Enemas involve instillation of a solution into the rectum and the colon, usually to stimulate peristalsis by mechanically distending the colon and stimulating rectal wall nerves. There are several types of enemas. A nonretention cleansing enema is the instillation of a large volume of liquid to remove flatus and feces from the rectum; it is usually expelled within 15 minutes. Another type, the retention enema, is introduced into the bowel and retained for approximately 30 minutes to 1 hour. For example, the oil retention enema is given to lubricate the rectum and anal canal and to soften hardened stool. The retention enema is also used to introduce medications that are absorbed through the rectal mucosa. A return flow enema, also called a Harris flush, is given to relieve flatulence.

Purpose
• To clean the lower bowel before diagnostic or surgical procedures
• To relieve constipation

- To relieve distention and promote expulsion of flatus
- To deliver medications by the rectal route
- To lubricate the rectum and lower bowel.

Indications

Enemas are indicated when diet, exercise, and laxatives fail to relieve constipation. They are sometimes used after barium studies to prevent impaction from retained barium and before diagnostic and surgical procedures that require cleaning of the bowel.

Certain enemas, such as the Harris flush, relieve gas or distention from paralytic ileus. The retention enema acts as an emollient, soothing irritated tissues of the colon. It also facilitates medication administration by the rectal route. For example, patients with hepatic coma may receive neomycin sulfate enemas to reduce blood ammonia levels by decreasing intestinal flora.

Enemas are contraindicated after recent colon or rectal surgery and in patients with an acute abdominal condition of unknown etiology or recent myocardial infarction. Enemas should be administered cautiously to patients with cardiac arrhythmias.

Procedure

An enema is administered by a nurse or nursing assistant, or may be administered at home by the patient or the family caregiver.

For a therapeutic enema, the patient should be positioned on his left side with the right knee flexed (Sims' position). This will enhance the flow of enema solution into the sigmoid colon. The patient who has poor sphincter tone may be placed on a bedpan in a supine position. To allow for easier insertion into the rectum, the tip of the enema tube is lubricated with a water-soluble lubricant. Then, using a clean glove, the nurse separates the patient's buttocks and inserts the tube 2″ to 4″ (5 to 10 cm) toward the umbilicus. For a child, the tube is inserted only 2″ to 3″ (5 to 7.6 cm) and for an infant, 1″ to 1½″ (2.5 to 3.8 cm). The solution should be infused slowly to avoid cramping. To obtain optimum hydrostatic pressure, the solution should be hung 12″ to 18″ (30 to 45 cm) above the adult patient's abdomen. A retention enema is administered at the slowest possible rate to avoid stimulating peristalsis and to promote retention.

After most of the prescribed amount of solution has been administered, the tubing is clamped. Stopping the flow before the container empties completely avoids introducing air into the bowel. The tube is then gently removed.

If a cleansing enema is administered, the patient is instructed to try to retain the solution for 5 to 15 minutes, if possible, before he empties his bowel. If the patient is receiving a retention enema, he is advised to avoid defecation and retain the solution for 30 minutes or as otherwise prescribed; lying flat for the prescribed retention time helps to prevent stimulation of peristalsis. When the solution has remained in the colon for the prescribed time or for as long as the patient tolerates it, he is assisted onto the bedpan or to the commode or bathroom, as required.

A Harris flush enema is administered similarly, but the flow is stopped by lowering the solution container below bed level and allowing gravity to siphon the enema out of the colon. Raising and lowering the container continues until gas bubbles cease or the patient feels more comfortable and abdominal distention ceases.

Commercially prepared small-volume enemas are administered according to the instructions provided with the package.

Complications

Enema administration is usually a safe procedure. However, use of a solution containing too much soap may irritate the rectal mucosa. Improper administration may cause rectal abrasions or perforation. Enemas may also produce dizziness or faintness due to fluid and electrolyte loss; electrolyte imbalances, such as hyponatremia and hypokalemia, may follow repeated administrations of hypotonic solutions. Hypervolemia or water intoxication may follow prolonged retention of hypotonic solutions. Cardiac arrhythmia may result from vasovagal reflex stimulation after insertion of the rectal catheter.

Care considerations

Before the procedure

• Explain the procedure to the patient, including why it has been prescribed.
• Obtain the necessary equipment.
• If the patient has difficulty retaining enemas, consider using a plastic rectal tube guard, indwelling urinary catheter, or a rectal catheter with a balloon.
• Prepare the prescribed type and amount of solution. The volume for an irrigating enema is usually 750 to 1,000 ml (26 to 34 oz) for an adult; 500 (about 18 oz) to 1,000 ml for a school-aged child; 250 (9 oz) to 500 ml for a toddler or preschooler; and 50 (about 2 oz) to 250 ml or less for an infant. A retention enema requires 50 to 250 ml or less. Because the ingredients may irritate the mucosa, make sure the proportions are correct and the agents are thoroughly mixed.
• Warm the solution to reduce patient discomfort. In the absence of a doctor's order, administer an adult's enema at 100° to 105° F (37.8° to 40.5° C) and a child's at 100° F.
• Clamp the tubing; and fill the solution bag with the prescribed solution. Unclamp the tubing; flush the solution through the tubing; then reclamp it.

• Assure privacy and place linen-saver pads under the patient's buttocks.

During the procedure

• Monitor the patient's tolerance frequently during instillation. If the patient complains of discomfort, cramps, or the need to defecate, stop the procedure until the cramps subside by pinching the clamp on the tubing. After a few minutes, when the discomfort passes, resume administration at a slower flow rate.
• Before leaving the room, place a call light and bedpan within the patient's reach in case he is unable to retain the solution.

After the procedure

• Provide the patient with materials for perianal cleaning and hand washing.
• Note fecal color, amount, and consistency. Observe for rectal tissue, blood, worms, or any other unusual matter.
• Send specimens to the laboratory if ordered.

Home care instructions

• Provide appropriate instruction if the patient will be receiving enemas at home.
• Explain the procedure. Warn family caregivers and patients against administering an enema to the patient in a sitting or standing position because this may cause abrasions or perforations to the anterior rectal wall.
• Teach methods of preventing constipation, such as exercise, adequate dietary fiber, adequate fluid intake, and establishing a regular time for elimination.

ENTERAL NUTRITION

Enteral nutrition delivers pureed food or a special liquid enteral formula directly into the stomach, duodenum, or jejunum via a feeding tube. The most common access sites for enteral nutrition include nasogastric, nasoduodenal, nasojejunal, gastrostomy, and jejunostomy.

Nasogastric feedings involve insertion of a feeding tube nasally and passage into the stomach. Nasogastric feedings are often used for patients who require enteral nutrition support. However, this access route should not be used for patients at risk for pulmonary aspiration of gastric contents or for those with severe vomiting or gastroesophageal reflux.

Nasoduodenal and nasojejunal feedings, which involve insertion of feeding tubes nasally and passage into the duodenum or jejunum, may be used for patients with stomach pathology or who are at risk for aspiration. However, transpyloric tube placement may be difficult, and dumping syndrome may occur if the feeding rate is not controlled.

Gastrostomy or jejunostomy is placement of a feeding tube through the patient's abdominal wall into the stomach or jejunum. These procedures may be performed during intra-abdominal surgery. In contrast, percutaneous endoscopic gastrostomy (PEG) or percutaneous endoscopic jejunostomy (PEJ) tubes may be inserted endoscopically without the need for surgery or general anesthesia. Gastrostomy or jejunostomy requires stoma care. Gastrostomy is commonly selected when the transnasal route is not available or prolonged enteral nutrition is anticipated; the patient should have normal gastric and duodenal emptying and should not be at risk for aspiration. Jejunostomy is commonly selected when access in the upper GI tract is not possible, when there is potential for pulmonary aspiration, and when prolonged enteral feeding is anticipated.

Special tubes, such as the Moss tube, may be used after abdominal surgery to accomplish both enteral feeding into the duodenum or jejunum and gastric suction.

Purpose

• To provide necessary nutrition in patients who can't maintain adequate nutrition by the oral route.

Indications

Enteral nutrition is indicated for patients who cannot or will not consume an adequate oral intake but whose GI system is at least partially functioning, permitting safe delivery of nutrients. This may include, for example, patients with hypermetabolism; oral or esophageal obstruction or injury; some patients with neurologic disease, such as a cerebrovascular accident; unconscious patients; and some patients with psychological disorders.

Tube feedings are contraindicated in patients who have no bowel sounds or who have suspected intestinal obstruction.

Procedure

Enteral feedings may consist of pureed foods or commercially prepared formulas. Many commercial tube feeding formulas are available. Selection depends on the individual patient's nutrient, fluid, and fiber needs. When tube feedings are initiated, the rate should be slow and should be gradually advanced with patient tolerance; initiate continuous feedings at a rate of 30 to 50 ml (1 to 1½ oz) hourly and progress to the desired volume, as tolerated. Also, the concentration of the feeding formula may be gradually increased to the desired level over 2 days, according to patient tolerance.

Enteral nutrition is administered either through intermittent or continuous feedings. Continuous feedings, the most common method, are preferred for initiation of enteral feeding, for critically ill patients, for patients who have not received oral nutrition for 3 days or longer, and for duodenal or jejunal feedings. Continuous feedings may be administered by gravity or pump. However, pump administration is most common.

Intermittent feedings are commonly administered to ambulatory patients receiving gastric tube feedings. This permits greater freedom of movement and more closely simulates meal patterns. Such feedings may be administered 5 to 8 times a day. Intermittent feedings may be delivered by gravity, pump, or syringe. However, syringe feedings are less desirable because they are often associated with too-rapid administration. Patients selected for intermittent feedings often begin with continuous feedings and then change to intermittent. If this is not possible, initial intermittent feedings should be administered in small volumes and at a slow rate. Intermittent feedings are tolerated best when no more than 250 ml (about 8 oz) of formula is delivered over about 30 minutes.

For syringe feedings, a 50- or 60-ml bulb or catheter-tip syringe is used to slowly administer the ordered amount of formula every 3 to 4 hours. The height at which the syringe is held determines the flow rate. After the flow is started, remove the bulb. Never use the bulb to force the formula through the tube. To avoid introducing air into the patient's GI tract, do not allow the syringe to empty completely.

When a feeding bag is used, pour the appropriate type and amount of formula into the bag and remove any air from the system. Connect the feeding bag tubing to the feeding tube. If an infusion controller or pump is used, thread the tube from the formula container through the device according to the manufacturer's instructions. After the system is purged of air, attach the tubing to the patient's feeding tube. For gravity feedings, the regulator clamp on the feeding bag tubing is used to control the rate. When a pump or controller is used, the manufacturer's instructions explain how to set the infusion rate. The feeding bag is usually hung on an I.V. pole during administration.

After delivering an intermittent feeding, flush the feeding tube with up to 60 ml of 0.9% sodium chloride solution or water to maintain patency. To discontinue feedings (depending on the type of equipment), close the regulator clamp on the feeding bag tubing, disconnect the syringe from the feeding tube, or turn off the infusion controller. Cover the end of the feeding tube with its plug or cap. Leave the patient who has received a gastric feeding in semi-Fowler's or high Fowler's position for at least 30 minutes.

For continuous feedings, flush the feeding tube every 4 hours to help prevent tube occlusion. For continuous gastric feedings, monitor gastric emptying every 4 hours. For intermittent gastric feedings, check gastric residual before administering each feeding.

Complications

Complications of enteral nutrition may be mechanical, GI, or metabolic. Fortunately, most can be managed without removing the feeding tube (see *Correcting complications of tube feedings*).

Care considerations

Before therapy

• Explain why enteral nutrition is necessary and how it will be provided.
• Obtain necessary equipment. Allow the formula to warm to room temperature. Then position the patient. If he has a gastric tube, put him in a semi-Fowler's or high Fowler's position. For a duodenal or jejunal tube, you don't need to elevate the bed; since the formula is infused beyond the cardioesophageal and pyloric sphincters, gastric reflux is unlikely.
• Before delivering a gastric feeding, check tube placement and position.

During therapy

• Assess the patient and the progress of feeding frequently. For continuous feedings, check the flow rate at least

Correcting complications of tube feedings

COMPLICATION	INTERVENTIONS
Aspiration of gastric secretions	• Discontinue feeding immediately. • Perform tracheal suction of aspirated contents if possible. • Notify doctor; prophylactic antibiotics and chest physiotherapy may be ordered. • To prevent aspiration: Keep head of bed elevated during and after gastric feeding. Check tube placement before feedings, and check gastric residuals regularly. Reduce the infusion rate if there is evidence of delayed gastric emptying. Suggest duodenal or jejunal feedings for patients at high risk.
Tube obstruction	• Flush tube with warm water or cranberry juice. If necessary, replace tube. • Flush tube with 50 ml of water after each feeding (or every 4 hours for continuous feedings) to remove excessive sticky formula, which could occlude the tube.
Nasal or pharyngeal irritation or necrosis	• Use small-caliber feeding tubes when possible. • Provide frequent oral and nasal hygiene using lemon and glycerin swabs. Offer mouthwash. Apply petroleum jelly to cracked lips. • Tape feeding tube carefully to avoid pressure on nostril. Re-tape the tube daily. Alternate taping the tube toward the inner and outer side of the nose. • If necessary, replace tube.
Vomiting, bloating, diarrhea, or cramps	• Reduce flow rate. • Administer formula at room temperature. • For 30 minutes after gastric feeding, keep patient on his right side with head elevated to facilitate gastric emptying. • Notify doctor to reduce the amount of formula being given during each feeding or to change or dilute the formula.
Constipation	• Provide additional fluids if the patient can tolerate them. • Administer a bulk laxative. • Increase fruit, vegetable, and fiber content of formula.
Electrolyte imbalance	• Monitor serum electrolyte levels. • Have formula content adjusted to correct deficiency.
Hyperglycemia	• Begin feedings at slow rate. • Monitor blood glucose levels. • Notify doctor of elevated blood glucose levels. • Administer insulin, if ordered. • Doctor may change formula to correct sugar content.
Congestive heart failure	• Monitor patient's intake, output, and respiratory status. • Reduce flow rate and notify doctor. • Administer diuretics and digoxin, as prescribed. • Decrease patient's fluid intake and enforce bed rest.

hourly. Monitor bowel sounds and observe for abdominal distention. If the patient vomits, promptly discontinue the feeding and notify the doctor.
• Record the amount of ingested formula.
• Weigh the patient daily at the same time, in the same type of clothing, and on the same scale to assess the results of therapy.
• Monitor laboratory studies, including blood urea nitrogen, serum electrolytes, serum creatinine, hematocrit, hemoglobin, serum protein levels, and serum triglycerides and cholesterol.
• Monitor urine and blood glucose levels to assess glucose tolerance. Monitor blood glucose every 6 hours or as otherwise ordered for patients with glucose intolerance.
• Measure fluid intake and output, and monitor vital signs at least every 8 hours.
• Provide meticulous mouth care. If nasal tube insertion is used, provide nasal hygiene daily and change the anchoring tapes daily. Provide skin care to gastrostomy or jejunostomy sites.
• If tube feedings will be given at home, refer the patient (before discharge) to a social worker to make arrangements for home feeding and follow-up care by a home health care nurse.

Home care instructions
• Have the patient and family caregiver observe administration of tube feedings. Coach them a step at a time until they can perform the feedings independently under supervision.
• If the patient will have an enteral feeding pump, show how to operate it and how to detect and correct problems.
• Help the patient and caregiver understand how to obtain equipment, how to use and care for the feeding tube, and how to safely prepare and store feeding formula. Also teach them how to troubleshoot problems with tube position and patency.

• Tell the patient and caregiver to weigh the patient three times a week at the same time of day and in the same type of clothing.
• Instruct the patient and caregiver about signs and symptoms to report to the doctor or home health care nurse as well as measures to take in an emergency.
• Explain how to care for the tube insertion site.
• Explain the importance of keeping follow-up appointments.

ERGOT ALKALOIDS

This group of adrenergic blocking agents, which includes *dihydroergotamine mesylate* and *ergotamine tartrate*, provides relief from vascular (migraine and cluster) headaches. When given in the prodromal phase of such a headache, these drugs effectively constrict dilated cerebral vessels and relieve pain.

Ergotamine tartrate, considered the more effective of the two ergot alkaloids, is available in oral, inhalant, and sublingual forms; the latter two forms provide more rapid action in treating acute episodes. Ergotamine also serves as an ingredient in products containing various mixtures of the belladonna alkaloids, phenobarbital, and caffeine.

Dihydroergotamine mesylate, administered I.M. or I.V., produces fewer and less serious adverse GI reactions than ergotamine and may be indicated for patients prone to GI reactions.

Purpose
• To cause cerebral vasoconstriction, counteracting the pain-producing vasodilation of a vascular headache.

Indications
Ergot alkaloids are indicated for treatment of vascular headaches, such as migraine and cluster headaches.

Because the ergot alkaloids cause vasoconstriction, they're contraindicated in severe hypertension, peripheral or occlusive vascular disease, coronary artery disease, phlebitis, impaired renal or hepatic function, and other debilitating diseases. Patients over age 40 should have a complete cardiovascular evaluation, including an electrocardiogram, before starting ergot alkaloid therapy.

Adverse reactions

Adverse reactions may include localized edema; pruritus; numbness and tingling of fingers, toes, or face; red or violet blisters on skin of hands or feet; pale or cold hands or feet; painful extremities; vision changes; anxiety; confusion; chest pain; transient sinus tachycardia or bradycardia; shortness of breath; nausea and vomiting; diarrhea; abdominal pain; fatigue; and weakness in legs. Increased frequency or severity of headache may indicate tolerance to the antimigraine effect.

Care considerations

• During ergot alkaloid therapy, observe for adverse reactions and carefully monitor the results of cardiac and renal function tests, complete blood count, and erythrocyte sedimentation rate. Report any abnormal test findings or adverse reactions to the doctor, who may change the patient's drug regimen.
• Because of these drugs' vasoconstrictive effects, be especially alert for signs of reduced peripheral circulation: coldness, numbness, tingling, muscle pain and weakness, and localized edema in the extremities.
• Review the patient's drug regimen for possible interactions. For example, propranolol or other beta blockers and vasopressors can dangerously intensify the vasoconstrictive effects of ergot alkaloids. If the patient is taking these drugs concurrently, carefully monitor pulse rate, blood pressure, and

respirations. Immediately report bradycardia or tachycardia, hypertension or hypotension, chest pain, or shortness of breath.

Home care instructions

• Tell the patient to take the drug during the prodromal stage of a headache or as soon as possible after onset. To help him relax, which will enhance the drug's effectiveness, advise him to lie down in a quiet, darkened room, if possible.
• Teach the patient how to use the sublingual or inhalant forms of ergotamine, if appropriate.
• Warn against increasing drug dosage without first consulting the doctor.
• To reduce the frequency and severity of vascular headaches, help the patient identify possible precipitating factors, such as stress or the ingestion of caffeine, chocolate, or alcohol.
• Instruct the patient on long-term therapy to report any coldness, numbness, tingling, or pain in his hands and feet; leg cramps; or chest or flank pain. Show him how to assess for peripheral edema, and tell him to report this effect as well.
• Tell the patient to avoid overexposure to cold temperatures, which may increase drug adverse effects.
• If the patient experiences nausea, vomiting, or other GI effects, tell him to take the drug with food or milk.
• Explain to the patient that ergotamine rebound – increased severity and frequency of headaches – may occur after discontinuing therapy.

ESCHAROTOMY

Escharotomy is an incision made through burn eschar down to superficial fat. It does not remove the eschar, but relieves constriction of a body part.

Normal skin is soft, supple, elastic, and able to adjust to tissue expansion.

Burned tissue, which forms eschar, is leathery, thick, and inelastic. When eschar completely surrounds a body part, it does not permit tissue expansion. As a result, tissue swelling beneath the eschar can compromise circulation and interfere with tissue perfusion. Circumferential eschar in the thorax can impede chest wall expansion and impair ventilation.

The need for escharotomy may be assessed by the use of a Doppler ultrasound stethoscope every hour for 42 hours after circumferential burns to detect small-vessel blood flow. If the patient has weak or absent distal peripheral pulses, escharotomy is indicated. Other assessment criteria that support the need for escharotomy include impaired capillary filling in the nail beds; paresthesias or motor weakness; cyanosis of distal, uninjured skin; pain on passive movement; and pallor, indicating tense edema. Impaired chest wall movements may warrant thoracic escharotomy.

Purpose

• To accommodate tissue expansion in order to permit unrestricted blood flow, thereby preventing ischemia and necrosis in remaining viable tissue
• To accommodate unrestricted chest wall movement and permit adequate ventilation.

Indications

Escharotomy is most often indicated for patients with full-thickness or third-degree circumferential burns of the thorax or an extremity.

Procedure

Escharotomy is a surgical procedure that is always performed by a doctor, frequently at the bedside. An anesthetic is not usually required because the burn injury has destroyed the nerve endings. However, some patients require sedation with morphine, a local anesthetic, or a single I.M. injection of ketamine.

Dressings are removed and the operative site is thoroughly cleaned. An electrocautery unit or heated scalpel is used to make linear incisions. The incisions are placed to avoid scar contracture bands and extend to the proximal and distal limits of the burn eschar. As the tissues are released, the subcutaneous fat bulges through the incisions, tissue tension is relieved, and effective blood flow is restored. Blood loss is usually minimal because the eschar is avascular and cutting of viable tissue should not occur.

Complications

Bleeding or excessive fluid loss may occur as a major complication after escharotomy. It may occur when clotting mechanisms are dangerously low preoperatively.

Care considerations

Before the procedure

• Reinforce the doctor's explanation of the procedure.
• Administer an analgesic, if ordered.
• Check results of coagulation tests, especially in patients with large-surface burns. Report abnormal levels.
• Ensure that a consent form has been signed.

After the procedure

• Apply the ordered topical antibacterial agent and sterile dressings to the site.
• Perform neurovascular assessments at least every hour for the first 24 hours.
• Check dressings over the escharotomy area at least hourly to assess bleeding.
• Tell the patient to report any numbness or tingling sensation in the affected site.
• If the escharotomy was performed on an extremity, elevate that extremity.

Home care instructions

• Advise the patient to contact his doctor if he notices signs of wound infection.
• Teach the patient how to assess the pulse distal to the wound site. Tell him to notify his doctor if this pulse disappears, if nail beds appear blue, or if he feels numbness or tingling.

ESOPHAGEAL SURGERY

Esophageal surgery is infrequently performed for adults and has major potential for serious complications. It may be performed to manage an emergency or to relieve serious symptoms associated with underlying pathology. Typically, esophageal surgery is attempted only after conservative measures or dilatations fail to produce results. Esophageal cancer is usually far advanced at diagnosis. Therefore, palliation is usually the goal of therapy and is usually accomplished by laser treatment and radiation treatment. Radical surgery, while uncommon, is the only hope for cure.

Purpose

• To remove an esophageal obstruction
• To repair traumatic esophageal tissue damage
• To correct an esophageal reflux problem
• To relieve severe esophageal stricture.

Indications

In an adult, esophageal surgery may be indicated to treat esophageal perforation, usually from a traumatic injury. This is a surgical emergency. Esophageal surgery may also be warranted to treat motility disorders, such as achalasia; esophageal diverticula, especially when severe symptoms occur; esophageal reflux of gastric secretions; and caustic injuries, such as those caused by ingestion of lye. Radical surgery to attempt a cure for esophageal cancer may be performed on selected patients.

Procedure

Esophagocardiomyotomy involves an incision of the muscle wall of the lower esophagus and cardiac sphincter. This surgery is performed to treat achalasia when pneumatic dilatations have been unsuccessful. A thoracic or abdominal approach may be used. This surgery is often combined with an antireflux procedure.

To perform a cricopharyngeal myotomy, the surgeon makes an incision along the lower anterior border of the left sternocleidomastoid muscle. Then he partially dissects the cricopharyngeal muscle (upper esophageal sphincter) to remove a Zenker's diverticulum, or he severs it to relieve cricopharyngeal spasm. Aspiration is a significant postoperative risk.

Antireflux surgery may be performed when esophageal reflux of gastric contents resulting from an incompetent lower esophageal sphincter causes esophagitis or stricture. Nissen fundoplication, the most common technique, involves wrapping and suturing the gastric fundus around the esophagus to anchor the lower esophageal sphincter area below the diaphragm and reinforce the high-pressure area. The Belsey Mark IV operation and the Hill posterior gastropexy are similar surgical methods. Rate of reflux recurrence is significant even with surgery.

Esophagectomy, which involves resection of diseased or damaged esophageal tissue with anastomosis of remaining segments, may be warranted to excise esophageal cancer, constriction, or diverticula or to correct congenital atresia. Radical esophageal surgery is most often attempted to remove tumors in the lower and middle esophagus. If insufficient esophageal tissue remains after massive resection, several procedures may be used to restore esophagogastric continuity. In esophagogastrostomy, the most common procedure, the diseased portion of the esophagus is removed and the remaining esophageal segment is anastomosed to the stomach, which is brought up into the chest cavity. This procedure requires both abdominal and thoracic incisions. In another procedure, the surgeon replaces resected esophageal tissue with a resected segment of the jejunum, colon, or a tube. The segment is brought up into the thorax and is attached to the distal end of the esophagus and proximal end of the stomach.

Complications

Esophageal surgery has the potential for causing serious complications. For example, radical surgery may result in leakage at the anastomosis site. Mediastinitis may result from leakage of esophageal contents into the thorax. Severe inflammation can produce obstruction of the mediastinal structures, such as the superior vena cava, the tracheobronchial tree, and the esophagus. Hemorrhage, respiratory infection, and wound infection may also occur. Postoperative reflux, hypersalivation, and impaired clearance of secretions put the patient at risk for aspiration pneumonia.

Care considerations

Before surgery

• Reinforce the surgeon's explanation. Explain preoperative and postoperative care. Emphasize measures to prevent complications, especially respiratory complications.
• In nonemergency situations, focus preoperative care on evaluating and, if necessary, improving the patient's nutritional status; many patients who require esophageal surgery have a long history of dysphagia, anorexia, or other eating problems. Maintain the patient on a high-protein, high-calorie, soft diet.

If he can't tolerate oral feedings, provide gastrostomy tube feedings or parenteral nutrition, as appropriate.
• Check laboratory results for serum protein, glucose, and electrolyte levels. Also check results of renal function studies, such as blood urea nitrogen and serum creatinine. If necessary, provide I.V. fluid and electrolyte replacement.
• Ensure that the patient or a responsible family member has signed a consent form.
• Provide psychological support and encourage the patient to discuss concerns and fears.

After surgery

• Monitor respiratory status. Place the patient in semi-Fowler's position to help minimize esophageal reflux, reduce the risk of aspiration pneumonia, and support ventilation. Encourage turning, coughing, and deep-breathing exercises. To minimize pain from these exercises, teach the patient how to splint the incision, and administer analgesics, as prescribed. Perform chest physiotherapy and administer oxygen, if ordered. Provide appropriate care for patients with chest tubes and water-seal drainage.
• Watch for developing mediastinitis, especially if surgery involved extensive thoracic invasion (as in esophagogastrostomy). Note and report fever, dyspnea, signs of shock, and complaints of substernal pain. If prescribed, administer antibiotics to help prevent or correct this complication.
• Watch for leakage at the anastomosis site. Check the drainage tubes for blood, test for occult blood in stool and drainage, and monitor hemoglobin levels for evidence of slow blood loss.
• If surgery involving the upper esophagus produces hypersalivation, the patient may be unable to swallow excess saliva. Control drooling by using gauze wicks to absorb secretions or by suctioning frequently. If the patient can spit, place an emesis basin within reach.

• If the patient has a nasogastric tube in place, avoid manipulating the tube because this may damage the internal sutures or anastomoses. For the same reason, avoid deep suctioning in a patient who has had extensive esophageal repair.

• Administer ordered I.V. therapy and enteral nutrition. Give the patient nothing by mouth after surgery, as ordered; after extensive surgery involving anastomoses, this restriction may last 4 to 5 days. Then, carefully assess his response to ingestion of small amounts of water. Progress diet as ordered and as tolerated. Watch carefully for signs of leakage.

• Initiate referrals to community or home health agencies, as needed, especially after extensive surgery. When appropriate, inform the patient and family about supportive organizations, such as the American Cancer Society.

Home care instructions

• Advise the patient to sleep with his head elevated to prevent reflux. He can use a wedge under his mattress or raise the head of his bed on blocks.

• Teach the patient and caregiver how to change dressings, inspect for signs of infection, and provide wound care. Tell them about signs of anastomosis leakage and the need to report them immediately.

• If the patient smokes, encourage him to stop. Explain that nicotine has a detrimental effect on the lower esophageal sphincter.

• Advise the patient to avoid alcohol, aspirin, and effervescent over-the-counter products (such as Alka-Seltzer) because they may damage the tender esophageal mucosa.

• Advise the patient to avoid heavy lifting, straining, and coughing, which could rupture the weakened mucosa.

• Instruct the caregiver to assist the patient with ambulation and chest physiotherapy when warranted. Ask the caregiver to report any respiratory symptoms, such as wheezing, coughing, or nocturnal dyspnea.

• Encourage a high-protein, high-calorie, soft diet in frequent, small feedings after extensive surgery. If warranted, instruct the caregiver and patient on management of tube feedings or parenteral nutrition.

• For patients awaiting reconstructive surgery while the area heals, also teach management of the esophagostomy (surgical formation of opening into esophagus). Frequently, drainage requires good skin care. The patient also requires parenteral nutrition. After several weeks, esophagogastric continuity can be restored.

ESOPHAGOGASTRIC TAMPONADE

In this emergency treatment, insertion of a multilumen esophageal tube with subsequent inflation of its gastric and esophageal balloons helps to control esophageal or gastric hemorrhage resulting from ruptured esophageal or gastric varices. The most commonly used esophageal tubes include the Minnesota esophagogastric tamponade tube, the Linton tube, and the Sengstaken-Blakemore tube (see *Types of esophageal tubes*, page 282). Esophagogastric tamponade requires close monitoring in an intensive care setting. Ancillary procedures to temporarily control bleeding may include irrigation with tepid or iced 0.9% sodium chloride solution and drug therapy with a vasopressor.

Purpose

• To provide temporary control of esophageal or gastric hemorrhage and prevent excessive blood loss.

Indications

Esophagogastric tamponade may be warranted when endoscopy confirms

Types of esophageal tubes

When working with a patient who has an esophageal tube, remember the advantages of the most common types.

Sengstaken-Blakemore tube
This triple-lumen, double-balloon tube has a gastric aspiration port, which allows for drainage and medication administration.

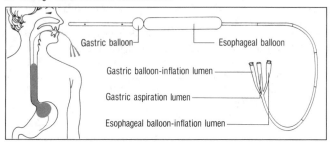

Linton tube
This triple-lumen, single-balloon tube has a port for gastric aspiration and one for esophageal aspiration. Additionally, the Linton tube reduces the risk of esophageal necrosis because it doesn't have an esophageal balloon.

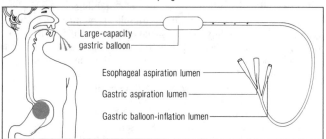

Minnesota esophagogastric tamponade tube
This esophageal tube has four lumens and two balloons. The device provides pressure-monitoring ports for both balloons without the need for Y-connectors. One port is used for gastric suction, the other for esophageal suction.

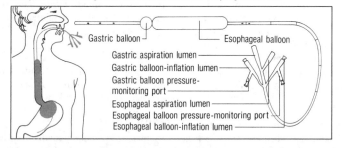

that hemorrhage is due to esophageal or gastric varices.

Procedure

Ordinarily the doctor inserts and removes the esophageal tube, but a nurse may remove it in an emergency situation. The doctor inserts the tube through the patient's nostril, or sometimes through his mouth, and then passes it through the esophagus into the stomach. Inflation of the tube's gastric and, depending on the type of tube, esophageal balloons exerts pressure on the varices and stops bleeding. The desired esophageal pressure is typically 30 to 40 mm Hg.

A foam nose guard is secured to minimize pressure on the nostril. To maintain tube position, traction may be applied to it, either by using a pulley and 1-lb (0.4-kg) weight or by pulling the tube gently and taping it securely to the face guard of a football helmet.

The Linton and Minnesota esophagogastric tamponade tubes each have two suction lumens that allow esophageal and gastric contents to be aspirated. The Sengstaken-Blakemore tube has a gastric aspiration lumen but does not have an esophageal aspiration lumen. Therefore, a nasogastric (NG) tube is inserted into the other nostril and passed into the esophagus to the point where the balloon is inflated. This is then connected to suction to aspirate swallowed secretions that can't pass into the stomach and to check for bleeding above the esophageal balloon.

The esophageal balloon may be deflated by the doctor after 24 hours, or it may be deflated in increments of 5 mm Hg every 30 minutes for several hours. The tube may be left in place for another 12 to 24 hours to check for any renewed bleeding.

Complications

Esophageal rupture, the most life-threatening complication associated with esophageal balloon tamponade, can occur at any time but is most likely during intubation or inflation of the esophageal balloon. Balloon inflation for more than 24 hours may cause pressure necrosis, which can produce further hemorrhage or perforation. Asphyxia may result if the balloon moves up the esophagus and blocks the airway. Tissue necrosis may also develop at the nasal insertion site.

Care considerations
Before the procedure
• Explain to the patient (or to his family, if the patient is unable to communicate) that this treatment aims to stop bleeding from the esophagus and stomach. Provide reassurance and emotional support.
• Emphasize the importance of relaxing and cooperating during intubation.
• Administer a sedative, as ordered, to help the patient relax.
• Place the patient in semi-Fowler's position to aid gastric emptying and prevent aspiration of vomitus. However, if the patient is unconscious, position him on his left side with the head of the bed raised about 15 degrees.
• Gather and prepare the necessary equipment. Keep emergency resuscitation equipment available. Tape a pair of scissors to the head of the bed for cutting the tube in case of acute respiratory distress. Be sure to check the balloons for air leaks by inflating them and holding them under water. If you don't detect any bubbles indicative of leaks, deflate the balloons and clamp their lumens so that they remain deflated during intubation. Run water through the esophageal and NG tubes to test patency. Also check the patency of all aspiration lumens, and make sure they're labeled properly.
During the procedure
• Never leave the patient unattended during esophagogastric tamponade. Closely monitor his condition and the tube's lumen pressure. Check vital signs

every 5 to 60 minutes, as ordered. A change may indicate bleeding or other complications.

• Maintain drainage and suction on the esophageal and gastric aspiration ports to prevent fluid accumulation. Document drainage on the intake and output record. Irrigate the gastric aspiration port with 0.9% sodium chloride solution, as ordered, to prevent clogging.

• Watch for signs of asphyxia while the esophageal tube is in place. If it develops, have someone else notify the doctor. Then release traction. Hold the tube firmly at the patient's nose and cut all lumens distally to where you are holding it. This causes the balloons to deflate. Then remove the tube gently and carefully.

• Keep the patient warm and comfortable, and instruct him to remain in bed and to be as still and quiet as possible; if ordered, administer a sedative to help him relax. Provide frequent mouth and nose care, applying a water-soluble ointment to the nostrils to prevent tissue irritation and pressure ulcers.

• Be sure that the traction weights hang from the foot of the bed at all times. Never rest them on the bed.

• When bleeding has been controlled, assist with tube removal.

After the procedure

• Monitor for signs of renewed bleeding.

• Offer mouth care.

Home care instructions

• The patient who undergoes esophagogastric tamponade is discharged only after his condition is stable and doesn't require instructions for home care.

ESTROGENS

Estrogens are naturally occurring hormones or synthetic steroidal and nonsteroidal compounds that possess estrogenic activity. The steroidal estrogens include the natural estrogens, such as *estradiol, conjugated estrogens, esterified estrogens*, and the semisynthetic estrogen *ethinyl estradiol*. The nonsteroidal estrogens include *chlorotrianisene, dienestrol, diethylstilbestrol*, and *quinestrol*.

Estrogens are administered orally, parenterally, intravaginally, or topically. Short-acting oral and parenteral forms are typically used for cyclic hormonal replacement therapy (3 weeks on and 1 week off the drug, for example).

Purpose

• To restore normal hormonal balance by replacing absent or deficient endogenous hormones.

Indications

Natural and synthetic estrogens help treat various conditions associated with endogenous estrogen deficiency, such as female hypogonadism, primary ovarian failure, vasomotor symptoms in menopause, atrophic vaginitis, and kraurosis vulvae. Conjugated estrogens also help treat abnormal uterine bleeding caused by hormonal imbalance. Short-acting forms of these synthetic agents are used with increased calcium intake and physical therapy to retard bone loss and the progression of osteoporosis in postmenopausal women. Longer-acting preparations help treat breast cancer.

Estrogens are contraindicated in patients with thrombophlebitis, thromboembolic disorders, or abnormal or undiagnosed vaginal bleeding. They should be used cautiously in patients with hypertension, gallbladder disease, blood dyscrasias, migraine headaches, seizure disorders, diabetes mellitus, amenorrhea, heart failure, hepatic and renal dysfunction, or a family history of breast or genital tract cancer.

Adverse reactions

Adverse reactions to estrogens commonly include gynecologic changes such as breakthrough bleeding, spotting, change in menstrual flow, dysmenorrhea, premenstrual-like syndrome, amenorrhea during and after treatment, increase in size of uterine fibromas, vaginal candidiasis, change in cervical secretion and degree of cervical erosion, cystitis-like syndrome, hemolytic uremic syndrome, and endometrial cystic hyperplasia. GI, dermatologic, ophthalmic, and central nervous system reactions (mood change, insomnia) may also occur.

Care considerations

• Before giving estrogens, review the patient's history for any disorders that may contraindicate their use.
• During administration, be alert for adverse effects. Also watch for changes in vaginal bleeding patterns, such as amenorrhea, spotting, breakthrough bleeding, or persistent bleeding.
• To administer the drug I.M., give the injection slowly and deeply into a large muscle, such as the upper outer quadrant of the buttock.

Home care instructions

• Review the package insert with the patient and answer any questions she may have. Patients often ask if they can get cancer if they use estrogens. Tell the patient that it's generally considered safe to take these hormones if she's had a complete physical examination before therapy begins and if she performs monthly breast self-examination. Explain that the doctor will prescribe the lowest possible effective dose and periodically evaluate the drug's effects. Tell the patient that estrogen dosage is usually reduced or the hormone discontinued after a few months.
• Instruct the patient to seek emergency treatment immediately if she experiences sudden or severe headache; sudden loss of coordination or change in vision; pains in her chest, groin, or leg (especially her calf); shortness of breath; sudden slurring of speech; or weakness or numbness in an arm or leg.
• Advise the patient to report swollen ankles or feet, changes in vaginal bleeding, breast lumps or discharge, abdominal or flank pain, rash, yellow skin or eyes, or dark urine.
• Suggest taking the drug with food if the patient develops nausea during the first few weeks of therapy. Explain that nausea usually disappears with continued therapy.
• Instruct the patient to take a missed dose as soon as she remembers. Tell her to stop taking the drug and to check with her doctor if she suspects she's pregnant.
• If the patient is using the transdermal form of estradiol, instruct her to apply the patch to a clean section of her abdomen (not to her breasts or to any areas where the patch may be rubbed loose). Tell her to apply the patch twice weekly and to wait at least a week before applying a patch to the same area.
• If the patient is receiving cyclic therapy for postmenopausal symptoms, explain that withdrawal bleeding may occur during the week off the drug. Tell the patient that spotting is a common adverse effect of estrogen therapy. Explain that the spotting is a sign that the body is responding to the drug just as it once did to its own estrogen supply.
• If the postmenopausal patient asks if she can get pregnant while on estrogen therapy, tell her that it's not possible because she hasn't ovulated.
• If the patient smokes, encourage her to stop. Warn her that smoking during estrogen therapy increases the risk of serious cardiovascular effects, especially if she's over age 35.
• Teach the patient how to perform a breast self-examination. Advise her to perform this examination monthly and

to report any abnormalities to the doctor.
• Instruct the patient to schedule an annual pelvic and breast examination and a Papanicolaou test.
• Tell the patient to have an annual eye examination because estrogen can cause a worsening of myopia or astigmatism.

ETHMOIDECTOMY

The ethmoidal sinuses consist of multiple thin-walled cavities located between the middle turbinates and the medial wall of the orbit. An ethmoidectomy is the removal of all or part of the mucosal lining and the bony partitions within the ethmoidal sinuses. The surgical approach may be intranasal or external.

Purpose
• To remove extensive nasal polyps
• To remove diseased mucosal tissue.

Indications
Ethmoidectomy is usually indicated when the nasal airway has been obstructed due to nasal polypoid disease resulting in chronic mucosal thickening of the ethmoidal sinuses. External ethmoidectomy may be performed to excise tumors of the frontal, ethmoidal, and sphenoidal sinuses or to search for or repair a cerebrospinal fluid leak in the cribriform, ethmoidal, or sphenoidal regions.

Procedure
Depending on the patient's condition and cooperativeness, he'll receive a local or general anesthetic. Then the surgeon performs the procedure using an external, frontal, or intranasal approach, as needed.

In an external ethmoidectomy, the surgeon makes a curved incision around the inner canthus of the eye,

exposing the bony wall of the ethmoidal area. He then removes the ethmoidal cells, diseased tissue, and the lateral wall of the nose medial to the ethmoidal area. If the sphenoidal sinuses are involved, he may also remove some of the sphenoidal mucosal lining.

In a frontoethmoidectomy, the surgeon makes a similar incision but extends it to the eyebrow, exposing portions of the frontal sinus. He then removes the ethmoidal cells and the mucosal lining of the frontal sinus. He may also remove some of the bony floor of the frontal sinus to create a pathway for drainage into the nose.

In an intranasal ethmoidectomy, which is typically performed under local and topical anesthesia, the surgeon fractures the middle turbinate medially toward the nasal septum or partially removes it to gain access to the ethmoidal sinus. He then removes the ethmoidal cells and diseased tissue through the nose. Depending on the extent of disease, he may also remove the medial wall of the orbit or the floor of the frontal sinus to promote drainage into the nose.

After any of these procedures, the surgeon inserts nasal packing.

Complications
The most common complication of ethmoidectomy is bleeding. Airway obstruction may result from dislodged nasal packing. Blindness has been reported in several cases because of the proximity of the optic nerve and of the blood vessels that supply the orbit.

Care considerations
Before surgery
• Reinforce the surgeon's explanation of the surgery, and answer any questions. Tell the patient what type of anesthesia to expect and its implications.
• Explain preoperative testing. A computed tomography (CT) scan of the sinuses should be completed before surgery. The scan will detect any bony de-

struction as well as the nature and the location of the disease.

• Anticipate a preoperative ophthalmology consultation if the CT scan shows diseased orbital walls or if the patient has any visual changes or complaints.

• Inform the patient that nasal packing will be inserted directly after surgery to help reduce bleeding and swelling. Explain that the packing will cause him to breathe through his mouth and may give him a sensation of facial fullness but that analgesics will reduce discomfort. Warn against pulling or otherwise moving the packing.

• Before the procedure, ensure that the patient or a responsible family member has signed a consent form.

After surgery

• Closely monitor for airway obstruction because the nasal packing may become dislodged and fall into the nasal pharynx. If the patient begins to choke on the dislodged packing, remove it gently and promptly notify the doctor. Also be sure to watch for bleeding from the patient's nose or blood in vomitus.

• Elevate the head of the bed 45 degrees to help minimize facial swelling. Apply ice packs, as ordered.

• Instruct the patient to sneeze or cough with his mouth open.

• Administer ordered analgesics to help relieve discomfort from the nasal packing. Because the patient's mouth may be uncomfortably dry from mouth breathing, perform oral care every 2 hours after the anesthetic's effects wear off. Assist with gentle rinses, using tepid water and dilute mouthwash. Offer ice chips and fluids unless the patient is nauseated.

• When the doctor removes the nasal packing (usually within 24 to 48 hours after surgery), encourage the patient to take regular deep breaths through his mouth. Also provide him with a basin so he can expectorate any blood. Explain that his eyes may tear when the doctor removes the packing but that this is normal.

Home care instructions

• Tell the patient to expect some oozing of blood-tinged fluid from his nose for 1 to 2 days after surgery. However, tell him that he should report any frank, heavy bleeding or any discharge that persists for more than 3 days.

• Instruct the patient to avoid bending, strenuous exercise, and heavy lifting (over 10 lb [4.5 kg]) for at least 10 days.

• Tell the patient to avoid blowing his nose or sneezing for 10 days. If he needs to clear his nostrils, he should sniff gently. If he can't avoid sneezing, he should keep his mouth open when he does.

• Advise the patient to eat a high-fiber diet and to increase fluid intake to prevent the constipating effects of the pain medication. Tell the patient to avoid straining because it may trigger nasal bleeding.

• Explain that a feeling of nasal congestion is normal postoperatively and may last for 2 to 3 weeks until the intranasal swelling subsides.

EXCHANGE TRANSFUSION

Exchange transfusion is the replacement of a patient's blood with an equal amount of donor blood. The treatment may be used for neonates and certain individuals with sickle cell anemia.

Purpose

• To lower excessive serum bilirubin levels caused by Rh incompatibility to prevent kernicterus

• To remove sensitized red blood cells (RBCs) and replace them with healthy donor cells

• To correct the anemia resulting from Rh incompatibility

• To correct severe anemia or break a cycle of frequently recurrent crisis in sickle cell anemia.

Indications

Exchange transfusion is the treatment of choice for erythroblastosis fetalis. It is used for extreme hyperbilirubinemia only after phototherapy has been tried and has been unsuccessful in reducing bilirubin levels. This treatment replaces Rh-positive RBCs damaged by Rh antibodies with Rh-negative cells, which aren't harmed by the antibodies. It also removes bilirubin and, to a lesser degree, antibodies from the neonate's circulation.

Procedure

The doctor inserts a catheter into the neonate's umbilical vein (although a central venous catheter can be used) and threads it into the inferior vena cava. Stopcocks are attached to the catheter. During the exchange procedure (which usually takes 1 to 2 hours) and depending on the neonate's weight, 5 to 20 ml of blood is withdrawn within 15 to 20 seconds and the same volume of donor blood is infused over 60 to 90 seconds. This technique prevents cardiac overload or stress. Transfusion results in the removal of about 85% of the neonate's RBCs and replacement with donor cells. Discarded blood flows through outflow tubing into a bag below the exchange site; donor blood flows through inflow tubing from a bag above the exchange site.

After the procedure, the doctor may remove the umbilical catheter unless further transfusions are anticipated; in that case, he'll flush the catheter with 0.9% sodium chloride solution and leave it in place.

Complications

Exchange transfusion carries many risks. Necrotizing enterocolitis may result from compromised bowel circulation or a misplaced or clogged catheter; hypoglycemia may result from increased insulin production in response to glucose in the donor blood; cardiac arrest may result from cardiac overload; hypocalcemia may develop from calcium depletion by sodium citrate in the donor's blood; and, with massive transfusions, hyperkalemia may result from RBC lysis. Hemorrhage and infection at the catheter site may also occur.

Care considerations

Before the procedure

• Explain the procedure to the parents (see *Questions parents ask about exchange transfusion*). Make sure that the parents have signed a consent form.

• Assure that the neonate has had nothing by mouth to prevent aspiration.

• If ordered, insert a feeding tube to empty the stomach.

• Turn on the radiant warmer and set the temperature as prescribed by hospital policy. Place a cardiac monitor at the bedside, along with the transfusion equipment ordered by the doctor. Check suction and resuscitation equipment, and place it at the bedside. Label laboratory tubes for blood samples.

• Obtain and verify the ordered blood as prescribed by hospital policy (see the entry "Blood Transfusion" for recommended identification procedures).

• Position the neonate under the radiant warmer to maintain a stable body temperature and provide an accessible working surface. If phototherapy is being used during the procedure to reduce bilirubin levels, place eye pads and shields over the neonate's eyes to prevent retinal damage from the phototherapy lights.

• Restrain the neonate as necessary. Tape a skin or rectal thermometer in place to continuously monitor temperature. Take his baseline vital signs; obtain a blood sample from his finger and test it for glucose. Don't take blood samples from below the neonate's waist to avoid masking signs of a malposi-

Questions parents ask about exchange transfusion

Exchange transfusion is the treatment of choice for erythroblastosis fetalis and neonatal sepsis. Review these answers to common questions from parents, and be prepared to offer them your support.

Is it safe?
Specially trained doctors will perform the procedure, and trained nurses will assist and constantly monitor your baby's progress. As a result, fewer than 1% of children develop complications. Erythroblastosis fetalis, however, poses a great risk to your child; if untreated, it would cause nerve damage and mental retardation.

How will my baby survive if you take out all of his blood?
Only a small amount—about a tablespoon—is removed at any one time, and it's replaced immediately with an equal quantity of donor blood. This process is repeated until about 85% of the blood has been replaced.

Will my baby get AIDS from the transfusion?
Blood donors are carefully screened and all blood is tested for acquired immuno-deficiency syndrome (AIDS) before it's used. Since the development of the blood test for AIDS, the risk of acquiring AIDS from a transfusion is extremely low.

  If the father's blood type is compatible, he may donate a unit of blood for his child. Similarly, other relatives or friends may be encouraged to donate blood, since the baby will need several units.

---

tioned catheter, such as mottling of the lower extremities.

• Remove all of the neonate's clothing except his diaper to allow easy access to the umbilical area. Connect the cardiac monitor to the neonate.

During the procedure
• Maintain the temperature of the blood at 98.6° F (37 ° C).

• If ordered, inject albumin to bind with and remove bilirubin from the neonate's tissues.

• As the neonate's blood begins to flow through the outflow tubing, draw a blood sample. Place it in the appropriate tube, label it, and send it to the laboratory. Be careful to keep the specimen away from the phototherapy unit to prevent bilirubin decomposition.

• Take the neonate's vital signs and measure blood glucose levels every 15 minutes during the procedure. Record the time and amount of collected or transfused blood on the exchange transfusion sheet. Repeat each amount after the doctor specifies it.

• Alert the doctor each time 100 ml of blood have been exchanged so he can consider whether to give calcium gluconate.

• During administration of calcium gluconate, monitor the neonate's heart rate and watch the cardiac monitor for arrhythmias. Document the administration time and amount on the transfusion record.

• After the prescribed amount of blood has been exchanged, draw the last blood samples and send them to the laboratory.

After the procedure
• Continue to observe the neonate for signs of hypothermia, hypoglycemia, hypocalcemia, acidosis, circulatory overload, cardiac arrhythmias, and sepsis. Take vital signs every 30 minutes for 12 to 24 hours, then every hour for 4 hours until he stabilizes, unless hospital policy dictates otherwise.

• Check bilirubin levels every 4 to 8 hours.

• Check dextrose level and pH 1 hour after the exchange.

• If the doctor leaves the umbilical catheter in place, begin the prescribed I.V. infusion to maintain catheter patency and provide hydration and nourishment. Follow the health care facility's policy for cord care while the catheter is in place.

• If the catheter has been removed, apply a sterile dressing and check the umbilical area for bleeding or infection.

Home care instructions

• Instruct the parents to keep all follow-up appointments with the doctor.

• Tell them to call the doctor immediately if the neonate develops fever, malaise, or jaundice.

EXERCISES, RANGE-OF-MOTION

Range-of-motion (ROM) exercises are isotonic exercises that contract and shorten muscles. They are designed to move the patient's joints through as full a range of motion as possible. Each joint of the body has a normal range of motion. When they're performed properly, ROM exercises help to improve or maintain joint mobility, improve circulation, enhance muscle tone, and prevent contractures and subsequent deformity.

ROM exercises may be active, active-assistive, or passive. Active ROM exercises are performed by the patient himself. Active-assistive ROM exercises are performed by the patient with the assistance of a nurse or physical therapist. Passive ROM exercises are performed manually by a nurse, a physical therapist, a member of the patient's family or another caregiver, or with the aid of a continuous passive motion machine (see *Continuous passive motion*).

Purpose

• To maintain or restore normal joint movement and muscle tone, preventing stiffness and contractures, improving circulation, and, possibly, speeding return of function.

Indications

ROM exercises are indicated during prolonged physical inactivity, provided that there are no contraindications. Active ROM exercises are indicated for patients who have good neuromuscular function. Passive ROM exercises are indicated for patients with temporary or permanent loss of function, paralysis, or decreased level of consciousness.

Contraindications to ROM therapy include severe arthritic joint inflammation, septic joint, recent trauma with possible occult fracture or internal injuries, thrombophlebitis, severe pain, and a stiff or immovable joint. Forced passive stretching — movement of a joint that's immobile because of disuse, disease, or injury — must be specially ordered and performed by a doctor or physical therapist.

Procedure

Depending on the type, mobility, and condition of the joints being exercised, ROM therapy will include some or all of the following movements: flexion and extension, internal and external rotation, abduction and adduction, supination and pronation, dorsiflexion and plantar flexion, and eversion and inversion (see *Pictorial glossary of joint movement*, page 292).

To perform passive ROM exercises, support the extremity at the joint and move the joint slowly, smoothly, and gently through its normal range of motion. If the joint is painful to the touch, as in arthritis, support the extremity as close to the joint as possible without causing pain. To help prevent complications, follow these three cardinal rules of ROM therapy: Exercise only

Continuous passive motion

Continuous passive motion (CPM) uses an electrically powered machine to automatically move a joint through its normal range of motion for an extended duration. CPM is most commonly used in patients recovering from total hip or knee replacement, internal fixation of knee or ankle fractures, or removal of the synovial membrane in the knee or other major joints. The use of the CPM machine prevents the development of scar tissue and facilitates rehabilitation. However, it may cause bleeding in some patients, especially if used immediately after surgery.

Nursing responsibilities for patients undergoing CPM therapy include setting up the machine and properly positioning the patient's extremity, monitoring therapy, assessing response, and ensuring patient comfort and safety.

Performing CPM therapy
- Attach the machine to the patient's bed, and set the prescribed degree of flexion and extension and cycles per minute.
- Fasten the patient's extremity securely in the frame. Use sheepskin padding to protect the skin.
- Remain with the patient for at least one cycle, and double-check the degree of flexion and extension. Adjust as necessary.
- Continue operation for the prescribed duration, which varies from continuously to 8 to 20 hours/day.

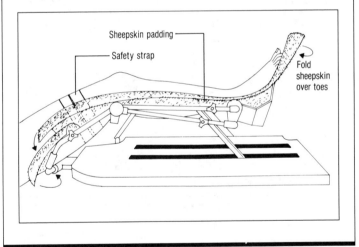

Sheepskin padding

Safety strap

Fold sheepskin over toes

one extremity at a time, never force any movement, and stop the exercise at once if the patient complains of pain.

To perform active ROM therapy, the patient must understand the prescribed exercises and their recommended frequency. The patient must move the involved joints slowly and smoothly through their range of motion and must stop and report any unusual pain or stiffness. Each joint is moved through its range of motion typically about three to five times twice daily.

Complications

Potential complications of active ROM exercises include exacerbation of inflammation from overmanipulation and joint or muscle injury from forced or

Pictorial glossary of joint movement

Below is a guide to the joint movements produced during range-of motion exercises.

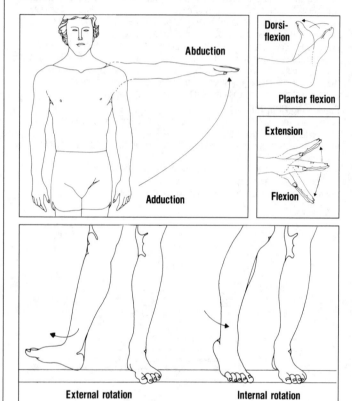

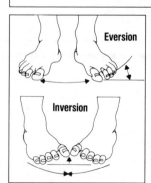

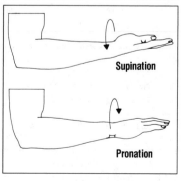

excessive movement. Possible complications of passive ROM therapy include joint instability and effusion from hyperextension and joint dislocation or bone fracture from excessively vigorous exercise.

Care considerations
Before therapy
• Assess the patient for disability and weakness in the involved extremity, and compare findings against a baseline neuromuscular assessment. If you note any deterioration in neuromuscular function, consult the doctor or physical therapist, who may order changes in the exercise regimen.
• Explain the exercises to the patient or whomever will be the patient's primary caregiver after discharge.
• For passive ROM therapy, explain that you'll move the patient's extremities, one at a time, through their normal range of motion in a prescribed pattern to maintain function and prevent stiffening.
• Describe and demonstrate the prescribed exercises if the patient is to perform active ROM exercises. Explain that he will perform the exercises at least twice a day, but warn against overextension or overexertion, which can lead to complications.
• Before passive ROM therapy, raise the patient's bed to a comfortable working height and position the patient properly—if possible, flat on his back, without a pillow, with hands at his sides and his feet together.
During therapy
• Assess for degree of mobility in the joint and for the level of pain elicited. Stiffness, immobility, or pain may indicate joint irritation. If these occur, consult the doctor or physical therapist, who may need to reevaluate therapy.
• Observe the patient performing active ROM exercises to ensure correct movement and that the patient performs all the prescribed exercises.

• For passive ROM exercises, support the joint throughout the range of motion.
After therapy
• Document the joints exercised, the presence of edema or pressure areas, pain resulting from the exercises, and the patient's tolerance.
• Position the patient comfortably in bed and encourage him to relax after passive ROM exercises.
• Administer analgesics, as provided, if pain develops.

Home care instructions
• Before discharge, make sure the patient and a family member or caregiver, if appropriate, fully understand each aspect of the prescribed exercise program and the need for strict compliance. Provide written, illustrated, or tape-recorded instructions, if possible, to enhance their understanding and improve compliance.
• To demonstrate understanding and the ability to do the exercises, have the patient or caregiver perform each aspect of prescribed ROM therapy before discharge.
• Instruct the patient or caregiver to report any complications associated with ROM exercise, such as increased joint or muscle pain, stiffness, or immobility.
• Stress the need for regular follow-up examinations to evaluate the patient's progress and the effectiveness of the exercise program.

EXERCISES, STRENGTHENING

Using exercise to strengthen weakened muscles is probably one of the most commonly used rehabilitation procedures. Strength can be defined as the maximum force that can be exerted by a muscle. Significant muscular inactivity can result in weakness, and forceful muscular activity can lead to strength gains. Exercises to increase strength depend on muscular contraction. Three different modes of exercise are commonly used to increase muscle strength—isotonic, isometric, and isokinetic exercise.

Isotonic exercise is the movement of a fixed load through the allowed joint range of motion. This is the most common form of strengthening exercise and usually involves the use of simple equipment, such as weights and pulleys, as well as specialized exercise units.

Isometric exercise involves the contraction of muscle without joint movement. In contrast to isotonic and isokinetic exercise, which are dynamic forms, this is a static form of exercise. Isometric exercise may be used to help maintain strength when a joint is immobilized.

Isokinetic exercise is movement performed at a fixed speed against resistance supplied by specialized equipment that accommodates to the specific force exerted by the individual muscle. This accommodation extends throughout the entire range of motion, making this form of strengthening exercise the most efficient. It allows the maximum amount of muscular exertion that can be performed throughout the joint's range of motion. However, this method involves the use of expensive equipment. Isokinetic equipment is also used for testing muscle groups.

Purpose
• To increase muscle strength, endurance, and power
• To improve functional ability.

Indications
Virtually everyone can benefit from a properly designed strengthening exercise program. Rehabilitative strengthening exercises are often prescribed for individuals with muscle weakness associated with inactivity due to disease, in-

jury, or life-style habits, provided there are no contraindications.

Strengthening exercises may be contraindicated after certain surgical procedures, such as skin grafting, in which the body part may need to be immobilized for a time. They may also be contraindicated in the presence of muscle or joint inflammation or pain during exercise. Strengthening exercises may also be contraindicated or may require careful adjustment and close supervision for patients with unstable angina, recent myocardial infarction, uncontrolled ventricular arrhythmia, aortic stenosis, congestive heart failure, thrombophlebitis, pulmonary embolism, or acute sepsis.

Procedure
Strengthening exercise programs may be designed by doctors, physical therapists, occupational therapists, or athletic trainers. These individuals, as well as nurses and physical therapist assistants, may administer these exercise programs. Strengthening programs are frequently conducted and supervised in hospitals, therapy clinics, and athletic training facilities.

An effective strengthening program must be individually designed to meet the patient's needs. Consideration must be given to the method of exercise to be used. Isotonic exercise, the most common form, may use several different approaches. The patient may exercise with the maximal weight that can be used for 5 to 10 repetitions, commonly using barbells, pulleys, and cuff-strap weights.

For isometric exercise, the patient is instructed to contract the muscle, hold for 6 seconds, and then relax and repeat. This is performed while keeping the affected part in a fixed position.

Isokinetic exercise involves the use of specialized equipment that supplies resistance. However, unlike isotonic exercise, this resistance is able to accommodate to the force exerted by the individual muscle throughout the entire range of motion.

Complications

Complications may include muscle soreness and fatigue. Cardiovascular complications are possible.

Care considerations

Before therapy
• Assess which muscles need to be strengthened.
• Identify any predisposing factors that might contraindicate exercise or require modification of the strengthening program.

During therapy
• Closely monitor the patient's performance and response to exercise.

After therapy
• Modify the program as needed.

Home care instructions

• Teach each exercise to the patient, and be certain that it is accurately performed.
• Emphasize the need to breathe during exercise activity and to exhale during the exertional phase of each exercise maneuver.
• Provide written and illustrated exercise instructions.
• Encourage the patient to continue the exercise program at home.
• Advise the patient not to overexercise.
• Encourage the patient to contact the physical therapist if problems or questions arise.

EXTRACORPOREAL MEMBRANE OXYGENATION

Extracorporeal membrane oxygenation (ECMO), a special form of life support, is an adaptation of cardiopulmonary bypass methods used during open-heart surgery; it is mainly used for neonates. By diverting cardiac output from the lungs and decreasing the potentially damaging adverse effects associated with mechanical ventilation, ECMO gives severely compromised lungs a chance to rest and to heal. During this therapy, a machine removes the patient's venous blood, passes it through a membrane oxygenator, and then returns it to the circulation. (See *How ECMO works,* pages 296 and 297.) Patients can usually remain on ECMO support for several days (up to 17 days have been reported), perhaps long enough for their lungs to heal.

Purpose

• To provide oxygenation while allowing the lungs to recover and heal
• To "buy time" in reversible life-threatening respiratory failure.

Indications

ECMO is used only after maximal ventilatory support has failed to improve oxygenation. Candidates must have a condition that is considered potentially reversible within 2 to 3 weeks.

Candidates for ECMO must have a partial pressure of oxygen in arterial blood (PaO_2) level below 40 mm Hg and optimal positive end-expiratory pressure (PEEP) for at least 2 hours.

ECMO has been most successful in neonates with persistent pulmonary hypertension. It is not often used for infants older than 10 days. Pediatric indications include hyaline membrane disease, meconium aspiration, persistent fetal circulation, sepsis, pneumonia, and cardiac failure secondary to congenital or acquired problems.

ECMO has not been greatly successful in adults but has been tried in adult respiratory distress syndrome (ARDS), bacterial and viral pneumonia, pulmonary emboli, and inhalation injuries.

ECMO is contraindicated in patients with central nervous system damage, irreversible shock, pulmonary fibrosis,

(Text continues on page 298.)

How ECMO works

Extracorporeal membrane oxygenation (ECMO) diverts pulmonary blood flow, decompresses the pulmonary circuit, and supports systemic circulation. It can be carried out using venovenous or venoarterial bypass.

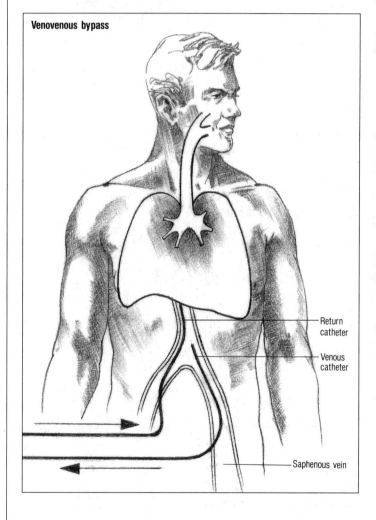

Venovenous bypass

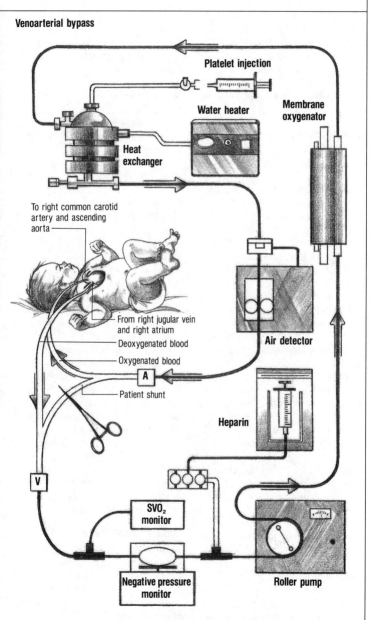

Venoarterial bypass

Platelet injection

Water heater

Membrane oxygenator

Heat exchanger

To right common carotid artery and ascending aorta

From right jugular vein and right atrium
Deoxygenated blood
Oxygenated blood

Air detector

A

Patient shunt

Heparin

SVO₂ monitor

Negative pressure monitor

Roller pump

V

Reprinted, by permission from the ECMO Department at Thomas Jefferson University Hospital, Philadelphia multiple organ failure, intracranial bleeding, congenital anomalies not compatible with life, cardiac anomalies, and coagulopathies, and in patients who have been receiving mechanical ventilation for more than 10 days. Infants of less than 35 weeks' gestation and those weighing less than 4.4 lb (2,000 g) are excluded as candidates for ECMO because they have the greatest risk of intracranial hemorrhage.

Procedure

The two approaches to ECMO are venoarterial (VA) and venovenous (VV). Insertion is a surgical procedure and is usually performed at an intensive care bedside by an operating room team. When used to treat neonates, this procedure should be performed only in a Level III neonatal center. Patients receiving ECMO require invasive hemodynamic monitoring and mechanical ventilation with systemic heparinization to prevent thrombus formation in the circuit.

The venoarterial ECMO approach is more common. In this technique a doctor inserts a large-bore catheter into the right atrium via the right internal jugular vein. The blood is drained into a membrane oxygenator. While blood travels this extracorporeal circuit, oxygen is infused and carbon dioxide is removed. After passing through the circuit, the blood is returned to the aortic arch via the right common carotid artery. In VA bypass, which bypasses the heart, the pump provides arterial perfusion pressure as cardiac support.

In venovenous ECMO, blood is drained by gravity into the extracorporeal circuit. After blood is oxygenated and carbon dioxide is removed, the blood is reinfused into the venous system rather than the arterial system. Unlike VA bypass, the VV bypass does not provide cardiac support but provides total respiratory support. Some advantages of the VV approach are that no major artery is catheterized and the risk of embolism is decreased.

When the patient is ready for discontinuation of ECMO, the operating room team is called to the intensive care unit for removal of the catheter. Afterward, the great vessels used are ligated.

Complications

ECMO can cause mechanical and physiologic complications, including hemorrhage and sepsis, the two most common physiologic complications. Patients may hemorrhage internally (thoracic hemorrhage) or externally from a dislodged catheter or as a result of anticoagulant therapy. There may also be bleeding from the catheter insertion sites. Intracranial bleeding is the most serious hemorrhagic complication. Sepsis may result from the presence of a large invasive catheter or from any of the many other invasive devices used during ECMO.

Mechanical difficulties can be life-threatening. Although such malfunctions are uncommon, the results are significant. Among them are thrombus formation in the membrane and air embolism in the return infusion line. Thrombi can interfere with adequate gas exchange and can also embolize. Catheter malposition inside the vein can impair the drainage of blood into the circuit and the return of blood from the circuit. Dislodgment of the catheter from the patient's body or perforation of the catheter outside the vein may interfere with gas exchange or lead to massive hemorrhage.

Care considerations
Before the procedure
• Patients receiving ECMO are critically ill. Therefore, clear, appropriate explanations of the procedure and emotional support of the patient and family are essential.
• Obtain a baseline assessment of the patient.

• Assure proper calibration of monitoring devices for accurate hemodynamic readings.
• Ensure aseptic technique.
• In neonates, ultrasonography of the head is performed to rule out intracranial bleeding before initiating ECMO.
• Ensure that the endotracheal tube is taped securely and that I.V. lines are patent.
• Make sure a consent form has been signed by the patient or his family.

During the procedure
• Assist the operating room team and surgeon as needed during insertion of the catheter.
• Monitor vital signs closely.
• Monitor respiratory status every 2 hours (and whenever a change of condition occurs) by auscultating all lung fields and by monitoring arterial blood gas results and pulmonary artery and pulmonary artery wedge pressures.
• Neonates require two nurses during ECMO support: one takes care only of the ECMO and the other provides nursing care.
• Suction the patient thoroughly.
• Watch closely for signs of infection. Observe all catheter insertion sites for redness, swelling, or drainage. Culture drainage when indicated.
• Clean the site daily according to hospital policy, and apply sterile dressings.
• Throughout ECMO support, be especially careful not to dislodge the catheters.
• Because the patient will receive heparin throughout ECMO, observe for signs of bleeding.
• Administer drugs and draw blood samples only from access ports on the equipment.
• Maintain accurate intake and output records.
• Provide emotional support to the patient and family. Patients are sedated during therapy to decrease movement.

Home care instructions
• Instruct the patient or the patient's family to promptly notify the doctor of fevers, bleeding, bruising, changes in mental status, shortness of breath, or chest pains. Signs of respiratory distress include cyanosis, increased respiratory rate, and congestion.
• Activity levels should follow the doctor's instructions or the assigned rehabilitation program.
• Other home care instructions depend on the underlying cause for ECMO.

EYE MUSCLE SURGERY

Eye muscle surgery corrects defects in the strength or placement of the eye muscles. Such defects cause misalignment of the eye, disruption of the visual axis, and possible diplopia (double vision). Eye muscle surgery adjusts the pull that the muscles exert on the affected eye, thereby realigning the visual axis, and may help in restoring binocular vision.

Two types of eye muscle surgery may be performed. Resection, which is the most common procedure, shortens and strengthens eye muscles. Recessive surgery weakens the muscles by repositioning them. One or both techniques may be used to carefully position the eye back into proper alignment.

Eye muscle surgery is most commonly performed in children, but it may also be therapeutic for adults. It's usually successful in restoring binocular vision, but may be repeated if the corrected eye drifts out of alignment.

Purpose
• To correct strabismus
• To straighten the eyes for cosmetic reasons.

Indications

Eye muscle surgery is one of three basic methods used to correct strabismus.

Procedure

The patient receives deep general anesthesia. This allows the eyes to return to their primary position before surgery begins.

In recessive surgery (a weakening procedure), the surgeon detaches the muscle from the eye, frees any attachments, and allows the muscle to retract. Then he reattaches the muscle to the eye at a measured distance behind the original insertion site.

In resection surgery (a strengthening procedure), the surgeon detaches the muscle from the eye, stretches it larger by a measured amount, and then reattaches the muscle to the eye at the original insertion site.

The greatest advance in eye muscle surgery in the last 10 years is "adjustable sutures." During eye muscle surgery, the muscles are reattached with a special knot in the suture that can be tightened or loosened to change the eye position as necessary when the patient is awake. The surgeon concludes either procedure by closing the conjunctiva and applying antibiotic ointment.

Complications

Complications of eye muscle surgery are rare but may include minor infection and minor bleeding.

Care considerations

Before surgery

• Inform the patient that the surgery will be performed under general anesthesia. Explain all preoperative care and the anticipated length of stay. Same-day surgery may be performed.
• If the patient is a child, take special measures to reduce his anxiety. Also let him know if he should expect an eye patch after surgery. (*Note:* Many

doctors no longer use patches on children's eyes after the surgery.)
• If the patient is a child, be sure his parents understand how to administer any preoperative medications.
• Instruct the patient or parents that the patient must have nothing to eat or drink for 8 to 12 hours before surgery.
• Tell the patient that after surgery the doctor may order orthoptic exercises to help train the eyes to work together and enhance restoration of binocular vision.
• Before surgery, ensure that the patient or a responsible family member has signed a consent form.

After surgery

• If the patient is a child, make sure that he doesn't pull at the eye patch or scratch the eye after surgery. Apply an arm splint, if necessary, to prevent disruption of the surgical site.
• Watch for and report excessive discharge from the eye.
• Tell the patient that he may return to normal daily activities when fully recovered from the anesthesia.

Home care instructions

• If appropriate, teach the patient or his parents how to instill antibiotic or corticosteroid eyedrops.
• Tell the patient or parents to expect that the conjunctiva will be red for 1 to 2 weeks. Emphasize the importance of notifying the doctor if increased redness, fever, or eye discharge occurs.
• Advise the patient to shield his eyes from light by wearing sunglasses or a wide-brimmed hat or cap.
• Explain that double vision may persist for several months. Stress the importance of keeping appointments with the doctor to monitor this condition.
• Review the prescribed orthoptic exercises and make sure the patient or parents understand the importance of practicing them as ordered.
• Warn the patient to avoid vigorous sports until the doctor gives permission.

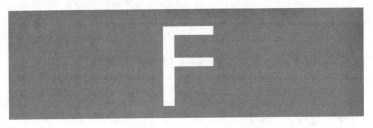

FACTOR REPLACEMENT

Factor replacement is the I.V. infusion of blood clotting factors to treat coagulation disorders. Various blood products are used, depending on the disorder being treated.

Purpose
• To correct clotting factor deficiencies and thereby stop or prevent hemorrhage.

Indications

Factor replacement is indicated for various disorders. Each blood product treats a specific clotting disorder. *Fresh frozen plasma* (FFP), for instance, helps treat clotting disorders whose causes aren't known, clotting factor deficiencies resulting from hepatic disease or blood dilution, and deficiencies of clotting factors (such as factor V) for which no specific replacement product exists.

Cryoprecipitate, which forms when FFP thaws slowly, helps treat von Willebrand's disease, fibrinogen deficiencies, and factor XIII deficiencies. In addition, it's used for young hemophilia patients or patients with mild hemophilia.

Factor VIII (antihemophilic factor) concentrate serves as the long-term treatment of choice for hemophilia A because the amount of factor VIII that it contains is less variable than with cryoprecipitate. It's administered I.V. whenever the hemophilia patient has sustained an injury.

Prothrombin complex, which contains factors II, VII, IX, and X, can be given to treat hemophilia B, severe liver disease, and acquired deficiencies of the factors it contains.

Procedure

Factor replacement products are administered I.V. Before the transfusion, the patient receives medication (for example, with diphenhydramine [Benadryl] and methylprednisolone [Solu-Medrol]). The nurse should practice universal precautions whenever blood products are handled, including wearing gloves, double-bagging empty blood product containers, and properly disposing of needles and venipuncture equipment. These universal precautions should be clearly designated by the individual institution.

A filter is always used when administering blood products. Different-sized filters are used for different blood components. Additional filters can be applied if the patient tends to develop transfusion reactions. The mechanisms of action vary among the different factor replacement components; so do the specific guidelines for administration. (See *Administering clotting factor replacements,* page 302.)

Complications

A transfusion reaction can result from a single or massive transfusion of blood or blood products.

Reactions generally occur during or within 96 hours of the transfusion. Infections, such as those caused by the human immunodeficiency virus, hepatitis virus, and cytomegalovirus (CMV)

Administering clotting factor replacements

Although all clotting factors are derived from whole blood, they're administered differently. Here's a summary of important pointers for administering these products.

Fresh frozen plasma
- Use fresh frozen plasma within 60 minutes of thawing.
- Administer only with 0.9% sodium chloride solution. Use an appropriate-sized filter.
- Infuse as rapidly as the patient will tolerate it — usually, 250 ml can be given over 30 to 45 minutes in patients without causing symptoms of circulatory overload.

Cryoprecipitate
- Don't refrigerate; use within 6 hours of thawing.
- Administer only with 0.9% sodium chloride solution. Use an appropriate-sized filter for cryoprecipitate infusion.
- Infuse rapidly (10 to 12 units in 30 minutes).
- Watch for symptoms of hepatitis.

Lyophilized factor VIII
- Reconstitute vials of factor VIII according to the manufacturer's directions.
- Administer by slow I.V. push through a butterfly set, at a rate of 1 reconstituted vial every 5 minutes.
- Don't use a glass syringe because factor VIII binds to ground glass surfaces.
- Watch for symptoms of hepatitis.

Prothrombin complex
- Prothrombin complex carries a high risk of transmitting hepatitis because it's collected from large donor pools.
- Give by slow I.V. push through a butterfly set, at a rate of 1 vial every 5 minutes.

may also be transmitted during a transfusion and can go undetected for weeks or months until they cause signs and symptoms. Prothrombin complex carries a special risk of transmitting hepatitis because it's collected from large pools of donors.

Care considerations
Before therapy
- Explain the procedure and ensure that the patient or a family member has signed a consent form.
- Gather equipment necessary to administer the appropriate blood product.
- Obtain the plasma fraction from the blood bank or pharmacy. Check the expiration date and the blood bank and patient identification numbers, and then carefully inspect the plasma fraction for cloudiness and turbidity. Most health care facilities require that two registered nurses check blood products before administration.
- Take the patient's vital signs to establish a baseline. If an I.V. line isn't in place, perform a venipuncture and infuse 0.9% sodium chloride solution at a keep-vein-open rate.

During therapy
- Observe for signs of anaphylaxis, other allergic reactions, and fluid overload.
- Monitor the infusion site for pain or swelling.
- Take vital signs, especially temperature, as required per protocol.

• Notify the doctor of adverse reactions.

After therapy

• Continue to monitor for transfusion reaction.

• Observe for signs of bleeding.

• Closely monitor partial thromboplastin time.

• Notify the doctor of any complications.

Home care instructions

• Increasingly, the patient or his family provides factor replacement therapy at home; in fact, children as young as age 9 can be taught how to do so. If ordered, demonstrate correct venipuncture and infusion techniques to the family or patient. Tell them to keep the factor replacement and infusion equipment available and to begin treatment immediately if the patient experiences a bleeding episode.

• Tell the patient and family to watch for signs of anaphylaxis, allergic reactions, or fluid overload. Instruct them to call the doctor immediately if such reactions occur.

• Also tell the patient and family to watch for signs of hepatitis, which may appear 3 weeks to 6 months after treatment with blood components.

FASCIOTOMY

Fasciotomy is a surgical incision into the fascia when swelling creates increased pressure within a muscle compartment. This increased pressure is identified by pain, paresthesias, paralysis, pallor, and pulselessness in the involved area.

Fascia is a sheet or a band of inelastic fibrous tissue that encloses muscles, nerves, and circulatory structures of the musculoskeletal system; fascia separates these structures into compartments that have entrance and exit points large enough to permit only the passage of blood vessels and nerves.

Fasciotomy is usually considered an emergency procedure because it must be performed within 6 to 12 hours of the onset of symptoms to prevent ischemic injury. If performed within this time the prognosis is good for functional return to the extremity. If performed after this time, the rate of complication is higher and functional return is less likely.

Purpose

• To relieve pressure in the involved compartment, reducing swelling and increasing blood flow.

Indications

Fasciotomy is primarily used as treatment for compartment syndrome, an orthopedic emergency. The musculoskeletal compartments in which the syndrome most commonly occurs are those located in the legs and the arms, but the syndrome can also develop in the shoulder, hand, buttocks, foot, and thigh.

To prevent ischemic injury, fasciotomy, an emergency procedure, must be completed within 6 to 12 hours after onset of compartment syndrome. Elevated tissue pressure (measured by the orthopedist) ranging from 10 to 30 mm Hg of the patient's diastolic pressure is an indication for fasciotomy.

Procedure

The orthopedic surgeon makes an incision through the skin and into the fascia that encloses the involved compartment, and extends the incision the length of the compartment to ensure relief of pressure in all the tissues involved. If necrotic tissue or hematomas have developed in the involved compartment, the surgeon may debride the necrotic tissue or remove the hematomas. The incision is then left open, covered only by a sterile dressing, until swelling has subsided (usually 3 to 7 days). After the swelling has subsided, the skin is closed by sutures or split-thickness skin grafts.

Complications

Complications of fasciotomy can include soft-tissue and bone infections resulting from an open wound, amputation of the extremity related to extensive muscle necrosis and compromised blood flow, renal failure related to myoglobinuria, loss of function of the involved area, and death resulting from sepsis.

Care considerations

Before surgery

• Notify the surgeon immediately of symptoms of compartment syndrome (pain, paresthesias, pallor, pulselessness in the involved area, or paralysis).
• If the patient is at high risk for development of compartment syndrome, the orthopedist may insert a needle or catheter into the compartment and connect the needle or catheter to a manometer to monitor the compartment pressure. If such a device is in place, monitor the pressure closely. Normal compartment pressure is 0 mm Hg. If the pressure is 30 mm Hg or greater, fasciotomy is usually necessary. Report elevated compartment pressure immediately.
• If compartment syndrome occurs in an extremity, position the extremity no higher than the heart.
• Loosen or remove all splints and constricting dressings. If the patient has a cast, split the cast and the padding to relieve pressure. Immobilize the extremity with nonconstricting splints.
• Monitor the involved area closely. If the neurovascular status improves within an hour after releasing constricting dressings or casts, a fasciotomy may not be necessary. If pressure increases or is unrelieved, fasciotomy must be performed.

After surgery

• Reassure and support the patient and his family because the incision is left open and bed rest must be maintained. Reinforce explanations and answer any questions about the procedure and the care required.
• Monitor dressings for drainage, and observe the incision for signs of infection when changing the dressing. Report increased drainage to the doctor immediately.
• Monitor vital signs because elevated temperatures could be a precursor to shock. Report any fever immediately.
• Monitor the involved area for pulse, pallor, and paresthesia to check return of normal function and blood flow.
• Administer prescribed analgesics as needed, and note their effectiveness.
• Monitor the patient's blood counts, especially white blood cell count, for indications of infection or sepsis, and administer antibiotics as ordered.
• Keep the affected extremity at heart level to increase perfusion.

Home care instructions

• At discharge, the wound will be closed either by sutures or skin graft. Teach the patient suture or graft care as recommended by the surgeon.
• Teach the patient the signs and symptoms of infection, such as redness, drainage, fever, warmth at incision site, and edema, and tell him to notify the doctor if these occur.
• Teach the patient how to monitor the pulse in the affected extremity and to be alert for numbness and tingling.
• Emphasize the importance of taking antibiotics exactly as prescribed.

FERTILITY DRUGS

Fertility drugs, used to induce ovulation, include *clomiphene, gonadorelin acetate, menotropins,* and *human chorionic gonadotropin* (HCG). The synthetic steroid clomiphene enhances secretion of follicle-stimulating hormone (FSH) and luteinizing hormone (LH), which stimulate follicular maturation in the ovary. Drug dosages may begin at 50 mg/day, increasing up to 250 mg/day if ovulation doesn't occur. Typically, ovulation occurs 4 to 10 days after the last day of treatment.

If clomiphene fails to induce ovulation after three trials, menotropins (human menopausal gonadotropin) and HCG may be given. Menotropins must be used with HCG to stimulate ovulation, which should occur within 18 hours after administration. HCG may also be used 7 to 10 days after clomiphene therapy.

Women with primary hypothalamic amenorrhea may receive gonadorelin acetate. This analogue of gonadotropin-releasing hormone (GnRH) is administered every 90 minutes for 21 days with a special portable I.V. infusion pump.

The use of fertility drugs may lead to multiple births. The incidence varies from 5% with clomiphene to 20% with HCG.

Purpose

• To stimulate follicular maturation in the ovary (clomiphene)
• To promote growth and maturation of ovarian follicles (menotropins)
• To stimulate ovulation of a menotropins-prepared follicle (HCG)
• To induce ovulation in women with primary hypothalamic amenorrhea (gonadorelin acetate).

Indications

Fertility drugs are used to stimulate ovulation in an anovulatory patient who wishes to become pregnant.

Fertility drugs are contraindicated in patients with undiagnosed vaginal bleeding, fibroid tumors, ovarian cysts, hepatic dysfunction, or thrombophlebitis. They should be used cautiously in patients with asthma, seizure disorders, or heart disease.

Adverse reactions

HCG and menotropins may cause ovarian hyperstimulation, ovarian enlargement, and hypersensitivity reactions. They may also cause such central nervous system effects as depression, insomnia, and restlessness. Clomiphene may also cause ovarian enlargement as well as ovarian cyst formation, uterine fibroid enlargement, and premenstrual syndrome. Other adverse reactions include blurred vision or diplopia, hot flashes, dizziness or lightheadedness, nervousness, restlessness, and insomnia. Gonadorelin acetate also may cause ovarian hyperstimulation. Local irritation, inflammation, and phlebitis may occur at the injection site.

Care considerations

• Starting 1 week after treatment begins, measure estrogen levels daily to help detect excessive ovarian stimulation. In addition, the doctor may perform a pelvic examination to evaluate ovarian size when estrogen levels begin to rise. Enlargement indicates excessive ovarian stimulation, requiring a decreased dosage or discontinuation of the drug for several days to weeks with a dosage reduction during the next course of therapy.
• Be alert for and report signs of severe ovarian hyperstimulation, such as ascites, pleural effusion, electrolyte imbalance, and hypovolemia with oliguria and hypotension. Also be alert for signs of mild ovarian hyperstimulation, such as abdominal distention and weight gain.

Home care instructions

• Instruct the patient to immediately report bloating or abdominal pain, indicating excessive ovarian stimulation.
• Teach the patient the signs and symptoms of hypersensitivity reactions (hives, wheezing, difficulty breathing), and instruct her to report them immediately.

• Encourage the patient to adhere to the monitoring schedule required by this therapy. Regular pelvic examinations, midluteal phase serum progesterone determinations, and multiple ovarian ultrasound scans are necessary.

• Inform the patient that the fertility drug may cause visual difficulties, dizziness, or light-headedness. Tell her to avoid driving until response to the drug is established.

• Advise the patient that the possibility of multiple births increases if she becomes pregnant while taking a fertility drug.

• If the patient is taking oral therapy, tell her to take a missed dose as soon as she remembers or to double the dose if she doesn't remember until the time of her next dose. Tell her to inform the doctor if she misses more than one dose.

• If the patient is taking gonadorelin, instruct her about proper aseptic technique and I.V. site care. Provide available written instructions. Catheter and I.V. site should be changed every 48 hours.

• Reinforce the importance of having intercourse as often as the doctor prescribes (usually every day or every other day during the patient's fertile period).

• Teach the patient to take her basal body temperature and to chart it on a graph. Suggest that she also use an ovulatory predictor test kit.

• Instruct the patient to bring a first-voided morning urine specimen for testing at each follow-up visit.

• Explain the importance of keeping follow-up appointments to monitor response to therapy.

FLUID RESUSCITATION

Fluid resuscitation is the administration of I.V. solutions to replace total body intracellular or extracellular water and electrolytes. It is undertaken when a patient has a deficit in water or electrolytes.

The fluids infused can be crystalloids, colloids, or blood. Crystalloids include standard I.V. solutions such as lactated Ringer's, 0.9% sodium chloride, and dextrose solutions. With the exception of dextrose solutions, these solutions expand extracellular space (both plasma volume and interstitium). Dextrose 5% solution expands total body water and intracellular fluid. These solutions take effect quickly but last only a short time in plasma, so they must be administered more frequently. They are less expensive than colloids and can restore both intravascular and interstitial fluid losses.

Colloids include dextran, plasma protein fraction (Plasmanate), albumin, and hetastarch (Hespan). If the patient's capillary endothelium is intact, colloids will remain in the bloodstream for several days and will draw additional fluid in from the interstitial space by osmosis.

Fluid resuscitation must be monitored very carefully in patients with preexisting heart or kidney disease to prevent heart failure from overload.

Purpose
• To replace depleted intravascular, interstitial, or intracellular volume
• To maintain blood flow to brain and vital organs
• To replace electrolytes.

Indications
A patient may need fluid resuscitation when severe vomiting and diarrhea cause dehydration or when blood loss from trauma or surgery causes hypovolemia. After major surgery, fluid resuscitation becomes necessary because of intraoperative fluid loss or fluid shift from the intravascular space to the interstitial space. Fluid volume deficit varies. The type of fluid resuscitation administered depends on the amount

of fluid lost and the patient's clinical status.

Procedure

The doctor will order the type of fluid and rate of administration. The nurse is responsible for inserting the peripheral I.V. catheters, administering the infusion, and monitoring the patient.

One or two I.V. lines are placed, preferably in the antecubital space. If a central line is the only site available for access, fluids can be infused through that line as well. The length of central lines greatly increases resistance, however, so short, large-bore peripheral I.V. catheters (14G to 16G) are preferred for rapid infusion. Once the lines are in place, fluid administration begins.

If the patient's condition requires rapid replacement of large fluid volume, the fluid should be warmed to prevent hypothermia. Ideal fluid temperature is 98.6° F (37° C). Equipment is available to both warm the fluid and infuse it rapidly. Pressure cuffs can be wrapped around plastic bags to increase flow rate.

Complications

Patients receiving fluid resuscitation are at risk for fluid overload. This is especially true of patients with cardiac or kidney disease. After blood replacement, the patient is at risk for transfusion reaction and blood-borne diseases. Complications of colloid or crystalloid administration are related to the specific type of infusion. Use of crystalloid solutions may lead to volume overload, congestive heart failure, pulmonary edema, and interstitial edema. Some patients receiving colloids have allergic reactions, including fever, chills, and even anaphylactic shock.

Care considerations

Before therapy

• Explain procedures as appropriate.
• Insert an indwelling urinary catheter, if ordered, to allow adequate monitoring of urine output.
• Check serum electrolyte levels to detect imbalances early.
• Provide nursing interventions to address the source of fluid depletion.

During therapy

• Assess and record vital signs at regular intervals based on the patient's condition; preferably, the patient will be connected to an automatic blood pressure cuff or have an arterial catheter in place.
• Monitor for fluid overload, which may cause restlessness, dyspnea, tachypnea, hypoxemia, pulmonary congestion, frothy sputum, jugular vein distention, and a gallop rhythm (see *Do's and don'ts of fluid resuscitation*, page 308).
• Monitor for adequate fluid replacement. Watch for normal pulse pressure (approximately 40 mm Hg), urine output of at least 50 ml/hour, heart rate of 60 to 100 beats/minute, normal mental status for patient, and capillary refill time of less than 2 seconds.
• Monitor the patient's temperature for hypothermia. Provide blankets to maintain body temperature, if necessary.
• Frequently observe the I.V. site to detect early signs of extravasation.
• Change the site promptly if the infusion line does not function properly.
• Monitor the I.V. flow rate to ensure accurate intake and be sure fluid resuscitation is ended when total volume is infused.
• Do not auscultate blood pressures in the arm used for infusion.

Home care instructions

• Teach the patient and family members early signs and symptoms of fluid depletion, and instruct them to notify their health care provider if these occur. This is especially important for home care of elderly and very young

Do's and don'ts of fluid resuscitation

Follow these guidelines to help prevent complications of fluid resuscitation.

Do establish peripheral I.V. access with a short, large-gauge catheter.

Do use the shortest length of tubing possible.

Do elevate the I.V. container so gravity can assist rapid infusion.

Do place I.V. bags in pressure bags and inflate as high as 300 mm Hg to increase the infusion rate.

Do assess the patient every 10 minutes for signs of fluid overload.

Don't encourage the doctor to place a central I.V. catheter for fluid resuscitation unless no other I.V. access is available. (In emergencies, central-line insertion is associated with a 15% complication rate.)

Don't administer fluid through a central line if a short, large-gauge peripheral line is available. If a central line is already in place, use it to monitor the patient's hemodynamic response to treatment.

Don't allow I.V. tubing to loop beneath the patient's bed. The flow rate will slow because of increased resistance from the tubing.

Don't use colloid solutions in patients who may have capillary leak syndrome; for example, those with adult respiratory distress syndrome or septic shock.

Don't use dextrose 5% in water (D_5W) or 0.45% sodium chloride solution to replace large-volume intravascular deficits.

Don't use D_5W or any other hypotonic solution in patients at risk for increased intracranial pressure or third-space fluid shifts (for example, patients suffering from burns, trauma, or low serum protein levels).

Don't insert a needle through a heparin lock for rapid-volume resuscitation. This procedure increases resistance and slows the flow rate.

Don't warm I.V. fluids in a microwave.

---

patients, who can quickly become dehydrated from vomiting and diarrhea.

FOOT CARE

An effective foot care regimen restores or maintains skin integrity and enhances circulation to rejuvenate or maintain peripheral sensory function and, if necessary, to aid healing.

Purpose

• To maintain cleanliness, control odor, prevent infection, and improve circulation in the feet.

Indications

Foot care is indicated for patients with peripheral vascular disease, diabetic neuropathy, traumatic injury, or prolonged immobilization.

Procedure

If the patient is in bed, place a pillow under his knees to provide support, and position the edge of a towel over the rim of a basin to cushion his lower legs. Then, immerse one of the patient's feet in water, wash it with soap, and allow it to soak for 5 to 10 minutes. If the patient is permitted to sit up and dangle his legs over the side of the bed, he may place his foot in a basin on a small footstool or the floor. Then rinse the foot, remove it from the basin, and pat it dry. Avoid rubbing because it could damage the skin. Apply lotion or oil to the foot immediately after drying to prevent evaporating water from drying the skin. If moisture remains between the toes, apply a mild foot powder to that area. Repeat the procedure on the other foot.

Next, clean the toenails with a cotton-tipped applicator or cotton ball. Gently remove dirt or debris from under the nails with an orangewood stick, taking care to avoid injuring the delicate subungual skin. The toenails should be trimmed if necessary by cutting straight across (to prevent ingrown nails) and then filing the nails even with the ends of the toes. Special care should be taken with diabetic patients or those who have reduced sensation in the feet.

Complications

Potential complications include damage to ungual tissue and cuticles as well as infection. Diabetic patients and others with reduced sensation in the feet may be at higher risk for complications.

Care considerations

Before therapy

• Discuss the purpose of foot care with the patient, and explain all the steps. If the patient will be performing foot care after discharge, instruct him to pay close attention and to ask questions.

• Inspect the patient's feet for blisters, bruises, cracks, open lesions, corns, calluses, and areas of dry, reddened skin. Observe areas of bony prominences, which are subject to rubbing from ill-fitting shoes.

• Note the color, shape, and texture of toenails; document any abnormalities.

During therapy

• Ensure the patient's safety and privacy.

• Make sure the patient is comfortable and does not become cold during the therapy.

After therapy

• Watch for and report any redness, bruising, drying or cracking, blisters, open wounds or other lesions, and ingrown or abnormal toenails, especially if the patient has impaired peripheral circulation. Such a patient is especially susceptible to infection and gangrene and requires prompt attention.

• If the patient will be performing regular foot care at home, be sure to review all the steps before discharge and have him demonstrate each step.

Home care instructions

• Warn against soaking the feet longer than 5 to 10 minutes because this may increase the risk of infection and skin damage.

• Encourage the patient to see his podiatrist regularly.

• Teach the patient the importance of wearing well-fitting and protective footwear (leather shoes) and tell him to avoid going barefoot.

• Instruct the patient to avoid tight shoes or tight-fitting socks or garter belts, which reduce the circulation to the feet.

• Instruct the patient to always test the temperature of the water before immersing his feet. A patient who has poor peripheral circulation could immerse his feet in water hot enough to cause burns without feeling pain.

• Instruct the patient to use an extra sheet in place of the bath blanket and a plastic bag to protect his bed linens.

• Tell the patient to check the skin of his feet daily for cuts, cracks, blisters, or red, swollen areas.

• Advise the patient to avoid using heating pads and hot-water bottles to warm cold feet. Recommend wearing warm, dry socks and using an extra blanket in bed.

FOREIGN BODY REMOVAL, EYE

Foreign body removal from the eye removes any object from within the eye, eyelid, or conjunctiva. Dust, dirt, eyelashes, and airborne particles can come in contact with the conjunctiva or cornea, causing the patient to have a foreign body sensation. Removing it is a first-aid procedure that can be performed by the nurse and sometimes by the patient. However, if the foreign body is embedded in the cornea, removal must be done by an ophthalmologist.

Purpose

• To remove a foreign body from the eye, thereby decreasing pain, preventing damage by abrasion, and reducing the risk of infection.

Indications

This procedure is indicated any time a foreign body contacts the conjunctiva or cornea. The patient complains of foreign body sensation, tearing, or photophobia.

Procedure

If a foreign particle is lying on the surface of the conjunctiva, instruct the patient to tilt his head back and to move his eyes away from the site of the particle. Hold the patient's eyelids open to prevent blinking. Then gently touch the particle with the tip of a wet cotton-tipped applicator and lift it from the eye, taking care not to drag the applicator across the surface of the cornea.

If the foreign body is not visible, evert the lid by having the patient look downward as you grasp the eyelashes of the upper lid and gently exert pressure in the midportion of the upper lid with a wet cotton-tipped applicator. If a foreign body is present, it can be easily seen and removed with the applicator.

Corneal foreign bodies can frequently be removed by irrigation. This can be accomplished by holding the eye open and irrigating or flushing the cornea with a steady stream of sterile ophthalmic irrigating solution. Aim the stream at the inner canthus (corner) of the eye and allow it to run over the cornea. Repeat the irrigation until the foreign body is removed. Then dry the eye with a cotton ball, wiping from the inner to the outer canthus of the eye.

Embedded foreign bodies should be removed by an ophthalmologist after instillation of topical anesthetic eyedrops. Iron and steel foreign bodies will leave a rust ring around the foreign body site. This is removed by using a speed spatula or appropriate instrument. Antibiotic eyedrops should be instilled and continued for several days to discourage infection of the damaged cornea. The eye is patched for several hours as well.

Complications

Deeply imbedded corneal foreign bodies can leave corneal scars that can cause impaired vision. Corneal infections can lead to ocular infections. Using topical anesthetic eyedrops for pain control after the foreign body is removed may delay healing.

Care considerations

Before the procedure

• After obtaining a thorough history, including the circumstances of the injury and description of symptoms, assess and document the patient's visual acuity.
• Explain the procedure to the patient.
• If the foreign body is lodged in the cornea, tell the patient that an anesthetic will be placed in his eye to reduce discomfort.
• Warn the patient not to rub his eye because this will cause further damage, making removal more difficult. Consider placing a protective shield over the eye to prevent the patient from

rubbing it until he can be examined by the ophthalmologist.

During the procedure
• Verify that the anesthetic has taken effect immediately before removal of the foreign body by gently touching the eye with a wet cotton-tipped applicator and asking about any sensation.
• Assess the patient's comfort during the procedure and administer additional anesthetic eyedrops as needed.

After the procedure
• After removal of an embedded particle, instruct the patient to sit quietly for a few minutes with his eyes closed. Warn him not to rub the eye because this will aggravate the abraded area.
• If the patient's eye requires a patch, tell him the length of time the patch may be needed.
• Advise the patient to wear glasses, goggles, or safety glasses when working.

Home care instructions

• Teach the patient how to correctly apply the antibiotic ointment by pulling down the lower lid and applying the ointment along the entire length of the conjunctival sac. Warn against touching the tip of the tube to the eye or lid.
• Show the patient how to apply an eye patch. Explain that the patch is a comfort measure that will be necessary only for 24 hours.
• Tell the patient to contact the doctor if his eye pain doesn't decrease in 24 hours or if his vision deteriorates.
• Tell the patient to contact his ophthalmologist if he notices increased redness of the eye, discharge from the eye, blurred vision, or photophobia.
• Instruct the patient to wear sunglasses for comfort.

FRACTURE REDUCTION, CLOSED

Closed fracture reduction is manual manipulation of a fractured bone into alignment without breaking the skin barrier. A closed reduction should be attempted as soon as possible because swelling, which tends to increase for 6 to 12 hours after injury, can inhibit adequate reduction. After alignment is achieved, the method of maintaining it may include casting, splinting, percutaneous pinning, or traction.

Because complete anatomical reduction is virtually impossible without actually visualizing the bone, an open reduction with internal fixation may be necessary after a closed reduction has been attempted.

The advantage of a closed reduction is that the skin barrier remains intact. The fracture site therefore is less likely to develop infection, osteomyelitis, or delayed union; local tissue damage also is kept to a minimum.

Maintaining alignment after closed reduction can be achieved by several different methods: Casting and splinting stabilize the joint above and below the fracture; traction maintains alignment by creating a continuous pull on the limb to hold the fragmented ends in place and decrease muscle spasms; and percutaneous pinning involves inserting a pin below the skin surface and using wire to maintain alignment.

Purpose
• To realign a fractured bone while keeping the skin over the site intact.

Indications
Closed reduction of a fracture may be indicated when the bone is displaced and can be realigned with external manipulation.

Procedure

After radiologic assessment of the fracture, the orthopedic surgeon manually manipulates the site to align the distal fragment to the proximal fragment of the fractured bone. This is achieved by applying pressure to the long axis of the bone and reversing the mechanism that initiated the fracture. Because the main obstacle to achieving adequate reduction is muscle spasm, the patient usually receives analgesia or anesthesia. X-rays are repeated throughout the procedure to assess alignment of the bone.

Complications

The usual complication of closed reduction is increased bleeding into the tissue around the fracture site caused by the manipulation of the bone. Specific complications are associated with each method of maintaining alignment. With percutaneous pinning, there is the potential for infection at the insertion sites. The use of skin traction may result in an excoriated area when the adhesive tape is removed. Casting is associated with several complications: pressure ulcers may form from either the initial trauma or folds in the case padding, compartment syndrome may result from increased intracompartmental pressure and insufficient space within the cast to accommodate edema, and joint stiffness may result from immobilization of the joints above and below the fracture.

Care considerations

• Elevate the extremity and apply ice to decrease swelling.
• Perform neurovascular checks to assess for any compromise of nerve or blood flow.
• Assess the placement of traction and the integrity of the cast or splint. Observe for increased drainage on the cast or splint, which may indicate bleeding and impending shock.

• Assist the patient with activities of daily living as needed.
• Administer prescribed pain medication to keep the patient comfortable. Teach diversion techniques as needed.
• Change the patient's position every 2 hours to ease muscle fatigue and relieve pressure point areas.
• Massage pressure point areas to minimize skin breakdown.

Home care instructions

• Instruct the patient to keep the cast or splint dry to prevent its deterioration.
• Teach the patient how to do range-of-motion exercises to keep joints flexible and maintain muscle tone.
• Discuss pain management, and instruct the patient on the correct use of prescribed analgesics, including possible adverse reactions.
• Tell the patient to report any change in sensation of the affected extremity (numbness or tingling), fever, increased drainage or pain, or a change in temperature of the affected extremity.
• Arrange referral for physical therapy to maintain muscle strength.

FRACTURE REDUCTION, OPEN

Open fracture reduction is the surgical restoration of the normal position and alignment of bone fragments or a dislocated joint. It is followed by insertion of internal fixation devices—pins, screws, nails, wires, rods, or plates—to maintain positioning until healing occurs. When closed reduction of a fracture or dislocation is impossible or inadvisable, open reduction and internal fixation may be necessary.

This procedure is most often performed in adults and adolescents. It's usually avoided in children because the handling of bones and placement of fixation devices can disrupt normal epiphyseal closure and interfere with bone growth and development.

Timing is critical to the success of this operation. Best results are obtained when the bones are set and fixation performed as soon as possible after injury, before the bones have had a chance to set improperly. If necessary, skeletal traction may precede open reduction and fixation to reduce severe muscle spasm and help realign grossly angulated fracture fragments or dislocations. Typically, a cast or splint is applied after surgery to immobilize the injury site and aid healing. If severe tissue damage accompanies fracture or dislocation, application of a cast may be contraindicated and skin or skeletal traction may be used instead.

Purpose
• To restore normal alignment to bone segments and maintain positioning during healing with screws, rods, pins, plates, or other fixation devices.

Indications
Open reduction with internal fixation is indicated for compound fractures, comminuted fractures (with the bone shattered into three or more fragments), impacted fractures (with one bone fragment), or a fracture or dislocation that has caused serious nerve or circulatory impairment.

Procedure
With the patient under general anesthesia, the surgeon makes an incision through the skin and soft tissue and spreads the muscle to expose the fragments or dislocated joint segments. Then he inserts one or more screws or another type of fixation device to immobilize the fragments in proper alignment. Next, he closes the incision and applies a cast, a splint, or traction, if necessary, to protect the surgical site and maintain alignment. (See *Reviewing internal fixation methods*, page 314.)

Complications
Potential complications associated with open reduction and internal fixation include infection, hypovolemia, compartment syndrome, and fat embolism. A patient with a severe open fracture of a large bone, such as the femur, is at particular risk for hypovolemic shock. Fat embolism is a potentially fatal complication that follows the release of fat droplets from the bone marrow or the release of catecholamines after trauma, which mobilizes fatty acids. Fat emboli can lodge in the lungs or the brain. They typically develop within 24 hours after a fracture but may be delayed up to 72 hours.

Care considerations
Before the procedure
• Immobilize the fracture site, if appropriate, to reduce pain and swelling.
• Prepare the patient for X-rays to visualize the fracture.
• Control bleeding in a severe fracture by applying direct pressure and administering fluid or blood products to prevent hypovolemia.
• Observe for complications such as compartment syndrome, which can develop within 6 hours of injury. Be alert for intense cramping pain, extreme muscle tension, and swelling in the fracture area, as well as numbness, erythema, and loss of pulse in the limb.
• Administer narcotic analgesics, sedatives, and prophylactic antibiotics as ordered preoperatively.
• Briefly explain the procedure to the patient as time permits.
• Restrict food after midnight on the night before surgery.
After the procedure
• Provide routine cast care postoperatively, and observe for drainage, foul odors, and signs of skin irritation. Report any of these signs, which may indicate infection.
• Monitor the patient's vital signs.
• Begin antibiotic therapy as ordered to prevent or treat infection.

Reviewing internal fixation methods

Choice of a specific fixation device depends on the location, type, and configuration of the fracture.

In a trochanteric fracture, the surgeon may use a hip pin or nail with or without a plate. A pin or plate with extra nails stabilizes the fracture by approximating the bone ends at the fracture site.

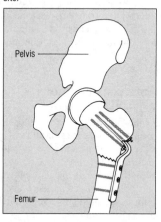

In an uncomplicated fracture of the femoral shaft, the surgeon may use an intramedullary rod, as shown. This device permits early ambulation with partial weight bearing.

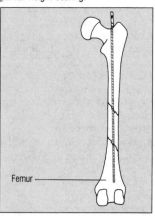

Another choice for fixation of a long-bone fracture is a screw plate, shown here on the tibia.

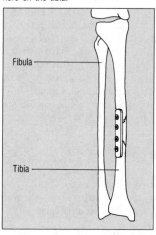

In an arm fracture, the surgeon may fix the involved bones with a plate, rod, or nail. Most radial and ulnar fractures may be fixed with plates, whereas humeral fractures may be fixed with rods.

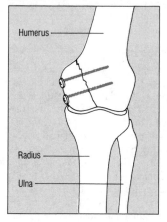

• Maintain the affected body part in proper alignment, and, if possible, support and elevate it to reduce swelling and the risk of circulatory impairment. Check for and report signs of impaired circulation in distal areas: skin mottling or discoloration and numbness, tingling, or coldness in the extremities. Such complications may require cast adjustment.

• If the patient has suffered a major fracture that requires long-term immobilization with traction, reposition him often to prevent pressure ulcers and enhance comfort. Encourage coughing and deep-breathing to prevent pulmonary complications and adequate fluid intake to prevent urinary stasis and constipation.

• As instructed by the doctor or physical therapist, assist with active or passive range-of-motion exercises to prevent muscle atrophy and contractures. Encourage the patient to get out of bed and move about as soon as possible after surgery; assist with ambulation as necessary.

• Be alert for signs of possible hypovolemic shock: hypotension; narrowed pulse pressure; tachycardia; decreased level of consciousness (LOC); rapid and shallow respirations; and cold, pale, and clammy skin.

• Watch for signs of fat embolism: diaphoresis, cyanosis, and a characteristic petechial rash on the patient's chest and shoulders associated with a decreased LOC, apprehension, fever, dyspnea, or overt seizure activity.

Home care instructions

• Review prescribed activity restrictions with the patient. Focus on weight-bearing restrictions for the affected limb. As appropriate, demonstrate correct use of crutches.

• Encourage compliance with prescribed physical therapy to maintain muscle tone and promote mobility.

• Instruct the patient to watch for and report signs of wound infection, including fever, fatigue, increased pain at the incision site, redness, purulent drainage, or separation of wound edges.

• Inform the patient that pain in the affected bone may persist for several months; advise him to take analgesics as prescribed.

• If the patient is discharged with a cast in place, make sure he understands all aspects of cast care. Tell him to watch for signs of skin irritation around the cast edges and to report severe irritation, foul odor, or discharge. Also instruct him to immediately report signs of impaired circulation, such as numbness or coldness. Warn him against getting the cast wet or inserting objects under it to scratch itching skin.

• If the patient is discharged with a removable splint, teach him how to apply and remove the device.

• To promote healing, instruct the patient to maintain a balanced diet with generous amounts of protein, calcium, and vitamin C, and tell him to drink plenty of fluids.

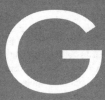

GALLBLADDER SURGERY

Gallbladder surgery is the removal of the gallbladder or gallstones in patients with gallbladder or biliary duct disease that fails to respond to drug therapy, dietary changes, and supportive treatments. Surgery is necessary to restore biliary flow from the liver to the small intestine.

Cholecystectomy is surgical removal of the gallbladder. It is typically performed along with common bile duct exploration to treat cholecystitis (inflammation of the gallbladder) and cholelithiasis (gallstones). The third most commonly performed surgery in the United States, cholecystectomy can relieve symptoms in roughly 95% of patients with gallstone disease. In the remaining 5% of patients and in those who aren't considered good candidates for this surgery, cholecystostomy or choledochotomy may be performed.

If the patient's condition contraindicates general anesthesia, cholecystostomy can be performed under local anesthesia. A catheter is inserted into the gallbladder to drain and decompress it and thereby control the disease without removing gallstones. For such patients, a cholecystectomy can be done later when the patient's condition improves.

Biliary obstruction may require duct resection and either cholecystoduodenostomy (joining the gallbladder to the duodenum) or cholecystojejunostomy (joining the gallbladder to the jejunum).

Laparoscopic cholecystectomy is rapidly gaining favor in this country. Some experts estimate that by the end of the 1990s, laparoscopic procedures will replace about 80% of traditional abdominal surgeries.

Extracorporeal shock-wave lithotripsy is an alternative procedure that utilizes a computer and an ultrasound monitor along with a shock-wave generator (lithotriptor), which fragments the gallstones until they are small enough to pass through the biliary system.

Relative contraindications to laparoscopic cholecystectomy are acute pancreatitis and cholecystitis, a history of abdominal (gastric) surgery with resultant scar tissue, and extreme morbid obesity (because available instruments aren't long enough). Absolute contraindications include severe acute cholecystitis with empyema, jaundice, portal hypertension, and pregnancy.

Purpose

• To correct biliary tract obstruction and restore biliary flow from the liver to the small intestine.

Indications

Gallbladder surgery is performed most frequently for patients with cholecystitis and cholelithiasis, and less frequently for patients with cancer of the gallbladder. Other indications include gallstone pancreatitis, symptomatic (bleeding) gallbladder polyps, a nonfunctioning gallbladder, gallstones in patients with sickle cell disease, gallstones that are larger than 3 cm even if they are asymptomatic, and a calcified gallbladder.

Procedure

After the patient receives general anesthesia (local anesthesia for a cholecystostomy), the surgeon will make an abdominal incision and remove the gallbladder in one of several ways. (See *Understanding gallbladder surgeries*, pages 318 and 319.) After completion of the surgery and, if necessary, implantation of a T tube, the surgeon removes blood and debris from the abdomen, closes the incision, and applies a dressing.

Complications

Although complications of gallbladder surgery are relatively rare, they can be serious. Peritonitis, for instance, may occur from obstructed biliary drainage and resultant leakage of bile into the peritoneum. Postcholecystectomy syndrome, marked by fever, jaundice, and pain, may occur. And, as in all abdominal surgeries, postoperative atelectasis may result from hampered respiratory excursion.

Complications associated with laparoscopic cholecystectomy include injury to adjacent structures (such as the bowel or bladder, blood vessels, or the bile duct) as well as hemorrhage, sepsis, and biliary peritonitis.

Care considerations

Before surgery
• Explain the planned surgery. Inform the patient about the purpose of and care associated with any tubes that may be in place after surgery, including a nasogastric (NG) tube, abdominal drain, or T tube.
• Teach the patient how to perform coughing and deep-breathing exercises. Tell him that an analgesic can be administered before these exercises to relieve discomfort.
• Ensure that the patient or a responsible family member has signed a consent form.

• Monitor and, if necessary, help stabilize the patient's nutritional status and fluid balance. Such measures may include administering vitamin K, blood, or dextrose and protein supplements.

After surgery
• When the patient returns from surgery, place him in low Fowler's position. As ordered, attach the NG tube to low intermittent suction. Monitor the amount and characteristics of drainage from the NG tube as well as from any abdominal drains. Check the dressing frequently and change it as necessary.
• If the patient has a T tube in place, frequently assess the position and patency of the tube and drainage bag. The drainage bag should be level with the abdomen to allow controlled drainage and prevent excessive drainage.
• Also note the amount and characteristics of T-tube drainage; Bloody drainage or blood-tinged bile typically occurs for only the first few hours after surgery. Subsequently, bile will be clear yellow. Provide meticulous skin care around the tube insertion site to prevent irritation.
• After a few days, expect to remove the NG tube and begin to introduce foods: first liquids, then soft solids. As ordered, clamp the T tube for 1 hour before and 1 hour after each meal to allow bile to enter the intestine and to aid digestion.
• Be alert for signs of complications, especially obstructed bile drainage. For several days after surgery, monitor vital signs and record intake and output every 8 hours.
• Assist the patient with ambulation on the first postoperative day, unless contraindicated. Have him cough, deep-breathe, and perform incentive spirometry every 4 hours; as prescribed, provide analgesics to ease discomfort during these exercises. Assess respiratory status every 3 hours to detect hypoventilation and signs of atelectasis.

(Text continues on page 320.)

Understanding gallbladder surgeries

Gallbladder surgeries include cholecystectomy and several less commonly performed procedures.

Cholecystectomy and common bile duct exploration
Performed under general anesthesia, this surgery begins with a right subcostal or paramedial incision. The surgeon then surveys the abdomen and uses laparotomy packs to isolate the gallbladder from the surrounding organs. After biliary tract structures have been identified, cholangiography or ultrasonography may help identify gallstones. Using a choledoscope, the surgeon directly visualizes the bile ducts and inserts a Fogarty balloon-tipped catheter to extract biliary tract stones.

The surgeon ligates and divides the cystic duct and artery, removes the entire gallbladder, and typically inserts a T tube into the common bile duct to compress the biliary tree and prevent bile peritonitis during healing. A small sump drain is sometimes inserted to drain the suphepatic space.

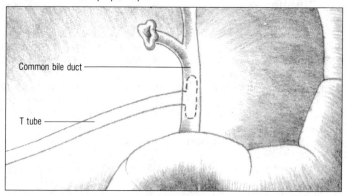

Cholecystoduodenostomy or cholecystojejunostomy
In these procedures, performed under general anesthesia, the surgeon makes a right subcostal incision and anastomoses the gallbladder to the duodenum or jejunum. These bypass procedures prevent further jaundice from an obstruction in the distal end of the common bile duct.

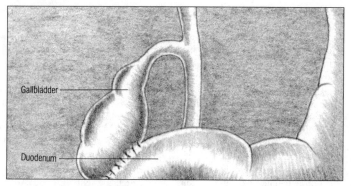

Cholecystostomy

After administering a local anesthetic, the surgeon inserts a trocar with suction through a small incision in the fundus of the gallbladder to decompress and aspirate the gallbladder and, using forceps, removes any retained gallstones or inflammatory debris. A large tube drain is inserted into the gallbladder and secured with pursestring sutures. Usually an emergency procedure, cholecystostomy is indicated when bile flow is completely obstructed, empyema or rupture is suspected, or the patient is a poor surgical risk. This procedure typically controls pain and fever sufficiently so that a cholecystectomy can be performed later.

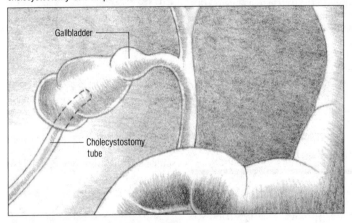

Choledochotomy

This procedure includes an incision into the common bile duct for exploration and re-moval of stones or other obstructions. It does not usually require T-tube implantation. Instead, the duct is irrigated and closed.

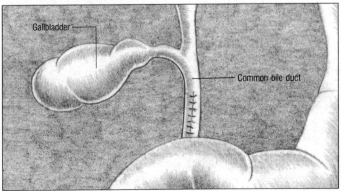

• The patient who has had a laparo-scopic cholecystectomy will be discharged the next day if there are no complications.

Home care instructions

• If the patient is being discharged with a T tube in place, emphasize the need for meticulous tube care.
• Tell the patient to immediately report any signs of biliary obstruction: fever, chills, tremors, jaundice, pruritus, pain, dark urine, and clay-colored stools.
• Instruct the patient to maintain a diet low in fats and high in carbohydrates and protein. Explain that as bile flow to the intestine increases, so will the ability to digest fats; when this happens, typically within 6 weeks, fats may gradually be added to his diet.
• Stress the importance of keeping follow-up appointments.

GASTRIC LAVAGE

Gastric lavage involves flushing the stomach and removing ingested substances through a nasogastric (NG) tube. It requires intubation with a large-bore single- or double-lumen tube, instillation of irrigating fluid, and aspiration of gastric contents.

Gastric lavage with ice water or iced 0.9% sodium chloride solution is an emergency treatment for GI hemorrhage caused by peptic ulcer disease or ruptured esophageal or gastric varices. In some cases, continuous irrigation and the use of a vasoconstrictor such as norepinephrine may be used to control the bleeding.

Some experts question the effectiveness of using an iced irrigant for gastric lavage to treat GI bleeding. The iced irrigating solutions stimulate the vagus nerve, which triggers increased hydrochloric acid secretion. In turn,

this stimulates gastric motility, which can irritate the bleeding site.

Some clinicians prefer using unchilled 0.9% sodium chloride solution (which may prevent rapid electrolyte loss) or water if the patient must avoid sodium. No research data supports the use of chilled irrigant to stop acute GI bleeding.

Correct NG tube placement is essential for patient safety because accidental misplacement (in the lungs, for example) followed by lavage can be fatal.

Purpose

• To flush the stomach to remove ingested substances
• To control upper GI hemorrhage.

Indications

Gastric lavage may be used with tepid or iced water or with 0.9% sodium chloride solution to treat patients with gastric or esophageal bleeding associated with esophageal varices or peptic ulcer. It is also used to treat poisoning or drug overdose, especially in patients with central nervous system depression or an inadequate gag reflex.

Gastric lavage is contraindicated after ingestion of a corrosive substance (such as lye, ammonia, or mineral acids) because the NG tube may perforate the already compromised esophagus.

Procedure

Gastric lavage is performed in an emergency department or intensive care unit by a doctor, a specialist such as a gastroenterologist, or a nurse; the wide-bore lavage tube is almost always inserted by a gastroenterologist. After the tube is inserted and correct placement has been verified, the irrigating solution is instilled into the stomach and then removed by either a double inflow and outflow tube setup or by a bulb syringe. The irrigating procedure is continued until the return fluid is clear, indicating that the bleeding has stopped or the harmful substances have been removed. On completion of therapy, the tube is removed or secured, as ordered.

Complications

Complications of iced gastric lavage are rare but may be serious if untreated. The most common complication is vomiting of gastric fluids and subsequent aspiration. Other complications include fluid overload, electrolyte imbalance, or metabolic alkalosis, which are especially likely in elderly or debilitated patients. Bradyarrhythmias may result from vagal stimulation and lowered body temperature.

Additionally, with the use of large-bore tubes, excessive aspiration pressure may cause damage to gastric mucosa.

Care considerations

Before therapy

• Explain the therapy to the patient or his family. Warn that he may experience some discomfort during intubation, but reassure him that the procedure isn't usually painful. Stress the importance of his relaxation and cooperation during treatment.
• Assemble the necessary equipment at the patient's bedside. Make sure a suction machine with catheter is available and that emergency equipment is available in case of airway obstruction caused by vomiting or excessive oral secretions.
• Place the patient in high Fowler's position, and help him relax. If he's wearing dentures, remove them.
• If iced lavage is ordered, chill the irrigating solution in a basin of ice.

During therapy

• If the doctor has ordered a vasoconstrictor added to the irrigating fluid, wait for a prescribed time before withdrawing the fluid to allow the drug to be absorbed into the gastric mucosa.
• Carefully measure and record fluid return, and document the character of the aspirate. Abdominal distention and

vomiting will occur if the volume returned doesn't at least equal the amount of fluid instilled. If it doesn't, reposition the tube. If this doesn't increase return, stop lavage and notify the doctor.
• Never leave the patient alone during gastric lavage. Observe continuously for developing complications, such as vomiting and aspiration.
• If you must restrain the patient during the procedure, avoid restraining him in a "spread eagle" position so that he can turn and avoid aspiration if vomiting occurs.
• Suction the patient's mouth as necessary to prevent aspiration and airway obstruction.
• When aspirating stomach contents for ingested poisons, be sure to save the contents in a labeled container to send to the laboratory for analysis.
• If ordered after lavage to remove poisons or drugs, mix charcoal tablets with the irrigant (whether it's water or 0.9% sodium chloride solution) and administer the solution through the NG tube.
• Obtain serum electrolyte or arterial blood gas levels (or both), as ordered, during or at the end of the lavage if the patient has large volumes of fluids instilled and withdrawn.

After therapy

• Continue to monitor vital signs every 30 minutes until the patient's condition stabilizes. Stay alert for bradyarrhythmias, hypothermia, and signs of hypovolemia, such as hypotension and an increased respiratory rate.
• Watch for other indicators of fluid volume deficit: decreased level of consciousness, dry skin and mucous membranes, and poor skin turgor. As appropriate, provide I.V. fluid replacements or blood transfusions to correct any volume deficit.

Home care instructions

• The patient who undergoes gastric lavage is discharged only after his condition has stabilized and doesn't require treatment-related instructions for home care.

GASTRIC RESECTION

Gastric resection can take various forms, depending on the location and extent of the disorder. Names of gastric surgeries (other than vagotomy) usually refer to the stomach portion removed. A partial gastrectomy (removal of the stomach) may be performed to reduce the amount of acid-secreting mucosa lining the stomach. A vagotomy may be performed to relieve ulcer symptoms by eliminating vagal nerve stimulation of gastric secretions. A pyloroplasty may be performed to improve drainage and prevent obstruction. Most commonly, gastric resection combines two procedures, such as vagotomy with gastroenterostomy or vagotomy with antrectomy.

Gastric resection for cancer depends on the extent of tumor involvement. For example, an antral lesion may be treated with antrectomy with Billroth I or Billroth II anastomosis. Tumors in the proximal part of the stomach or other extensive tumors (such as linitis plastica) may be treated with total gastrectomy with splenectomy. The spleen is also removed because the splenic lymph nodes are a major site of metastasis. A Roux-en-Y esophagojejunostomy is performed to restore the alimentary tract. The alternative, formation of a Hunt-Lawrence pouch (gastric pouch from the intestine) to act as a food reservoir, is less favorable because of immediate complications.

For cancer of the cardia, the distal esophagus is resected, as is the proximal stomach and spleen. An anastomosis of the esophagus to the distal stomach depends on how much of the stomach is resected. A palliative resection may be performed if the tumor is obstructing the pylorus or the patient is elderly, but most resections are

curative. Overall 5-year survival rate after gastric resection for cancer is about 12%.

Purpose
• To control an upper GI bleeding site by repairing the vessel or removing a bleeding lesion
• To excise areas of gastric ulceration or cancer
• To reduce acid secretion by removing portions of the gastric mucosa or severing vagal innervation
• To relieve gastric obstruction.

Indications
Gastric resection may be necessary to remove diseased tissue and prevent recurrence of ulcers if the disease doesn't respond to drug and dietary therapy and rest. Gastric resection may also be used to excise cancer or relieve an obstruction. In an emergency, it may be performed to control severe GI hemorrhage resulting from a perforated ulcer. Additionally, gastric resection may be performed to remove foreign bodies or gastric polyps (if they cannot be removed endosurgically).

Procedure
With the patient under general anesthesia, the surgeon will make an abdominal incision to expose the stomach and part of the intestine. Total gastrectomy, the removal of the entire stomach, requires a more extensive incision.

The rest of the procedure varies depending on the type of surgery. (See *Understanding common gastric surgeries*, pages 324 and 325, for descriptions of these and other gastric surgeries.) To complete the operation, the surgeon inserts abdominal drains, closes the incision, and then applies a dressing.

Complications
Gastric surgery carries a risk of serious complications, including hemorrhage, obstruction, paralytic ileus, vitamin B_{12}

deficiency, anemia, atelectasis, chronic gastroparesis (delayed emptying of the stomach contents), and dumping syndrome (see *Dumping syndrome*). Alkaline gastritis can result from reflux of duodenal contents on gastric or esophageal mucosa; duodenal stump leakage can occur after a Billroth II anastomosis.

Care considerations
Before surgery
• Preoperative preparation depends on the nature of surgery. If emergency surgery is necessary, preparation may be limited to immunohematologic studies and measures to control acute hemorrhage.
• Patients with gastric outlet obstruction may require several days' preparation to correct dehydration and fluid and electrolyte imbalance and to clean out residual gastric contents by nasogastric (NG) suction or gastric lavage.
• Before planned surgery, evaluate and stabilize the patient's fluid and electrolyte balance and nutritional status. Monitor intake and output, and draw serum samples for hematologic studies. As prescribed, begin I.V. fluid replacement and parenteral nutrition.
• On the night before surgery, administer cleansing laxatives and enemas as necessary.
• As time permits, discuss and describe postoperative care with the patient, including the insertion of an NG tube or indwelling urinary catheter. Be sure to explain the need for postoperative deep-breathing exercises and coughing to prevent pulmonary complications.
• To ease anxiety, explain that successful surgery should allow a near-normal life with few activity restrictions.
• Discuss how surgery will affect the patient's diet. Explain that an I.V. line will be in place for several days after surgery and that oral feeding will gradually resume, starting with clear

---

Dumping syndrome

After gastric resection, rapid emptying of gastric contents into the small intestine produces dumping syndrome.

Early dumping syndrome, which may be mild or severe, occurs a few minutes after eating and lasts up to 45 minutes. Onset is sudden, with nausea, weakness, sweating, palpitations, dizziness, flushing, borborygmy, explosive diarrhea, and increased blood pressure and pulse rate.

Late dumping syndrome, which is less serious, occurs 2 to 3 hours after eating. Symptoms include profuse sweating, anxiety, fine tremor of the hands and legs accompanied by vertigo, exhaustion, lassitude, palpitations, throbbing headache, glycosuria, and marked decrease in blood pressure and blood sugar.

These symptoms may persist for 1 year after surgery or for the rest of the patient's life.

---

liquids and progressing slowly to solid foods. After extensive gastric resection, parenteral nutrition may continue for a week or longer.
• Ensure that the patient or a responsible family member has signed a consent form.

After surgery
• After the patient has recovered from anesthesia, place him in low or semi-Fowler's position – whichever is more comfortable. Either position will ease breathing and prevent aspiration if vomiting occurs.
• Check the patient's vital signs every 2 hours until his condition stabilizes. Watch especially for hypotension, bradycardia, and respiratory changes, which may signal hemorrhage and shock. Periodically check the wound site, NG tube, and abdominal drainage tubes for bright red blood.

Understanding common gastric surgeries

Besides treating chronic ulcers, gastric surgeries help remove obstructions and cancer. Names of gastric surgeries (other than vagotomy) usually refer to the stomach portion removed. Most procedures combine two types of surgery.

Vagotomy with pyloroplasty
In this procedure, the surgeon resects the vagus nerves and refashions the pylorus to widen the lumen and aid gastric emptying.

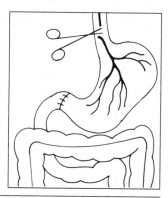

Vagotomy with antrectomy
After resecting the vagus nerves, the surgeon removes the antrum. Then he anastomoses the remaining stomach segment to the jejunum and closes the duodenal stump.

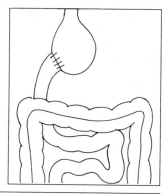

Vagotomy with gastroenterostomy
In this procedure, the surgeon resects the vagus nerves and creates a stoma for gastric drainage. He'll perform selective truncal or parietal cell vagotomy, depending on the degree of decreased gastric acid secretion required.

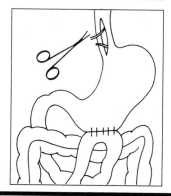

Understanding common gastric surgeries *(continued)*

Billroth I
In this partial gastrectomy with a gastroduodenostomy, the surgeon excises the distal third to half of the stomach and anastomoses the remaining stomach to the duodenum.

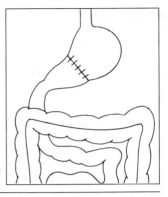

Billroth II
In this partial gastrectomy with a gastrojejunostomy, the surgeon removes the distal segment of the stomach and antrum. Then he anastomoses the remaining stomach and the jejunum and closes the duodenal stump.

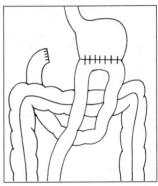

• Maintain parenteral nutrition and I.V. fluid and electrolyte replacement therapy as appropriate.
• Take care not to move the position of the NG tube because of its proximity to suture lines.
• Monitor blood studies daily. Watch for signs of dehydration, hyponatremia, and metabolic alkalosis, which may result from gastric suctioning. Weigh the patient daily; monitor and record intake and output, including NG tube drainage.
• Auscultate the patient's abdomen daily for the return of bowel sounds. When they return, the doctor will order clamping or removal of the NG tube and gradual resumption of oral feeding. During tube clamping, watch for nausea and vomiting; if they occur, unclamp the tube immediately and reattach it to suction.
• Throughout recovery, encourage the patient to cough, deep-breathe, and change position frequently. Provide incentive spirometry, as necessary. Assess breath sounds frequently to detect atelectasis.
• Assess for other complications, including vitamin B_{12} deficiency anemia (especially common in patients who have undergone total gastrectomy) and dumping syndrome, a potentially serious digestive complication marked by

weakness, nausea, flatulence, and palpitations that occur within 30 minutes after a meal.

Home care instructions

• Instruct the patient to call the doctor immediately if he develops nausea, vomiting, or pain because these may indicate possible life-threatening complications, such as hemorrhage, obstruction, or perforation.
• Instruct the patient about the possibility of vitamin B_{12} deficiency, and tell him to promptly report any fatigue, numbness, tingling of the extremities, and any other central nervous system changes to the doctor.
• Explain dumping syndrome and ways to avoid it. Advise the patient to eat small, frequent meals at regular intervals throughout the day; to chew food thoroughly and drink fluids *between* meals, not *with* meals; to decrease intake of carbohydrates and salt while increasing fat and protein; and to lie down for 20 to 30 minutes after a meal.
• If the doctor has prescribed a histamine-2 receptor antagonist, such as cimetidine, to reduce gastric acid secretion, instruct the patient to take the drug 30 minutes to 1 hour before meals.

GOLD COMPOUNDS

Gold compounds slow the degenerative course of arthritis and may even induce remission.

Three gold compounds are used for treating arthritis: *aurothioglucose* and *gold sodium thiomalate*, which are administered I.M., and *auranofin*, a recently developed oral compound. All three drugs are equally effective, but auranofin appears to be the least toxic.

Treatment with gold salts can only prevent additional damage to bone and cartilage; it doesn't repair existing damage. Therefore, gold therapy is most beneficial in the early stages of disease before irreversible joint changes have occurred. Beneficial effects develop slowly. Some patients experience improvement after 6 weeks of therapy; others, after 6 months.

Purpose

• To reduce inflammation in rheumatoid arthritis.

Indications

Gold compounds serve as antirheumatic agents for both juvenile and adult rheumatoid arthritis. Less commonly, they're used to treat psoriatic arthritis.

Gold compounds shouldn't be used in patients with blood dyscrasias, uncontrolled diabetes, compromised cerebral or cardiovascular circulation, colitis, renal or liver disease, urticaria, eczema, or a hypersensitivity to gold or the heavy metals.

Adverse reactions

Adverse reactions to gold therapy range from mild effects to potentially life-threatening complications. Short-term effects include anaphylaxis and arthralgia; adverse reactions after long-term use may include stomatitis, metallic taste, dermatitis, and GI upset (especially with auranofin). The most common adverse reaction is diarrhea. Rarely, blood dyscrasias, hepatitis, renal impairment, encephalopathy, and pulmonary complications occur.

Care considerations

• Before beginning treatment with gold compounds, obtain a baseline complete blood count and urinalysis. Throughout therapy, monitor these studies to detect blood dyscrasias, proteinuria, or hematuria.
• Review the patient's medication regimen for possible interactions. Concurrent use of penicillamine can cause severe hematologic and renal effects.
• If the patient will be receiving I.M. injections, record their location so that

sites can be rotated. After injection, tell the patient to lie down for 10 to 20 minutes. During this period, observe for signs of anaphylaxis and ask the patient if he's experiencing joint pain. If so, notify the doctor.

Home care instructions

• Tell the patient to be alert for toxic effects, which may occur at any time during therapy or even several months after its discontinuation. The patient should call his doctor immediately if he experiences pruritus (a sign of emerging dermatitis), shortness of breath, a metallic taste (a sign of impending stomatitis), coughing, unusual bleeding or bruising, nausea, vomiting, diarrhea, or abdominal pain.

• Warn the patient that arthralgia may occur for 1 to 2 days after an injection, but explain that this reaction usually disappears after the first few injections.

• Tell the patient that the benefits of therapy may not be apparent for 6 weeks or longer. Instruct him to record the date that he first notices any relief from stiffness and pain or improvement of joint function.

• Warn the patient that gold compounds may predispose to mouth ulcers and a sore throat. To help forestall these problems, tell him to brush his teeth and use a mouthwash after every meal.

• Urge the patient to avoid exposure to sunlight, which can worsen gold-induced dermatitis.

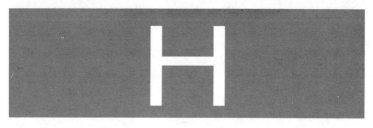

Harrington Rod

The Harrington rod is a form of spinal instrumentation that involves the surgical placement of one or two (twin) metal rods to straighten or stabilize the spine through internal fixation. (See *Types of spinal instrumentation*.) This rigid instrument contains hooks that attach to the vertebral laminae at designated levels above and below the curvature.

The major advantage of using the Harrington rod is its longstanding proven reduction of lateral curvatures of the spine. Other advantages include the relative simplicity of application and a low rate of neurologic complication. A major disadvantage is that it requires prolonged postoperative casting. Like other spinal implants, the Harrington rod is contraindicated in patients who have significant osteoporosis. (For more information about another technique, see the entry "Cotrel-Dubousset Spinal Instrumentation.")

Purpose

• To maintain alignment of the vertebrae after a fusion of the spinal column.

Indications

Indications for Harrington rod placement include a spinal curvature too severe for correction by a brace, an angle of the spinal column greater than 60 degrees, or conditions for which a brace is not a feasible alternative.

Harrington rod spinal instrumentation is the standard treatment for scoliosis. The rod may be used for correction of other deformities such as kyphoscoliosis, thoracic kyphosis, or lumbar lordosis. It is also used for metastatic spinal tumors, thoracolumbar spine injuries, and spondylolisthesis.

Procedure

Using a posterior approach, the orthopedic surgeon places the Harrington rod in the concavity of the spinal curve from the lowest to the highest vertebra to be fused and bends it to conform to the curvature. The rod is attached to the vertebral column by placing the upper hook in the thoracic facet joint and the lower hook over the laminar edge at the lowest vertebra to be fused. The rod then becomes fixed in two areas and may be used on both sides of the vertebral column. The rod maintains alignment, which allows the bone grafts to heal and the vertebra to fuse solidly. Immediately postoperatively, the patient is placed in a Risser cast for 6 months and afterward uses a brace for another 3 to 6 months, depending on his healing ability.

Complications

Complications after placement of a Harrington rod may include pain, inflammatory reaction (due to a foreign body), local wound infection, and meningeal infection.

Surgical intervention may be required if the spinal attachments holding the rods move or if the instrumentation breaks or requires repair. Prolonged use of the body cast or brace or surgical intervention may be necessary if the bone grafts, required for cor-

Types of spinal instrumentation

Review the selected spinal instrumentation systems described here. Explain the procedure fully, and be prepared to support the patient and his caregivers through a long recovery period.

Luque rod instrumentation

The surgeon uses Luque rod instrumentation (LRI) for patients with neuromuscular curves. Unlike Harrington rod instrumentation, LRI rods are custom-contoured and are segmentally fixated with sublaminar wires that are threaded at each vertebral level. An advantage of LRI is that postoperative casting and bracing are avoided. The main disadvantage is a higher neurologic risk because wires must be threaded under the vertebral laminae near the neural elements.

Harri-Drummond instrumentation

Harri-Drummond instrumentation (HDI) uses a Harrington rod on the concave side of the curve and a contoured Luque rod on the convex side. It achieves the segmental fixation capabilities of the Luque rod without increasing the incidence of neural complications. A disadvantage of HDI is the need for postoperative casting or bracing.

Cotrel-Dubousset instrumentation

This technique involves placing a series of rods and hooks to distract, compress, and derotate the spine. Cross-linking devices provide further stability. Tell the patient that this apparatus can be adapted to normal sagittal spinal alignment and lumbar lordosis. Because the surgeon attaches it to many points, the patient may not need to wear a brace after the operation.

Zeilke instrumentation

Similar to Cotrel-Dubousset instrumentation in construction and function, Zeilke instrumentation may be used alone or combined with the second stage of the operation to treat a double spinal curve. Advise the patient that he may have to wear a brace for about 7 months after this surgery.

The Kaneda device

This is a new type of spinal instrumentation. It provides a treatment option for thoracolumbar burst fracture. It addresses such potential problems of spinal injury as the treatment of bone fragments in the spinal canal and repair of anterior decompression of the spine followed by posterior fusion with extensive surgery.

rection of the curvature, do not unite solidly. Although the risk of neurologic complications is low with Harrington rod placement, all spinal surgery carries some risk of neurologic deficit and paralysis.

Care considerations

Before surgery

• Explain the procedure to the patient. Provide an opportunity for an adolescent patient to speak with a contemporary who has undergone the same procedure to minimize fear and anx-

iety about the surgery and postoperative casting.
• Perform a preoperative neurologic evaluation.
• During the preoperative period the patient may be in halo femoral traction or an upper body cast to stretch contracted muscles and will need assistance with activities of daily living.
• Perform neurovascular checks every 4 hours or according to hospital policy to assess circulation.
• Clean the skin thoroughly to prevent infection at pressure points and pin sites of traction.

• Offer pain medication, as prescribed, to diminish discomfort.

• X-rays will be required to assess spinal and respiratory status.

• As appropriate, obtain urinalysis and blood studies to monitor for infection and provide a preoperative baseline.

• Intermittent positive-pressure breathing treatments should be given every 4 hours postoperatively to enhance respiratory function and loosen secretions.

• Give the patient an enema to clear the lower bowel.

• Insert an indwelling urinary catheter.

After surgery

• On the 1st postoperative day, maintain the patient in flat position and log-roll him every 2 hours to decrease pressure on bony prominences.

• Gradually increase activity as recommended by the doctor and as tolerated. Encourage self-care and range-of-motion exercises for arms and legs.

• Offer pain medications, as prescribed, to diminish discomfort and antibiotics to prevent infection.

• Continue to perform frequent neurovascular checks to assess circulation.

• Instruct the patient about coughing and deep-breathing as well as use of an incentive spirometer, if available.

• Reinforce the dressing as needed, and document any continued or increased drainage.

• Observe for return of normal bowel function by auscultating for bowel sounds. Monitor for flatus and abdominal distention to determine advancement in diet.

• Start the patient on clear liquids, and advance his diet as tolerated to prevent nausea and vomiting.

Home care instructions

• Tell the patient to expect confinement in a Risser body cast for 6 months, followed by a brace for 3 to 6 months. The patient can increase physical activity after the cast is removed but must avoid contact sports and gymnastics.

• Instruct the patient and family about placement of the brace and the necessity for wearing it, and teach cast care and complications.

• Inform the patient that muscle aches and pains will decrease with increased activity.

• Warn the patient against sudden position changes.

• Instruct the patient and family about consumption of a well-balanced diet to expedite bone growth, muscle strength, and return to normal bowel function.

• Tell the patient and family to notify the doctor of fever over 101° F (38.3° C) that persists longer than 24 hours; increased pain, redness, swelling, or drainage; or numbness or tingling of extremities.

HEARING AIDS

A hearing aid is an electronic device that, when placed in the ear, improves hearing in individuals with certain types of hearing loss. Powered by a replaceable battery, a hearing aid consists of a microphone, an amplifier, a receiver, and an ear mold. The microphone picks up sound and converts it to electrical energy. The amplifier magnifies this energy electronically, and the receiver converts it back to sound waves, which the ear mold directs into the patient's ear.

Four types of hearing aid are commonly available: behind-the-ear, eyeglass, in-the-ear, and body aids. A behind-the-ear hearing aid, the most commonly used type, consists of a short curved plastic tube that connects the unit (which rests behind the ear) to an acrylic ear mold. In an eyeglass hearing aid, a similar unit, the components are contained in the eyeglass temple. An in-the-ear hearing aid, the most compact device, consists of a single piece fashioned like an ear mold, which houses the microphone, amplifier, and receiver. A body hearing aid, most suitable for the patient with severe or profound hearing loss or with limited manual dexterity, has a larger microphone, amplifier, and power supply than the other types of hearing aid and produces less distortion. It's built into a case that can be clipped to the patient's pocket or worn on the body. A long wire connects the unit to an ear mold.

A bone-conduction aid, which delivers sound waves to the mastoid process, may be used when an acrylic mold can't be inserted into the patient's ear. This aid comes in all styles, including the eyeglass type.

An estimated 22 million Americans with hearing disorders wear some sort of hearing aid. Other hearing "aids" are available, including amplified telephone receivers, flashing lights instead of doorbells and telephones that ring, vibrators that respond to sound, headphones for television sets, and teletypewriters.

Purpose
• To amplify sound for persons with hearing loss.

Indications
Hearing aids are indicated for hearing dysfunction. They are used to treat the sensorineural hearing loss caused by presbycusis, an otologic effect of aging that results from a loss of hair cells in the organ of Corti.

Procedure
Typically, an audiologist administers hearing tests and, after determining the type and extent of hearing loss, selects the appropriate hearing aid. The hearing aid is placed in position and the patient is instructed about its use.

Complications
Hearing aids are usually beneficial and have few disadvantages. The body hearing aids pick up the sound of the patient's clothing rubbing against his body. Behind-the-ear hearing aids eliminate this problem but are less durable and more prone to acoustic feedback. All hearing aids require a period of adjustment because the patient may hear background noises that he hasn't heard in years. All types that depend on batteries require that the patient keep an extra supply of batteries on hand.

Care considerations
Before therapy
• Reinforce the audiologist's explanation of the hearing aid and its use.
• Advise the patient that the device will improve hearing but will require some adjustment to the amplification. Initially, the patient may find background noise, such as traffic or the chirping of birds, uncomfortably loud.
During therapy
• Encourage consistent use of the hearing aid at the prescribed setting.
• Advise the patient to increase amplification, if necessary, to improve hearing.

Home care instructions
• Encourage the patient's family to encourage his adjustment to the hearing aid. Instruct them to be patient and to speak in a normal voice. They should get the patient's attention before speaking and, if possible, eliminate background noise. They should repeat messages, if necessary, and reword them.
• Teach the patient how to use the hearing aid's on-off switch and volume control and how to change the battery.
• Tell the patient to store the hearing aid in a dry place when he's not using it and to avoid getting it wet. Have him inspect the unit daily for a cracked case, corroded battery contacts, frayed wires, or an occluded ear mold. Except for an in-the-ear hearing aid, the ear mold can be cleaned with warm, soapy water after disconnection from the unit.

• Warn the patient against applying hairspray when wearing the aid because it may damage the microphone. Also warn against inserting sharp objects, such as needles or pencil points, into the unit.

• Inform the patient about organizations that offer help for the hearing-impaired, such as the Alexander Graham Bell Association for the Deaf. Also help him obtain additional devices, such as a loop system to clarify sound on the television set, a coupler for the telephone to improve clarity, and a battery tester.

• If the hearing aid seems to be malfunctioning, instruct the patient and family to check the battery first, if appropriate. Instruct the patient to contact the audiologist or hearing-aid dealer if the hearing aid continues to malfunction.

• Teach the patient to routinely check the ears for excessive earwax, which may muffle sounds. If the patient has excessive earwax, his ears may have to be irrigated by a doctor or nurse.

HEART SURGERY FOR CONGENITAL DEFECTS

Congenital heart defects vary in severity. Mild defects allow children to grow normally without surgical intervention. However, most congenital heart defects eventually require surgical repair, usually during infancy or childhood. Corrective surgery and its timing depend on the type and extent of the defect. Recent advances in technology allow repair of certain smaller congenital heart defects in a cardiac catheterization laboratory instead of in an operating room.

Congenital heart defects are classified as acyanotic or cyanotic. In children with acyanotic defects, unoxygenated blood does not enter the systemic circulation; in those with cyanotic defects, unoxygenated blood enters the bloodstream. The prognosis for repair of acyanotic defects is excellent; prognosis is good for cyanotic defects but depends on the size of the defect and prompt detection of the problem. (See *Reviewing common congenital heart defects*.)

Purpose

• To improve blood flow and subsequent oxygenation of tissues by surgical or catheter-based correction of congenital heart defects.

Indications

Surgical correction is indicated for those congenital heart defects that cause inadequate oxygenation, failure to thrive, and poor quality of life; it is sometimes recommended for asymptomatic defects. For example, coarctation of the aorta requires correction because it causes persistent hypertension with a risk of further complications, such as intracranial hemorrhage, aortic aneurysm, and endocarditis of the aortic and mitral valves.

The incidence of congenital heart defects is slightly less than 1%. Infants at high risk for congenital heart defects include those with Down's syndrome, Turner's syndrome, and Holt-Oram syndrome. Certain defects, such as patent ductus arteriosus, may result from intrauterine rubella.

Procedure

Before surgical repair of a congenital heart defect, the patient will have a thorough diagnostic workup, which includes a physical examination, detailed family history, and diagnostic tests (chest X-ray, electrocardiogram [ECG], echocardiogram, and usually cardiac catheterization).

A specialized surgeon performs the procedure, which depends on the type, size, and location of the defect. Such procedures require general anesthesia and intensive postoperative care. The

Reviewing common congenital heart defects

DEFECT	PATHOPHYSIOLOGY
Ventricular septal defect	One or more abnormal openings in the ventricular septum allow shunting of blood from the left to the right ventricle. This defect results from incomplete closure of the ventricular septum by the 8th week of gestation; it varies in size from a pinhole to complete absence of the entire septum. This defect causes recirculation of some oxygenated blood through the lungs, which may lead to congestive heart failure (CHF).
Atrial septal defect	One or more openings between the left and right atria (includes ostium secundum, ostium primum, and sinus venosus) allows shunting of blood left to right between the chambers. This defect results from delayed or incomplete closure of the foramen ovale or atrial septum. Small defects are usually asymptomatic and may be undetected in children; they may lead to CHF and pulmonary vascular disease in adults.
Patent ductus arteriosus	A patent ductus arteriosus between the pulmonary artery bifurcation and the descending aorta allows left-to-right shunting of blood from the aorta to the pulmonary artery, resulting in recirculation of arterial blood through the lungs. This defect is caused by failure of the ductus to close after birth; it may produce no clinical effects initially, but eventually can cause CHF, pulmonary vascular disease, and infective endocarditis.
Coarctation of the aorta	Constriction of the aorta, usually below the left subclavian artery near the junction of the ligamentum arteriosum and pulmonary artery. The defect is often classified as preductal (above the ligamentum arteriosum) or postductal (below it) and may result from spasm and constriction of smooth muscle in ductus arteriosus during normal closure or from abnormal development of the aortic arch. The defect causes altered perfusion pressure.
Tetralogy of Fallot	A complex of four defects: ventricular septal defect, overriding aorta, pulmonary stenosis, and right ventricular hypertrophy. Blood shunts from right to left through the ventricular septal defect, permitting mixing of unoxygenated and oxygenated blood and causing cyanosis. The defect is caused by incomplete development of the ventricular septum and pulmonary outflow tract.
Transposition of the great arteries	Reversal of normal position of the great arteries; the aorta arises from the right ventricle and the pulmonary artery from the left ventricle, producing two noncommunicating circulatory systems. Unoxygenated blood flows through the right atrium and ventricle and out the aorta to systemic circulation; oxygenated blood circulates through the left side of the heart and back to the lungs. It results from faulty embryonic development (mechanism unknown).

following brief descriptions review treatment of the most common congenital heart defects.

For a small *ventricular septal defect,* close monitoring is recommended because many such small defects close spontaneously. For a medium-to-large defect, medical therapy includes oxygen, digoxin, diuretics, antibiotics to prevent infective endocarditis, and fluid restrictions for acute congestive heart failure (CHF). Surgical correction of medium to large ventricular septal defects closes the septal defect by suturing or by covering it with a Dacron patch. This surgery requires cardiopulmonary bypass.

Medical management for the symptomatic patient with an *atrial septal defect* is similar to that for a patient with a ventricular septal defect. Surgical correction usually occurs during the preschool years. Again, depending on its size, the defect is closed by sutures or by placement of a Dacron patch. This surgery requires cardiopulmonary bypass.

Medical therapy for *patent ductus arteriosus* involves treatment of CHF. Administration of indomethacin is about 80% effective in closing the duct in premature infants. Surgical correction is performed between ages 1 and 2. Repair of a patent ductus arteriosus requires a thoracotomy approach. The ductus is divided in two, and the divided ends are litigated.

Surgical repair of *coarctation of the aorta* is performed in all symptomatic infants and in asymptomatic children at age 4. This defect can be corrected by a thoracotomy approach, and resection and anastomosis; occasionally, it is treated by tubular vascular prosthesis.

Medical intervention for *tetralogy of Fallot* relieves cyanosis with knee-to-chest positioning; administration of oxygen, morphine, and possibly propranolol; and prophylactic antibiotics to prevent endocarditis. Because te-

tralogy of Fallot causes numerous clinical problems, surgical management depends on the patient's signs and symptoms; its purpose is to enhance pulmonary circulation and relieve hypoxia. Corrective surgery to relieve pulmonary stenosis and close the ventricular septal defect can be performed on a neonate or older child.

For *transposition of the great vessels,* medical management includes treatment of CHF and prevention of infective endocarditis. The current trend supports surgical repair of transposition of the great arteries before age 12 months. Surgery (Mustard operation or Senning operation) attempts to redirect venous return to the appropriate ventricle.

Complications

Surgical repair of heart defects can cause severe complications, including cardiogenic shock, CHF, hypoxemia, hypercapnea, arrhythmias (particularly heart block), cerebrovascular accident (CVA), renal insult, pulmonary embolism, hypotension, hemorrhage, cardiac tamponade, and cardiac arrest. As in any surgical procedure, infection poses a constant threat. Neonates are also particularly susceptible to alterations in thermoregulation after such surgery.

Care considerations
Before surgery
• Unless the congenital heart defect is completely nonthreatening, the infant should be examined every 1 to 2 weeks for the first 6 weeks of life to monitor for complications such as CHF.
• Help the child and his family cope with their anxieties by providing comprehensive preoperative teaching and emotional support with careful explanations of all treatments and diagnostic procedures.
• Adjust explanations to the child's level of understanding.

• To help decrease postoperative anxiety, prepare the child and his family for the sights and sounds of the intensive care unit (ICU). Tell them about expected I.V. lines, monitoring equipment, and endotracheal and chest tubes. If possible, arrange for them to meet the ICU staff. Encourage them to ask questions and express their concerns.

• Prepare the child, and have him practice an alternative method of communication (pointing to pictures, using a writing pad) to use during ventilation.

• Make sure that the patient fasts 6 to 8 hours before surgery.

• Ensure that the parents have signed a consent form.

After surgery

• The patient awakening from anesthesia will be anxious when confronted with the tubes, monitors, and alarms of the ICU. Help decrease his anxiety by speaking in a soft, soothing voice and by touching the child gently. Encourage the parents to visit as much as possible.

• Monitor the patient's hemodynamic status. Watch particularly for severe hypotension, decreased cardiac output, and shock.

• Monitor vital signs every 15 minutes until they are stable, then as frequently as ordered.

• Frequently evaluate the child's peripheral pulses, capillary refill time, and skin temperature and color, and auscultate heart sounds. Notify the doctor of any abnormalities.

• Evaluate tissue oxygenation by monitoring breath sounds, pulse oximetry, chest excursion, and symmetry of chest expansion. Check the child's arterial blood gas levels every 2 to 4 hours, and adjust ventilator settings as needed.

• Monitor the ECG for alterations of heart rate and rhythm, such as bradycardia, ventricular tachycardia, and heart block. Such disturbances may result from myocardial irritability or ischemia, fluid and electrolyte imbalance, hypoxemia, or hypothermia. If you detect serious abnormalities, notify the doctor and prepare to assist with epicardial pacing.

• To ensure adequate myocardial perfusion, maintain the patient's arterial pressure within prescribed guidelines. Also monitor pulmonary artery and left atrial pressure.

• Maintain chest tube drainage at the prescribed negative pressure. Maintain patency of chest tubes.

• Monitor regularly for hemorrhage and excessive or insufficient drainage; keep the chest drainage system below the level of the child's heart.

• As prescribed, administer antiarrhythmics and other medications needed to maintain normal hemodynamic status.

• Carefully monitor intake and output, noting electrolyte imbalances, especially hypokalemia.

• Administer prescribed pain medication before pain becomes severe. As the patient's incisional pain increases, provide analgesics, as prescribed. Because an infant or very young child may not be able to express the degree of pain he's experiencing, watch for physiologic signs of severe pain: diaphoresis, pallor, tachycardia, elevated blood pressure, and chest splinting on inspiration.

• Be especially alert for symptoms of CVA (altered level of consciousness, pupillary changes, weakness and loss of movement in the extremities, ataxia, aphasia, dysphagia, sensory disturbances), pulmonary embolism (dyspnea, cough, hemoptysis, chest pain, pleural friction rub, cyanosis, and hypoxemia), and impaired renal perfusion (decreased urine output and elevated blood urea nitrogen and serum creatinine levels).

• After weaning the patient from the ventilator and removing the endotracheal tube, promote chest physiotherapy. Start incentive spirometry and encourage the child to cough, turn, and deep-breathe frequently. Also assist with range-of-motion exercises, as ordered, to enhance peripheral circulation and to prevent thrombus formation.

Home care instructions

• Instruct the parents to notify the doctor immediately if the child develops chest pain, fever, muscle or joint pain, or weakness.

• Warn the parents that prolonged hospitalization may cause behavioral changes and that separation anxiety and changes in dietary habits and sleep patterns may persist for some time after discharge. Encourage them to relate to their child in a loving, consistent manner and to offer the child opportunities to express feelings and concerns through conversation and play.

• Make sure the patient or parents understand the dosage, schedule, administration technique, and possible adverse effects of all prescribed medications. If the doctor has prescribed digoxin, emphasize the importance of reporting early signs of toxicity promptly.

• Instruct the patient or parents to inform all health care providers about the heart surgery before any dental or other surgical procedure because antibiotic prophylaxis is usually needed.

• Encourage the patient and family to take special precautions to avoid exposure to infection during flu season and other viral epidemics. The patient may need prophylactic antibiotics and influenza immunization.

• Teach the parents how best to meet the child's special nutritional needs.

• Inform parents about requirements for rest and activity restrictions.

• Stress the importance of regular checkups to monitor health status.

HEART TRANSPLANTATION

The first heart transplantation in the United States was performed in 1968. This complex procedure replaces a diseased heart with a donated healthy heart. (Alternatively, the diseased heart may be replaced with an artificial heart—a more controversial procedure.) The donor patient must be certified as brain dead and screened for cardiac abnormalities and terminal illnesses. Preferably, male donors should be younger than age 35 and female donors should be younger than age 45. Because of improvements in technique and immunosuppressant therapy (notably cyclosporine), the number of heart transplantations performed is steadily increasing. Its use is limited largely by its high cost and the scarcity of donor hearts.

Transplantation may represent the only means available to prolong a patient's life, but it is by no means a certain cure.

Purpose

• To restore cardiac function in patients with end-stage cardiac disease.

Indications

Heart transplantation is limited to patients with end-stage cardiac disease. It offers a valid treatment for survival after more conservative medical or surgical therapies have failed. Candidates for heart transplantation must meet several strict criteria, including previous medical compliance and emotional stability.

Most candidates for this surgery have severe coronary artery disease with widespread left ventricular dysfunction caused by myocardial infarction and associated fibrosis. Others have idiopathic hypertrophic subaortic stenosis, myotonic muscular dystrophy, or cardiomyopathy caused by viral infection.

Clinical conditions that contraindicate heart transplantation include irreversible pulmonary hypertension, severe peptic ulcers, unresolved pulmonary embolism, acute infection, carcinoma, severe hepatic or renal dysfunction, or insulin-dependent diabetes. Patients with irreversible pulmonary hypertension may be candidates for heart-lung transplantation. Relative contraindications to heart transplantation include advanced age, extreme cachexia, and mental disability.

Procedure

The two methods of heart transplantation are orthotopic and heterotopic transplantation. In orthotopic transplantation, the recipient's heart is removed and the donor heart is implanted in its place by connecting (anastomosing) its left and right atria to the remnants of the recipient's atria. In heterotopic transplantation, the recipient's heart is left in place; the donor heart is positioned to the right of the recipient's heart and the left of the right atria, aorta, and pulmonary artery. Presently, the orthotopic approach is preferred.

A specialized surgeon performs the heart transplantation while the patient is under general anesthesia. The donor heart must continue beating when it is removed from the brain-dead donor because severe physiologic damage can result after 20 to 30 minutes of anoxia. Immunosuppressant therapy to prevent or delay rejection of the donor heart begins preoperatively and continues into the postoperative period.

Complications

Serious postoperative complications of heart transplantation include infection and tissue rejection; most transplant recipients can expect to experience one or both of these complications. Rejec-

tion, caused by the patient's immune response to foreign antigens from the donor heart, usually occurs within the first 6 weeks after surgery. It's treated with potent immunosuppressants, such as azathioprine, corticosteroids, and cyclosporine – sometimes in massive doses. However, the resulting immunosuppression leaves the patient vulnerable to potentially life-threatening infection.

Other postoperative complications resemble those associated with any open-heart surgery. Among them are pulmonary embolism, impaired renal perfusion, hemodynamic compromise, cerebrovascular accident (CVA), and such pulmonary complications as pneumonia and failure to wean from mechanical ventilation. Psychological problems also are common after heart transplantation and include depression, mood alterations, increased stress, difficulty returning to work, alterations in body image, and problems with compliance; such complications may occur during initial hospitalization or later during recovery.

Care considerations

Before surgery

• Provide emotional support for the patient and family on the waiting list for a donor heart; this waiting period is stressful. Provide emotional support to the heart donor's family as they deal with the donor's death.

• Discuss the procedure, possible complications, and the impact on the lives of the patient and his significant others.

• Explain that transplantation requires prolonged recovery, which may cause changes in family functioning.

• Encourage the patient and family to ask questions, and refer them to psychological counseling as necessary.

• Make sure the patient and family understand that heart transplantation doesn't guarantee a life free from medical problems and that it requires life-long follow-up care.

• Explain what to expect before surgery, including food and fluid restrictions and the need for intubation and mechanical ventilation. Prepare the patient and family for the sights and sounds of the recovery room and intensive care unit. If possible, arrange for a tour of these facilities and an opportunity to meet the staff.

• Describe postoperative isolation procedures, if ordered, and the tests used to detect tissue rejection and other complications. Explain the expected immunosuppressant regimen necessary to combat rejection.

• Ensure that the patient or a responsible family member has signed a consent form.

After surgery

• Maintain reverse isolation as required by the hospital's protocol (typically for 1 to 2 weeks).

• Administer immunosuppressants, as ordered. These drugs typically mask obvious signs of infection. Watch for more subtle signs, such as fever above 100° F (37.8° C). Expect to administer prophylactic antibiotics, and maintain strict asepsis when caring for incision and drainage sites.

• Assess for signs of hemodynamic compromise, such as severe hypotension, decreased cardiac output, and shock. Check and record vital signs every 15 minutes until the patient's condition stabilizes and as needed.

• Monitor the patient's electrocardiogram (ECG) for disturbances in heart rate and rhythm, such as bradycardia, ventricular tachycardia, and heart block. Such disturbances may result from myocardial irritability or ischemia, fluid and electrolyte imbalance, hypoxemia, or hypothermia. Notify the doctor of any abnormalities.

• Be aware that because the recipient's atria remain in place, the patient's ECG tracing may show two P waves.

• Ensure adequate myocardial perfusion. Maintain arterial pressure within the prescribed guidelines. Usually, mean arterial pressure below 70 mm Hg results in inadequate tissue perfusion. Also monitor pulmonary artery, central venous, and left atrial pressure, as ordered.

• Evaluate peripheral pulses, capillary refill time, and skin temperature and color, and auscultate heart sounds. Notify the doctor of any abnormalities.

• Evaluate tissue oxygenation by assessing breath sounds, chest excursion, and symmetry of chest expansion. Check arterial blood gas levels every 2 to 4 hours, and adjust ventilator settings as needed to maintain them within prescribed limits.

• Maintain chest tube drainage at the prescribed negative pressure (usually −10 to −40 cm H_2O). Maintain patency of chest tubes according to hospital policy. Regularly assess for hemorrhage, excessive drainage (greater than 200 ml/hour), or sudden decrease or cessation of drainage (less than 50 ml/hr).

• As ordered, administer antiarrhythmic, inotropic, pressor, and analgesic medications as well as I.V. fluids and blood products. Monitor intake and output, and assess for hypokalemia or other electrolyte imbalances.

• Evaluate for the effects of the denervation that occurs during heart transplantation. Absence of variation in heart rate in response to changes in position, Valsalva's maneuver, or a carotid massage indicates complete denervation. The patient may be unable to feel anginal pain. Look for an elevated resting heart rate or a sinus rhythm unaffected by respirations. Remember that atropine, anticholinergics, and edrophonium may have no effect on a denervated heart and that the effects of quinidine, digoxin, and verapamil may vary.

• Watch especially for symptoms of CVA (altered level of consciousness, pupillary changes, weakness and loss of movement in the extremities, ataxia, aphasia, dysphagia, and sensory disturbances).

• After weaning the patient from the ventilator and removing the endotracheal tube, promote chest physiotherapy. Start incentive spirometry and encourage the patient to cough, turn frequently, and deep-breathe. Also assist with range-of-motion exercises, as ordered, to enhance peripheral circulation and prevent thrombus formation and other complications of prolonged immobility.

Home care instructions

• Explain that the doctor will schedule frequent (weekly to monthly) myocardial biopsies to check for signs of tissue rejection. Stress the importance of keeping these appointments, and reassure the patient that biopsy doesn't require hospitalization.

• Instruct the patient to immediately report any signs of rejection (fever, weight gain, dyspnea, lethargy, weakness) or infection (chest pain; fever; sore throat; or redness, swelling, or drainage from the incision site).

• Explain that postpericardiotomy syndrome often develops after openheart surgery. Tell the patient to call the doctor if he experiences its characteristic symptoms: fever, muscle and joint pain, weakness, and chest discomfort.

• If the patient shows signs of cardiac denervation, advise him to rise slowly from a sitting or lying position to minimize orthostatic hypotension.

• Make sure the patient knows the dose, schedule, and effects of prescribed drugs.

• Encourage the patient to follow his prescribed diet, especially noting sodium and fat restrictions.

• Instruct the patient to maintain a balance between activity and rest. Tell him to try to sleep at least 8 hours a night, to rest briefly each afternoon, and to take frequent breaks during tiring physical activity. As appropriate, tell the patient he can climb stairs, engage in sexual activity, take baths and showers, and do light housework and other chores but should avoid lifting heavy objects (heavier than 20 lb [9 kg]), driving, and work such as mowing the lawn or vacuuming until the doctor approves. Encourage the patient to follow the prescribed exercise program.

• Recommend appropriate support groups and counseling services to deal with any postoperative psychological problems, such as depression, mood alterations, and overeating.

HEART VALVE REPLACEMENT

Heart valve replacement removes a diseased or dysfunctional heart valve and replaces it with a mechanical or biological prosthesis. This procedure is often necessary in severe valvular disease when a heart valve cannot open fully, preventing the passage of blood from one heart chamber to another (valvular stenosis), or when the valve cannot fully close, allowing back flow of blood into a heart chamber (valvular insufficiency or regurgitation). Valvular heart disease most commonly affects the mitral and aortic valves because of the high pressure generated by the left ventricle.

Purpose

• To improve cardiac circulation in severe valvular disease.

Indications

Indications for heart valve replacement depend on the severity of the patient's symptoms and on the amount of damage to the affected valve. Mitral valve replacement may be required for mitral stenosis and mitral insufficiency; aortic valve replacement for

Comparing prosthetic valves

Both mechanical and biological prosthetic valves are commonly used. The mechanical valve, such as the Starr-Edwards caged-ball valve (by Baxter-Edwards), can withstand considerable stress. However, its large size makes it sometimes difficult to implant. And because blood flow is turbulent through the valve, the patient usually requires long-term anticoagulant therapy to prevent thrombus formation.

The biological prosthetic heart valve, such as the Carpentier-Edwards valve (by Baxter-Edwards), doesn't obstruct blood flow as much as a mechanical valve and is less likely to cause thrombus formation; in addition, it doesn't require prolonged anticoagulant therapy. However, this valve is difficult to insert and less durable (prone to degeneration or calcification, especially in patients with renal disease) than its mechanical counterpart. Despite these disadvantages, the surgeon will probably implant a biological prosthetic valve if the patient appears unlikely to comply with anticoagulant therapy. Other types of biological prosthetic heart valves include human and animal valves.

Starr-Edwards valve

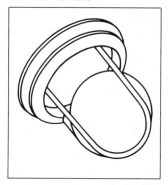

Carpentier-Edwards valve

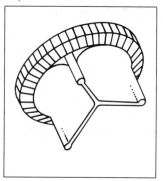

aortic stenosis and aortic insufficiency. (See *Comparing prosthetic valves*.)

Procedure

Heart valve replacement requires open-heart surgery with cardiopulmonary bypass and is performed by a surgeon who specializes in cardiology.

The surgeon performs a medial sternotomy (an opening into the chest through the sternum for access to the heart) and initiates cardiopulmonary bypass. He then exposes and excises the diseased heart valve. Next, the surgeon sutures around the margin of the valve annulus (ring area around the

valve that is left intact when the valve is removed), threading the sutures through the sewing ring of the prosthetic valve, positions a valve holder in place, and secures the sutures to hold the prosthetic valve in correct position. When the new valve is securely in place, he disconnects the patient from cardiopulmonary bypass, restarts the heart, inserts a chest tube and mediastinal tube, closes the incision, and applies a sterile dressing.

Complications

Valve replacement surgery carries a low mortality rate but can cause serious complications. Hemorrhage may result from unligated vessels, anticoagulant therapy, or coagulopathy from cardiopulmonary bypass during surgery. Cerebrovascular accident (CVA) may result from thrombus formation due to turbulent blood flow through the prosthetic valve or from poor cerebral perfusion during cardiopulmonary bypass. Bacterial endocarditis can develop within days of implantation or months later. Valve dysfunction or failure may occur as the prosthetic device wears out. Other complications include pulmonary embolism and impaired renal perfusion.

Care considerations

Before surgery

• Reinforce the doctor's explanation of the procedure and listen to the patient's and family's concerns. Encourage them to ask questions. Tell the patient he'll awaken from surgery in an intensive care unit (ICU) or recovery room. If appropriate, arrange a preoperative tour of the ICU so the patient will not be unduly frightened by his surroundings after surgery.

• Mention to the patient that he'll be connected to a cardiac monitor and have I.V. lines, an arterial line and, possibly, a pulmonary artery or left atrial catheter in place. Explain that he'll breathe through an endotracheal (ET) tube that's connected to a mechanical ventilator and will have a chest tube in place.

• As ordered, begin cardiac monitoring before surgery and expect to assist with insertion of an arterial line and possibly a pulmonary artery catheter.

• Ensure that the patient has signed a consent form and that necessary laboratory studies and blood typing and crossmatching have been performed.

After surgery

• Closely monitor hemodynamic status for signs of compromise. Watch especially for severe hypotension, decreased cardiac output, and shock.

Check and record vital signs every 15 minutes and as needed until the patient's condition stabilizes.

• Frequently monitor heart sounds; report distant heart sounds or new murmurs, which may indicate prosthetic valve failure.

• Monitor the electrocardiogram for disturbances in heart rate and rhythm, such as bradycardia, ventricular tachycardia, and heart block. Such disturbances may point to injury of the conduction system, which may occur during valve replacement because of the proximity of the atrial and mitral valves to the atrioventricular node. Postoperative arrhythmias may also result from myocardial irritability or ischemia, fluid and electrolyte imbalance, hypoxemia, or hypothermia. Notify the doctor of any abnormalities, and be prepared to assist with temporary epicardial pacing.

• To ensure adequate myocardial perfusion, maintain mean arterial pressure within the prescribed guidelines. For adults, this range is usually between 70 and 100 mm Hg. Also monitor pulmonary artery and left atrial pressure, as ordered.

• Frequently check the patient's peripheral pulses, capillary refill time, and skin temperature and color, and auscultate for heart sounds.

• Evaluate tissue oxygenation by monitoring breath sounds, chest excursion, and symmetry of chest expansion. Report any abnormalities.

• Check arterial blood gas levels every 2 to 4 hours, and adjust ventilator settings as needed.

• Maintain chest and mediastinal tube drainage at the prescribed negative pressure (usually -10 to -40 cm H_2O for adults). Maintain chest tube patency, and assess regularly for hemorrhage, excessive drainage (more than 200 ml/hour), and sudden decrease or cessation of drainage (less than 50 ml/hour).

• As prescribed, administer analgesic, anticoagulant, antibiotic, antiarrhythmic, inotropic, and pressor medications as well as I.V. fluids and blood products, and note patient response.

• Monitor intake and output, and assess for electrolyte imbalances, especially hypokalemia. Evaluate the effectiveness of anticoagulant therapy by monitoring partial thromboplastin time or prothrombin time daily.

• Observe the patient carefully for complications throughout the recovery period. Watch especially for symptoms of CVA (altered level of consciousness, pupillary changes, weakness and loss of movement in the extremities, ataxia, aphasia, dysphagia, and sensory disturbances), pulmonary embolism (dyspnea, cough, hemoptysis, chest pain, pleural friction rub, cyanosis, and hypoxemia), and impaired renal perfusion (decreased urine output and elevated blood urea nitrogen and serum creatinine levels).

• After weaning the patient from the ventilator and removing the ET tube, promote chest physiotherapy. Start incentive spirometry and encourage the patient to cough, turn frequently, and deep-breathe. Gradually increase the patient's activities, as appropriate.

Home care instructions

• Teach the patient how to care for the sternal incision. Tell him to immediately report chest pain; fever; or redness, swelling, or drainage at the incision site.

• Tell the patient to notify the doctor about symptoms of possible valve problems: fatigue, dyspnea, irregular heart rate, palpitations, and dizziness.

• Explain that postpericardiotomy syndrome – fever, muscle and joint pain, weakness, and chest discomfort – often develops after open-heart surgery. Tell the patient to report these symptoms to the doctor.

• Make sure the patient understands the dosage, schedule, and adverse effects of all prescribed drugs. Advise him to wear a medical identification bracelet and carry a card with information and instructions about his anticoagulant and antibiotic therapy.

• Encourage the patient to follow the prescribed diet, noting especially sodium and fat restrictions.

• Offer suggestions for maintaining a balance between activity and rest: to try to sleep at least 8 hours a night; to schedule a short rest period each afternoon; and to rest frequently during tiring physical activity. As appropriate, tell him he can climb stairs, engage in sexual activity, take baths and showers, and do light housework and other chores, but should avoid lifting heavy objects (more than 20 lb [9 kg]), driving a car, or doing heavy work (such as mowing the lawn or vacuuming) until his doctor approves. Encourage the patient to follow a prescribed exercise program.

• Instruct the patient to inform the dentist or any other doctors about the prosthetic heart valve before undergoing any invasive procedures because prophylactic antibiotics are usually needed. Such procedures, including dental work, are usually delayed for 6 months after surgery.

• Warn the patient that he may experience postoperative depression, which may begin after he's discharged. Reassure him that such depression is usually temporary.

• Encourage the patient to keep follow-up medical appointments.

HEAT TREATMENTS

Applying heat directly to a patient's body raises tissue temperature and enhances inflammation by causing vasodilation, increasing nutrition to the cells, and facilitating the elimination of waste products, such as bradykinin, histamine, and prostaglandins, from muscle. Heat increases local circulation and tissue metabolism, reduces pain, provides comfort by promoting muscle relaxation, and decreases congestion in deep visceral organs. It also raises the pain threshold of sensory nerve endings and thus may break the pain-spasm-pain cycle with its analgesic effects. Heat increases the extensibility of connective tissue, thereby preparing stiff joints and tight muscles for activity.

Heat treatments can be superficial or deep. Superficial heat can be applied in many forms, such as *chemical hot packs, paraffin, heat lamps, hot-water bottles, heat pads,* and *warm packs,* and can be moist or dry. Dry heat can be delivered at a higher temperature and for a longer time. Moist heat penetrates more deeply than dry heat, doesn't dry the skin, produces less perspiration, and is usually more comfortable for the patient.

Deep-heat treatments include *ultrasonography* and *diathermy.* Ultrasonography directs sound waves that are absorbed by various tissues and converted into heat energy. Diathermy uses high-frequency electric current. Both ultrasonography and diathermy penetrate deeply and significantly elevate tissue temperature. They are valuable for delivering heat to injured soft tissue such as muscle. Ultrasonography is currently used more often than diathermy, but both modalities can be useful.

Purpose

• To relieve pain and stiffness, relax muscles, increase range of motion, and promote tissue healing.

Indications

Heat treatments are commonly used to treat muscle spasms and arthritis and to restore mobility after muscle or joint injury or surgery. They may also be used as an adjunct to other therapies.

Heat treatments should be used cautiously in patients with sensory impairment, heat intolerance, or impaired renal, cardiac, or respiratory function. Patients with impaired arterial or venous circulation have a decreased ability to dissipate heat effectively, thereby reducing their tolerance and increasing the risk of heat-induced injury. Ultrasound heat treatments should be not be applied over the heart, eye, or a pregnant uterus.

Because heat causes vasodilation, it is contraindicated in bleeding disorders and should be avoided after traumatic injury. It should be used with caution in steroid-dependent patients because of increased capillary fragility. Deep-heat therapy shouldn't be used in patients with metal implants because of the risk of local tissue damage.

Procedure

Superficial heat treatments may be self-administered or provided by a physical therapist or technician.

With chemical hot packs, the size and shape of the pack used depends on the area being treated. The packs are made of canvas and contain a heat-sensitive chemical. Towels are wrapped around the packs before they are applied. The pack is then placed on the patient. (The patient should not lie on the pack to avoid overheating of skin.) The pack is removed when it becomes cool.

Paraffin wax is melted and mixed with mineral oil and then maintained at a temperature between 118.4° and 131° F (48° and 55° C). The patient's hands or feet are then dipped in and out of the paraffin tank 8 to 10 times to form a solid coating. Then, a plastic bag and toweling are wrapped around the part to retain heat. When the paraffin is cool, it is removed.

With a heat lamp, the heat output is determined by the wattage and the distance of the lamp from the area being treated. For most cases, allow 14″ (35 cm) between the bulb and the patient's skin for a 25-watt bulb, 18″ (46 cm) for a 40-watt bulb, and 24″ to 30″ (61 to 76 cm) for a 60-watt bulb. Only one body part should be heated at a time, and the lamp should be turned off after

10 to 15 minutes for the first treatment and after 20 to 30 minutes for subsequent treatments.

Hot-water bottles are filled one-half to two-thirds full with water that has been heated to 115° to 125° F (46.1° to 51.7° C). The bottle is covered with an absorbent protective cloth and applied to the area to be heated.

Heat pads may be moist or dry. The temperature should not exceed 131° F (55° C). The pad should not be left on the patient longer than 20 to 30 minutes unless ordered.

A warm pack may be nonsterile material, such as an absorbent towel or a few abdominal pads. Soak the towel or pads in water that has been heated to 131° F (55° C), and apply them to the affected area. Cover with a hot-water bottle or chemical hot pack to maintain the temperature.

Deep-heat treatments require specially skilled personnel and equipment.

Ultrasound therapy is delivered to the patient through a transducer. A coupling medium, such as mineral oil, water, or a commercial ultrasound gel, is applied to the area to be heated and then the ultrasound transducer is applied and activated. Ultrasound heat treatments typically last 5 to 10 minutes.

Diathermy supplies heat through a cable electrode. A layer of toweling is placed between the patient's skin and the coils that are wrapped around the desired body part.

Complications

Any of the superficial heat treatments can cause redness, blistering, burns, maceration, or vasoconstriction of the treated area if it is exposed to excessive heat or the treatment is continued too long (over 45 minutes).

Care considerations
Before therapy
• For superficial heat treatments, explain the purpose and effects of treatment.
• Assess the patient's pain level, activity level, circulation, and need for analgesics.
• Position the patient comfortably.
• Expose only the area to be treated.
• Assemble and check the required equipment.
• Make sure that the patient's skin is clean, dry, and free of oils and creams.
During therapy
• For ultrasound therapy, apply a coupling medium between the transducer and the patient's skin.
• Monitor the patient's skin condition every 5 minutes for signs of intolerance (excessive redness, blistering, or maceration).
• Monitor debilitated patients for cardiovascular or respiratory effects (dizziness, unconsciousness, shortness of breath, or dyspnea).
• Monitor vital signs until the patient's response to treatment is clear.
• Stay with an elderly, neurologically impaired, or confused patient during treatment, as necessary.
• Don't use an electric heating device near oxygen or near liquids (or for a patient who is incontinent).
• Avoid using safety pins to secure heating devices.
• Monitor the treated area for burns and response to treatment.
• Dry or wipe off the patient's skin as necessary.
After therapy
• Be sure to allow at least 1 hour between treatments to avoid vasoconstriction.
• Assess the patient's response to therapy and the effectiveness of therapy.

Home care instructions
• If the patient will be performing heat treatments at home, provide clear in-

structions and have him demonstrate the correct technique.

• Teach the patient safety measures, such as checking equipment carefully before use. Caution him against lying or sleeping on or near the heating device to prevent burns. Also instruct him to secure the device with gauze – never with safety pins; heated metal can cause burns or electric shock. Warn him against exposing electrical heating devices to water because of the risk of electric shock.

• Instruct the patient to follow the doctor's orders precisely for the duration and frequency of treatment and not to alter treatment.

• Tell the patient to check his skin every 5 minutes during treatment. (Sensory-impaired patients should be especially cautious.) He should report any unusual redness or blistering to the doctor. Also have him report any increase in pain or skin breakdown.

HEMODIALYSIS

Hemodialysis removes toxic wastes and other impurities from the blood of a patient with renal failure. This potentially lifesaving procedure removes blood from the body, circulates it through a purifying dialyzer, and then returns the blood to the body. The underlying mechanism in hemodialysis is differential diffusion across a semipermeable membrane, which extracts byproducts of protein metabolism, such as urea and uric acid, as well as creatinine and excess water.

Various access sites can be used for dialysis (see *Hemodialysis access sites*, pages 346 and 347). The most common access device for long-term treatment is an arteriovenous (AV) fistula.

For those patients who have fluid overload but do not require hemodialysis, continuous AV hemofiltration is

---

Continuous arteriovenous hemofiltration

A relatively new procedure, continuous arteriovenous hemofiltration (CAVH) is used to treat patients who have fluid overload but don't require dialysis. CAVH filters fluid, solutes, and electrolytes from the patient's blood and infuses a replacement fluid.

The hemofilter, composed of about 5,000 hollow fiber capillaries, filters blood at a rate of 250 ml/minute and is driven by the patient's arterial blood pressure (a systolic blood pressure of 60 mm Hg is adequate for the procedure). Some of the ultrafiltrate collected during CAVH is replaced with filter replacement fluid. This fluid can be lactated Ringer's solution or any solution that resembles plasma. Because the amount of fluid removed is greater than the amount replaced, the patient gradually loses fluid (12 to 15 liters daily).

---

rapidly gaining acceptance (see *Continuous arteriovenous hemofiltration*).

Purpose

Hemodialysis extracts toxins, notably byproducts of protein metabolism – urea and uric acid – as well as creatinine, potassium, and excess water. It helps to restore or maintain acid-base and electrolyte balance and prevent the symptoms and complications associated with uremia.

Indications

Hemodialysis is one of the forms of dialysis indicated in end-stage renal disease, evidenced by hyperkalemia, hypervolemia, azotemia, and acidosis. (See also the entry "Peritoneal Dialysis.") Hemodialysis may be indicated in acute renal failure and less commonly in acute poisoning, such as barbiturate or analgesic overdose.

(Text continues on page 348.)

Hemodialysis access sites

Hemodialysis requires vascular access. The site and type of access may vary, depending on the expected duration of dialysis, the surgeon's preference, and the patient's condition.

Subclavian vein catheterization
Using the Seldinger technique, the surgeon inserts an introducer needle into the subclavian vein, inserts a guide wire through the introducer needle, and removes the needle. Using the guide wire, he then threads a 5″ to 12″ (12.7- to 30.4-cm) plastic or Teflon catheter (with a Y-connector) into the patient's vein.

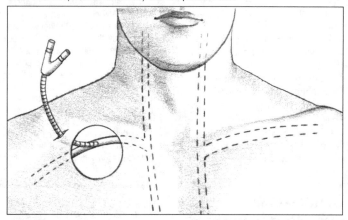

Femoral vein catheterization
Using the Seldinger technique, the surgeon inserts an introducer needle into the left or right femoral vein. He then inserts a guide wire through the introducer needle and removes the needle. Using the guide wire, he then threads a 5″ to 12″ plastic or Teflon catheter with a Y-connector or two catheters, one for inflow and another placed about ½″ (1.3 cm) distal to the first for outflow.

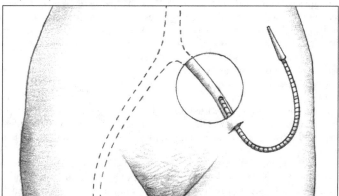

Arteriovenous fistula

To create a fistula, the surgeon makes an incision into the patient's wrist or lower forearm, then makes a small incision in the side of an artery and another in the side of a vein. He sutures the edges of these incisions together to make a common opening about 1″ to 3″ (3 to 7 cm) long.

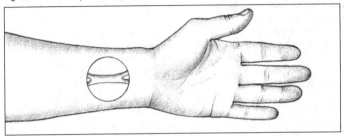

Arteriovenous shunt

To create a shunt, the surgeon makes an incision in the patient's wrist, lower forearm, or (rarely) an ankle. He then inserts a 6″ to 10″ (15.2- to 25.4-cm) transparent Silastic catheter into an artery and another into a vein. Finally, he tunnels the catheters out through stab wounds and joins them with a piece of Teflon tubing.

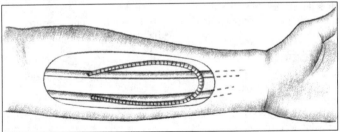

Arteriovenous graft

To create a graft, the surgeon makes an incision in the patient's forearm, upper arm, or thigh. He then tunnels a natural or synthetic graft under the skin and sutures the distal end to an artery and the proximal end to a vein.

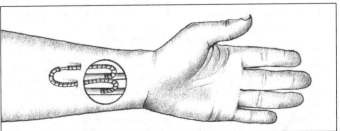

Procedure

Specially prepared personnel usually perform this procedure in a hemodialysis unit. However, if the patient is acutely ill, hemodialysis can be done at the bedside. Special hemodialysis units are also available for home use.

A surgeon creates a vascular access. The blood lines from the dialyzer are then connected to the access site. Blood samples are drawn for analysis. The hemodialysis unit is turned on at a flow rate of 90 to 120 ml/minute and, depending on the patient's condition, the flow rate is gradually increased to 300 ml/minute. Dialysis usually continues for 3 to 6 hours. At the end of the procedure, additional blood samples are drawn and the patient is disconnected from the dialysis unit.

For patients with chronic renal failure, dialysis is commonly prescribed for three times a week, 4 hours each treatment. This may vary in chronic renal failure, depending on the patient's condition and response to hemodialysis.

Complications

Common complications of hemodialysis include hypotension, nausea and vomiting, muscle cramps, and disequilibrium syndrome (rapid fluid removal and electrolyte changes can cause seizures, muscle twitching, and headache). Other complications include internal bleeding (apprehension, restlessness, clammy skin, thready pulse, increased respirations, and decreased body temperature), air embolism (dyspnea, chest pain, and cyanosis), excessive external bleeding at the vascular access site, and infection from vascular access or pathogens in the dialysate or equipment.

Care considerations

Before therapy

• Assure that the blood tubing and dialyzer have been primed and prepared according to unit policy.

• Explain the purpose and duration of treatment, associated complications, and required aftercare.

• Weigh the patient before each treatment to evaluate fluid retention.

• Monitor vital signs, including sitting and standing blood pressure.

• Place the patient in a supine position, with the vascular access site well supported.

• Recheck the prepared hemodialysis equipment and place the appropriate needles in the patient's access site, or attach tubing to the hemodialysis catheter.

• Draw required blood specimens as necessary.

• Connect patient to the dialysis unit.

During therapy

• Begin hemodialysis at a blood flow rate of 90 to 120 ml/minute.

• If heparin is being used, inject prescribed loading dose into the port of the atrial line.

• Monitor vital signs routinely. Frequently monitor blood pressure.

• Increase blood flow rate according to protocol and the patient's condition.

• Monitor closely for complications.

• Draw blood samples for clotting time as required.

• Administer 0.9% sodium chloride solution into venous return line as necessary to relieve complications associated with rapid fluid removal (extreme hypotension or rapidly falling blood pressure, muscle cramps, nausea, and vomiting).

• Notify the doctor if signs of internal bleeding, air embolism, or disequilibrium syndrome occur.

After therapy

• After hemodialysis is complete, monitor the venous access site for bleeding. If bleeding is excessive, maintain pressure on the site and notify the doctor.

• To prevent clotting or other problems with blood flow, make sure that the arm used for venous access isn't used for any other procedure, including I.V. line insertion, blood pressure

monitoring, and venipuncture. At least four times a day, assess circulation at the access site by auscultating for the bruit and palpating for the thrill (vibration).
• If the patient is treated in an outpatient dialysis center, be sure his vital signs are stable and his level of consciousness is adequate before discharge. Check for orthostatic symptoms.

Home care instructions
• Teach the patient how to care for the vascular access site: to keep the incision clean and dry to prevent infection and to clean it with hydrogen peroxide solution daily until healing is complete and the sutures are removed (usually 10 to 14 days after surgery).
• Tell the patient to notify the doctor of pain, swelling, redness, or drainage in the accessed arm. Teach correct use of a stethoscope to auscultate for the bruit (an unusual sound) and show the patient how to palpate for the thrill (vibration).
• Explain that the arm may be used freely once the access site has healed. Exercise is considered beneficial because increased blood flow stimulates vein enlargement. Remind the patient not to allow any treatments or procedures on the accessed arm, including blood pressure monitoring or needle punctures; to avoid putting excessive pressure on the arm; not to sleep on it or wear constricting clothing over it; nor to lift heavy objects or strain with it. Tell the patient to avoid showering, bathing, or swimming for several hours after dialysis.
• Make sure the patient who will be performing hemodialysis at home understands all aspects of the procedure. Give the phone number of the dialysis center, and encourage the patient to call with any questions about the treatment.
• Encourage the patient to contact the American Association of Kidney Pa-

tients or the National Kidney Foundation for additional information and support.
• Tell the patient to keep an accurate record of food and fluid intake, and encourage compliance with prescribed restrictions, such as limited protein, potassium, and sodium intake; increased caloric intake; and decreased fluid intake.

HEMORRHOIDECTOMY

Hemorrhoidectomy is the surgical removal of hemorrhoidal varicosities by cauterization or excision. Hemorrhoids are swollen or distended veins in the anorectal region that can be internal or external. Internal hemorrhoids are not visible on inspection of the anal region unless they enlarge and fall through the anal sphincter (prolapse); typically, they lie above the anal sphincter. External hemorrhoids, which lie below the anal sphincter, are visible at inspection. Patients can have either internal or external hemorrhoids or both types.

Hemorrhoids can be extremely painful, can become thrombosed or inflamed, and can bleed. They require surgical extirpation if they cause severe symptoms and conservative treatment is ineffective. Hemorrhoidectomy is performed in approximately 10% of patients with problematic hemorrhoids. Hemorrhoids can also be removed by rubber band ligation, sclerotherapy, cryosurgery, anal dilatation, and laser surgery (see *Ligating hemorrhoidal tissue*, page 350).

Although the patient is usually discharged after hemorrhoidectomy on the day of surgery, postoperative healing of delicate anorectal tissues can be slow and painful. For this reason, postoperative care focuses on measures to promote comfort and speed healing: pain control, sitz baths, frequent dress-

Ligating hemorrhoidal tissue

Large internal hemorrhoids can sometimes be removed in the doctor's office by rubber band ligation. In this surgical technique, the doctor inserts an anoscope to dilate the anal sphincter, then uses grasping forceps to pull the hemorrhoid into position. He then inserts a ligator through the anoscope and slips a small rubber band over the pedicle of the hemorrhoid to bind it and cut off blood flow. Ischemia within the hemorrhoid causes it to slough off naturally, usually within 5 to 7 days. Patients who undergo this therapy often experience a pressure sensation or the urge to void for 24 to 48 hours after the ligation. Rarely, this therapy may be complicated by pelvic sepsis.

Grasping the hemorrhoid

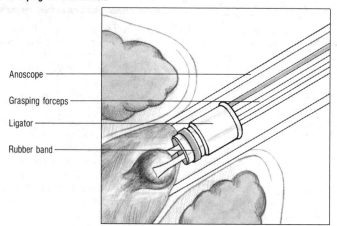

Anoscope

Grasping forceps

Ligator

Rubber band

Ligating the hemorrhoid

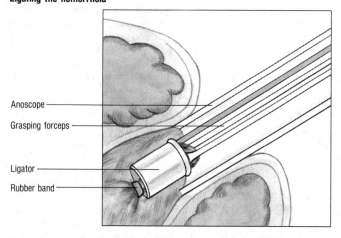

Anoscope

Grasping forceps

Ligator

Rubber band

ing changes, and maintenance of a regular elimination schedule.

Purpose

• To remove hemorrhoidal varicosities from the anus and rectum.

Indications

Hemorrhoidectomy is indicated for internal hemorrhoids that are large, that prolapse but cannot be reduced, or are associated with symptomatic external hemorrhoids and skin tags. Hemorrhoidectomy is also recommended for hemorrhoids that are ulcerated, thrombosed, gangrenous, or associated with hypertrophied papillae or fissures.

Hemorrhoidectomy is contraindicated in patients with blood dyscrasias or certain GI cancers, and during the first trimester of pregnancy because of the risk of hemorrhage.

Procedure

Hemorrhoidectomy is performed in the operating room under local, regional, or general anesthesia. After administration of anesthesia, the surgeon digitally dilates the anal sphincter, excises the hemorrhoidal tissue, and ligates the connecting blood vessels. Absorbable sutures may be used to close the incisions because this may allow faster wound healing and a lower incidence of anal stricture after surgery. The surgeon may place a small, lubricated tube in the patient's anus to drain air, fluid, blood, and flatus or may pack the area with petroleum gauze.

Complications

Complications of hemorrhoidectomy include hemorrhage, urine retention, anal stricture, and infection that can lead to abscess and development of anal skin tags. The risk of hemorrhage, the most serious complication, is greatest during the first 24 hours after surgery and then again 7 to 10 days after surgery when the sutures slough off. Mucosal prolapse can develop if excess rectal mucosa was not adequately removed during surgery. Pruritus ani can result from mucous discharge or aggressive anal hygiene. In older patients, hemorrhoidectomy sometimes requires sphincter stretching or sphincterotomy that can cause fecal incontinence.

Care considerations

Before surgery

• Explain that the surgery will remove hemorrhoids and relieve pain and bleeding.
• Explain to the patient the details of postoperative care, including frequent dressing changes and regular perianal cleaning. Reassure the patient that his privacy will be respected during these procedures.
• Prepare the patient for surgery by administering an enema (usually 2 to 4 hours before surgery) and by shaving and cleaning the perianal area, as ordered.
• Ensure that the patient or a responsible family member has signed a consent form.

After surgery

• Promote patient comfort. Pain is the most common and most severe problem after surgery. Position the patient comfortably in bed. The side-lying position is usually the most comfortable; support the patient's buttocks with pillows if necessary. Encourage the patient to shift position regularly and, if able, to assume the prone position for 15 minutes every few hours to reduce edema at the surgical site. Administer analgesics as prescribed.
• Keep alert for acute hemorrhage and hypovolemic shock. Check the dressing regularly and immediately report any excessive bleeding or drainage. After vital signs have stabilized, monitor them every 2 to 4 hours until the patient is discharged; also check and record intake and output while the patient is in the hospital. If bleeding is excessive, you may be asked to insert

a balloon-tipped catheter into the rectum and inflate it to exert pressure on the hemorrhagic area and reduce blood loss.

Home care instructions

• Tell the patient to check the dressing regularly and to report any increased bleeding or drainage immediately.
• Tell the patient that pain is most severe the first 2 days after surgery. Be sure the patient understands the medications that are ordered for pain.
• Encourage the patient to take sitz baths three to four times daily and after each bowel movement to reduce swelling and discomfort and to help maintain perineal hygiene. Teach the patient how to take a sitz bath (see the entry "Sitz Bath").
• Teach correct perianal hygiene: wiping gently with soft, white toilet paper (the dyes used in colored paper may cause irritation), cleaning with mild soap and warm water, and applying a sanitary pad.
• Encourage the patient to void within the first 24 hours after surgery. If this is a problem, he should try to stimulate voiding with measures such as massages and warm sitz baths. If these measures fail, the patient should notify the doctor.
• Tell the patient to report increased rectal bleeding, purulent drainage, fever, constipation, or rectal spasm.
• Emphasize the importance of regular bowel habits. Offer suggestions for avoiding constipation, including regular exercise and adequate intake of dietary fiber and fluids (eight to ten 8-oz glasses [1,920 to 2,400 ml] of water a day).
• Warn against overusing stool-softening laxatives. Explain that a firm stool is necessary to dilate the anal canal and prevent stricture formation.
• Tell the patient to keep follow-up appointments to check the operative site for infection and abscess formation.

HERNIA REPAIR

A hernia repair corrects the protrusion of a tissue or an organ through a weak area of tissue or muscle by herniorrhaphy or hernioplasty. Herniorrhaphy, the surgery of choice for inguinal and other abdominal hernias, returns the protruding intestine to the abdominal cavity and repairs the abdominal wall defect. Hernioplasty, used to correct more extensive hernias, reinforces the weakened area around the repair with plastic, steel, or tantalum mesh or wire.

Hernias of the abdominal wall may be inguinal, femoral, epigastric, umbilical, or incisional. Inguinal hernia, protrusion of part of the intestines through the inguinal canal (where the testicles descend to the scrotum), occurs in about 2% of adult males. Femoral hernia is protrusion of part of the intestine through the area where the femoral artery and vein pass from the abdomen to the thigh. Epigastric hernia results from a weakness in the upper abdominal muscles that allows the intestine to protrude through an area between the umbilicus (navel) and the breastbone. An umbilical hernia causes the intestine to protrude through the abdominal wall near the umbilicus. Incisional hernias may appear after surgery involving the abdominal wall.

The protruding intestine may become trapped and twisted within the hernia and its blood supply may be diminished or cut off. This condition is known as a strangulated or incarcerated hernia and can lead to gangrene if not corrected surgically.

Hernia repairs may be performed on an outpatient basis with local anesthesia. Performed as an inpatient procedure, hernia repair usually requires a hospitalization of 3 to 5 days.

Purpose
• To return herniated tissue to its original position and to repair the underlying musculofascial wall defect.

Indications
Surgical repair is indicated when the herniated tissue is painful and cannot be pushed back into place or if the intestine becomes strangulated or incarcerated, requiring emergency surgery.

Procedure
Herniorrhaphy is performed under local, regional, or general anesthesia, depending on the patient's condition. After the surgeon makes an abdominal incision, the herniated tissue is pushed back into the abdomen and the weakened area of the abdominal wall is repaired and strengthened by suturing. A large hernia may require a hernioplasty. In this procedure, the abdominal wall is reinforced with plastic, steel, or tantalum mesh or wire. After the repair, the surgeon closes the incision and applies a dressing.

Complications
Hernia repair is typically done quickly and produces few complications and minimal postoperative pain and bleeding. Recurrence occurs in 10% to 20% of repaired hernias.

Care considerations
Before surgery
• Describe the surgery and explain that it will relieve the discomfort. Assure the patient who's having outpatient surgery that recovery is usually rapid and that he may return home on the day of surgery if no complications occur.
• Ensure that preoperative laboratory work and procedures are complete.
• Ensure that the patient or a responsible family member has signed a consent form.
• Prepare the patient for surgery as ordered (by shaving the surgical site and administering a cleansing enema and a sedative).

After surgery
• Monitor vital signs until the patient is stable.
• Help the patient reduce pressure on the incision site. For example, teach the patient how to get up from a lying or sitting position without straining the abdomen and how to splint the incision when coughing or sneezing. Reassure him that coughing or sneezing won't cause the hernia to recur.
• Encourage early ambulation, but warn against bending, lifting, or other strenuous activities.
• Make sure the inpatient voids within 12 hours after surgery. If swelling interferes with normal urination, insertion of an indwelling urinary catheter may be necessary. The outpatient must void before discharge.
• Monitor for excessive bleeding, swelling, and inflammation at the incision site, and report them to the surgeon as required.
• Provide analgesia, as prescribed, and provide comfort measures.
• Administer a stool softener, as prescribed, to prevent straining during defecation.

Home care instructions
• Instruct the patient to avoid lifting, bending, and pushing or pulling movements as indicated by the surgeon.
• Tell the patient to watch for and report signs of infection, including fever, chills, diaphoresis, malaise, and lethargy as well as pain, inflammation, swelling, and drainage at the incision site.
• Emphasize the importance of regular follow-up examinations to evaluate wound healing and the success of hernia repair.
• Typically, the patient is encouraged to resume previous activities within 4 to 6 weeks.

HISTAMINE-2 RECEPTOR ANTAGONISTS

The treatment of choice for ulcer disorders, the histamine-2 (H$_2$) receptor antagonists include *cimetidine, nizatidine, ranitidine,* and *famotidine.*

The H$_2$-receptor antagonists, which are usually given orally, are much preferred over surgery. Typically, they help heal ulcers within 6 to 8 weeks. Because these drugs can be effective in a once-daily dosage form, they provide a good alternative for patients who are noncompliant with prolonged antacid therapy.

Purpose

• To block the histamine-receptor sites on the parietal cells of the stomach, reducing gastric acid secretion.

Indications

H$_2$-receptor antagonists are used for prophylactic and short-term treatment of duodenal and gastric ulcers. These drugs are also used to treat disorders that produce peptic ulcers, such as Zollinger-Ellison syndrome, systemic mastocytosis, and multiple endocrine adenomas. In addition, they are commonly administered I.V. to prevent stress ulcers and GI bleeding in critically ill patients. These drugs also provide relief from gastroesophageal reflux disease in patients who do not respond to conventional therapy (lifestyle changes, diet modification, and antacids).

Adverse reactions

Cimetidine and ranitidine may produce headache, dizziness, malaise, myalgia, nausea, diarrhea or constipation, skin rashes, and pruritus. Famotidine and nizatidine produce few adverse reactions but may cause headache and less often constipation, diarrhea, and skin rash.

Reversible confusion, agitation, depression, and hallucinations can result, most commonly in patients receiving cimetidine, especially in severely ill or elderly patients. These reactions, which usually are associated with decreased renal function, also may occur with overdose.

When given by rapid I.V. injection, H$_2$-receptor antagonists can produce profound bradycardia and other cardiotoxic effects. Occasionally, pain occurs at the injection site.

H$_2$-receptor antagonists rarely cause hypersensitivity reactions or increased hepatic enzyme levels. Cimetidine interferes with hepatic microsomal drug-metabolizing enzymes and may alter the pharmacokinetics of other drugs given concurrently.

Care considerations

Before therapy

• Review the patient's medication regimen for possible interactions, especially with cimetidine therapy. For example, cimetidine decreases the metabolism of theophylline and of most benzodiazepines, possibly causing toxic effects. Because antacids interfere with absorption of H$_2$-receptor antagonists, separate doses of the two drugs by at least 1 hour.

During therapy

• If you're administering cimetidine I.V., rotate injection sites to reduce discomfort. During the infusion, carefully monitor the patient's vital signs to prevent adverse cardiac reactions. Continue to check vital signs for 2 hours after administration.

• Regularly monitor hematologic studies, especially platelet count and prothrombin time, to detect granulocytopenia or thrombocytopenia. Also watch for signs of hemorrhage: bloody or tarry stools, hematemesis, unusual bleeding or bruising, and signs of shock. Be especially alert for these signs in patients with bleeding ulcers.

• Observe for other adverse reactions to H$_2$-receptor antagonists. If adverse central nervous system (CNS) reactions occur, take safety precautions and notify the doctor, who will probably change the administration schedule or, if severe reactions persist, discontinue the drug.

Home care instructions

• Emphasize the need to complete the full course of therapy. If the patient has chronic peptic ulcers, explain that abrupt discontinuation of the drug can cause perforation, a life-threatening emergency.

• Instruct the patient to make up a missed dose as soon as he remembers. However, if it's almost time for his next dose, the patient should omit the missed dose and resume the regular schedule with the next dose. Tell the patient not to double-dose.

• Tell the patient to watch for and immediately report any signs of bleeding disorders: easy bruising, bloody stools, or bloody vomitus. Also advise the patient to report any other adverse reactions, including sexual dysfunction.

• Warn the patient who experiences dizziness or other CNS reactions to avoid driving or other hazardous activities that require good coordination and alertness.

• Tell the patient who's taking antacids not to take them within 1 hour of taking an H_2-receptor antagonist.

• Encourage the patient to avoid smoking because it interferes with drug action.

• Instruct the patient to prevent GI irritation by avoiding spicy foods, alcohol, hot drinks, caffeine-containing products, and aspirin.

HYDROCELECTOMY

Hydrocelectomy is the surgical removal of a hydrocele—a collection of fluid in the tunica vaginalis of the testicle or along the spermatic cord. Hydrocelectomy is typically reserved for males older than age 1; in infants, a hydrocele usually regresses spontaneously. Hydrocelectomies are usually performed on an outpatient basis.

Purpose

• To remove a persistent hydrocele by surgical excision or plication.

Indications

Hydrocelectomy is necessary when needle aspiration fails to remove the fluid that has collected around the tunica vaginalis, when the hydrocele becomes large and uncomfortable, or when swelling caused by the collected fluid compresses testicular tissue, interfering with circulation to the testicles and causing loss of testicular function.

Procedure

The hydrocele is excised or plicated by the surgeon through a small scrotal incision after the patient receives a local anesthetic. The surgeon follows excision with ligation and fulguration (use of electric sparks generated by a high-frequency current to destroy tissue) of the involved vessels and may then insert a small incisional drain before closing the incision.

Alternatively, the surgeon may plicate the hydrocele, permanently collapsing its walls and preventing refilling. No incisional drain is required after plication.

After the incision is closed, the surgeon applies a dressing and a scrotal support or suspensory.

Complications

Hydrocelectomy rarely causes complications if meticulous wound care is provided. Occasionally, infection, frank bleeding from the incision or drainage site, and internal scrotal hemorrhage may occur.

Care considerations

Before surgery

• Teach the patient (or the child's parents) about the procedure. If the patient will have a drain after the surgery, explain that it prevents fluid buildup and helps to prevent infection and promote healing.

• Teach the patient or his parents about the importance of wearing a scrotal support after the procedure. Tell them that such support relieves swelling and pain and helps to keep the dressing in place.

• As appropriate, reassure the patient that his privacy will be respected at all times and that the surgery will not impair sexual or reproductive function but may actually enhance it by eliminating discomfort and a possible cause of low sperm production.

After surgery

• Administer prescribed analgesics as necessary to decrease pain. Keep in mind that the amount of pain experienced by each patient having this procedure varies widely. Most patients experience moderate pain for the first 24 hours, but the pain should begin to rapidly decrease in severity.

• Check the dressing regularly, usually every 2 to 4 hours for the first 24 hours after surgery. Expect moderate-to-heavy serosanguineous drainage during this period. Change the dressing as necessary.

• Observe for frank bleeding from the drain or the suture line. Assess for signs of internal scrotal hemorrhage: increased pain, swelling, and tenderness as well as systemic signs of infection.

• Keep the patient's scrotum elevated to minimize swelling and snugly supported to enhance comfort. Change the scrotal support when it becomes saturated with drainage. Administer anti-inflammatory drugs as prescribed to reduce scrotal swelling.

Home care instructions

• If the patient is discharged on the day of surgery, be sure to teach him or a family caregiver how to change the dressing using sterile technique, how much and what kind of drainage to expect, and how to change the scrotal support. Also teach about any prescribed medications. Be sure the patient understands when and how to administer them.

• Inform the patient that scrotal swelling may persist for up to a month after surgery but will gradually subside.

• Instruct the patient or a family member to watch for and report signs of infection, including fever, chills, and worsening scrotal pain, tenderness, or swelling. Also tell the patient to notify the doctor of any obvious bleeding from the incision or from the drain if one was inserted.

• Tell the patient to shower but avoid taking baths until all wound drainage has ceased and healing is complete.

• Warn the patient to avoid heavy lifting or straining for at least 6 weeks to reduce the risk of incisional hernia.

• Also warn the adult patient to refrain from sexual activity as advised by his doctor (usually for 6 weeks).

• Encourage the patient to keep follow-up visits with the surgeon to evaluate healing of the wound.

HYDROTHERAPY

Hydrotherapy is the external use of water to promote relaxation, increase circulation, alter body temperature, strengthen muscles, improve joint mobility, and aid the cleaning of wounds. The beneficial effects of water are well-known, and it has been used as a therapeutic modality for thousands of years. The buoyancy of water allows the patient to achieve greater range of motion and to have fuller use of the extremities with less discomfort. Hydrotherapy can be performed in whirlpools, tanks, Hubbard tanks, and swimming pools.

The benefits of whirlpool therapy are derived from the increase in tissue temperature and mechanical stimulation of the agitation of the water. The Hubbard tank allows immersion of the entire body; smaller tanks are used for treating extremities or for immersion of the lower body.

Purpose
• To aid cleaning of a wound and the removal of necrotic tissue
• To assist in the strengthening of muscles
• To increase joint mobility
• To promote relaxation
• To reduce pain
• To increase or decrease body tissue temperature.

Indications
Hydrotherapy is indicated for various conditions. Whirlpool and Hubbard tank treatments are most commonly administered for wound cleaning. The therapeutic swimming pool may be used to promote relaxation and relieve pain. Patients with arthritis, chronic pain, low back pain, and other painful conditions typically enjoy the pool for these sedative effects and for the ease of performing strengthening and mobility exercises. The buoyancy of the water may be used to assist with exercises for weakened muscles. Conversely, strengthening exercises may be performed in the pool, using the water to provide resistance to specific muscles. The buoyancy of the water can be used to aid gait training, especially for patients with painful joints or significant weakness.

Finally, the therapeutic swimming pool can be psychologically and physically beneficial for patients with spinal cord injuries. The buoyancy of the water allows them some control of body movement that is impossible out of water.

Contraindications for hydrotherapy depend on the form of hydrotherapy selected and the condition for which it is used. Water temperature should not exceed 95° F (35° C) for patients with circulatory insufficiency. Patients with cardiac disorders may not be candidates for therapeutic activities in the swimming pool or may need to have close monitoring. Patients who are incontinent or have open draining wounds should not use the swimming pool to avoid bacterial cross-contamination, nor should patients with excessively high, low, or unstable blood pressure. Patients with multiple sclerosis may react adversely in warm, humid conditions and will need close monitoring.

Hydrotherapy is also contraindicated if the patient's status reflects sudden changes, such as fever, electrolyte or fluid imbalance, or unstable vital signs. Immersion isn't recommended for patients with mending fractures, endotracheal tubes, or tracheostomy tubes (or other respiratory aids) or for patients with skin grafts less than 5 days old.

Procedure
Hydrotherapy is usually administered by a physical therapist or a physical therapy assistant in a hospital setting or physical therapy clinical setting. Other health care professionals who can provide hydrotherapy treatment include athletic trainers, recreation therapists, occupational therapists, and nurses. Hydrotherapy treatments are usually performed in whirlpools, Hubbard tanks, or swimming pools. (See *Positioning the burn patient for hydrotherapy*, page 358.)

Most whirlpool treatments are performed with water temperature at 98° to 104° F (36.6° to 40° C).

If the therapy involves total immersion, the patient is slowly lowered into the tank by a hoist. He is positioned so that his head is supported by a headrest. Smaller tanks may be used if only

Positioning the burn patient for hydrotherapy

To perform hydrotherapy for the burn patient, you'll immerse the patient in a tub or a Hubbard tank as shown. Alternatively, you may spray the patient's wounds with water as he lies on a special shower table. Either way, hydrotherapy is traumatic and painful for the burn patient. Provide continual support and encouragement as you proceed.

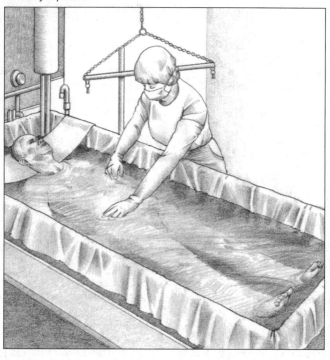

one body part, such as an arm or leg, requires therapy. During immersion, certain other treatments can be accomplished, such as debridement and passive or active range-of-motion exercises. Hydrotherapy usually lasts 20 minutes, after which the patient is slowly removed from the tank, dried, and covered with a warm sheet or blanket.

Complications

Cardiac or respiratory arrest are possible complications of hydrotherapy if water temperature is not given careful consideration. High water temperatures and humid conditions place a significant demand on the body's cardiovascular and pulmonary systems. Therefore, patients with cardiac and pulmonary disorders need close assessment to evaluate the risk of hydrotherapy. Thermal injury is also a potential complication of hydrotherapy; to avoid it, water temperature should never exceed 110° F (43° C).

Infection is another complication of hydrotherapy. To prevent it, antibacterial agents must be added to the water.

Care considerations

Before therapy

• Determine the status of the patient's circulation, and set the temperature of the water accordingly.
• Add an appropriate antibacterial solution to the water to prevent cross-contamination. Sodium hypochlorite 5.25% (bleach) and povidone-iodine solution are commonly used for whirlpools. A dilution ratio of 1:120 is recommended for sodium hypochlorite. Povidone-iodine in approximately 4 to 5 parts per million should be added to whirlpools.
• Determine which exercises should be performed in the water, and provide clear instructions to the patient.

During therapy

• Patients who have vascular insufficiency should be treated with the water temperature between 92° and 95° F (33.3° and 35° C).
• Monitor the patient's response to hydrotherapy, and modify the program as needed.
• Assure the patient's safety at all times. Provide assistance when the patient is entering and leaving the hydrotherapy facility.
• Maintain the patient's privacy.

Home care instructions

• Teach the recommended exercise program to supplement the exercises performed in hydrotherapy.
• Provide clear instructions and supplies for wound care at home (if needed).

HYPERBARIC OXYGEN THERAPY

Hyperbaric oxygen therapy increases tissue oxygenation by exposing the patient to oxygen that is at a much higher pressure than normal atmospheric pressure. The patient is placed inside a chamber and breathes 100% oxygen while the pressure within the chamber is increased to up to three times normal atmospheric pressure. This markedly increases partial pressure of oxygen in the patient's arterial blood, commonly achieving arterial oxygen pressures of 1,000 to 1,900 mm Hg. The additional oxygen is physically dissolved within the plasma, which enhances oxygen delivery to tissues.

Purpose

• To enhance and improve oxygen delivery to tissues.

Indications

Hyperbaric oxygen therapy is widely recognized as a treatment for patients with decompression sickness or arterial gas embolism and is also the primary treatment for severe carbon monoxide poisoning. Additionally, it aids the treatment of gas gangrene. Adjunctive hyperbaric oxygen can optimize therapy outcomes in other properly selected cases. (See *Investigative indications for hyperbaric oxygenation,* page 360.)

An untreated pneumothorax poses the only absolute contraindication to hyperbaric oxygen therapy. Other conditions that require specific precautions include upper respiratory infections, chronic sinusitis, seizure disorders, emphysema with carbon dioxide retention, and uncontrolled high fever as well as a history of spontaneous pneumothorax, thoracic surgery, reconstructive ear or eye surgery, pulmonary lesions on routine X-ray or computed tomography scan, viral infections, congenital spherocytosis, and optic neuritis.

Procedure

Hyperbaric oxygen therapy is provided in either a one-person (monoplace) or a multiplace chamber that can

Investigative indications for hyperbaric oxygenation

Review this list of indications for hyperbaric oxygenation that are currently under investigation.

- Acute (central) retinal artery insufficiency
- Brain abscesses (mixed aerobic and anaerobic)
- Carbon tetrachloride poisoning (acute)
- Head injury (cerebral edema)
- Healing of fractures and bone grafts
- Hydrogen sulfide poisoning
- Lepromatous leprosy
- Meningitis
- Cerebrovascular accident (acute-thrombotic or embolic)
- Radiation myelitis, enteritis, and proctitis
- Multiple sclerosis
- Selective refractory mycoses
- Sepsis (chronic), intra-abdominal
- Sickle-cell crisis
- Spinal cord injury
- Spider bite (brown recluse, *Loxosceles reclusa*)

accommodate up to 10 patients simultaneously. In a monoplace chamber, the patient lies on a cart that slides inside the chamber; its hull, made of clear acrylic plastic, allows the patient to see outside of the chamber. The chamber is filled with compressed oxygen, and the patient breathes from the environment surrounding him.

In multiplace chambers, oxygen is supplied from the wall via a mask, hood, or endotracheal tube. Oxygen delivery is not always 100%, but the fraction of inspired oxygen (FIO_2) is increased to enhance delivery. Patient care attendants oversee use of the special equipment modified for use in the chamber.

Treatment pressures commonly vary from 2.0 to 6.0 absolute atmospheres (14.7 to 73.5 psi), and duration of treatment is typically 2 to 6 hours. The treatment schedule provides intermittent periods of air breathing to help prevent oxygen toxicity.

Complications

Hyperbaric oxygen therapy may be associated with barotrauma (rupture of the tympanic membrane, sinus barotrauma, lung barotrauma, and air embolism), oxygen toxicity (chronic lung fibrosis or seizures), visual acuity changes (worsening myopia and has-

tened maturation of cataracts), and paresthesias.

Care considerations

Before therapy

- Provide adequate teaching to minimize confinement anxiety or other concerns about therapy.
- Because of the different pressures inside and outside the chamber, equipment must be able to operate with this pressure gradient. For example, an I.V. pump outside the chamber must have the capability to pump against the pressure inside the chamber. Check with the manufacturer of support equipment such as I.V. lines, ventilators, and monitors to ensure they have the ability to overcome a variable gradient of 0 to 30 psi.
- Administer mild sedation if necessary.
- Demonstrate techniques of ear clearing, such as yawning, swallowing, or chewing motions, and evaluate the patient's ability to ventilate the middle ear.
- An ear, nose, and throat consultation is recommended if ear problems are anticipated. In emergencies, a myringotomy can be performed to allow airflow across the tympanic membrane to prevent painful barotrauma.

• Emphasize the importance of discontinuing smoking, which causes vasoconstriction and makes treatment less effective.

During therapy

• Strictly observe fire safety precautions because the environment within the chamber can contain up to 100% oxygen.

• Use grounded electrical outlets; decrease static electricity by having the patient wear proper attire, including sneakers; and increase the relative humidity.

• Watch for signs and symptoms of oxygen toxicity: facial pallor, sweating, apprehension, confusion, loss of visual acuity, ringing in ears, nausea, vomiting, facial twitching, and seizures.

• Protect the patient from injury if seizures occur.

• Pay close attention to I.V. infusions during pressure changes within the multiplace chamber. The amount of fluid in the drip chamber will vary, requiring manual adjustment. Any glass I.V. bottles must be vented during pressure changes. Gas expansion during decompression must be vented to avoid injecting air into the patient.

• Adjust the volume of air in endotracheal tube cuffs during pressure changes to maintain an adequate but minimally occlusive seal by withdrawing air until auscultation at the neck detects a minimal leak at peak inspiration.

• When administering drugs, consider the following: Absorption of I.M. and S.C. injections administered before hyperbaric oxygen therapy will be delayed by normal vasoconstriction in response to elevated Po_2. These drugs' effects will be minimal until the patient's Po_2 returns to normal. Drugs administered in the chamber should be given I.V. or orally. This avoids I.M. accumulation of the drug because of altered absorption and subsequent rebound when the patient returns to the normal vasoactive state.

Home care instructions

• Instruct the patient to notify the staff if he experiences any adverse reactions, especially apprehension, sweating, confusion, visual changes, ringing in ears, nausea, vomiting, or twitching.

• Advise patients who have had a myringotomy to avoid getting water in their ears.

• Inform the patient that a small amount of bleeding from the ears is normal.

HYPOPHYSECTOMY AND ADENECTOMY

Microsurgical methods have dramatically reversed the high mortality once associated with removal of pituitary and sella turcica tumors. As a result, hypophysectomy (surgical removal of the pituitary gland) and adenectomy (surgical removal of a pituitary adenoma) is the treatment of choice for many pituitary tumors.

Hypophysectomy and adenectomy can be performed transsphenoidally (entering from the inner aspect of the upper lip through the sphenoid sinus) or transfrontally (approaching the sella turcica through the cranium [transfrontal craniotomy]). The transsphenoidal approach, which uses powerful microscopes and improved radiologic techniques to allow removal of microadenomas, is most commonly used because it causes fewer complications. The transfrontal approach carries a high risk of mortality and of such complications as loss of smell and taste and permanent, severe diabetes insipidus. As a result, the transfrontal craniotomy is used rarely, only if the tumor is too large or inaccessible by the transsphenoidal approach. (For a discussion of craniotomy and patient care required, see the entry "Craniotomy.")

Transsphenoidal hypophysectomy

When a pituitary tumor is confined to the sella turcica, the neurosurgeon will perform transsphenoidal hypophysectomy. For this procedure, the patient is placed in a semi-sitting position and given a general anesthetic. The surgeon incises the upper lip's inner aspect so that he can enter the sella turcica through the sphenoidal sinus to remove the tumor.

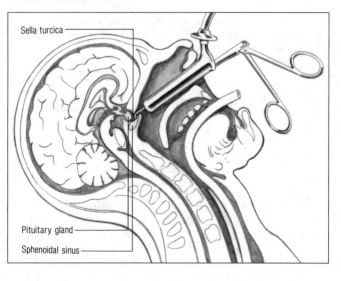

Sella turcica

Pituitary gland

Sphenoidal sinus

Purpose

• To remove pituitary tissue that is secreting excessive levels of pituitary hormones or that is causing pressure on adjacent structures (hypophysectomy)
• To remove a pituitary adenoma (adenectomy).

Indications

Hypophysectomy and adenectomy are the treatments of choice for pituitary tumors, which can cause acromegaly, gigantism, and Cushing's disease.

Contraindications to this surgery include anatomic anomalies barring access to the pituitary, sphenoidal infection, and nasal infection.

Procedure

Transsphenoidal hypophysectomy is performed with the patient in a semi-sitting position, under general anesthesia. The neurosurgeon makes an incision on the inner aspect of the upper lip and enters the sella turcica through the sphenoidal sinus, places a speculum through the incision into the sella turcica, and removes the pituitary gland, part of the gland, or the tumor, using instruments passed through the speculum (see *Transsphenoidal hypophysectomy*).

Before wound closure, the surgeon may apply hemostatic agents, or he may use the patient's own subcutaneous fat or a muscle plug from the thigh as intersellar graft tissue to prevent the leakage of cerebrospinal fluid (CSF) through the opening. In addition, the floor of the sella turcica may be sealed off with a small piece of bone or cartilage. Finally, the surgeon inserts nasal stents with petroleum gauze packed around them, closes the initial incision inside the upper lip, and applies a dressing under the nose to prevent the packing from dislodging.

Complications

Even mild trauma to the pituitary stalk may interrupt secretion of vasopressin; therefore, transient diabetes insipidus frequently occurs postoperatively. Other complications may include infection, CSF leakage, hemorrhage, and visual defects. Total removal of the pituitary gland causes a hormonal deficiency that requires monitoring and hormonal replacement therapy.

Care considerations

Before surgery

• Explain the surgery and provide preoperative teaching. Tell the patient to expect some headaches and discomfort at the graft site after surgery and the presence of nasal packing for 2 to 3 days after the surgery, which will require him to breathe through his mouth. Also tell the patient to expect a moustache dressing under the nose and possibly an indwelling urinary catheter.
• Arrange for and explain preoperative tests and examinations, as appropriate. For example, a patient who has acromegaly will need thorough cardiac evaluation for incipient myocardial ischemia. All patients should have visual field tests to serve as a baseline.
• Review the patient's preoperative medication, if appropriate. If he has a prolactin-secreting tumor, find out if he has been taking bromocriptine mesylate (Parlodel) for 6 weeks before surgery to help shrink and soften the tumor.

• Most patients will also receive a steroid such as hydrocortisone during surgery even if they did not have hormone deficiency before because removal of all or part of the pituitary gland causes cortisol deficiency.
• Ensure that the patient or a responsible family member has signed a consent form.

After surgery

• Keep the patient on bed rest for 24 hours after surgery, then encourage ambulation. Keep the head of the bed elevated to avoid placing tension or pressure on the suture line. Tell the patient not to brush his teeth, sneeze, cough, blow his nose, or bend over for several days to avoid disturbing the muscle graft.
• Administer mild analgesics, as prescribed, for headache caused by loss of CSF during surgery or for paranasal pain. Typically, paranasal pain subsides when the catheters and packing are removed — usually 24 to 48 hours after surgery.
• Perform neurovascular checks to evaluate intracranial pressure.
• Monitor for transient diabetes insipidus (increased thirst and increased urinary volume with a low specific gravity), which usually occurs within 24 hours after surgery. If diabetes insipidus occurs, replace fluids and administer aqueous vasopressin or sublingual desmopressin acetate, as ordered. With these measures, diabetes insipidus usually resolves within 72 hours.
• Tell the patient to report postnasal drip, which may indicate a CSF leak.
• Remind the patient to deep-breathe frequently. Provide frequent mouth rinses because the patient will be breathing through his mouth.
• Be alert for signs of infection, especially for signs of meningitis such as headache and nuchal rigidity. As prescribed, administer prophylactic antibiotics.

• Arrange for visual field testing as soon as possible because visual defects can indicate hemorrhage.
• Collect a serum sample to measure thyroid and adrenal hormone levels, and evaluate the need for hormone replacement.

Home care instructions

• Instruct the patient to report signs of diabetes insipidus immediately. Explain that he may need to limit fluid intake or take prescribed medications.
• If ordered, tell the patient not to brush his teeth for 2 weeks to avoid suture line disruption. Mention that he can use a mouthwash and dental floss. Reinforce warnings to avoid bending and nose blowing.
• The patient may need hormonal replacement therapy as a result of decreased pituitary secretion of thyroid-stimulating hormone. Teach the patient who needs cortisol or thyroid hormone replacement to recognize the signs of excessive or insufficient dosage. Advise him to wear a medical identification bracelet.
• Tell the patient with hyperprolactinemia that follow-up visits are required for several years because relapse is possible. Explain that bromocriptine may be prescribed if relapse occurs.

HYSTERECTOMY

Hysterectomy is the excision of the uterus. It can be performed using a vaginal or an abdominal approach, but the latter approach allows better visualization of the pelvic organs and a larger operating field.

Hysterectomy may be classified as subtotal, total, panhysterectomy, or radical. A *subtotal hysterectomy,* which is performed rarely, is the removal of all of the uterus except the cervix. In *total hysterectomy,* the surgeon removes all of the uterus, including the cervix, by a vaginal or abdominal approach. In *panhysterectomy,* which requires the abdominal approach, the surgeon removes all of the uterus (hysterectomy) as well as the ovaries and the fallopian tubes (bilateral salpingo-oophorectomy). *Radical hysterectomy* is the removal of the uterus, ovaries, fallopian tubes, adjoining ligaments and lymph nodes, the upper third of the vagina, and surrounding tissues (parametrium).

Purpose

• To remove the uterus and, if necessary, accompanying organs and surrounding tissues.

Indications

Hysterectomy may be indicated for malignant and nonmalignant growths of the uterus, cervix, and adnexa; control of uterine bleeding and hemorrhage; irreparable uterine rupture or perforation; life-threatening pelvic infection; treatment of endometriosis when conservative treatment has failed; and correction of problems involving pelvic floor relaxation, such as rectocele and cystocele.

Procedure

A hysterectomy is usually performed with the patient under general anesthesia. Using an abdominal approach, the surgeon makes a midline (vertical) incision from the umbilicus to the symphysis pubis or a horizontal incision in the lower abdomen and removes the uterus and necessary accompanying structures. Then, the surgeon closes the abdomen and applies an abdominal dressing and a perineal pad.

The vaginal approach does not require an external incision. The surgeon makes an incision above and around the cervix and removes the uterus. He then closes the opening to the peritoneal cavity with sutures and applies a perineal pad. This approach is not used in panhysterectomy or radical hysterectomy.

Complications

Possible complications of hysterectomy include wound infection, urine retention, abdominal distention, thromboembolism, atelectasis, pneumonia, hemorrhage, ureteral injury, and bowel injury. Abdominal hysterectomy may also be complicated by wound dehiscence, pulmonary embolism, and intestinal obstruction caused by paralytic ileus. Psychological complications may include depression, loss of libido, and a perceived loss of femininity.

Care considerations
Before surgery

• Reinforce the surgeon's explanation of the procedure, and make sure the patient has signed a consent form.
• Review the preparation that may be required: a douche, enema, shower with an antibacterial soap, and shaving the site.
• Review the preoperative laboratory tests that are performed as a baseline. These may include blood tests, electrocardiogram, chest X-ray, and urinalysis.
• Review any drug therapy, such as prophylactic antibiotics and atropine.
• Provide routine postoperative teaching about turning, coughing, and deep-breathing; using an incentive spirometer; performing range-of-motion (ROM) exercises; and early walking. Tell the patient that after surgery (on the day of surgery) she'll lie supine or in low to mid-Fowler's position but will have to turn from side to side. On the day after surgery, she will be encouraged to walk to prevent venous stasis.
• Explain to the patient that urine retention is common after surgery and will require an indwelling urinary catheter.
• Tell the patient to expect some abdominal cramping and moderate perineal drainage that will require a perineal pad.

After surgery

• Encourage the patient to cough, deep-breathe, and turn frequently—at least every 2 hours—and listen to breath sounds to note any respiratory complications. Administer and regulate prescribed I.V. fluids. Monitor intake and output and vital signs. Monitor the patient for bowel sounds to note presence of peristalsis and to detect any GI problems.
• Change the patient's perineal pad frequently. Note the characteristics and amount of drainage.
• Administer prescribed analgesics to relieve pain, and note their effectiveness. Offer a heating pad to relieve abdominal pain.
• As ordered, change dressings after the abdominal hysterectomy. The incision should be intact without signs of infection, such as redness and edema.
• Monitor postoperative bleeding by noting the amount of drainage on the perineal pad and the abdominal dressing. Bleeding should not saturate more than one pad in 4 hours.
• If the patient has an indwelling urinary catheter, provide catheter care and maintain patency.
• Encourage the patient, and help her to perform leg ROM exercises to maintain adequate circulation and help prevent thromboembolism.

Home care instructions

• Be sure that the patient understands that she should avoid driving; heavy lifting; heavy housework; and heavy exercise, including jogging, aerobics, dancing, and active sports, for the period prescribed by her doctor—usually at least 1 month. Tell her to avoid sexual intercourse, douching, and use of tampons as prescribed by her doctor—usually for 3 to 6 weeks.
• Tell the patient that moderate exercise such as walking is helpful. She

should try to increase the distance she walks a little each day.

• Teach the patient the signs of complications: fever, increased bleeding, and difficulty with urination or bowel movements. Tell her to report such findings to her doctor.

• Tell the patient to eat foods high in protein, vitamin C, and iron to aid healing.

• Explain to the patient and her family that she may feel depressed or irritable temporarily because of abrupt hormonal fluctuations. Encourage family members to respond calmly and supportively.

IMMOBILIZATION

Commonly used to maintain proper alignment and limit movement, immobilization devices also relieve pressure and pain. These devices include plaster and synthetic casts, splints, slings, skin or skeletal traction, braces, and cervical collars. All types of immobilization devices help heal injured bones and surrounding soft tissue.

Purpose
• To maintain alignment, limit movement, or provide support in management of musculoskeletal injuries or disorders.

Indications
Immobilization devices are indicated for various skeletal injuries. Casts are applied after closed or open reduction of fractures or after other severe injuries; splints are used to immobilize fractures, dislocations, or subluxations; slings are used to support and immobilize an injured arm, wrist, or hand, to support the weight of a splint, or to hold dressings in place; skin or skeletal traction, using a system of weights and pulleys to reduce fractures, is used to treat dislocations, correct deformities, or decrease muscle spasms; braces are used to support weakened or deformed joints; and cervical collars are used to immobilize the cervical spine, decrease muscle spasms and, possibly, relieve pain.

Procedure
The doctor usually applies the immobilization device. In certain situations, a nurse may apply a splint. Slings and braces may also be applied by a nurse or other trained individual. Application procedures vary depending on the type of immobilization device. (See *Understanding types of immobilization*, pages 368 to 370, for details on common devices.)

Complications
Neurovascular compromise is the major complication related to immobilization devices and can result in loss of a limb or limb function. Traction, casting, and splinting may result in perineal nerve palsy (lower extremity device), compartment syndrome, and constrictive edema. Additionally, complications of long-term immobility may include constipation, thrombophlebitis, urinary stasis, hypostatic pneumonia, and depression. Skin irritation or breakdown may also occur with any device. Osteomyelitis is a complication of skeletal traction.

Care considerations
Before therapy
• Explain to the patient the purpose of the immobilization device the doctor has chosen. If possible, show him the device before application and demonstrate how it works. Explain associated care measures. Tell the patient approximately how long the device will remain in place.
• Reassure the patient that initial discomfort will resolve as he becomes accustomed to the device.

(Text continues on page 371.)

Understanding types of immobilization

Use this chart as a guide to immobilization devices and the interventions they require.

Braces

Description
Braces are support devices made of metal, leather, and hard plastic and are typically worn externally; common types include the Milwaukee brace, Parvis brace, and Somi brace.

Indications
• To limit movement and enhance stability of an injured or weakened joint
• To help correct neuromuscular defects in patients with cerebral palsy, other spastic disorders, and scoliosis

Nursing considerations
• Check the condition of the brace daily for worn or malfunctioning components.
• Frequently assess the skin under the brace for breakdown and abrasions.
• Check carefully for proper fit, keeping in mind that any fluctuation in the patient's weight may change the fit.

Casts

Description
Casts are made of plaster or synthetic material and may be applied to any body part, covering a single finger or the whole body; types of casts include the Minerva jacket, hip-spica, and extremity fixation with plaster of paris.

Indications
To maintain correct alignment and immobilization during healing; casts are used for traumatic injuries and correction of congenital deformities; examples include severe ligament rupture, extremity or spinal fractures, club foot, and congenital hip dysplasia; if necessary, casts may be used with traction to enhance immobilization

Nursing considerations
• Support a plaster cast with pillows while it's drying (for up to 72 hours, depending on cast size) to maintain proper shape. Keep the cast dry at all times.
• Demonstrate proper body mechanics for movement with larger casts.
• Perform regular neurovascular checks.
• Tell the patient to report extreme pain or pressure beneath the cast. Observe for drainage or fever, which may point to infection under the cast.
• Check the skin along the edges of the cast, and protect it as necessary.

Collars

Description
Made of soft foam or metal and plastic components, collars fit around the neck and under the chin; common types include the Philadelphia collar, doll's collar, Camp Victoria collar, and soft or hard cervical collar.

Understanding types of immobilization *(continued)*

Collars *(continued)*

Indications
To support an injured or weakened cervical spine and maintain alignment during healing; common indications include cervical osteoarthritis, muscle strain, herniated disk, cervical spondylosis, and torticollis

Nursing considerations
- Check carefully for proper fit. You should be able to slip only one finger beneath the edge of the collar.
- Regularly inspect the skin under the collar for abrasions and breakdown.
- Keep the collar clean.
- Because the collar will restrict the patient's head movement, assist with eating and other activities as necessary.
- Remove a Philadelphia collar one-half at a time, with the patient lying flat.

Skeletal traction

Description
Skeletal traction involves placing a pin through the bone to which the traction apparatus is attached; common types include Gardner-Wells and Crutchfield tongs, halo vest, Kirschner wire, Steinmann pin, and pin placement through the femur, lower tibia, calcaneus, ulna, radius, or wrists.

Indications
To immobilize bones and allow healing of fractures, correction of congenital abnormalities, or stabilization of spinal degeneration

Nursing considerations
- Perform pin care daily with water and 0.9% sodium chloride solution or hydrogen peroxide.
- Observe the pin insertion site for signs of infection.
- Check the pin for proper fit, making sure that it doesn't move in the bone.
- Teach the patient how to use the trapeze to lift himself off the bed if permitted.
- If cervical traction is being used, frequently check the patient's occipital area for skin breakdown.
- When caring for a patient in a halo vest, bathe under the vest daily. *Never* move the patient by grasping the tongs. Instead, stabilize him on his back before opening the vest. Then open it one side at a time.
- Teach the patient how to ambulate with an altered center of gravity, and show him how to adapt his clothes to fit over the vest. Remind him not to bend over, but to use an assistive device for reaching. Also tell him to change the vest liner as necessary.

Skin traction

Description
Applied to the skin and soft tissue, skin traction indirectly pulls on the skeletal system and typically consists of weights, ropes, pulleys, and slings; common types include Buck's traction, Alvik traction, Hamilton-Russell traction, Bryant's traction, and Cotrel's traction.

(continued)

Understanding types of immobilization *(continued)*

Skin traction *(continued)*

Indications
- To relieve muscle spasms
- To restrict movement and provide correct alignment in cervical disk disease, pelvic fractures of the extremities, and spinal deformities

Nursing considerations
- Periodically check to ensure that weights, ropes, and pulleys are functional and in proper alignment. Check for proper skin placement.
- Do not manipulate the weights yourself; consult the doctor if you suspect the need for adjustment.
- Show the patient how to move in bed without disturbing the traction.

Slings

Description
Slings are composed of a soft fabric material or elastic adhesive fabric; common types include the Gisson sling, Snyder sling, and Velpeau bandage.

Indications
- To support an injured arm, hand, or wrist
- With other types of immobilization to treat other upper extremity problems, such as fractures of the scapula or clavicle and shoulder dislocation

Nursing considerations
- Check placement to ensure support of the weakened or injured area.
- Perform frequent neurovascular checks to detect circulatory or nerve impairment.
- Stress the need to wear the sling for the prescribed period to prevent further injury or delayed healing.
- Regularly perform passive range-of-motion exercises, as ordered.

Splints

Description
Splints are made of leather, metal, and hard plastic components; common types include the Denis Brown splint, McKibbee splint, Thomas splint, Bell-Grice splint, Shrewsbury splint, Foster-Brown splint, Girdlestone mermaid splint, Nissen splint, Hodgen splint, and Brain-Thomas working splint.

Indicatons
- To provide support for injured or weakened limbs or digits
- To help correct deformities such as mallet finger
- To help treat spinal tuberculosis, hip dislocation or dysplasia, long-bone fractures, scoliosis, footdrop, and inflammatory lesions of the hip, spine, or shoulder

Nursing considerations
- Check to ensure proper fit and alignment of the device. Frequently inspect the splint for cleanliness and overall condition.
- Regularly assess for skin breakdown under the splint.
- Clean leather components daily with saddle soap to keep them soft and supple.

• If the patient is in pain, give analgesics and muscle relaxants, as ordered.
• Obtain a baseline neurovascular assessment, and note the condition of the patient's skin.

After therapy
• Monitor neurovascular status. When assessing an immobilized extremity, compare findings bilaterally. Palpate distal pulses, and assess color, temperature, and capillary refill of fingers or toes (whichever is appropriate). Assess sensory and motor function of immobilized and nonimmobilized extremity, and report any abnormalities promptly.
• To enhance comfort and prevent pressure ulcers, frequently reposition the patient who's in traction or who requires long-term bed rest. Maintain proper body alignment.
• As ordered, assist with active or passive range-of-motion exercises to maintain muscle tone and prevent contractures.
• Encourage regular coughing and deep-breathing to prevent pulmonary complications and adequate fluid intake to prevent urinary stasis and constipation.
• Provide analgesics, as ordered.

Home care instructions
• Teach the patient and family caregiver how to care for the device. As needed, arrange for assistance with daily activities.
• Instruct the patient to promptly report signs of complications, including increased pain, inability to move fingers or toes, drainage, or swelling in the involved area.
• Emphasize the need for strict compliance with activity restrictions while the immobilization device is in place.
• Make sure the patient who has been given crutches understands how to use them. Make sure the environment is safe to prevent falls.
• Make sure the patient who has a removable device, such as a knee immobilizer, knows how to apply it correctly.
• Advise the patient to keep scheduled medical appointments to evaluate healing.

IMMUNOSUPPRESSANTS

The immunosuppressants, a chemically distinct group of drugs that suppress the immune system, include *azathioprine, cyclosporine, levamisole hydrochloride, lymphocyte immune globulin,* and *muromonab-CD3.* The idea of using drugs to suppress the body's immune response was considered nearly 100 years ago, but the actual development and use of such drugs is recent, coinciding with the development of organ transplantation. In combination with corticosteroids, the immunosuppressants have been used to prevent and treat organ transplant rejection. Immunosuppressants have also been used experimentally to treat many autoimmune diseases.

Purpose
• To block humoral and cell-mediated immune responses.

Indications
Azathioprine treats severe refractory rheumatoid arthritis and is also used preoperatively for kidney transplantation. Cyclosporine helps prevent rejection in various organ transplants, graft-versus-host disease after bone marrow transplantation, and chronic rejection in patients receiving other immunosuppressants. When used with corticosteroids, it reduces inflammation in rheumatoid arthritis. Levamisole is used to aid treatment of colon cancer after surgical resection. Muromonab-CD3 and lymphocyte immune globulin are used to prevent acute renal allograft rejection.

Immunosuppressants should not be used in patients with recent or existing chicken pox or herpes zoster infection because of the potential risk of severe generalized disease. These drugs also should not be used in patients exposed to live-virus vaccines and must be used cautiously in patients with hepatic or renal impairment.

Adverse reactions

Azathioprine commonly produces GI adverse reactions—nausea, vomiting, diarrhea, and mouth ulcerations—as well as leukopenia or thrombocytopenia from bone marrow depression.

Cyclosporine causes significant nephrotoxicity, evidenced by increased blood urea nitrogen (BUN) and serum creatinine levels. Common adverse reactions include hyperkalemia, hypertension, tremor, gingival hyperplasia, hirsutism, and GI complaints (nausea, vomiting, diarrhea, abdominal distention). Occasionally it causes sinusitis, gynecomastia, hearing loss, tinnitus, hyperglycemia, muscle pain, and edema.

Care considerations

• Review the patient's drug regimen for possible interactions. Allopurinol, for instance, greatly enhances the action and toxic effects of azathioprine. If these drugs must be given concurrently, the azathioprine dosage should be reduced by two-thirds to three-quarters.
• To monitor bone marrow function, a complete blood count (CBC) and platelet count should be performed at least every other day at the beginning of therapy or whenever the patient is receiving high doses. In addition, a CBC and platelet count should be performed at least weekly for the first 2 months of therapy. Closely monitor the results of these studies as well as BUN, creatinine, and alkaline phosphatase levels. Also, watch for any changes in urine output or signs of jaundice. Report any abnormalities to the doctor immediately.

• Watch for signs of infection, such as fever and sore throat. Report these symptoms to the doctor immediately.
• If the patient develops thrombocytopenia, watch for bruises, hematuria, hematochezia, or other signs of bleeding.
• Avoid giving I.M. injections, if possible, to prevent bleeding.

Home care instructions

• Emphasize the importance of following the prescribed medication schedule. If the patient is taking cyclosporine, tell him to take a missed dose as soon as possible, unless it's almost time for the next dose (in which case he should simply continue the regular schedule). If the patient is taking azathioprine several times a day, he should take a missed dose as soon as possible. If it's time for the next dose, he should take two doses. If a patient misses two consecutive doses of either of these drugs, he should notify his doctor immediately.
• Recommend safety precautions to prevent infection: avoiding crowds and people suffering from colds, flu, and other contagious illnesses; not receiving any immunizations, especially with live-virus vaccines such as poliovirus vaccines; avoiding contact with anyone who has recently received a live-virus vaccine; and washing hands before handling food.
• Teach the patient to recognize the early signs of infection, such as sore throat, fever, chills, or malaise. Stress the importance of informing the doctor at the first sign of an infection.
• Tell the patient to watch for signs of bleeding, such as melena, hematuria, or easy bruising, and to report them to his doctor. Warn him to avoid aspirin and aspirin-containing compounds, and encourage him to use an electric shaver rather than a razor.
• Inform the patient that immunosuppressants often cause temporary hair loss.

• Also inform the patient that the prescribed drug may cause loss of appetite, nausea, and vomiting. If GI effects occur, tell him to take the drug with meals. If they persist, the doctor may prescribe an antiemetic.

• Explain that symptoms of refractory arthritis may not improve for up to 12 weeks.

• Instruct the patient who's taking cyclosporine to report symptoms of hypertension, such as frequent headaches or dizziness. Also tell him to watch for signs of hepatic impairment, such as clay-colored stools, pruritus, or yellowing of the skin or sclera, and to inform the doctor of such signs immediately.

IMPLANTABLE CARDIOVERTER DEFIBRILLATOR

The implantable cardioverter defibrillator (ICD) is a surgically implanted device used for the treatment of life-threatening ventricular tachycardia (VT) or ventricular fibrillation (VF). It consists of a set of leads and a pulse generator. The defibrillator monitors cardiac rhythm. When it detects a life-threatening arrhythmia, it delivers an electric shock directly to the heart within 10 to 35 seconds to reestablish a normal sinus rhythm. If this shock does not convert the patient's heart rhythm, the device will recycle and deliver up to four more shocks, depending on the specific model.

The ICD generator weighs less than ½ lb (0.2 kg) and has a battery life of 3 to 5 years, with the ability to deliver 200 to 300 shocks.

Purpose
• To detect and terminate sustained VT or VF.

Indications
The ICD is used for treatment of patients with documented, spontaneous sustained VT or VF. It is also an appropriate treatment for survivors of sudden cardiac death not related to an acute myocardial infarction (MI). Patients with syncope who have inducible sustained VT or VF by electrophysiologic testing may also be candidates for an ICD. Because implantation of the device requires open-heart surgery, it's usually reserved for patients unresponsive or intolerant to conventional antiarrhythmic therapy and for patients with a life expectancy of at least 1 year. In patients with severe left ventricular dysfunction (especially those in whom antiarrhythmics have a smaller effect on reducing mortality), the ICD may be considered earlier.

The ICD is not indicated for patients with syncope of unknown origin, nor for the treatment of bradyarrhythmias, supraventricular tachycardia, or nonsustained VT. Newer devices have been developed that combine the ICD with pacemaker therapy for the treatment of bradyarrhythmias and tachyarrhythmias.

Procedure
The implantation procedure, typically combined with coronary artery bypass surgery, is performed under general anesthesia through either a sternotomy or a thoracotomy incision. (A new generation of devices that are implanted transvenously, without the need for thoractomy, have been approved by the Food and Drug Administration and are available for use.)

The Ventak defibrillator has four leads. Two leads end in coil electrodes that the surgeon places on or in the left ventricle, and two end in patch electrodes that the surgeon places over the left and right ventricles. These two are connected to the pulse generator, which is implanted in the abdominal wall. VT or VF is induced during surgery to evaluate appropriate arrhythmia detection and termination by the device.

The ICD continuously monitors heart rate through a system of rate sensing leads. When the device detects ventricular tachyarrhythmias, the capacitor-charging cycle begins, and the ICD commits to deliver either a low-energy cardioversion or high-energy defibrillation shock. Some devices are "non-committed"; before delivering the shock, they reevaluate the rhythm after charging to make certain that the arrhythmia is sustained. Because most devices deliver shocks based on heart rate, care must be taken to set the ICD detection rate above the patient's exercise heart rate. *Note:* ICDs do not prevent arrhythmias; therefore, most patients must continue antiarrhythmic therapy to reduce the need for defibrillator shocks.

Complications

Patients requiring ICD implantation are subject to the same risks as those associated with open-heart surgery. In addition, death—caused by the inability to terminate an arrhythmia induced during surgery—is an uncommon but potential risk of the implantation procedure. Infection in the ICD pocket or the leads' sites is especially significant for these patients. Infections may occur during hospitalization or several months postoperatively. Erosion of the device through the skin may occur.

Patients may also develop device-related complications. Inappropriate shocks may be delivered for sinus or supraventricular tachycardia rates above the ICD detection rate. Nonsustained VT can cause the device to unnecessarily commit to deliver a shock, which is then delivered after spontaneous conversion to normal sinus rhythm. Inappropriate shocks during sinus rhythm may actually induce ventricular arrhythmias. The ICD may interact adversely with permanent pacemakers. Lead or patch dislodgment may cause oversensing from random noise or undersensing because of loss of the signal from the heart by the ICD. The ICD may fail to terminate a ventricular arrhythmia. External defibrillation may be rendered more difficult because patches electrically "shield" the heart muscle.

Care considerations
Before surgery
• Reinforce the surgeon's explanation of the procedure and describe the preoperative, postoperative, and home care measures that will be needed.
• Make certain that the patient has signed a consent form.
• Obtain a baseline assessment.
After surgery
• Provide routine postoperative care.
• Determine whether the ICD has been activated. Sometimes the doctor inactivates the device during the immediate postoperative period to prevent response to transient supraventricular arrhythmias, which are common after surgery.
• Monitor the patient for arrhythmias and appropriate ICD function. Be prepared to initiate standard advanced cardiac life support protocol for ventricular arrhythmias not terminated by the ICD. Paddle placement may need to be modified from standard chest position to anterior-posterior placement.
• Monitor for signs of local or systemic infection.
• Schedule the patient for repeat electrophysiologic testing and exercise stress testing before discharge to tailor detection and therapy to his individual needs.
• Explain to the patient that antiarrhythmics are almost always prescribed to limit the frequency of shocks.
• Give concise instructions to the patient and his family about ICD function before the patient's discharge.

• Teach the patient about appropriate care of the surgical site, and describe the signs and symptoms of infection.

• Arrange the patient's follow-up appointment.

• Assist members of the patient's family to obtain training in cardiopulmonary resuscitation (CPR).

• Prepare the patient for the sensation of an ICD shock, commonly described as a "punch" or "kick" in the chest. Because detection and delivery of definitive therapy may take up to 30 seconds, the patient may become dizzy or light-headed, and even lose consciousness before a shock is delivered. Explain that a family member touching the patient at the time of shock delivery may experience a mild tingling sensation, which is not harmful.

• Assist the patient in obtaining a medical identification bracelet; stress the importance of wearing the bracelet or carrying an identification card. A temporary card is supplied before hospital discharge; a permanent card is mailed to the patient in 4 to 8 weeks.

Home care instructions

• Emphasize the importance of follow-up appointments to maintain proper ICD function.

• Advise the patient to notify the doctor after receiving a shock. Tell the patient that if he receives multiple shocks within a short time, he should go to a hospital emergency room.

• Tell members of the patient's family that CPR should be initiated if the patient becomes unconscious and pulseless.

• Instruct the patient to observe for signs of infection and to inform the doctor immediately if they occur.

• Review the recommended activity restrictions. Typically, patients should avoid activities that involve rough, physical contact or that would be dangerous if the patient lost consciousness (for example, driving an automobile or operating heavy machinery).

• Instruct the patient to keep a diary of symptoms and related events.

• Instruct the patient to avoid exposure to strong magnetic fields (such as power plants, large running engines, or magnetic resonance imaging scanners) because they may inactivate the patient's ICD.

• Explain that the ICD will trigger the metal detector at an airport. This will not cause the device to discharge. Most patients who show their identification card to airport personnel are permitted to bypass the security checkpoint. A patient who has an ICD should never be frisked with magnets.

INCENTIVE SPIROMETRY

Incentive spirometry gives a patient immediate feedback, encouraging him to take deep breaths to increase lung expansion. Many doctors now consider it safer and more effective than intermittent positive-pressure breathing for volume enhancement.

Normally, a person sighs every 6 to 10 minutes. But when deep breaths cause pain, a natural tendency to override the process leads to a pattern of taking shallow breaths that do little to open the airways. Incentive spirometry enhances natural sighing, inducing the patient to take a deep breath and hold it. In addition, the spirometer measures the amount of air inhaled to provide feedback on performance.

Purpose

• To encourage the patient to take deep breaths, especially postoperatively, to help prevent pulmonary complications such as atelectasis or pneumonia.

Indications

Incentive spirometry is indicated when a patient needs guided breathing exercises for volume enhancement. Frequently, this includes postoperative patients who don't take deep breaths due to pain, anesthesia, or narcotic analgesia. It is also indicated in patients with rib fractures who are reluctant to breathe deeply because of pain and in patients with neuromuscular disease who have weak respiratory muscles.

Procedure

The patient performs the procedure himself but initially receives direction from the nurse or respiratory therapist. Spirometers vary in incentive design.

To perform incentive spirometry, the patient first exhales normally. He then places his lips tightly around the mouthpiece of the incentive spirometer and inhales slowly and deeply. The patient attempts to reach the goal, which is visually apparent. Depending on the specific spirometer used, this may be accomplished by forcing the ball to the top of the chamber, compressing the bellows, or lighting up the different color panels. The patient who has difficulty achieving this goal is told to suck in as if he were sipping through a straw. Inspiring slowly ensures an even distribution of air to the alveoli.

After inspiration, the patient holds his breath for 3 seconds and then removes the mouthpiece and exhales normally. A 60-second rest between consecutive deep breaths helps prevent fatigue and dizziness. This exercise should be repeated 5 to 10 times per hour; therefore, the patient may require frequent reminders and encouragement.

Complications

Hyperventilation may occur if breathing exercises are performed too quickly.

Care considerations

Before therapy
• Briefly explain the procedure to the patient.
• Auscultate breath sounds to establish a baseline.

• Place the patient in a sitting position to promote optimal lung expansion.

During therapy
• Note the maximum volume of air the patient inhales, called the inspiratory capacity. (Some machines will automatically record the highest level reached.)

After therapy
• If appropriate, help the patient splint his incision before he coughs.
• Observe the patient's sputum, and document amount and color if indicated.
• Note any changes in breath sounds.

Home care instructions

• If indicated, inform the patient about the need to continue therapy at home using a disposable unit until he is able to deep-breathe normally without pain and no longer requires narcotic analgesics.
• Instruct the patient with neuromuscular disease to continue therapy as directed by the doctor. Tell the patient to notify the doctor if inspiratory capacity declines.

INCISION AND DRAINAGE

This procedure, called an I and D, drains accumulated pus from an infected area through a surgically created incision.

Purpose

• To treat localized suppurative infections.

Indications

An I and D is indicated when a localized infection fails to resolve, and the timing of the procedure is critical. If induration is just beginning, more pus is likely to form, so the procedure should be postponed. In that case, the area should be treated with moist heat until the pus consolidates, thereby allowing an I and D to be most effective.

Procedure

The doctor performs the procedure, commonly in the office. The doctor begins by anesthetizing the area. Using sterile technique, he then makes an incision directly over the suppurative area, spreading its edges to allow drainage of pus. The doctor may obtain a culture sample. After the pus drains, the doctor leaves the cavity open to promote healing. If the cavity is large, he may pack it with gauze to provide further drainage and to ensure healing from within. Finally, he applies a sterile dressing.

Complications

Complications rarely occur, but infection may become problematic.

Care considerations

Before the procedure
• Explain the procedure to the patient.
• Assemble sterile equipment to perform the procedure and, if needed, the equipment for obtaining a culture.
• Prepare the skin with antiseptic solution, and cover the area with sterile drapes.

During the procedure
• Support the patient and assist the doctor, as needed.

After the procedure
• Change the patient's dressings as needed using sterile technique. Record the appearance and amount of drainage, and check for signs of infection.
• Give analgesics, as ordered, and assess any complaints of excessive pain. Typically, local pain should diminish soon after the I and D.
• Observe for signs of systemic infection: fever, malaise, and chills. Check culture results.

Home care instructions

• Tell the patient to report redness, warmth, swelling, excessive pain, fever, or changed appearance of drainage.
• If the doctor orders warm soaks to promote further drainage, teach the patient to perform this procedure.

• If the patient must change the dressings at home, teach him how to perform this procedure. Explain the importance of cleanliness, hand washing, and proper disposal of soiled dressings.
• Inform the patient about ordered analgesics and antibiotics.

INFERTILITY MANAGEMENT

Infertility is defined as the inability to conceive and carry a pregnancy to viability after 1 year of regular intercourse without contraception. Almost one-fifth of all couples in the U.S. have difficulty conceiving. The causes of infertility are varied. Female causes account for about 40% of all cases, male causes account for about 40% of all cases, and interactive or unexplained causes account for 20%.

Once the cause of the infertility is known, treatment can be initiated. Several types of treatment are available, depending on the diagnosis. Drug therapy and surgery are commonly used to restore normal reproductive function. Other treatments include artificial insemination, in vitro fertilization (IVF), gamete intrafallopian transfer (GIFT), and zygote intrafallopian transfer (ZIFT). (See also the entry "Fertility Drugs.") Couples have about an 18% to 25% chance of conception through IVF and GIFT, respectively, in reputable programs. ZIFT, the newest option for infertile couples, has a success rate of approximately 40% among certain couples.

Purpose
• To achieve fertilization of a healthy ovum by viable sperm.

Indications

Infertility management may be indicated for cervical abnormality, such as a cervical environment hostile to sperm;

cervical incompetence; uterine abnormality, such as a bicornuate uterus or uterine myomas or leiomyomas; tubal abnormality, such as adhesions related to pelvic inflammatory disease or endometriosis; and ovarian abnormality, such as anovulation. In the male, indications may include inadequate sperm production, inadequate motility of the sperm, blockage of the sperm within the reproductive system, and problems in ejaculation. Interactive causes of infertility include sexual dysfunction or female antibody reaction to healthy sperm. Unexplained infertility is possible.

Procedure

Treatments vary depending on the cause of infertility, and even when the cause is unknown, various therapeutic approaches might be tried. Therapy might consist of changing habits. For example, treatment of oligospermia might consist of eliminating environmental hazards that are decreasing sperm production (tight underclothes, hot tubs, or saunas). The workup may indicate the need for sexual counseling. Surgery might be warranted if, for example, the male has a varicocele. Advances in tubal microsurgery have offered treatment of various tubal problems. Medications may be needed, such as drugs used to induce ovulation.

Sophisticated techniques may now be able to help infertile couples more than ever before, but there is a significant physical, emotional, and financial cost.

Artificial insemination is instillation of seminal fluid into the vaginal canal, cervix, or, in cases where the cervical mucus is not conducive to the sperm's survival, directly into the uterus. The partner's sperm or, in cases of male infertility, donor sperm may be used.

IVF may be performed when infertility is due to fallopian tube problems. This procedure bypasses the fallopian tubes by harvesting mature ova from the ovary, fertilizing them in a test tube, and then implanting the fertilized ova in the woman's uterus.

GIFT is a newer technique in which ova are similarly retrieved from the ovary and implanted into the fallopian tube, along with sperm; the goal is for fertilization to occur naturally.

ZIFT is a new technique in which ova are harvested from the ovary and fertilized in a test tube. The fertilized egg is then placed directly into the fallopian tube, the natural site for conception.

Complications

Infertility management causes few complications other than emotional stress. There may be complications associated with drug therapy or secondary to surgery. Reputable sperm banks test donors for antibodies to the human immunodeficiency virus to avoid spreading acquired immunodeficiency syndrome. Sperm banks also use frozen semen to ward off the problem.

Care considerations
Before the procedure
• Explain the appropriate procedure to the couple, and answer any questions they may have. Develop written procedures and provide patient information for the treatments.
• Administer an antianxiety agent, as ordered. Teach stress-reduction techniques.
• If appropriate, ensure that consent forms are signed.
• Coordinate the patient's care with the rest of the health team.
During the procedure
• Offer emotional support throughout the diagnostic and treatment phase.
• Monitor for adverse effects of drug therapy.
After the procedure
• Instruct the patient to be still for 2 hours after GIFT or ZIFT.
• Tell the patient to remain in the knee-chest position after artificial insemination. Explain to her that the doctor

may apply a cervical cap to prevent leakage of semen into the vagina.
• Monitor for complications after surgery, and take measures to prevent them.

Home care instructions

• Encourage couples who are involved in lengthy fertility programs to get on with other aspects of their lives.
• Encourage counseling for couples who are having difficulty communicating their feelings or who express uncontrollable anger or grief.
• Advise the couple to return for follow-up appointments as necessary.
• Assist the couple who remains infertile to decide on other options, which may include adoption, choosing to remain childless, or use of a surrogate mother (if not legally prohibited).
• Provide referral to sources of support, such as Resolve, a national organization for infertile couples and individuals.

INOTROPICS

The inotropics provide emergency treatment for shock by increasing cardiac output and blood pressure. These drugs include *amrinone* and the adrenergic drugs *dobutamine, dopamine, epinephrine, isoproterenol,* and *norepinephrine.* (See *Comparing inotropic drugs,* pages 380 to 383, for specific mechanisms of action.) The digitalis glycosides, which are used to treat certain types of cardiogenic shock and congestive heart failure (CHF), are not discussed here. (See the entry "Digitalis Glycosides.")

The inotropics aren't a substitute for blood and fluid replacement. They should be given to patients in hypovolemic shock only after whole blood or plasma expanders have corrected hypovolemia.

Because extravasation of some ino-

tropics may lead to tissue sloughing, they should be administered through a central venous line or a large peripheral vein; a volumetric infusion pump should be used to ensure the correct infusion rate and prevent inadvertent delivery of a bolus of the drug. Infusions of certain inotropics—especially dopamine and dobutamine—must be tapered off gradually to prevent severe hypotension.

Purpose

• To increase myocardial contractility
• To produce vasodilation.

Indications

Because these drugs don't act by the same mechanism, their effects and indications differ. For example, amrinone and dobutamine provide short-term management of patients with CHF or cardiogenic shock who fail to respond to digitalis glycosides, diuretics, and other vasodilators. Dopamine boosts blood pressure and cardiac output in patients with cardiogenic shock, refractory CHF, or cardiac arrest. Epinephrine treats asystole and ventricular fibrillation as well as anaphylaxis and bronchospasm. The cardiac stimulant isoproterenol is used in patients with heart block or severe bradycardia who fail to respond to atropine. Norepinephrine, a potent vasopressor, treats hypotension and shock.

Adverse reactions

Inotropics may cause adverse central nervous system reactions such as restlessness, nervousness, anxiety, fear, dizziness, vertigo, headache, and insomnia. Cardiovascular reactions include pallor, palpitations, flushing, cardiac arrythmias, tachycardia, slow and forceful heartbeat, hypotension or hypertension, cerebrovascular accident, decreased peripheral circulation, and angina. Musculoskeletal reactions may include weakness or mild tremors. The most common GI reactions include nau-

(Text continues on page 382.)

Comparing inotropic drugs

Refer to this chart for information about administration of various inotropic drugs.

DRUG AND ACTION	CONTRAINDICATIONS AND CAUTIONS
amrinone This biperiden derivative inhibits the breakdown of cyclic adenosine monophosphate (AMP), which facilitates calcium influx into the cell. It has no adrenergic action and increases cardiac output by causing vasodilation, thus decreasing afterload; it may have some direct action to enhance myocardial contractility.	• Contraindicated in patients with severe aortic or pulmonary valvular disease. • Use cautiously in idiopathic hypertrophic subaortic stenosis (IHSS).
dobutamine This synthetic catecholamine acts as a strong beta$_1$ stimulant and a weak beta$_2$ and alpha stimulant. It enhances contractility and diminishes peripheral vascular resistance.	• Contraindicated in IHSS.
dopamine This precursor to norepinephrine directly stimulates alpha-, beta-, and dopaminergic receptors; enhances renal perfusion; increases myocardial contractility; and, in high doses, causes vasoconstriction.	• Contraindicated in uncorrected tachyarrhythmias, pheochromocytoma, and ventricular fibrillation. • Use cautiously in patients with occlusive vascular disease, cold injuries, diabetic endarteritis, or arterial embolism; in pregnant patients; and in those taking monoamine oxidase (MAO) inhibitors.
epinephrine A naturally occurring catecholamine, epinephrine stimulates beta$_2$-receptors in low doses and alpha-receptors in high doses; it increases contractility and vasodilation.	• Contraindicated in acute angle-closure glaucoma, shock (except anaphylactic shock), organic brain damage, cardiac hypertrophy, and coronary insufficiency. Also contraindicated during general anesthesia with halogenated hydrocarbons or cyclopropane and during labor (may delay second stage). • Use with extreme caution in patients with chronic obstructive pulmonary disease and degenerative cardiac disease. Also use cautiously in elderly patients and in those with hyperthyroidism, angina, hypertension, psychoneurosis, or diabetes.
isoproterenol A beta stimulant, isoproterenol acts on beta$_1$-receptors to increase contractility and conduction velocity and on beta$_2$-receptors to produce vasodilation.	• Contraindicated in digitalis-induced tachycardia, arrhythmias (especially tachyarrhythmias), and recent myocardial infarction. • Use cautiously in coronary insufficiency, diabetes, or hyperthyroidism.

INTERACTIONS	ADMINISTRATION GUIDELINES
digitalis: increased inotropic effect, excessive hypotension	• Don't dilute amrinone with dextrose solutions. Instead, use 0.9% or 0.45% sodium chloride solution. • Discard solutions after 24 hours.
anesthetics: arrhythmias *beta blockers:* diminished effect *MAO inhibitors, tricyclic antidepressants:* potentiate pressor effects	• Because dobutamine is incompatible with alkaline solutions, don't mix it with sodium bicarbonate injection.
ergot alkaloids: hypertension *furazolidone, phenytoin:* hypotension, bradycardia	• Don't mix dopamine with alkaline I.V. solutions.
anesthetics: arrhythmias *digitalis, guanethidine:* severe hypertension *tricyclic antidepressants, phentolamine:* hypotension *propranolol:* hypertension, bradycardia	• Don't mix epinephrine with alkaline solutions. Use dextrose 5% in water, 0.9% sodium chloride solution, or a combination of the two. Mix just before use. • Because an epinephrine solution deteriorates after 24 hours, discard it at that time or if the solution becomes discolored or contains precipitate. Store the solution in a light-resistant container until use. • Massage the site after injection to counteract possible vasoconstriction. To prevent tissue necrosis, rotate injection sites. Avoid I.M. injection into the buttocks. • If the patient experiences a sharp rise in blood pressure, give a rapid-acting vasodilator to counteract pressor effects.
propranolol: antagonistic effects *epinephrine:* additive effects *tricyclic antidepressants:* arrhythmias	• If the patient experiences angina, stop the isoproterenol immediately and notify the doctor. • If possible, don't give isoproterenol at bedtime because it may interrupt sleep patterns. *(continued)*

Comparing inotropic drugs *(continued)*	
DRUG AND ACTION	**CONTRAINDICATIONS AND CAUTIONS**
norepinephrine A naturally occurring catecholamine with potent alpha and beta, stimulation, norepinephrine produces vasoconstriction and increased contractility.	• Contraindicated in pregnancy, mesenteric or peripheral vascular thrombosis, profound hypoxia, hypercapnea, or hypotension from blood volume deficits, or during cyclopropane or halothane anesthesia. • Use cautiously in hypertension, hyperthyroidism, or severe cardiac disease.

sea, vomiting (which may be severe), and diarrhea.

Care considerations

• During administration of an inotropic, monitor the patient's blood pressure and heart rate frequently (as often as every 5 minutes). Check urine output hourly.
• Monitor the patient's electrocardiogram continuously to detect arrhythmias, particularly tachyarrhythmias. Assess the need for pulmonary artery catheterization, which provides information on cardiac filling pressures, cardiac output, and peripheral resistance. This information allows adjustment of dosage to help maintain maximum cardiac contractility.
• If the patient is receiving dopamine, epinephrine, or norepinephrine, regularly assess the extremities for strength and rhythm of peripheral pulses, color, capillary refill time, and skin temperature. These drugs may severely compromise peripheral circulation.

• Assess the I.V. site hourly for blood return and signs of infiltration, such as continued hypotension despite the infusion, swelling, erythema, and coolness over the infusion site. If infiltration occurs, inject 5 to 10 mg of phentolamine in 10 ml of 0.9% sodium chloride solution, as ordered.
• Carefully review the patient's drug regimen because many drugs interact with inotropics.

Home care instructions

• Use of inotropics is typically restricted to emergency situations with the hospitalized patient.

INSULIN INJECTION, SUBCUTANEOUS

Although the indications for insulin use have remained the same since its introduction in the 1920s, commercial preparations of this drug have under-

INTERACTIONS	ADMINISTRATION GUIDELINES

guanethidine, methyldopa,
  tricyclic antidepressants:
  possible severe hypertension
MAO inhibitors: increased
  pressor effects
general anesthetics: arrhythmias
	• Administer in dextrose and 0.9% sodium chloride solution.
	• Discard solutions after 24 hours.
	• During infusion, check blood pressure every 2 minutes until stabilized, then every 5 minutes. Also check pulse and color and temperature of extremities. Titrate infusion according to findings, using doctor's guidelines.
	• If prolonged I.V. therapy is necessary, change injection sites frequently. Check sites frequently for signs of extravasation.
	• Report decreased urine output to the doctor immediately.
	• Keep emergency drugs on hand to reverse effects of norepinephrine: atropine for reflex bradycardia, propranolol for arrhythmias, and phentolamine for increased vasopressor effects.
	• When stopping norepinephrine, slow infusion rate gradually. Monitor for severe hypotension, even after the drug is discontinued.

gone many changes. For instance, U-80 insulin has been replaced by U-100 insulin, by far the most commonly used strength today. And U-500 insulin is available for patients with severe insulin resistance.

Standard insulins, made primarily from beef or pork pancreas, have been supplemented by semisynthetic and recombinant deoxyribonucleic acid (DNA) human insulins and by "purified" insulins—beef or pork insulins with less than 10 parts per million (ppm) of the by-product proinsulin as compared with less than 25 ppm for conventional insulins. These newer insulins reduce the risk of allergic reactions.

Insulins also vary in their durations of action. (See *Comparing insulin preparations*, pages 384 and 385, for details.) They may also be prescribed in a "split-and-mix" regimen, in which the patient takes two or three types of insulin with different durations of action to improve control over blood glucose levels.

Continuous insulin infusion is also available. With its use, patients can very closely control their blood glucose levels. (See *Insulin infusion pumps*, pages 386 and 387.)

Purpose
• To regulate blood glucose levels.

Indications
Insulin injection is the treatment of choice for Type I (insulin-dependent) diabetes. The insulins also treat Type II (non-insulin-dependent) diabetes when affected patients experience acute infection or excessive stress. Semisynthetic and recombinant DNA human insulins and "purified" insulins are recommended for patients who have never received insulin, for Type II diabetic patients who need insulin during stress or illness, for patients with gestational diabetes, and for nondiabetic patients who are receiving total parenteral nutrition.

Comparing insulin preparations

Insulin is available in various types and purities, with various times of onset, peak effect, and durations of action. The doctor may prescribe any of the insulins listed below or a mixture of several.

PREPARATION	ONSET (hr)	PEAK EFFECT (hr)	DURATION OF ACTION (hr)
Rapid-acting insulins			
Insulin injection (regular, crystalline zinc)			
Regular Iletin I	½ to 1	2 to 4	6 to 8
Regular Insulin	½	2½ to 5	8
Pork Regular Iletin II	½ to 1	2 to 4	6 to 8
Regular (concentrated) Iletin II	½	1 to 5	24
Velosulin	½	1 to 3	8
Purified Pork Insulin	½	2½ to 5	8
Humulin R	½ to 1	2 to 4	6 to 8
Humulin B.R.	½ to 1	2 to 4	6 to 8
Novolin R	½	2½ to 5	8
Prompt insulin zinc suspension (semilente)			
Semilente Insulin	1½	5 to 10	16
Semilente Purified Pork Prompt	1½	5 to 10	16
Intermediate-acting insulins			
Isophane insulin suspension (NPH)			
NPH Iletin I	2	6 to 12	18 to 26
NPH Insulin	1½	4 to 12	24
Pork NPH Iletin II	2	6 to 12	18 to 26
NPH Purified Pork Isophane Insulin	1½	4 to 12	24
Insulatard NPH	1½	4 to 12	24
Humulin N	1 to 2	6 to 12	18 to 24
Novolin N	1½	4 to 12	24
Isophane (NPH) 70%, regular insulin 30%			
Humulin 50/50	½	2 to 12	18 to 24
Mixtard 70/30	½	4 to 8	24

Comparing insulin preparations *(continued)*

PREPARATION	ONSET (hr)	PEAK EFFECT (hr)	DURATION OF ACTION (hr)
Intermediate-acting insulins *(continued)*			
Isophane (NPH) 70%, regular insulin 30% *(continued)*			
Mixtard Human	½	4 to 8	24
Humulin 70/30	½	2 to 12	24
Novolin 70/30	½	4 to 8	24
Insulin zinc suspension (lente)			
Lente Iletin I	2 to 4	6 to 12	18 to 26
Lente Insulin	2½	7 to 15	24
Pork Lente Iletin II	2 to 4	6 to 12	18 to 26
Lente Purified Pork Insulin	2½	7 to 15	22
Humulin L	1 to 3	6 to 12	18 to 21
Novolin L	2½	7 to 15	22
Long-acting insulins			
Protamine zinc insulin suspension			
Protamine Zinc & Iletin I	4 to 8	14 to 24	28 to 36
Beef Protamine Zinc & Iletin II	4 to 8	14 to 24	28 to 36
Pork Protamine Zinc & Iletin II	4 to 8	14 to 24	28 to 36
Extended insulin zinc suspension (ultralente)			
Ultralente Insulin	4	10 to 30	36
Humulin U Ultralente	4	10 to 30	36

Adverse reactions

The most common adverse reactions to insulin therapy, hypoglycemia and hyperglycemia, are dose-related. Allergic reactions may occur at the start of therapy and may include urticaria, angioedema, lymphadenopathy, bullae, or even anaphylaxis. During therapy, the patient may experience fatty buildup at injection sites if these sites aren't properly rotated. Over time, insulin resistance may develop. Typically, such resistance can be overcome by changing insulins.

Care considerations

• Explain to the patient that S.C. insulin injection helps regulate his blood glucose levels (see *S.C. insulin injection: A guide to self-care,* pages 388 and 389). Make sure he understands that insulin treats diabetes but doesn't cure it. Emphasize that lifelong medical follow-up is necessary and that he should *never*

Insulin infusion pumps

By delivering basal (small) insulin doses every few minutes and bolus (large) doses at mealtimes, an insulin infusion pump helps a diabetic patient exert better control over blood glucose levels and minimizes long-term complications.

The MiniMed pump

The MiniMed insulin pump shown here is about the size of a deck of cards and resembles a beeper. Its case holds three disposable batteries to power the pump. The syringe inside holds regular insulin. A tiny computer inside the pump controls the action of the syringe and precisely regulates how much insulin the pump delivers. The pump can deliver up to four different basal rates in a 24-hour period. These rates

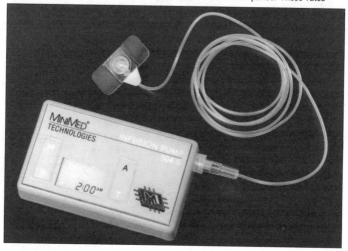

stop taking insulin because of the risk of life-threatening hyperglycemic coma.

• Review the patient's drug regimen for possible interactions. For example, concurrent use of beta blockers, clofibrate, fenfluramine, monoamine oxidase inhibitors, salicylates, or tetracycline prolongs insulin's hypoglycemic effects. Corticosteroids, oral contraceptives, and thiazide diuretics diminish these effects.

• Before giving an insulin injection, be sure that the insulin is of the correct type and strength. *Don't* substitute another type of insulin.

• If insulins must be mixed, follow the doctor's directions for their propor-

tions. After mixing NPH or Lente insulin in the same syringe with regular insulin, be sure to administer the mixture immediately to avoid binding.

• If giving insulin to a patient who hasn't received it previously or is changing brands, observe him carefully for allergic reactions.

• Closely monitor the patient's blood and urine glucose levels.

• Be alert for the Somogyi effect – hyperglycemia caused by insulin administration in patients who have received excessive doses of insulin for a prolonged period. Hyperglycemia persists in these patients because the hypoglycemia caused by excess insulin admin-

and their associated delivery times are called *profiles.* Insulin is delivered through an infusion set and exits through a needle inserted under the skin.

Waterproof tape holds the needle in place. The patient can also choose the needle-less (Sof-Set) system in which a tiny plastic tube with a needle is inserted into the skin. The needle is then removed, leaving only the tube in place. The Sof-Set can be placed in the abdomen, thigh, or flank and should be changed every 2 to 3 days.

Advantages over conventional insulin injection
Small, frequent insulin doses released automatically, with extra doses at mealtimes, permit better blood glucose level control, thus reducing long-term diabetic complications. Because the patient can adjust the insulin dosage as needed, he can be more flexible about what and when he eats. The best candidates for insulin pump therapy include:
- patients whose blood glucoses levels fluctuate widely despite optimal insulin and dietary regimens
- patients with variable work schedules or mealtimes
- pregnant women, who may have a healthier pregnancy with more precise blood glucose level control
- children or teenagers who aren't developing normally or who experience blood glucose fluctuations related to puberty.

Patient requirements
Insulin pump therapy requires that the patient know the basics of insulin pharmacology and blood glucose level self-monitoring. He must also adhere to appropriate diet and exercise regimens. Consequently, the doctor probably won't order insulin pump therapy for patients who:
- won't or can't comply with standard dietary, insulin, and self-monitoring regimens
- miss medical appointments
- can't recognize signs and symptoms of hypoglycemia.

Patients with severe diabetic complications, such as advanced renal disease, proliferative retinopathy, or severe autonomic neuropathy, may also be poor candidates.

istration stimulates the secretion of large amounts of epinephrine, glucagon, and glucocorticoids. These substances act to elevate blood glucose levels; the peak blood sugar after true hypoglycemia is typically about 150 to 160 mg/dl. When insulin levels are lowered, this response decreases and blood glucose levels fall.

Home care instructions
- Explain that insulin therapy is only part of the patient's care regimen—diet and regular exercise also contribute to good blood glucose control. Tell the patient to consult his doctor if his caloric intake or activity level changes or if he becomes ill because such conditions may

change insulin requirements. Reinforce the importance of effective blood glucose control, which may delay or prevent the vascular and neurologic complications of diabetes.
- Provide instructions for mixing, drawing up, and injecting insulin. If the patient's vision is impaired, explain that magnifying devices, such as a magnifying sleeve and the Cornwall syringe, are available to aid him.
- Show the patient how to rotate injections within a site on his abdomen, thighs, and upper arms: Full use of an injection site can allow for indefinite use of that area. (Remember that portable pumps typically inject insulin only

(Text continues on page 390.)

S.C. insulin injection: A guide to self-care

To inject insulin S.C., wash your hands thoroughly and remove your prescribed insulin from the refrigerator if it's stored there. Then follow these steps.

Warm and mix the insulin by rolling the vial between your palms. *Caution:* Never shake the vial. Check the expiration date; then read the label to make sure the medication is the correct strength and type. Use an alcohol sponge to clean the rubber stopper of the vial.

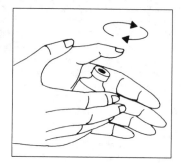

Select an appropriate site. (Refer to the guide your nurse gave you, showing how to rotate your injection sites correctly. To help you remember which site to use, write them on a calendar.) Pull the skin taut; then clean it with an alcohol sponge or a cotton ball soaked in alcohol, using a circular motion.

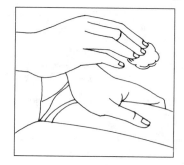

Before drawing up the insulin, inject an equal amount of air into the vial. That way, you won't create a vacuum in the vial, and it will be easier to withdraw your insulin.

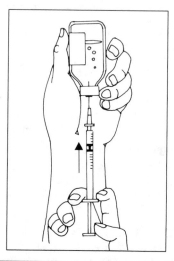

S.C. insulin injection: A guide to self-care *(continued)*

If air bubbles appear in the syringe after you fill it with insulin, tap the syringe lightly to remove them. Draw up more insulin if necessary.

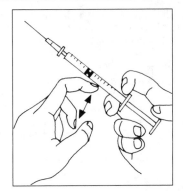

Using your thumb and forefinger, pinch the skin at the injection site. Then quickly plunge the needle up to its hub into the fat fold at a 90-degree angle. As you hold the syringe with one hand, pull back on the plunger slightly with your other hand to check for blood backflow. If blood appears in the syringe, discard everything and start again. If no blood appears, inject the insulin slowly, as shown here.

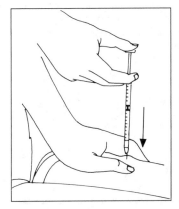

Place the alcohol sponge or cotton ball over the injection site; then press down on it lightly as you withdraw the needle. Snap the needle off the syringe, and dispose of both needle and syringe properly.
Important: When you travel, keep a bottle of insulin and a syringe with you at all times. The insulin doesn't need to be refrigerated as long as you keep it away from heat.

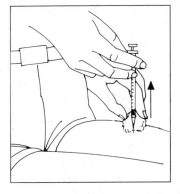

into the abdomen.) Advise the patient not to use the same site more than once every 2 months, and show him how to use a site rotation chart.

• Tell the patient to store insulin in a cool, dry place but never to freeze it. (Refrigeration isn't necessary, but it may be convenient.)

• If the patient will be testing his urine for glucose and ketones, show him how to use reagent strips following the manufacturer's guidelines. If he'll be using a home blood-glucose monitoring system, have him practice obtaining a drop of blood manually or with a blood-letting device. Advise testing glucose levels before insulin administration or meals.

• Tell the patient to inform the doctor if he misses an insulin dose or takes the incorrect amount or type.

• Suggest wearing a medical identification bracelet and carrying ample supplies of insulin and syringes with him on trips. Also recommend that he carry a fast-acting carbohydrate, such as hard candy or fruit juice, in case of a hypoglycemic episode.

INTRACRANIAL HEMATOMA, ASPIRATION

An intracranial hematoma—epidural, subdural, or intracerebral—commonly follows blunt head injury and usually requires lifesaving surgery to control bleeding and reduce intracranial pressure (ICP). Even if the patient's life isn't in immediate danger, surgery is usually indicated to prevent irreversible damage from cerebral or brain stem ischemia.

An epidural hematoma is the accumulation of blood in the potential space between the skull and the dura mater. About half of these patients (usually children) experience a lucid interval followed by rapid deterioration and possible death or serious morbidity;

therefore, emergency surgery is typically required. The epidural hematoma is evacuated through burr holes, and the bleeding vessels are ligated. Early intervention generally allows complete recovery to normal neurologic function.

A subdural hematoma is the accumulation of blood in the potential space between the dura mater and the arachnoid membrane. Acute subdural hematomas produce symptoms quickly (within 24 to 48 hours), are associated with more severe underlying brain contusion, and require prompt surgery because the brain is unable to tolerate rapid compression. Because these lesions are of jellylike consistency, a craniotomy is necessary to remove the clot. Subacute subdural hematomas produce symptoms within days of the injury; they are partially liquefied and may be removed through burr holes. Chronic subdural hematomas may not produce symptoms for weeks, perhaps for months; such lesions are liquefied and burr holes may therefore be used to evacuate them, reducing the risks associated with more complicated surgery. If the neurologic examination is stable and computed tomography (CT) demonstrates a small chronic clot, surgery may not be necessary.

An intracerebral hematoma involves bleeding in the brain parenchyma. Significant, accessible intracerebral hematomas associated with deteriorating neurologic status require surgical evacuation through a craniotomy.

Purpose

• To remove an intracranial hematoma, thereby relieving pressure on the intracranial vessels and tissues and preventing cerebral ischemia and brain tissue damage.

Indications

Aspiration of intracranial hematomas may be indicated for patients with acute or chronic epidural, subdural, or intracerebral hematomas.

Procedure

Depending on the type of hematoma, the surgeon gains access to the bleeding site through either a craniotomy or burr holes.

If the hematoma is liquid, the surgeon uses a twist drill to burr holes through the skull, most commonly in the frontoparietal or temporoparietal areas. He drills at least two holes to delineate the extent of the clot and allow complete aspiration. Once he reaches the clot, he inserts a small suction tip into the burr holes to aspirate the clot. He then inserts drains, which usually remain in place for 24 hours.

If the clot is solid (or, although liquid, can't be completely aspirated through burr holes), the surgeon performs a craniotomy, the more common approach. After exposing the hematoma, he aspirates it with a small suction tip or may use an irrigation of 0.9% sodium chloride solution to wash out parts of the clot. He then ligates any bleeding vessels in the hematoma cavity and closes the bone and scalp flaps. (If cerebral edema is severe, the craniotomy site may be left exposed and the flaps replaced only after edema subsides.) He may place a drain in the surgical site.

Complications

Aspiration of the hematoma carries a risk of severe infection and seizures as well as respiratory compromise and increased ICP if a craniotomy is performed.

Care considerations

Before surgery

• Briefly explain the procedure to the patient and family if time permits. Include preoperative and postoperative teaching.
• Prepare the patient as for a craniotomy. (See the entry "Craniotomy.")
• Ensure that the patient or a responsible family member has signed a consent form.

• Obtain a baseline neurologic assessment.

After surgery

• Perform a complete neurologic assessment. Watch for and immediately report signs of an elevated ICP, such as headache, altered respirations, deteriorating level of consciousness, and visual disturbances.
• Monitor vital signs and observe for signs of infection.
• As ordered, keep the head of bed elevated about 30 degrees to promote venous drainage from the brain. For subdural hematomas, however, some doctors order that the patient's head remain down for 24 hours postoperatively in an effort to allow the brain to reexpand or to prevent a clot from reforming.
• Accurately record intake and output.
• As ordered, administer an analgesic to relieve pain, antibiotics to prevent infection, and anticonvulsants to prevent seizures.
• Regularly check the surgical dressing and the surrounding area for excessive bleeding or drainage. Report any abnormal drainage from the incision. If a drain is in place, evaluate patency by noting the amount of drainage. Although the surgeon may set specific guidelines, drainage usually shouldn't exceed 125 ml during the first 8 hours after surgery, 100 ml during the following 8 hours, and 75 ml over the next 8 hours.
• To prevent formation of decubitus ulcers and to enhance circulation, turn the patient frequently and perform passive range-of-motion exercises for all extremities.
• Anticipate a follow-up CT scan 2 to 3 days postoperatively to check the operative site.

Home care instructions

• Teach the patient and his family proper suture care techniques. Tell them to observe the suture line for signs of infection, such as redness and swelling, and to report any such signs immediately.

• Also instruct the patient and family to watch for and report any neurologic symptoms, such as altered level of consciousness, sudden weakness, increased headaches, and visual disturbances.

• Suggest that the patient wear a wig, hat, or scarf until his hair grows back. Advise using a lanolin-based lotion to help keep the scalp supple and decrease itching, but warn against applying lotion to the suture line.

• Remind the patient to continue taking prescribed anticonvulsants to minimize the risk of seizures. Tell him to report any drug adverse effects, such as excessive drowsiness or confusion.

• Tell the patient he may take acetaminophen or another mild nonnarcotic analgesic for headaches and should inform the doctor if he doesn't get relief.

J

JOINT REPLACEMENT

Total or partial replacement of a joint with a synthetic prosthesis aims to restore mobility and stability and to relieve pain. Recent improvements in surgical techniques and prosthetic devices have made joint replacement increasingly common. Some centers now specialize in custom joint replacement; in this technique, a mold is taken of the patient's joint and then, using computer techniques, the prosthesis is custom-made to replicate within 99% the patient's joint. All joints except the spine can be replaced with a prosthesis; hip and knee replacements are the most common. The benefits of joint replacement include not only improved, pain-free mobility but also an increased sense of independence and self-worth. (Also see *Reconstruction alternatives*, page 394.)

Purpose
• To replace a diseased or damaged joint, thereby restoring or improving joint function and eliminating or reducing pain.

Indications
This procedure is indicated for severe joint destruction, such as in patients with arthritis, other degenerative joint disorders, and extensive joint trauma.

Procedure
Surgery is performed using general anesthesia. The details of the joint replacement procedure vary slightly depending on the joint and its condition.

In a total hip replacement, for instance, the surgeon replaces the head and neck of the femur and the acetabulum with a prosthesis. Several prostheses are available, but the femoral component is typically constructed of stainless steel or vitalium; the acetabular component, of polyethylene with metal backing. The surgeon may secure the device in place with methyl methacrylate adhesive, which fills the gap between the prosthesis and the bone. Prosthetic components may also be made of ceramic materials or porous coated metals that do not require adhesives. Bone ingrowth and repair allow fixation of these prostheses. To prevent infection, special precautions are taken during surgery, such as the use of impermeable operating room attire, laminar airflow, and prophylactic antibiotics. Blood loss is usually large and is monitored carefully. Large amounts of I.V. fluids are commonly infused, and whole blood or packed-cell transfusions are usually administered.

For total knee replacement, the surgeon replaces the patient's distal femur, proximal tibia, and patellar articulating surfaces with a prosthesis. As with total hip replacement, the surgeon may either use methyl methacrylate adhesive to secure the prosthesis or allow bone ingrowth to fixate prostheses that do not require adhesives. Strict infection precautions are needed; a pneumatic tourniquet may be used to control blood loss.

Reconstruction alternatives

Arthroplasty is a surgical technique intended to restore motion to a stiffened joint. Joint replacement is one option; other options include joint resection or interpositional reconstruction.

Joint resection involves careful excision of bone portions, creating a ¾" (2-cm) gap in one or both bone surfaces of the joint. Fibrous scar tissue eventually fills in the gap. Although this surgery restores mobility and relieves pain, it decreases joint stability.

Interpositional reconstruction involves reshaping the joint and placing a prosthetic disk between the reshaped bony ends. The prosthesis used for this procedure may be composed of metal, plastic, fascia, or skin. However, with repeated injury and surgical reshaping, total joint replacement may be necessary.

Complications

Complications of joint replacement include hypovolemic shock, fat embolism, thrombophlebitis, infection, dislocation of the prosthesis (with hip replacement), and the need for eventual revision.

Care considerations

Before surgery

• Clarify the surgeon's explanation of the procedure if necessary.
• Prepare the patient for a long period of rehabilitation.
• Warn that surgery may not relieve pain immediately and that pain may actually worsen for several weeks. Reassure the patient that analgesics will be available as needed.
• Inform the patient about postoperative measures, such as positioning, transfer techniques, assisted ambulation, and an exercise regimen. Explain that the exercise program will begin shortly after surgery, even while he is confined to bed.
• Ensure that the patient or a responsible family member has signed a consent form.
• Administer antibiotics, as ordered.
• Prepare the operative site as ordered.
• Begin discharge planning, including arranging for assistance with activities of daily living at home.

After surgery

• Keep the patient on bed rest for the prescribed period after surgery.
• Maintain the affected joint in proper alignment. For example, with total hip replacements, maintain abduction of the affected hip with abductor pillow, traction, or pillows. Do not elevate the bed more than 60 degrees to prevent acute flexion, which may cause dislocation.
• Assess the patient's level of pain, and provide analgesics, as prescribed.
• Apply antiembolism stockings precisely as ordered.
• Monitor for signs of hypovolemia, fat embolism (typically 72 hours after surgery), and thrombophlebitis.
• Inspect the incision site and dressing frequently for signs of infection. Monitor for temperature elevation. Change the dressing as necessary, maintaining strict aseptic technique. Administer antibiotics, as prescribed.
• Periodically assess neurovascular and motor status distal to the site of joint replacement. Immediately report any abnormalities.
• Reposition the patient often to enhance comfort and prevent pressure ulcers. Encourage frequent coughing and deep-breathing to prevent pulmonary complications and adequate fluid intake

to prevent urinary stasis and constipation.
• Encourage the patient to implement the recommended exercise program. (Some doctors routinely order physical therapy to begin on the day of surgery.) The doctor may prescribe continuous passive motion, which involves use of a machine or a system of suspended ropes and pulleys, or a series of active or passive range-of-motion (ROM) exercises. (For further details, see the entry "Exercises, Range-of-Motion.")
• Assist with progressive ambulation precisely as ordered. Make certain that the patient obtains and can correctly use prescribed supportive equipment, such as crutches, walker, or cane.

Home care instructions

• Encourage the patient to report for follow-up evaluation and testing.
• Review signs of complications. Tell the patient to promptly report signs of possible infection, such as persistent fever and increased pain, tenderness, and stiffness in the joint and surrounding area. Remind him that infection may develop even several months after joint replacement. Also tell the patient to report suddenly increased pain or decreased function, which may indicate dislodgment of the prosthesis.
• Reinforce the doctor's and physical therapist's instructions for the patient's exercise regimen. Remind him to adhere to the prescribed schedule of exercise and not to rush rehabilitation, no matter how well he feels.
• Review prescribed limitations on activity. Depending on the location and extent of surgery, the doctor may order the patient to avoid bending or lifting, extensive stair climbing, or sitting for prolonged periods (including long car trips or plane flights). He also will caution against overusing the joint—especially if it is a weight-bearing joint.
• The patient who has undergone knee replacement may be instructed to wear a knee brace or an immobilizer. If so, make sure he knows how to apply it correctly.
• After hip replacement, instruct the patient to keep his hips abducted and not to cross his legs when sitting in order to reduce the risk of dislocating the prosthesis. Tell him to avoid flexing his hips more than 90 degrees when rising from a bed or chair. Tell him to avoid sitting in low chairs or in a bathtub. Encourage him to sit in chairs that have high arms and a firm seat and to sleep only on a firm mattress.
• After shoulder joint replacement, tell the patient to keep his arm in a sling until postoperative swelling subsides, then to slowly begin the prescribed exercise program when healing is complete—usually about 6 weeks after surgery.
• Explain the possible need for prophylactic antibiotics for minor surgical procedures or dental procedures to prevent bacteremia. Tell the patient not to have magnetic resonance imaging studies because of the metal component of the prosthesis.

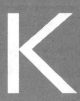

KERATOTOMY, RADIAL

This surgical procedure is performed to correct myopia, a refractive error in which light rays come to a focus in front of the retina. Radial keratotomy involves creation of small radial incisions in the cornea. These incisions flatten the cornea to help properly focus light on the retina.

The degree of myopia is measured in diopters (unit of measurement of refractive power of lenses or prisms). Because radial keratotomy can only reduce myopia by up to 4 diopters, this procedure will not help highly myopic patients.

Purpose
• To correct myopia by flattening the cornea, thereby reducing the corneal curvature and changing its refractive properties.

Indications
This procedure is an option for patients with myopia (ranging from -2 to -8 diopters) whose vision with glasses or contact lenses is unsatisfactory.

Disadvantages of this procedure are its unpredictability and instability. This procedure is controversial in the ophthalmic community for those reasons.

Procedure
Radial keratotomy is commonly performed in an outpatient surgical setting. The nurse typically is involved in the direct preoperative and postoperative care and teaching.

Sedation and topical anesthetic eyedrops are used for the surgery. Corneal thickness is measured using an ultrasonic pachometer. Then, using a calibrated diamond knife, the surgeon makes eight or more incisions into the cornea in a radial pattern. A topical antibiotic solution and a cycloplegic agent are then instilled. A pressure patch may be applied for 24 hours.

Complications
Because keratotomy has been widely used only since the 1970s, its long-term effects aren't known. Complications include overcorrection or undercorrection as well as corneal perforation (usually self-healing).

Care considerations
Before surgery
• The patient will have had an ophthalmologic examination to evaluate visual acuity and refraction, the thickness and curvature of the cornea, endothelial cell count, intraocular pressure, and axial length of the eye.
• As needed, explain the keratotomy procedure and answer any questions the patient may have.
• Tell the patient that his face will be cleaned with an antiseptic solution and that a sedative will be given to help him relax. He'll also have a drape placed over his face, supplemental oxygen will be provided, and a local anesthetic will be instilled in the affected eye. Explain that the procedure takes 3 to 8 minutes and that he must remain still until it's over. Inform him that the doctor may cover the eye with a dressing after surgery.

• Ensure that the patient has signed a consent form.

After surgery

• After the patient recovers from the local anesthetic, he may experience some discomfort for 10 to 18 hours. Administer the ordered analgesic. Warn the patient not to rub the eye, as this may damage the cornea.

• If the patient's eye isn't patched, lower the lights because sensitivity to bright lights may aggravate his discomfort.

Home care instructions

• If the doctor prescribes eyedrops, review their use with the patient. Emphasize the importance of instilling them as ordered.

• Explain that photophobia and foreign body sensation commonly follow keratotomy but usually subside in 1 to 2 months. Suggest that the patient wear dark sunglasses or glasses with polarizing lenses when he's in bright sunlight. Warn him to avoid night driving if he's bothered by glare from oncoming lights.

• Because the patient's vision may fluctuate, advise him to avoid any hazardous activity that requires clear vision until symptoms subside.

• Instruct the patient to protect the affected eye from soap and water when showering and bathing and to avoid contact and water sports until the doctor gives permission. Also advise the female patient to avoid wearing eye makeup until the cornea is healed (in approximately 1 month).

KIDNEY TRANSPLANTATION

Ranked as the most commonly performed and most successful of all organ transplants, kidney transplantation is an attractive alternative to dialysis for many patients with end-stage renal disease (ESRD). A successful transplant can allow the patient to resume a normal lifestyle.

The major obstacle to successful transplantation is rejection of the donated organ by the recipient's body. Histocompatibility testing, which measures the degree of antigenic compatibility between the recipient and donor, is performed to select the most histocompatible donor and prevent rejection. Transplant success rates have improved in recent years and may be attributed to improved tissue typing, immunosuppression, surgical techniques, and candidate selection. However, because donor kidneys are scarce, some patients remain on waiting lists for months or years.

Purpose

• To restore renal function by implanting a healthy donor kidney.

Indications

Kidney transplantations may be indicated for the ESRD patient after careful evaluation. Physiologic, psychological, and social parameters are taken into consideration. Complex rating systems are commonly used because of the inherent risks of surgery and scarcity of donor organs.

Although there are few absolute contraindications for kidney transplantation, they may include active cancer or another major organ or system disease such as liver failure. A history of substance abuse, severe psychiatric disorders, noncompliance with treatment, and a lack of support systems may also rule out the patient as a transplant candidate.

Procedure

In this procedure, a surgeon implants a healthy kidney that has been surgically removed from a living relative or cadaver donor into the recipient's iliac fossa. The organ's vessels are then connected to the internal iliac vein and internal iliac artery.

The donor ureter is connected to the bladder. The recipient's own kidneys typically aren't removed unless they're structurally abnormal, infected, greatly enlarged, or are causing intractable hypertension. They're left in place to increase circulating hematocrit levels, ease management of dialysis, and reduce blood transfusion requirements in case of transplant rejection.

Complications

Major complications include rejection, infection, increased incidence of cancer, and death.

Care considerations
Before surgery

• Review the transplant procedure, supplementing and clarifying the doctor's explanation as necessary. Tell the patient that the surgery is performed under general anesthesia.
• In conjunction with the transplant team, discuss the benefits and risks of transplantation with the patient and family. Make certain that the patient understands the meaning of rejection and what methods (including drugs) will be used to prevent it.
• Ensure that the comprehensive pretransplant evaluation is complete. It may include a thorough physical examination; a battery of laboratory tests; radiographic studies; an electrocardiogram; bowel preparation; and shaving of the operative area. Explain that dialysis is usually necessary the day before surgery and may be needed for a few days after surgery if the transplanted kidney fails to function immediately.
• As ordered, begin administration of immunosuppressants, such as azathioprine, cyclosporine, and corticosteroids.
• Ensure that the patient or a responsible family member has signed a consent form.
After surgery
• Monitor vital signs, I.V. lines, indwelling urinary catheter, arterial lines, and ventilator (if applicable), as ordered.
• Monitor for postoperative pain, and administer analgesics as ordered.
• Take precautions to reduce the risk of infection.
• Monitor laboratory work as ordered, especially creatinine and potassium levels.
• Carefully monitor urine output, and promptly report output below 100 ml/hour. With a living-donor transplantation, urine flow usually begins immediately after revascularization and connection of the ureter to the recipient's bladder. After a cadaver kidney transplantation, anuria may persist for from 2 days to as long as 2 weeks; dialysis will be necessary during this period. Observe urine color; expect it to be slightly blood-tinged for several days and then to gradually clear.
• Monitor and record the patient's weight daily.
• The patient may gradually resume a normal diet, with appropriate restrictions, as ordered.

Home care instructions

• Have the patient measure and record intake and output daily, weigh himself daily, and take temperature and blood pressure twice daily.
• Direct the patient to watch for and promptly report any signs and symptoms of transplant rejection, including tenderness or swelling over the graft site, fever exceeding 100° F (37.8° C), decreased urine output, weight gain, blood in the urine, general weakness, and elevated blood pressure. (See *Managing transplant rejection*.)
• Instruct the patient to report signs of infection promptly. Because the patient is at increased risk for infection, advise him to avoid exposure to crowds and persons with known or suspected infections for at least 3 months after surgery.

Managing transplant rejection

Transplant rejection can occur immediately after surgery or may develop years later. But whenever it occurs, rejection demands prompt intervention.

Hyperacute rejection

Hyperacute rejection occurs several minutes to hours after transplantation as the patient's circulating antibodies attack the donor kidney. Renal perfusion plummets, and the organ rapidly becomes ischemic and dies. If the patient experiences hyperacute rejection, prepare him for removal of the rejected kidney. Provide emotional support—to the patient and the donor—to help ease disappointment.

Acute rejection

This type of rejection may occur 1 week to 6 months after transplantation of a living donor kidney or 1 week to 2 years after transplantation of a cadaver kidney. Acute rejection is caused by an antigen-antibody reaction, which produces acute tubular necrosis.

Acute rejection may be reversible with prompt treatment. Be alert for its characteristic indicators: signs of infection (fever, rapid pulse, lethargy, elevated white blood cell count), oliguria or anuria, hypertension, or a weight gain of more than 3 lb (1.4 kg) in a day.

If the patient shows signs of acute rejection, reassure him that this complication is common and often reversible. As ordered, prepare him for dialysis.

Chronic rejection

This irreversible complication can start several months or years after transplantation. It is caused by long-term antibody destruction of the donor kidney. Typically, it is detected by serial laboratory studies that show a declining glomerular filtration rate accompanied by rising blood urea nitrogen and serum creatinine levels.

If the patient is experiencing chronic rejection, inform him that complete destruction of the donor kidney may not occur for several years. Prepare him for a renal scan, renal biopsy, and other tests, as ordered. Administer an increased dose of immunosuppressants, and adjust his dietary and fluid regimen; when necessary, prepare him for dialysis or another transplant.

• Emphasize the need for strict compliance with all prescribed medication.

• Encourage regular, moderate exercise. Tell the patient to begin exercise slowly and increase it gradually, and to avoid excessive bending, heavy lifting, and contact sports.

• Also warn the patient against activities or positions that place pressure on the new kidney—for example, long car trips and lap-style seat belts.

• Advise the patient to refrain from sexual activity for at least 6 weeks after surgery. Discuss family planning. Pregnancy poses an additional risk to a new kidney.

• Stress the importance of regular follow-up visits to evaluate renal function and the status of the transplant.

• Tell the patient to avoid exposure to strong sunlight and to use a sunscreen when outdoors because immunosuppressant therapy increases the risk of skin cancer.

LAMINECTOMY AND SPINAL FUSION

In laminectomy, the surgeon removes one or more of the bony laminae that cover the vertebrae.

After removal of several laminae, spinal fusion — grafting of bone chips between vertebral spaces — is often performed to stabilize the spine. Spinal fusion also may be done apart from laminectomy in some patients with vertebrae weakened by trauma or disease. (See *Alternatives to laminectomy*.)

Purpose
For laminectomy
• To repair spinal cord defects
• To provide spinal cord stimulation
• To allow insertion of infusion pumps for pain control.
For spinal fusion
• To strengthen and stabilize the spine.

Indications
Most commonly performed to relieve pressure on the spinal cord or spinal nerve roots resulting from a herniated disk, laminectomy may also be done to treat a compression fracture, dislocated vertebrae, or spinal cord tumor.

Spinal fusion may be needed to treat traumatic disruption of the vertebrae as well as ruptured disks that have resulted in unusual instability. Commonly, this procedure is performed when more conservative treatments prove ineffective.

Procedure
To perform a laminectomy, the surgeon makes a midline vertical incision and strips the fascia and muscles from the bony laminae. He then removes one or more sections of laminae to expose the spinal defect. For a herniated disk, the surgeon removes part or all of the disk. For a spinal cord tumor, he incises the dura and explores the cord for metastasis. Then he dissects the tumor and removes it, using suction, forceps, or dissecting scissors.

To perform spinal fusion, the surgeon exposes the affected vertebrae and then inserts bone chips obtained from the patient's iliac crest or, rarely, from a bone bank. To restore optimal strength to the vertebral column, the surgeon wires these bone grafts into several vertebrae surrounding the area of instability.

Complications
Complications may include recurrence of herniation, nerve root injury causing motor and sensory deficits, arachnoiditis, chronic neuritis caused by adhesions and scarring, vascular injury, and urine retention or paralytic ileus due to stimulation of the autonomic nervous system.

Care considerations
Before surgery
• Explain the procedure and answer the patient's questions.
• Discuss postoperative recovery and rehabilitation. Point out that surgery won't relieve back pain immediately and that pain may even worsen after the surgery. Explain that pain will be relieved only after chronic nerve irritation and swelling subside, which may take up to several weeks. Reassure the patient that

Alternatives to laminectomy

Microsurgical diskectomy, percutaneous automated diskectomy, and chemonucleolysis are alternative treatments for a herniated disk.

Microsurgical diskectomy
This treatment involves use of microsurgical techniques. Through a small incision, the involved area can be visualized and herniated disk material can be excised. Extruded fragments may also be removed. Blood loss is minimal, complications are less frequent, and the postoperative course is generally less painful.

Percutaneous automated diskectomy
In this technique for removal of lumbar herniated disks, the doctor uses a nucletome, an instrument with cutting and aspiration capabilities, to gently aspirate (through a small skin incision) only the disk portion that is causing pain. Typically used for small, less severe disk abnormalities, the procedure can be performed on an outpatient basis using local anesthesia. It is not effective for patients who have disk extrusion or fragments in the spinal canal.

Chemonucleolysis
This treatment involves injection of chymopapain or collagenase to reduce the nucleus pulposus of the herniated disk. Usually performed with radiographic visualization, it eliminates the need for major surgery. However, it has risks. Studies indicate disk space narrowing after chemonucleolysis, leading to irreversible osteoarthritis-like changes. Anaphylactic reactions are also possible.

---

analgesics and muscle relaxants will be available during recovery.

• Tell the patient that he'll return from surgery with a dressing over the incision and will maintain bed rest for the time prescribed by the doctor. Explain that he'll be turned often to prevent pressure ulcers and pulmonary complications. Show him the logrolling method of turning and the correct way to rise from a bed or chair.

• Perform a baseline assessment of motor function and sensation in the patient's lower trunk, legs, and feet. Assess complaints of pain, paresthesia, and muscle spasm. Carefully document the results for comparison with postoperative findings.

• Ensure that the patient has signed a consent form.

After surgery
• After lumbar laminectomy, keep the patient flat for the prescribed period, with 6″ (15-cm) blocks to elevate the head of the bed. Tell the patient not to sit up or raise his head. When he's able to assume a side-lying position, make sure he keeps his spine straight, with his knees flexed and drawn up toward his chest. Insert a pillow between his knees to relieve pressure on the spine from hip adduction. Use logrolling to turn the patient.

• After cervical laminectomy, teach the patient to avoid extreme flexion and extension of the neck and to wear a soft cervical collar.

• Give analgesics and muscle relaxants, as ordered.

• Inspect the dressing frequently for bleeding or cerebrospinal fluid leakage; report these signs immediately. The surgeon will probably perform the initial dressing change. If asked to perform subsequent changes, observe the incision for signs of infection.

• Assess vital signs and neurologic status. Assess movement, sensation, color, and temperature of upper extremities

following cervical laminectomy and lower extremities following lumbar laminectomy. Compare with baseline findings. Also assess urine output, and auscultate for the return of bowel sounds. If the patient doesn't void within 8 to 12 hours after surgery, notify the doctor and prepare to insert a catheter to relieve urine retention. If the patient can void normally, assist him in getting on and off a bedpan while maintaining proper alignment.
• Assess lung sounds. Ask the doctor if the patient should cough postoperatively.
• Anticipate physical therapy for the patient who is allowed out of bed. Encourage prescribed exercises.

Home care instructions

• Teach the patient and family caregiver how to perform meticulous care of the incision. Tell them to report signs of infection immediately. Instruct the patient to avoid tub baths until healing is complete and to shower with his back away from the stream of water.
• After lumbar laminectomy, advise the patient to gradually increase his activity; minimize sitting to decrease pressure on the disk space; support his lower back when sitting; bend at the knees, not the waist; allow rest periods between activities; wear a fitted corset or brace for 6 to 8 weeks postoperatively, as instructed; avoid lifting or pulling heavy objects; perform daily stretching exercises as directed; and maintain normal weight.

LAPAROSCOPY AND LAPAROTOMY

A laparoscopy is the endoscopic examination of the upper abdominal cavity and reproductive organs. A laparotomy includes any surgical incision into the peritoneal cavity.

After laparoscopic surgery, the patient may go home the next day; after laparotomy, the hospital stay will be the same as for any other abdominal surgery.

Purpose

• To allow visualization of the organs in the pelvis and upper abdominal cavity for diagnosis or further surgery.

Indications

Laparoscopic procedures may include tubal ligations, aspiration of ovarian cysts, cauterization of endometrial implants, lysis of adhesions, salpingectomy, adnexectomy, myomectomy, oophorectomy, salpingostomy, appendectomy, cholecystectomy, cancer staging, some liver biopsies and, possibly, removal of an ectopic pregnancy.

Laparoscopy may also help detect abnormalities such as cysts, adhesions, fibroids, and infection; identify the cause of pelvic pain by diagnosing endometriosis, ectopic pregnancy, or pelvic inflammatory disease; and evaluate pelvic masses or the fallopian tubes of infertile patients.

Laparotomy may be indicated for gynecologic conditions unsuited for treatment by laparoscopy; for example, to remove ovarian cysts containing endometrial tissue and thereby avert the risk of rupture or to remove endometrial implants that are too large for removal by laparoscopy.

Laparoscopy should be avoided in a patient with intestinal obstruction, abdominal cancer, acute abdominal tuberculosis, or ruptured ectopic pregnancy with massive hemorrhage.

Procedure

The patient will receive regional or general anesthesia for laparoscopy. The surgeon makes a small incision in the abdominal wall slightly below the umbilicus and introduces a trocar and a catheter into the incision. The trocar is then removed, and carbon dioxide gas is pumped into the abdominal cavity to distend the visual area. If additional instruments are needed, they may be inserted through another incision made below the initial one or they may be passed through the laparoscope. The laparoscope allows passage of surgical instruments such as laser, cryosurgical, or electrocautery devices. When the surgeon has completed the specific procedure, the carbon dioxide gas is removed, the incision is sutured with absorbable suture, and a dressing is applied.

Laparotomy is performed under general anesthesia. The surgeon makes an abdominal incision and explores the entire abdominal contents for disease. Any diseased organ is removed or repaired, the incision is closed, and a dressing is applied.

Complications

Possible complications of laparoscopic procedures include excessive bleeding, abdominal cramps, and shoulder pain. These effects may result from infection of the abdomen with carbon dioxide.

Complications of laparotomy may include infection or other complications associated with abdominal surgery.

Care considerations

Before the procedure or surgery

• Explain that laparoscopy can be both a test and a treatment.
• Describe the laparoscopic procedure, and answer any questions.
• If applicable, tell the patient to expect same-day discharge after recovery from the laparoscopic procedure.
• Instruct the patient to fast 6 to 8 hours before the procedure, and tell him that a general anesthetic will most likely be administered.
• Tell the patient who smokes to avoid smoking for about 12 hours before the procedure.

• Ensure that the patient has signed a consent form and that preoperative laboratory work (complete blood count, blood chemistry studies, urinalysis) has been completed.
• For laparotomy, prepare the patient as for abdominal surgery, following the prescribed preoperative regimen.

After the procedure or surgery

• Monitor vital signs.
• After laparoscopy, check for excessive vaginal bleeding, which may indicate hemorrhage; minor bleeding is normal.
• Ask the patient who has had a laparoscopy about abdominal cramps or shoulder pain, and provide analgesics, as ordered. If the patient complains of bloating or abdominal fullness, explain that this feeling will subside as the gas in the abdomen is absorbed into the bloodstream, exchanged in the lungs, and exhaled.
• After laparotomy, provide care as for any patient after abdominal surgery.

Home care instructions

• After laparoscopy, emphasize the importance of reporting bright red vaginal bleeding; fever of 100.4° F (38° C) or higher; severe abdominal pain; redness, puffiness, or drainage from the incision; or any nausea, vomiting, or diarrhea.
• Instruct the patient to wait until the day after laparoscopy to bathe or remove the bandage.
• Encourage the patient to eat lightly after laparoscopy because there may be residual abdominal gas.
• After laparoscopy, advise the patient to resume normal activities after 2 days and to avoid strenuous work and sports for 1 week or as recommended by the doctor.
• Encourage the patient to keep follow-up medical appointments.
• After laparotomy, encourage the patient to follow the prescribed activity restrictions.

LARYNGECTOMY

Laryngectomy is the removal of all or part of the larynx. The various types of laryngectomy differ mainly in the anatomical structures that are surgically removed, depending on the extent of underlying disease. For example, laryngofissure may be used to remove a glottic tumor limited to one vocal cord. However, radiation is now replacing this procedure because both treatments have similar survival rates and radiation leaves the patient with better voice quality. More widespread tumors may require a vertical hemilaryngectomy or a horizontal supraglottic laryngectomy. For a large glottic or supraglottic tumor with vocal cord fixation, a total laryngectomy may be needed.

The prognosis after laryngectomy, though generally good, reflects the extent of the disease at the time of surgery. After laryngectomy and radiation treatment, the 5-year survival rate is about 80% to 85% for lesions without vocal cord fixation; 75% for tumors with cord fixation; and 50% for tumors with metastases to the cervical lymph nodes.

Purpose
• To remove all or part of the larynx to treat laryngeal cancer.

Indications
A laryngectomy is the most common treatment for laryngeal cancer. It is indicated for tumors that are not treatable with radiation therapy alone. A partial laryngectomy may be indicated for smaller tumors. Total laryngectomy is indicated for advanced laryngeal cancer.

Procedure
The patient receives general anesthesia. The surgeon chooses the specific procedure type based on the type and site of the tumor, the extent and location of metastases, and vocal cord mobility. The most common procedures used are total laryngectomy, horizontal supraglottic laryngectomy, vertical hemilaryngectomy, and laryngofissure. (See *Understanding types of laryngectomy,* pages 406 and 407.)

Complications
Many complications can result from laryngectomy. Immediately after surgery, respiratory distress or, rarely, bleeding into the wound or hematoma formation may occur. There is also a risk of salivary fistulas with any surgery involving the esophagus or pharynx. Other complications include infection or empyema and edema. Later complications include pneumonia, atelectasis, and pharyngeal fistulas.

Care considerations
Before surgery
• Describe the surgery and its aftercare in detail, and answer any questions the patient and family (if applicable) may have.
• Explain the expected voice quality and extent of speech the patient will have postoperatively.
• Before surgery, help the patient develop a communication system for the postoperative period. If the patient will be unable to speak after surgery, suggest a communication system such as flash cards, paper and pencil, or a magic slate. Also, coordinate visits by a speech pathologist who will evaluate the patient, reinforce earlier information, and answer questions about reestablishing speech.
• If the patient will have a total laryngectomy, explain that he'll breathe through an opening in his neck after surgery. Inform him that he won't be able to smell, blow his nose, whistle, gargle, sip, or suck on a straw. Describe and show pictures of the laryngectomy stoma. Explain that he'll expectorate secretions through his stoma, which will

need suctioning periodically. Emphasize that he'll be able to perform stoma care and suctioning himself. If possible, arrange a meeting with a laryngectomy patient who has adjusted well to having a stoma.

• Inform the patient that he may have a laryngectomy tube after surgery (shorter and thicker than a tracheostomy tube but requiring the same care) and that it's usually removed after 7 to 10 days. Explain that he'll also have a nasogastric (NG) tube in place for 7 to 10 days; this will provide a route for nourishment until his suture line heals. Mention that he'll begin receiving oral feedings (thick, easy-to-swallow fluids, such as gelatin or ice cream) about 10 days after his surgery.

• Before a laryngectomy, make sure the patient has signed a consent form.

After surgery

• Keep emergency resuscitation equipment readily available.

• Elevate the head of the bed 30 degrees to prevent tension on the suture line, decrease neck edema, and prevent aspiration during feeding. Be sure to support the patient's head, neck, and back for 24 to 48 hours.

• Periodically auscultate the patient's lungs to detect pulmonary congestion. Also check the rate and depth of respirations, and observe for use of accessory muscles. If the patient has a tracheostomy tube, suction it gently using sterile technique. Provide humidification. If the patient experiences respiratory difficulty, notify the doctor immediately.

• Stress the importance of frequent coughing, turning, and deep-breathing. If the patient has a tracheostomy, suction regularly until he can do it himself.

• For 8 hours after surgery, check the incision site hourly for bleeding or signs of hematoma formation (swelling or bulging of the stoma under the skin flap). Monitor for evidence of saliva in the skin folds or of drainage from the incision because this may indicate a salivary fistula. If neck drains are in place, ensure their patency. Report any abnormalities. Perform tracheostomy care every 8 hours or as needed.

• Check the site for signs of drainage and tissue necrosis, and monitor the patient's temperature. Report any signs of infection to the doctor, who may order additional drains or antibiotics.

• As ordered, give I.V. fluids and nasogastric tube feedings and monitor intake and output. If the patient experiences discomfort, give analgesics and sedatives, as ordered, through the NG tube or I.V. line. Keep in mind, though, that narcotics depress respirations and inhibit coughing.

• Be alert for secretions leaking around the wound about 10 days after surgery because this may indicate a pharyngeal fistula. Notify the doctor immediately and discontinue oral feedings.

• To help relieve the patient's anxiety, use the communication system developed before surgery. Tell the patient who has had a partial laryngectomy not to use his voice until the doctor gives permission. Reassure him that speech rehabilitation will enable him to speak again.

• Notify the doctor immediately if you detect active bleeding. This could indicate carotid artery rupture, which can occur as long as a month after surgery.

Home care instructions

• Begin patient teaching as soon as possible because the patient must know how to perform stoma care himself before discharge. Call a home health care agency to arrange help for the patient at home, and, if possible, have one of the home health care nurses attend the teaching sessions. If the patient has had a total laryngectomy, explain that a speech pathologist will work closely with him.

• If appropriate, teach the patient how to perform tracheostomy care using clean technique. Instruct him to clean

(Text continues on page 408.)

Understanding types of laryngectomy

Although laryngoscopic surgery may be used to remove an early localized glottic tumor, other techniques must be used to excise more widespread tumors. These include total laryngectomy, horizontal supraglottic laryngectomy, vertical hemilaryngectomy, and laryngofissure.

Total laryngectomy

Used to excise a large glottic or supraglottic tumor with vocal cord fixation, this procedure involves removal of the true vocal cords, false vocal cords, epiglottis, hyoid bone, cricoid cartilage, and two or three rings of the trachea.

Neighboring areas may also be removed depending on the extent of the tumor. A permanent tracheotomy is performed, creating a laryngeal stoma that leaves the patient without speech.

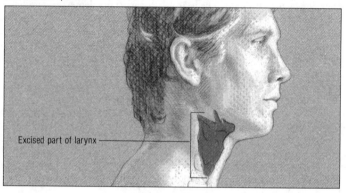

Excised part of larynx

Horizontal supraglottic laryngectomy

Performed to remove a large supraglottic tumor, this procedure excises the top of the larynx (the epiglottis, the hyoid bone, and the false vocal cords), leaving the true vocal cords intact. Although there's no laryngectomy stoma, a temporary tracheotomy may be performed to ensure a patent airway until edema subsides. The patient's voice is unaffected by this procedure, but removal of the epiglottis may cause swallowing difficulty.

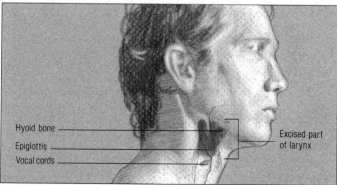

Hyoid bone

Epiglottis

Vocal cords

Excised part of larynx

Vertical hemilaryngectomy

Used to remove a widespread tumor, this procedure involves excision of half the thyroid and subglottis, one false vocal cord, and one true vocal cord. The area is then rebuilt with strap muscles. The patient doesn't have a laryngectomy stoma, but his voice may be hoarse postoperatively.

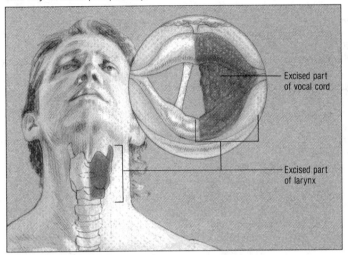

Excised part
of vocal cord

Excised part
of larynx

Laryngofissure

This procedure removes a glottic tumor limited to one vocal cord. To perform laryngofissure, the surgeon incises the thyroid cartilage and excises the affected vocal cord.

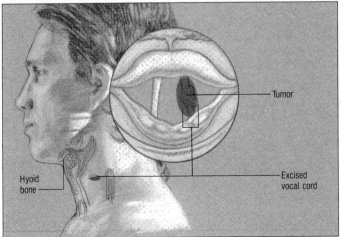

Tumor

Hyoid
bone

Excised
vocal cord

the inner cannula of his tube with hydrogen peroxide and water daily to help maintain a patent airway and prevent infection. Explain that he must suction the outer cannula to keep his airway patent whenever he feels congested or when his breathing sounds raspy or wheezy, or when excess mucus forms. Also, tell him to watch for bloody secretions, which may indicate local trauma. Finally, have him demonstrate correct cleaning and suctioning techniques.

• Emphasize the importance of daily stoma care using warm water to maintain a patent airway, promote healing, and prevent infection. Warn the patient not to use tissues, loose cotton, or soap during cleaning because these may obstruct his airway. Tell him to wear a bib or dressing over his stoma to act as a filter and to warm incoming air. Also instruct him to avoid swimming and getting water in his stoma. Mention that he'll need to humidify his home, especially during the winter.

• Alert the patient to signs and symptoms of later complications, such as pneumonia and atelectasis, wound infection, pharyngeal fistula formation, and hemorrhage.

• Instruct the patient to inform the doctor promptly if he develops symptoms of a respiratory infection, such as fever, cough, yellow or green drainage from the stoma, pain, or erythema around the stoma.

• Stress the importance of keeping follow-up medical appointments to monitor for recurrence of cancer.

• Provide emotional support, and help the patient adjust to his new self-image. Suggest that he contact organizations such as the International Association of Laryngectomees and the American Cancer Society to learn about support groups in his area.

LASER SURGERY

Laser is an acronym for light amplification by stimulated emission of radiation. An invaluable tool during surgery, a laser generates an intense beam of light. At times referred to as a "scalpel of light," the laser can cut, coagulate, or vaporize tissue. The intense beam can be focused to a very fine spot for extreme precision or defocused (the beam enlarged to affect a wider area) to coagulate or vaporize tissue.

The most common types of lasers are neodymium yttrium aluminum garnet (Nd:YAG), carbon dioxide, and argon lasers, although many new lasers, such as the Holmium, Excimer, and potassium-titanyl-phosphate (KTP), are being developed for new applications. The laser is named for the medium used. Each type of light beam has distinct characteristics that interact with tissue in various ways. The means of transmission and its application will determine selection of the laser. For example, the carbon dioxide laser, which can't penetrate liquids, is ineffective in a fluid-filled environment such as the bladder or an actively bleeding area; the Nd:YAG and argon lasers, however, readily pass through liquids and would prove useful in these areas.

Advantages of laser surgery include the following: noncontact capabilities, the assurance of dry fields (coagulation of the capillary beds prevents oozing into the field) and sterility (the intense heat generated by the laser provides constant sterilization), precise control of the spot size of the beam, and added accessibility (allowing the use of endoscopes to replace open surgical procedures). Laser tissue interaction also aids healing by minimizing swelling while decreasing postprocedural pain.

Purpose
- To cut, coagulate, or vaporize tissue
- To reduce or ablate tumors and lesions
- To seal a source of bleeding.

Indications
The numerous indications for laser therapy range from a simple wart removal to a complex intra-abdominal procedure. The following medical specialties are among those that apply laser techniques in treatment of various conditions.

Gynecology: cervical procedures, removal of condylomata, tubal microsurgery, endometrial ablation, endometriosis

General surgery: laparoscopic cholecystectomy, liver resections, other laparoscopic procedures, any incisional and excisional soft-tissue procedures

Gastroenterology: treatment of esophageal lesions, rectal lesions, bleeding, esophageal varices, and ulcers

Urology: treatment of urethral stenosis, superficial bladder tumors, and interstitial cystitis; transurethral resection and removal of condylomata

Pulmonary: treatment of endobronchial stenosis, removal of endobronchial lesions, photoradiation of endobronchial cancer

Otolaryngology: treatment of tracheal stenosis, vocal cord lesions, and pharyngeal papilloma; otoplasty; incisional and excisional work in head and neck surgery

Ophthalmology: posterior capsulotomy; vitrectomy; cytocoagulation; treatment of diabetic retinopathy, glaucoma, and retinal tears; iridectomy

Dermatology (including plastic and cosmetic surgery): removal of port wine stains, telangiectasia, hemangioma, and melanoma; tattoo removal; excision of skin tumors; incisional and excisional soft-tissue procedures

Cardiology: laser-assisted balloon angioplasty, many investigational procedures

Dentistry: frenectomy, gingivoplasty, treatment of aphthous ulcers, or vascular lesions

Neurosurgery: treatment of brain tumors (meningiomas, acoustic neuromas, hemangiomas, gliomas) and spinal cord tumors, percutaneous diskectomies

Orthopedics: methyl methacrylate removal, meniscectomy, investigational procedures in other joints

Oncology: investigational photoradiation of tumors.

Procedure
Laser procedures are performed by a trained doctor or dentist; they may not require anesthesia or any form of general or local anesthesia, depending on the type of laser used and the specific procedure being performed.

To cut tissue, the laser is focused in a precise beam. The size of the area and the tissue to be treated will determine the laser to be used. Laser technology can be used with or without microscopes and together with or separate from conventional surgical methods.

Lasers can deliver energy to tissues by contact and noncontact modes. In the noncontact mode, energy is emitted from the end of a silica or quartz fiber in a free beam, which interacts with tissue. The noncontact mode is used primarily for vaporization and coagulation. With the contact mode, the laser beam is passed through the fiber-optic device and focused on the tip of the fiber, which has been shaped into a point, ball, or wedge. The tip then contacts the tissue, and the intense heat generated causes the desired effect on the tissue. The contact mode is used primarily for incisional and excisional work. The Nd:YAG and argon lasers use both the contact and noncontact modes of delivery. The carbon dioxide laser, however, is always noncontact because the carbon dioxide wavelength cannot be transmitted through a fiber-optic device.

Complications

Laser surgery is associated with the same complications that follow conventional surgery (hemorrhage, infection, perforation) as well as some that are uniquely associated with lasers. Fire is a potential complication due to the intense heat from the laser beam. Airway fire and lung explosion, which can result from contact with a flammable endotracheal tube or oxygen, is a tragic complication that is avoidable when safety precautions are enforced. All personnel who work with lasers should have specific safety training. Eye damage from exposure to the laser beam can result in painful or permanent injury.

Care considerations

Before surgery

• Prepare the patient according to the policy of the health care facility for the scheduled surgery. For example, the patient who will receive general anesthesia receives nothing by mouth after midnight before the surgery. The laser procedure itself requires no specific preparations.
• Explain the procedure to the patient, and encourage questions from him and the family.
• Ensure that a consent form has been signed.

During surgery

• Safety is the main care consideration in laser use. Special eye wear is required because a laser aimed at the eye can cause damage.
• Nonreflective instrumentation must be used because reflected laser light is just as hazardous as a directed beam.
• Avoid using flammable substances, such as alcohol, because they present a significant fire hazard.
• Use only moistened sponges, drapes, and towels near the area of laser use and have water or sodium chloride solution available in case of a fire. Have an appropriate liquid chemical fire extinguisher, such as a Halon extinguisher, nearby.
• Post LASER WARNING signs at all entrances to the room to prevent inadvertent entry without protective eye wear.
• Smoke evacuation should be used to clear the room of potentially hazardous smoke plume from treated tissue.

After surgery

• Monitor vital signs, and observe for increased drainage and bleeding at the laser site.
• Monitor the patient as you would after the corresponding conventional surgical procedure. For example, after laser therapy to remove a brain tumor, appropriate monitoring resembles postcraniotomy care; it includes monitoring of neurologic status, elevating the head of the bed, and administering steroids and osmotic diuretics, as ordered.
• Administer analgesics, as ordered.

Home care instructions

• Inform the patient that the course of recovery is the same for laser surgery as after conventional surgery. However, healing may be faster with less pain.
• After a pulmonary or oral procedure, tell the patient to expect a smoky taste in the mouth; he may cough up small amounts of blackened tissue.
• Make sure that the patient understands that lasers are not a cure-all. It is important that he has realistic expectations because many laser procedures (such as malignant tumor ablation) are merely palliative.

LAXATIVES

Classified according to their mechanism of action, laxatives may be bulk-forming agents, saline laxatives, stool softeners, hyperosmolar agents, lubricants, or stimulants.

Bulk-forming laxatives (*psyllium, methylcellulose*) absorb water and expand, increasing the bulk and fluid content of stool. The increased bulk enhances peristalsis and evacuation.

Stool softeners *(docusate salts)* reduce the surface tension of bowel contents. This detergent activity promotes incorporation of additional liquid into the stool, forming a softer mass.

Hyperosmolar laxatives act in different ways. Glycerin draws water into the feces, increasing bulk and promoting peristalsis. Lactulose produces an osmotic effect, which draws water into the colon; the resulting bowel distention stimulates peristalsis.

The saline laxatives (*magnesium salts* and *sodium phosphates*) exert an osmotic effect in the small intestine, producing distention and enhancing peristalsis; they also promote secretion of cholecystokinin by the intestinal mucosa, which stimulates intestinal motility and inhibits fluid and electrolyte absorption in the jejunum and ileum.

Lubricant laxatives (*mineral oil*) create a barrier between the colonic wall and the fecal mass, preventing absorption of fecal water by the colon and promoting its retention in the stool.

Stimulant laxatives (*bisacodyl, cascara sagrada, castor oil, senna, phenolphthalein*) are thought to increase peristalsis by exerting a direct effect on intestinal smooth muscle, either by irritating the muscle or by stimulating the colonic intramural plexus. These drugs also promote fluid and electrolyte accumulation in the colon and small intestine.

Laxatives vary widely in their speed of action. Typically, bulk-forming laxatives and stool softeners produce elimination in 12 to 48 hours; hyperosmolar laxatives, in 30 minutes to 3 hours.

Purpose

• To ease the passage of feces through the colon and rectum, thereby relieving or preventing constipation.

Indications

Bulk-forming laxatives, such as methylcellulose and psyllium, help treat chronic constipation. Stool softeners, such as docusate salts, prevent constipation and straining during defecation. Hyperosmolar agents, such as glycerin and magnesium salts, treat constipation. Saline laxatives are used to prepare the bowel for diagnostic or surgical procedures. Lubricants, such as mineral oil, and stimulants, such as castor oil, are also used for constipation. These agents are usually avoided for bowel preparation because they may obscure visualization.

The use of all types of laxatives is contraindicated in patients with abdominal pain, nausea, vomiting or other symptoms of appendicitis, intestinal obstruction, or ulceration. High-sodium bulk-forming laxatives should not be given to patients on sodium-restricted diets. Stimulant laxatives are contraindicated in patients with anal or rectal fissures and in the presence of rectal bleeding. Stimulant and lubricant laxatives are contraindicated in patients with fecal impaction. Lubricant laxatives should be used cautiously in young children, in elderly or debilitated patients because of their susceptibility to lipid pneumonitis, and in patients with rectal bleeding. Hyperosmolar laxatives are contraindicated in patients with myocardial damage or heart block, and in pregnant patients in the final stages of labor.

Adverse reactions

Most laxatives can cause nausea, vomiting, and diarrhea, and excessive or long-term use may cause abdominal cramps and laxative dependence. Bulk-forming laxatives may cause flatulence; they can also cause esophageal obstruction when chewed or taken in dry form or may cause intestinal obstruction or fecal impaction. Hyperosmolar and stimulant laxatives may cause dehydration, electrolyte imbalance (in acute overdose or chronic misuse), and acid-base imbalance. Stimulant laxatives may cause intestinal cramps, increased mucus secretion, and fluid and electrolyte deficiencies (such as hypokalemia) that result from excessive catharsis (generally dose-related).

Care considerations

• When administering laxatives, monitor for adverse reactions and report them to the doctor.
• Monitor bowel movements, and note the amount, consistency, and color. Also note the degree of effort required for defecation.
• During long-term therapy, monitor the patient's fluid intake to ensure adequate hydration. (This is especially important with use of a bulk-forming laxative.) Regularly assess for signs of dehydration, including fever, tachycardia, hypotension, decreased urine output, poor skin turgor, and extreme thirst.
• Monitor serum electrolytes—especially potassium and sodium—and acid-base balance. Watch for signs of electrolyte and acid-base imbalances, such as weakness, diminished reflexes, twitching, vomiting, hypotension, and a rapid, thready pulse.
• Lubricant laxatives should not be given with or immediately after meals because they delay passage of food from the stomach. Give lubricant laxatives on an empty stomach.
• Do not give oral drugs within 2 hours of a hyperosmolar laxative.
• Store stool softeners at 59° to 86° F (15° to 30° C), and protect them from light.

Home care instructions

• Warn the patient not to take a laxative if he's experiencing abdominal pain, nausea, or vomiting because these symptoms may herald a serious condition that laxatives may worsen.

• Encourage the patient to drink 6 to 8 glasses of water a day while taking these drugs.
• Advise the patient to tell the doctor if he doesn't have a bowel movement after taking the laxative as prescribed.
• Reassure the patient that a daily bowel movement isn't essential to good health; it's more more important to maintain a consistent pattern of elimination. Warn against overusing laxatives, which can lead to dependence.
• Teach the patient alternative ways to prevent constipation, such as regular exercise and adequate fluid and fiber intake. Tell him that good dietary sources of fiber include bran and other cereals, fresh fruits, and vegetables.

LEUKAPHERESIS

Leukapheresis refers to the large-scale collection or removal of any of the three major types of white blood cells: monocytes, granulocytes, and lymphocytes. The primary function of monocytes and granulocytes is phagocytosis, whereas lymphocytes produce antibodies and play a key role in the immune system.

Typically, the leukocyte count (percent of white blood cells in total blood volume) is less than 1%, but some disorders can stimulate massive leukocyte production. When the leukocyte count exceeds 20%, significantly increased viscosity of the peripheral blood reduces pulmonary and cerebral blood flow. The leukocytes also compete with tissues for oxygen in the microcirculation. This condition, known as leukostasis, may result in tissue hypoxia and organ dysfunction.

Two methods can be used to achieve cell depletion: manual or automated apheresis. Manual apheresis is the removal of a volume of blood not exceeding 15% of the patient's total volume. It may be used for patients with extremely poor venous access or for children whose safe extracorporeal volume is less than the amount removed by an automated device. Manual removal is also an option when automated cell separators are unavailable.

Automated apheresis by computerized cell separators is safer and more efficient than manual apheresis; this method is also faster, removes more undesired cells and fewer desired cells, and reduces the risk of misidentification of blood components. However, venous access and the large volume of extracorporeal blood required to prime the disposable set can be limiting factors; the cost of automated apheresis, which is substantial, can also limit its use.

Purpose

• To remove leukocytes, reducing the complications of leukostasis
• To alter immune responsiveness.

Indications

The most common indication for leukapheresis is hyperleukocytic leukemias. The removal of leukocytes has little if any effect on the underlying pathologic process, but it can provide valuable and rapid adjunctive therapy. For example, a few patients with chronic myelocytic and lymphocytic leukemia have been maintained for prolonged periods without chemotherapy by a regular schedule of leukapheresis. Although disease manifestations such as adenopathy, splenomegaly, anemia, thrombocytopenia, and leukocytosis improve with leukapheresis, the long-term prognosis is unchanged. Leukapheresis is sometimes indicated for chronic leukemia during pregnancy when cytotoxic drugs are contraindicated.

In recent studies, leukapheresis has been used to achieve lymphocyte depletion in various autoimmune disorders. Leukapheresis-induced immunomodulation benefits some patients with rheumatoid arthritis and multiple sclerosis and has also been used to enhance allograft survival and reverse graft rejection.

Procedure

Leukapheresis must be performed by an apheresis specialist, typically a registered nurse or medical technologist. The procedure may be performed at the bedside or in the apheresis unit. After venous access is achieved in manual apheresis, the blood is aspirated into a syringe or allowed to flow by gravity into a plastic bag. The bag is disconnected from the patient and placed in a high-speed centrifuge for separation of plasma, red blood cells, platelets, and white blood cells. The white cell layer (buffy coat) is extracted manually, and the remaining portion of the blood is returned to the patient. This process can be repeated until a desired degree of depletion is obtained.

In automated apheresis, the blood is withdrawn by a large-gauge catheter (16 or 17) into a sterile plastic kit that has been placed in a blood cell separator. The blood flows into the device under negative pressure and enters a centrifuge, where separation of the blood elements takes place. The desired cell type (lymphocyte, monocyte, or granulocyte) is selectively removed and placed in a collection container. The remaining portion of the blood is returned to the patient.

The degree of cell depletion achieved with apheresis depends on the volume of blood processed. An automated apheresis procedure processing 5 liters of whole blood can reduce the white cell count by 20% to 50%. With an average blood flow of 50 to 60 ml per minute, this procedure would require 2 hours.

The patient will be monitored by the specialist during the procedure. Upon completion, the venipuncture sites are wrapped with a pressure dressing.

Complications

The most common complications of routine apheresis are vasovagal reactions (dizziness, hypotension, bradycardia, fainting, and seizures), hematoma formation at the venipuncture site, and discomfort. Leukemia patients with symptoms of leukostasis may develop complications associated with anemia and thrombocytopenia, which are common in these patients. These patients are critically ill and require careful assessment and constant monitoring during the procedure.

A frequent problem encountered in automated apheresis is inadequate venous access.

Care considerations

Before the procedure

• Provide a detailed explanation to the patient and family, including the method of cell removal, duration of the procedure, and expected outcome. Contact the apheresis specialist to obtain necessary information.
• Confirm that a medical order for the procedure is in the chart.
• Confirm that an informed consent document describing the procedure and potential risks has been signed.
• Unless contraindicated, serve the patient a balanced, low-fat meal within a few hours of the procedure. Encourage additional oral fluids.

After the procedure

• Observe the venipuncture site for several hours after leukapheresis. The patient who is thrombocytopenic has a significant risk of bleeding after venipuncture with large-gauge needles.
• Leave the dressing intact for 3 to 4 hours. If bleeding occurs, place pressure on the site and elevate the arm.
• Take and record vital signs. Report significant changes immediately.
• Encourage oral fluids for several hours unless contraindicated. The volume of blood removed is usually small, but additional fluids will ensure hemostatic balance.

• Advise the patient to report anything unusual. Most adverse reactions occur during apheresis, but the patient should be monitored closely for several hours afterward.

Home care instructions

Leukapheresis has no long-term effects; home care instructions are required only if the patient is released from care immediately after apheresis. Chronic leukemia patients or those having leukapheresis to modify immune responsiveness may be treated as outpatients; these patients should receive the following instructions before discharge.
• Tell the patient to leave the bandage in place for 2 to 3 hours. If bleeding occurs, tell him to apply pressure to the venipuncture site and elevate the arm until bleeding stops.
• Advise the patient to avoid lifting heavy objects and strenuous exercise for several hours.
• Tell the patient to drink extra fluids and eat a well-balanced meal after leukapheresis.
• Instruct the patient to report any adverse reactions to the doctor.
• Tell the patient to eat a low-fat diet before each leukapheresis procedure. (Fat consumption may cause cloudy, chylous plasma, which can cause malfunction of the optic sensor in the cell separator.)

LIGHT THERAPY

Light therapy, also called phototherapy, is therapeutic exposure to artificial light that contains all of the wave frequencies present in sunlight. Although ordinary indoor lighting will provide between 300 to 500 lux (unit of illumination), the recommended full-spectrum artificial light—available from several manufacturers—will provide 2,500 lux or more.

This is 5 to 10 times brighter than the light in a well-lit office.

The exact mechanism of light therapy is not well understood, but it is thought to reduce the hormonal activity of melatonin, which appears to inhibit numerous endocrine functions. When injected, exogenous melatonin causes drowsiness. Correctly used, light therapy has many beneficial effects.

Purpose
• To elevate the patient's mood
• To cause an antidepressant effect
• To reset and synchronize the human biological clock (circadian rhythm) with the solar clock during seasons of shortened sunlight.

Indications
Light therapy is primarily indicated for seasonal affective disorder (SAD). Seasonal changes and limited exposure to bright light may induce depression in sensitive persons. SAD is characterized by a mild depression during the shortened daylight seasons of fall and winter. Patients with SAD experience reduced symptoms or remission of symptoms as the days get longer with increased sunlight and warmth.

Light therapy may also be indicated for other conditions, including delayed sleep-phase syndrome (marked by difficulty in getting to sleep and waking up at conventional times), premenstrual syndrome, circadian disruption caused by shift work, and jet lag.

Procedure
A light box for phototherapy can be assembled by an electrician or purchased commercially. It consists of a box containing a high-lux lighting system. The patient should sit about 3′ (1 meter) away from the source and may read, write, or watch TV during treatment. The optimal time and duration of therapy remain controversial, but some clinicians recommend early-morning exposure to the bright light for 2 to 3 hours. The patient should glance at the light a few times every minute or so. Typically, patients who are going to respond to light therapy will experience improvement within 3 to 4 days. If the response is inadequate, evening hours may be substituted or added to the schedule.

Complications
No long-term adverse effects of phototherapy have been identified. However, people with eye problems might be at risk for visual reactions. Appropriate precautions should be taken to avoid eye trauma. The most common reactions are eyestrain, headache, and insomnia, which can be managed by decreasing the duration of exposure or increasing the distance from the light.

Care considerations
Before therapy
• Recommend mental health counseling, which may be beneficial to both the patient and the family.
• Inform the patient and family that antidepressants and other psychotropic drugs may be administered along with light therapy and that treatment will be closely monitored by a psychiatrist.
• Stress the importance of compliance.
• Provide emotional support. Allow the patient to express any anxiety or fears. Encourage and assist the development of coping skills.
• Inform patients and their families that SAD has a biochemical cause. This information may reduce their feelings of frustration and guilt.
During therapy
• Monitor the patient for headache, eyestrain, and insomnia.
• Set realistic goals with the patient during periods of depression.

Home care instructions
• Inform the patient that the seasonal variation of this disorder may require

adjustment of work and personal schedules.

• Encourage continued follow-up with the doctor or mental health professional to evaluate treatment and make recommendations in therapy.

• Advise the patients to contact the National Organization for SAD (P.O. Box 451, Vienna, Va. 22180) for information on a local support group.

LIPOSUCTION

Liposuction is the removal of fat cells by suction from various areas of the body. Body areas that can benefit from liposuction are the face, chin, neck, abdomen, breasts, thighs, hips, posterior upper arms, upper midback, knees, calves, and ankles.

The most frequently used method of liposuction is the wet technique. A new method, the tumescent technique requires less anesthesia and offers faster postoperative recovery. Like other cosmetic procedures, liposuction requires thorough assessment of the patient's attitude and expectation about the outcome. It should not be performed for patients with unrealistic expectations or for those who are 30% over ideal body weight; this procedure is not an alternative to weight loss.

Purpose

• To remove fat from body areas that are resistant to diet and exercise
• To reshape a part of the body.

Indications

Liposuction is a cosmetic procedure used to improve or enhance the appearance. It is not a treatment for obesity and will not remove cellulite. Patients who are in good physical condition with a history of rapid healing but who are unable to trim certain areas by dieting are good candidates for this procedure. Liposuction is frequently combined with soft-tissue surgery to reduce the skin envelope. Liposuction can remove lipomas, thus resulting in a much smaller scar.

Procedure

Typically, a dermatology surgeon or a cosmetic surgeon performs liposuction. Photographs of the patient are taken before and after the surgery to provide a record for the patient's chart. The wet technique is performed under general anesthesia or heavy sedation. The area to be suctioned is marked, and a local anesthetic is injected into the designated fatty area. An incision is made in the area and a catheter is introduced to remove the fat. The size of the catheter largely depends on the size of the area of fat to be removed. Suction is applied through the catheter to remove the fat.

The tumescent technique is performed under local anesthesia combined with preoperative sedation. A local anesthetic and a vasoconstrictor diluted with a large volume of sterile 0.9% sodium chloride solution are injected into the fatty tissue, producing an anesthetic effect that may last as long as 10 hours after the injection. One advantage of local anesthesia is that it allows the patient to stand during the procedure to facilitate comparison of liposuctioned areas with nonsuctioned areas.

Frequently, especially with the wet technique, patients need autologous blood transfusions (1 to 2 units for every 2,500 ml of fat that is aspirated). After the procedure, an elastic dressing is placed over the site to prevent swelling, bleeding, and fluid shifts.

Complications

Blood and fluid loss is possible with both liposuction procedures but is less common with the tumescent technique. Other complications may include hematoma, seromas, hypovolemic shock, nerve damage, dents or waviness over the surgical area, wound separation, and wound infection. Rarely, pulmonary fat embolus or thromboembolism may occur.

Care considerations
Before the procedure
• Aspirin and other anti-inflammatory agents should be discontinued 2 weeks before surgery. The patient must be adequately nourished and must avoid following a starvation diet, which will interfere with healing.
• The patient should stop smoking at least 2 weeks before surgery, because smoking increases the potential for skin sloughing.
• Caution the patient that a preoperative sunburn may lead to infection.
• Observe the patient's mental attitude and expectations about the surgery's outcome. The surgery may have to be deferred until the patient has had appropriate counseling about self-esteem.
• Teach the patient about the surgical procedure.
• Give complete instructions regarding procedures and care the patient can expect preoperatively, on the day of surgery, and postoperatively.
• Instruct the patient about the possible need for a touch-up procedure and about costs before the first liposuction procedure.
• Preoperative blood work must include screenings for serum human immunodeficiency virus and hepatitis and must confirm normal coagulation profile.
• Ensure that the patient has signed a consent form.
After the procedure
• Monitor vital signs, and observe for signs of hypovolemia.
• Monitor the patient's comfort level, and administer analgesics, as ordered.
• Be sure that the patient remains on bed rest for 24 to 48 hours after the surgery.
• Encourage fluid intake.

Home care instructions
• Inform the patient that bruising, swelling, numbness of surgical area, tenderness, fatigue, and redness at the incision site are normal after this procedure.
• Inform the patient that asymmetry may require a follow-up procedure.
• Tell the patient that pink-tinged drainage from the liposuctioned area is common. Absorbent dressings are used to collect the drainage. Tell the patient that sanitary pads are useful to collect abdominal drainage, which can be profuse.
• Instruct the patient to take antibiotics as ordered.
• Tell the patient to wear the prescribed compression garments.
• Instruct the patient about the recommended type and amount of activity and exercise. This will depend on the size of the area suctioned and the technique that was used.
• Tell the patient to inform the doctor about increased pain, fever, or bleeding.
• Inform the patient that ultrasound treatments to ecchymotic areas may be ordered two to three times weekly to smooth out irregularities and resolve ecchymosis.
• Emphasize the importance of keeping all follow-up appointments.

LITHOTRIPSY, EXTRACORPOREAL SHOCK WAVE

Extracorporeal shock wave lithotripsy (ESWL) uses high-energy shock waves to break up renal calculi and allow their normal passage from the body. Depending on the type of equipment used, the patient may be anesthetized and placed in a water tank. The affected kidney is positioned over an electric spark generator, which creates high-energy shock waves that shatter calculi without damaging surrounding tissue. Afterward, the patient is able to excrete the fine, gravel-like remains of the calculi.

The newer types of equipment used for ESWL do not require the patient's submersion in water and may not require general anesthesia. Instead, a membrane coupling device can be directly applied to the skin over the affected kidney. Additional treatments may be necessary for large or multiple calculi. ESWL is not as effective for cystine, uric acid, and some calcium oxalate stones.

Because ESWL is noninvasive, most patients can be discharged the same evening or the next day and can resume normal activity after a few days. ESWL also minimizes the risk of many potentially serious complications, such as infection and hemorrhage, associated with invasive methods of calculi removal.

Purpose

• To break obstructive renal calculi into small, more easily eliminated particles.

Indications

ESWL may be performed as a preventive measure in a patient with potentially obstructive renal calculi or as an emergency treatment for an acute obstruction; more often, a stent (retrograde or percutaneous) is inserted to ensure urine drainage and facilitate passage of calculi fragments. Renal calculi about 1″ (2 cm) or smaller are ideal targets for ESWL. The larger the calculi, the less likely is successful elimination of all calculi fragments.

ESWL may be contraindicated during pregnancy or in the presence of a urinary tract obstruction distal to the calculi, which would prevent passage of fragments. Other contraindications include unrelated infection, excessive obesity, history of bleeding or clotting disorder, renal cancer, and calculi that are attached to the kidney or ureter or located below the level of the iliac crest.

Still controversial, a new procedure known as cholelithotripsy has successfully removed biliary calculi.

Procedure

Before ESWL, the patient will receive some form of anesthesia because the shock waves can cause discomfort as they pass through the walls of the body. The type of anesthesia depends on the type of lithotriptor used. Some devices require general or epidural anesthesia; others, which pulverize calculi effectively while delivering energy less painfully, can be used with local anesthesia alone. An I.V. line and catheter are inserted and electrocardiograph (ECG) electrodes attached. For lithotripsy in water, the patient is placed in a semireclining position on the machine's hydraulic stretcher and is lowered into the water tank. In the tank, the patient's position is adjusted so that the shock-wave generator focuses directly on the calculi. Biplane fluoroscopy or ultrasonography can be used to enhance visualization of the calculus and confirm its position. The generator is then activated to direct high-energy shock waves through the water at the calculi. To prevent disruption of the patient's cardiac rhythm, the shock waves are synchronized to the patient's R waves and fired during diastole. The number of waves fired during treatment depends on the size and composition of the calculi but may range from 500 to 2,000 shocks. After the shocks are delivered, the patient is removed from the tub and the ECG electrodes are removed.

Complications

Complications of ESWL, occurring in about 1% of patients, include perirenal hemorrhage, urinary tract obstruction caused by calculi fragments, severe pain, and urinary tract infection. Recent reports indicate that patients who have undergone ESWL have an increased incidence of hypertension, although the clinical significance of this response has not been determined.

Care considerations
Before the procedure
• Review the ESWL procedure with the patient.
• If possible, arrange for the patient to see the ESWL device before the first scheduled treatment. Describe the procedure and answer any questions.
After the procedure
• Monitor vital signs every 4 hours for the first 24 hours after treatment or until discharge if the patient is released within 24 hours. Report any abnormal findings to the doctor.
• Maintain patency of the indwelling urinary catheter and I.V. line, and closely monitor intake and output.
• Instruct the patient to maintain fluid intake of at least 1,900 ml (about 2 qt) of water a day to aid passage of calculi fragments.
• Strain all urine for calculi fragments, and send them to the laboratory for analysis.
• Note the urine's color, and test its pH. Remember that slight hematuria is normal for several days after ESWL. However, notify the doctor of frank or persistent bleeding.
• Encourage ambulation as early as possible after treatment to aid passage of calculi fragments.
• To help remove any particles lodged in gravity-dependent kidney pockets, instruct the patient to lie facedown with his head and shoulders over the edge of the bed for about 10 minutes and to perform this maneuver twice a day. To enhance its effectiveness, encourage fluid intake 40 to 45 minutes before starting.
• Monitor for pain on the treated side, and administer analgesics, as ordered. Warn the patient that severe pain may indicate ureteral obstruction from new calculi and should be promptly reported to the doctor.

Home care instructions
• Instruct the patient to drink 3 to 4 qt (2,840 to 3,780 ml) of fluid each day for about 1 month after treatment. Explain that this will aid passage of calculi fragments and will help prevent formation of new calculi.
• Teach the patient how to strain his urine for fragments. Tell him to strain all urine for the 1st week after treatment, to save all fragments in the container provided, and to bring the container along on his first follow-up doctor's appointment.
• Teach the patient the expected adverse effects of ESWL, including pain on the treated side as fragments pass, slight redness or bruising on the treated side, blood-tinged urine for several days after treatment, and mild GI upset. Reassure the patient that these effects are normal and not a cause for concern. However, tell him to report severe unremitting pain, persistent hematuria, inability to void, fever and chills, or recurrent nausea and vomiting.
• Encourage the patient to resume normal activities, including exercise and work, as soon as he feels able (unless the doctor instructs otherwise). Explain that physical activity will promote the passage of calculi fragments.
• Emphasize the importance of compliance with any dietary or drug regimen designed to reduce the formation of new calculi.

LITHOTRIPSY, PERCUTANEOUS ULTRASONIC

In this lithotripsy technique, renal calculi are shattered by an ultrasonic probe inserted through a nephrostomy tube into the renal pelvis. Ultrahigh-frequency sound waves are generated to pulverize the calculi while continuous suctioning removes the fragments. Like extracorporeal shock wave lithotripsy (ESWL), percutaneous ultrasonic lithotripsy (PUL) greatly reduces the patient's recovery time as compared to open renal surgery. PUL may replace ESWL or may be performed after it to remove residual fragments. It's particularly useful for removing radiolucent calculi lodged in the kidney, which aren't treatable by ESWL.

Purpose

• To shatter renal calculi and remove their fragments by suction.

Indications

Lithotripsy techniques are used to remove kidney calculi that cannot pass through the urinary tract spontaneously. This procedure is principally used in patients with renal or upper ureteral calculi larger than 1″ (2.5 cm), including staghorn calculi and those within the upper ureter that cannot be manipulated back into the renal pelvis for extracorporeal lithotripsy. Typically, PUL is useful for radiolucent calculi not treatable by ESWL.

This procedure is contraindicated in patients with irreversible coagulopathies or active, untreated urinary tract infection.

Procedure

Because the shock waves can cause discomfort, the patient will receive general or epidural anesthesia. The surgeon establishes a nephrostomy tract with a needle puncture performed under fluoroscopic or ultrasound guidance, threads an angiographic wire through the needle, and passes various-sized nephrostomy tubes over the wire to progressively dilate the tract. When the tract is sufficiently dilated, he inserts a nephroscope to visualize the calculus.

Next (or 1 or 2 days later, if PUL is being performed in two stages), the surgeon inserts a working tube that resembles a small cystoscope through the nephrostomy tract and into the kidney's collecting system. He then passes an ultrasonic probe through the tube and positions it against the calculus. When the probe is in position, he turns on the device, producing ultrahigh-frequency sound waves that shatter the calculus into fragments. He then uses suction, irrigation, or a basketing instrument to remove the fragments. After treatment is complete, the surgeon withdraws the probe and the working tube and then reinserts the nephrostomy tube. The tube remains in place until nephrotomography confirms that all fragments of the calculi have been passed.

Complications

Potential complications include postoperative bleeding, pneumothorax, urinary tract infection, and extravasation of irrigating fluid. PUL may also lead to renal damage from insertion of the nephrostomy tube and ureteral obstruction from incomplete passage of calculi fragments.

Care considerations

Before the procedure

• Explain the procedure to the patient, including insertion of the nephrostomy tube and the lithotripsy technique. Some surgeons prefer to perform PUL in two stages, with nephrostomy tube insertion and dilation on the first day followed by lithotripsy 1 or 2 days later, after intrarenal bleeding has subsided and the calculi can be better visualized. If two-stage PUL has been scheduled, explain this to the patient.
• Tell the patient that he may experience discomfort from the nephrostomy tube but that the treatment should be otherwise painless.
• Reassure the patient that analgesics will be given if needed.
• Describe posttreatment care to the patient.
• The day before scheduled treatment, prepare the patient for intravenous pyelography or lower abdominal X-rays,

whichever is ordered, to locate the calculi.

• Ask about the patient's medication history, particularly his aspirin intake.

• Review results of laboratory studies to determine if the patient has abnormalities such as coagulopathies.

• Withhold all foods and fluids after midnight on the night before the procedure.

After the procedure

• Check the volume of nephrostomy tube drainage hourly for the first 24 hours and then every 4 hours thereafter.

• Report absent or decreased drainage, which could indicate obstruction by retained calculi fragments. Also note the urine's color, and test its pH.

• Slight hematuria is normal for several days after PUL; however, frank or persistent bleeding should be reported to the doctor.

• Strain all urine for calculi fragments, and send them to the laboratory for analysis.

• Monitor the patient for pain, and administer analgesics as needed. Keep in mind that severe pain accompanied by decreased drainage may indicate obstruction by retained calculi fragments; promptly report such findings to the doctor.

• Watch for and report signs of hemorrhage or infection.

• As ordered, gently irrigate the nephrostomy tube to ensure its patency. Maintain sterile technique and use no more than 10 ml of 0.9% sodium chloride solution. Never clamp the tube; the resultant pressure increase could cause renal damage.

• To aid passage of retained fragments and hinder formation of new calculi, maintain the patient's high fluid intake — up to 4,000 ml (about 4 qt) a day, as ordered. For the same reason, encourage early ambulation.

• Monitor serum electrolyte levels, and observe for signs of fluid overload.

• Prepare the patient for nephrotomography to check for retained fragments. This usually takes place 1 or 2 days after the procedure. If no fragments are revealed, the tube is clamped and removed the next day. Occasionally, a patient will be discharged with the tube in place.

• Tell the patient that the tract heals and closes within 24 hours after removal of the tube and that he can return to work within days.

Home care instructions

• If no complications develop, the patient may be discharged 2 to 4 days after treatment.

• Instruct the patient to drink 3 to 4 qt (or liters) of fluid each day for about a month after treatment. Explain that this will aid passage of any retained calculi fragments and help prevent formation of new calculi.

• Tell the patient to promptly report persistent bloody or cloudy and foul-smelling urine, an inability to void, fever and chills, or severe and unremitting flank pain. He should also report redness, swelling, or purulent drainage from the nephrostomy tube insertion site.

• Teach the patient how to strain his urine for calculi fragments. Tell him to strain all urine for the 1st week after treatment, to save all fragments in the container provided, and to bring the container along on his first medical follow-up visit.

• Encourage the patient to avoid strenuous exercise, sexual activity, heavy lifting, or straining until his doctor instructs otherwise. However, encourage him to take short walks. Explain that mild physical activity will help aid passage of any retained calculi fragments.

• Review any prescribed dietary or drug regimen to help prevent formation of new calculi.

• Outline proper nephrostomy tube care if the patient is discharged with a tube in place.

LIVER RESECTION

Resection of the liver is the excision of a significant portion of the organ. Partial or subtotal hepatectomy is excision of a portion of the liver. Lobectomy is the excision of an entire hepatic lobe.

Because liver cancer is often advanced at diagnosis, few such tumors are resectable. Before the decision is made to resect the liver, thorough assessment must ensure that at least 15% of healthy liver tissue will remain after surgery and that the blood and biliary systems will be functional postoperatively. Resection for a metastatic tumor requires that the primary tumor has been resected, that there are no other metastatic sites, and that the metastatic tumor does not involve the inferior vena cava or the portal vein. Probability of successful resection increases if the tumor is solitary and is confined to one lobe.

Purpose
• To excise diseased hepatic tissue
• To repair hepatic injury.

Indications
Resection or repair of diseased or damaged liver tissue may be indicated for various hepatic disorders, including cysts, abscesses, tumors (primary and secondary malignant and benign), lacerations, or crush injuries from blunt or penetrating trauma. Such surgery is usually performed only after conservative measures prove ineffective. For instance, if aspiration fails to correct a liver abscess, resection may be necessary.

Procedure
The patient will receive general anesthesia. The surgeon usually makes a vertical incision in the right upper quadrant and can quickly extend the incision if he finds more damage than suspected. For emergency surgery when a liver laceration or crush injury is suspected, the extent of resection is determined intraoperatively. The surgeon resects damaged liver tissue and sutures any lacerations; then he carefully explores the surrounding tissue and organs for additional injury. When all damage is repaired and bleeding controlled, the surgeon inserts a chest tube or abdominal drains and closes the incision.

In elective surgery, the technique depends on the location and extent of liver disease. (See *Types of hepatic resection*.) For a right lobectomy, the surgeon makes a thoracoabdominal incision or a right subcostal incision; for a left lobectomy, a large upper midline incision. In a right lobectomy, the surgeon inserts a chest tube through the right lateral chest wall and connects it to suction to remove accumulated blood, fluid, and air. Because a left lobectomy usually doesn't involve the pleural space, no chest tube is needed. Instead, the surgeon may insert one or more abdominal drains to remove fluid, blood, and air from the abdominal cavity. The incision is sutured and a dressing is applied.

Complications
The postoperative course is frequently complicated and becomes more difficult as the amount of liver resected increases. Because of the liver's anatomic location, surgery is typically performed through a thoracoabdominal incision and therefore carries many risks associated with both thoracic and abdominal surgery: atelectasis, ascites, renal failure, and infection. In addition, impaired liver function due to surgery can result in such diverse complications as hypoglycemia from decreased hepatic

Types of hepatic resection

The illustration below indicates the various types of hepatic resection.

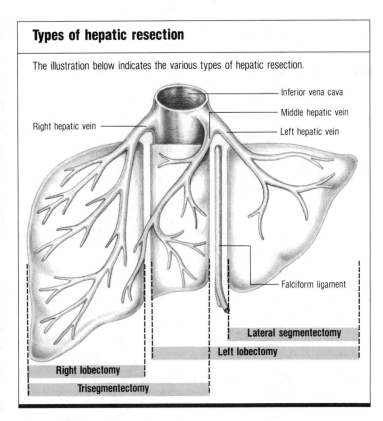

gluconeogenesis and hepatic encephalopathy from interference with hepatic conversion of ammonia to urea. Because of the liver's friability, acute hemorrhage remains a threat during and after surgery.

Care considerations
Before surgery
• If emergency surgery is necessary, briefly explain the procedure to the patient.
• If surgery is elective, the preparation may extend up to 6 weeks. During this time, explain the purpose of coagulation studies; blood chemistry tests, including serum ammonia and creatinine, aspartate aminotransferase (AST, formerly SGOT), alanine aminotransferase (ALT, formerly SGPT), blood urea

nitrogen (BUN), blood glucose, and serum electrolyte levels; arterial blood gas analysis; and blood typing and crossmatching.
• Depending on the results of these tests, give fluid and electrolyte replacements, transfuse blood or blood components, or provide protein supplements, as ordered.
• Prepare the patient for additional diagnostic tests that help locate and identify lesions. Such tests may include a liver scan, ultrasonography, computed tomography (CT), percutaneous needle biopsy, hepatic angiography, and cholangiography.
• Encourage adequate rest and good nutrition, and provide vitamin supplements, as ordered, to help improve liver function.

• Explain postoperative care, including the presence of a nasogastric (NG) tube, chest tube, and hemodynamic lines.

• Because of the liver's anatomic position, surgery often interferes with normal respiratory excursion, increasing the risk of postoperative atelectasis. To reduce this risk, encourage the patient to practice the coughing and deep-breathing exercises that he will perform postoperatively.

• Ensure that the patient or a responsible family member has signed a consent form.

After surgery

• Monitor the patient's vital signs, and evaluate fluid status every 1 to 2 hours. Report any signs of volume deficit, which could indicate intraperitoneal bleeding. Maintain I.V. line patency for possible emergency fluid replacement or blood transfusion. Administer analgesics, as ordered.

• Check laboratory test results for hypoglycemia, increased prothrombin time, increased ammonia levels, azotemia (increased BUN and creatinine levels), and electrolyte imbalances (especially potassium, sodium, and calcium imbalances). Promptly report any such findings, and take corrective actions, as ordered. For example, vitamin K may be given I.M. to decrease prothrombin time, or hypertonic glucose solution may be infused to correct hypoglycemia.

• Check the dressings often and change them as needed. Note and report excessive bloody drainage on the dressings or in the drainage tube. Also note the amount and characteristics of NG tube drainage; keep in mind that excessive drainage could trigger metabolic alkalosis.

• If the patient has a chest tube in place, maintain tube patency by milking it as necessary and according to hospital policy. Make sure the suction equipment is working.

• Encourage the patient to cough, deep-breathe, and change position frequently to prevent pulmonary complications. Periodically auscultate the lungs, and report any adventitious breath sounds.

• Watch for symptoms of hepatic encephalopathy: behavioral or personality changes, such as confusion, forgetfulness, lethargy or stupor, and hallucinations.

• Also observe for asterixis (hand-flapping tremor), apraxia (inability to manipulate objects), and hyperactive reflexes.

• Throughout recovery, take measures to enhance patient comfort.

• Promote rest and relaxation, and provide a quiet atmosphere.

• Assist with ambulation.

Home care instructions

• Encourage the patient to return for follow-up visits and examinations with the surgeon to evaluate liver function.

• Inform the patient that CT scans may be performed at some point during the first year after surgery to assess the liver's regeneration and detect any tumor recurrence.

• Inform the patient that adequate rest and good nutrition will conserve energy and reduce metabolic demands on the liver, thereby speeding healing.

• As ordered, instruct the patient to maintain a high-calorie, high-carbohydrate, high-protein diet during recovery to help restore the liver mass. However, if the patient has developed hepatic encephalopathy, recommend a low-protein diet with carbohydrates making up the balance of caloric intake.

LIVER TRANSPLANTATION

Liver transplantation replaces a diseased liver with a healthy liver removed from a donor. Liver transplantations are an accepted treatment for end-stage liver disease. Since introduction of the surgery in 1963, liver transplantation rates have improved remarkably. Before 1980 and the use of the immunosuppressant cyclosporine, only 38% of patients survived liver transplantation for 1 year. Today, many transplant programs are reporting survival rates of 80% or more.

There are three notable types of liver transplantation. In orthotopic transplantation, the surgeon removes the native liver and replaces it with a healthy donor liver (from a recently brain-dead individual); in the second type, heterotopic transplantation, a donor liver is inserted at an ectopic site while the native liver remains in place; in the third type, reduced-sized liver transplantation, the surgeon transplants a portion of a liver. This type of surgery is relatively new and is reserved for pediatric patients.

Liver transplantations are typically reserved for terminally ill patients who have a realistic chance of surviving the surgery and postoperative complications.

The most limiting factor in transplantation is the availability of donor organs, particularly for pediatric patients. Many qualified transplantation candidates are awaiting suitable donor organs. Often the wait proves fatal. And even if a compatible healthy liver is located and transplantation is performed, the patient faces many obstacles to recovery.

Purpose
• To replace a terminally diseased liver with a healthy donor organ.

Indications
Liver transplantations are indicated for children and adults with severe, irreversible liver disease that cannot be successfully treated by alternative medical and surgical approaches. The most common pediatric indication is biliary atresia; other major indications for liver transplantations in children and adoles-

cents are genetic diseases associated with liver failure, such as extrahepatic biliary atresia.

In adults, chronic active hepatitis and cirrhosis of nonviral etiology are indications for transplantation. Other indications in adults include primary biliary cirrhosis (nonalcoholic), sclerosing cholangitis, hepatic vein thrombosis, and hepatobiliary cancer. Note, however, that the survival rate in patients with liver cancer is low.

Contraindications may include a positive human immunodeficiency virus antibody test, advanced cardiopulmonary or cerebrovascular disease, and active substance abuse. In addition, any potentially dangerous sequelae of liver disease, such as hypertension, hepatic encephalopathy, coagulopathy, or hepatorenal syndrome, may disqualify the patient for liver transplantation.

Procedure
In an orthotopic transplantation, the liver is excised from the donor and then flushed by injecting an electrolyte solution through the portal vein; the organ is then placed on ice. The combination of cold storage and electrolyte solution preserves the liver for up to 10 hours. The organ is then transported in an ice-slush solution to the transplant center. Newer flush solutions containing high-molecular-weight sugars have extended the transportation time to approximately 36 hours.

To prepare the recipient for transplantation, the surgeon opens the abdomen, clamps and frees the vena cava and portal and hepatic vessels, and excises the diseased liver. During this critical stage, he decompresses venous return from the lower half of the body with a vascular pump connecting the iliac and axillary arteries. He then quickly positions the donor organ in place and anastomoses the upper and lower vena cava, portal vein, and hepatic artery to restore circulation. After controlling all bleeding, the surgeon reconstructs the common bile duct. Finally, abdominal drains are inserted, the incision is closed, and a dressing is applied.

After surgery, the patient will return to an intensive care setting with an endotracheal tube in place and on mechanical ventilation. The patient will also have in place a nasogastric tube, hemodynamic monitoring lines, cardiac monitor, I.V. lines, and abdominal drains.

Complications

Tissue rejection and infection are the two major complications of liver transplant. Tissue rejection results from antigenic differences between the donor and recipient; successful transplantation requires overcoming rejection. Renal dysfunction is common and is usually related to cyclosporine toxicity. Other complications include vascular thrombosis and biliary leakage. Psychological complications may arise as the chronically ill patient moves from overwhelming sickness to wellness.

Care considerations

Before surgery

• Preoperatively, the patient will have a complete workup, including a thorough physical examination, a barium swallow and enema, hepatic arteriography, and ultrasonography to determine suitability as a transplant candidate. In addition, the patient will undergo an extensive battery of tests designed to match him with a donor, including ABO blood group compatibility, histocompatibility studies, and lymphocyte crossmatching.
• The health care team will prepare the patient for surgery and will take steps to improve nutritional and fluid status in order to stabilize the metabolic state in preparation for the extreme physiologic demands of transplantation.
• Reinforce the doctor's explanation of the transplant procedure to the patient or, if the patient is a child, to his parents.
• Discuss the prospects of success and of postoperative complications. Point out that successful transplantation doesn't guarantee a life free from medical problems. Stress the need for lifelong follow-up care to minimize these problems.
• Discuss anticipated postoperative care.
• If possible, arrange for the patient and his family to visit the intensive care unit and meet staff members before the surgery.
• Explain expected fluid and food restrictions.
• As ordered, begin immunosuppressant therapy to decrease the risk of tissue rejection, using such drugs as cyclosporine and corticosteroids. Explain the need for lifelong therapy to prevent rejection.
• Also take time to address the patient's and family's emotional needs.
• Assure the patient that you and other members of the health care team will provide support through the difficult times. Offer to arrange referral to a staff psychologist or psychiatric clinical nurse specialist for further support both before and after the surgery.
• Ensure that the patient or a responsible family member has signed a consent form.

After surgery

• Although hospitalization after liver transplantation typically lasts 4 to 6 weeks, it can vary from 11 days to 5 months. Consequently, it is extremely important that care be individualized.
• Continue immunosuppressant therapy, as ordered, to combat tissue rejection.
• Monitor the patient for early signs of rejection and other complications.
• Try to prevent opportunistic infections, which can lead to rejection.
• Provide reassurance and emotional support throughout recovery.

Home care instructions

• Make sure the patient and family understand the early signs of tissue rejection: pain and tenderness in the right upper quadrant, right flank, or center of the back; fever; tachycardia; jaundice; and changes in the color of urine or stool. Stress the need to call the doctor immediately if any of these signs or symptoms develop.

• Tell the patient and family to watch for and report any signs of liver failure, such as abdominal distention, bloody stool or vomitus, decreased urine output, abdominal pain and tenderness, anorexia, or altered level of consciousness.

• To reduce the risk of tissue rejection, advise the patient to avoid contact with any person who has or may have a contagious illness.

• Emphasize the importance of reporting any early signs of infection, including fever, weakness, lethargy, and tachycardia.

• Stress the importance of strict compliance with the prescribed immunosuppressant regimen. Warn that noncompliance can trigger rejection, even of a liver that has been functioning well for years. Also warn the patient about potential adverse effects of immunosuppressant therapy, such as infection, fluid retention, acne, glaucoma, diabetes, or cancer.

• Emphasize the importance of regular medical follow-up examinations to evaluate the integrity of the surgical site and continued tissue compatibility.

• If appropriate, suggest that the patient and his family seek psychological counseling to help them cope with the effects on their lives of the patient's long-term and perilous recovery.

LUNG EXCISION

A lung excision, also known as a thoracotomy, is the surgical removal of part or all of a lung to spare healthy lung tissue from disease. Pneumonectomy, excision of an entire lung, is used only when a less radical approach cannot remove all the diseased tissue. After pneumonectomy, chest cavity pressures will stabilize; over time fluid will fill the cavity once filled by lung tissue, preventing significant mediastinal shift. Lobectomy is the removal of one of the five lung lobes. After lobectomy, the remaining lobes expand to fill the entire pleural cavity.

Segmental resection removes one or more lung segments; it preserves more functional tissue than lobectomy. Wedge resection, which removes a small portion of the lung without regard to segments, preserves the most functional tissue but can treat only a small, well-circumscribed lesion. Remaining lung tissue needs to be reexpanded after both segmental and wedge resection.

Purpose

• To remove diseased or damaged lung tissue.

Indications

Pneumonectomy is usually performed to treat bronchogenic cancer but may also be used to treat tuberculosis, bronchiectasis, or lung abscess. A lobectomy can treat bronchogenic cancer, tuberculosis, lung abscess, emphysematous blebs or bullae, benign tumors, or localized fungal infections. Segmental resection is commonly used to treat bronchiectasis. Finally, wedge resection is reserved for small, well-circumscribed lesions. All types of lung excision can also be performed for trauma when part of the lung is destroyed.

Procedure

After the patient receives general anesthesia, the surgeon makes a posterolateral incision through the fourth, fifth, sixth, or seventh intercostal space. Then he spreads the ribs and exposes the lung area. In a pneumonectomy, the surgeon

Four types of lung excision

Lung excision may be total (pneumonectomy) or partial (lobectomy, segmental resection, or wedge resection), depending on the patient's condition. The illustrations here show the extent of each of these surgeries for the right lung.

Pneumonectomy

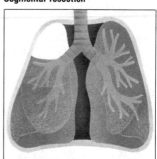

Segmental resection

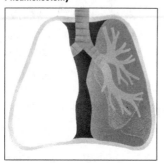

Lobectomy

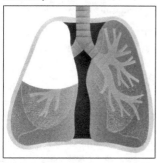

Wedge resection

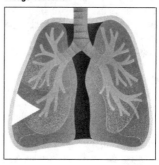

ligates and cuts the pulmonary arteries and veins, clamps the main stem bronchus leading to the affected lung, divides it, closes it with nonabsorbable sutures, and then removes the lung. To ensure airtight closure, the surgeon places a pleural flap over the bronchus and closes it. Then he severs or crushes the phrenic nerve on the affected side, causing the diaphragm to rise and reducing the size of the pleural cavity. After air pressure in the cavity stabilizes, he closes the chest.

In a lobectomy, the surgeon resects the affected lobe and ligates and cuts

the appropriate arteries, veins, and bronchial passages. In a segmental resection, the surgeon removes the affected segment and ligates and cuts the appropriate artery, vein, and bronchus. In a wedge resection, the surgeon clamps and excises the affected area and then sutures it. In both segmental and wedge resection, he inserts two chest tubes to drain fluid and aid lung reexpansion. After completing the excision, the surgeon closes the chest cavity and applies a dressing. (See *Four types of lung excision.*)

Complications

Complications of lung excision include hemorrhage, infection, and recurrent or tension pneumothorax. Additional complications include bronchopleural fistulas and empyema.

Care considerations

Before surgery

• Explain the procedure and postoperative course to the patient, and answer any questions. Also teach him about mechanical ventilation and what to expect in an intensive care unit, as appropriate.

• Prepare the patient psychologically, according to his condition. A patient with lung cancer, for example, faces the fear of dying as well as the fear of surgery and will need continuing emotional support. In contrast, a patient with a chronic lung disorder, such as tuberculosis or a fungal infection, may view the surgery as a cure for his ailment.

• Teach the patient coughing and deep-breathing techniques, and explain to him that he'll use these after surgery to facilitate lung reexpansion. Also show him how to use an incentive spirometer.

• Record preoperative inspiratory volumes to provide a baseline.

• As ordered, arrange for diagnostic studies, such as pulmonary function tests, electrocardiogram, chest X-ray, arterial blood gas analysis, bronchoscopy and, possibly, cardiac catheterization to assess cardiovascular function before pneumonectomy.

• Ensure that the patient or a responsible family member has signed a consent form.

After surgery

• Postoperatively, the patient may have chest tubes in place and may be receiving oxygen or be connected to a ventilator.

• If the patient has had a pneumonectomy, make sure he lies only on his operative side or his back until he's stabilized. This prevents fluid from draining into the unaffected lung if the sutured bronchus opens.

• The patient who has had a wedge or segmental resection will have chest tubes in place. Make sure the chest tubes are providing drainage, and monitor for signs of tension pneumothorax.

• Provide analgesics, as ordered.

• Encourage the patient to begin coughing and deep-breathing exercises as soon as he's stabilized.

• Auscultate the lungs, place the patient in semi-Fowler's position, and have him splint his incision to facilitate coughing and deep-breathing. Encourage him to cough every 2 to 4 hours until breath sounds are clear.

• Perform passive range-of-motion (ROM) exercises the evening of surgery and two or three times daily thereafter. Progress to active ROM exercises.

Home care instructions

• Tell the patient to continue coughing and deep-breathing exercises to prevent complications.

• Advise the patient to report any changes in sputum characteristics to his doctor.

• Instruct the patient to continue performing ROM exercises to maintain mobility of the shoulder and chest wall.

• Tell the patient to avoid smoking and contact with people who have upper respiratory tract infections.

• Provide instructions for wound care and dressing changes as necessary.

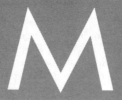

MAMMOPLASTY

Mammoplasty is a surgical procedure to change the size of the breast. Breast reduction mammoplasty removes excess breast skin and underlying tissue and reshapes the contour of large breasts. Breast reduction also includes repositioning the nipple and areola. Breast augmentation mammoplasty enlarges the size and shape of the breast. Breast reconstruction mammoplasty is performed to reconstruct the breast after cancer surgery.

These procedures are usually performed after breasts are fully developed, and they are not recommended for women who want to breast-feed. Breast reconstruction is contraindicated when metastasis is possible, if healing is impaired, or if the patient has unrealistic expectations of the effects of surgery.

Purpose

• To remove excess breast skin and tissue
• To reshape the breasts to a smaller size, in proportion with the rest of the body
• To enlarge the breasts
• To reconstruct the breasts after mastectomy.

Indications

Breast reduction is usually indicated because of physical discomfort, such as backache, shoulder aches, irritation, or fungal infections under the breasts. However, breast reduction or augmentation can also be performed for a woman who is self-conscious about the size of her breasts. The effect of breast surgery is permanent, but breast size can increase due to weight gain, use of birth control pills, or pregnancy.

Breast reconstruction can help relieve the emotional distress caused by mastectomy. It can improve the patient's self-image and restore her sexual identity.

Procedure

Mammoplasty is usually performed under general anesthesia and will take 3 to 4 hours, depending on the extent of the procedure. For breast reduction, incisions may be made around the edge of the nipple or in the crease below the breast, following the natural contour of the breast. A vertical incision may resemble the shape of a keyhole around the areola to allow the nipple to be repositioned. Excess tissue, fat, and skin are removed from the sides of the breast and around the areola. The nipple, areola, and underlying tissue are then repositioned to a normal location on the breast. If the breasts are extremely large, the nipple and areola may be completely detached and then relocated after the tissue is removed. The skin is brought together to re-form the breast.

In breast augmentation mammoplasty, the surgeon makes a small incision under the breast to insert an implant.

In breast reconstruction mammoplasty, the surgeon also places an implant under the skin. During the mastectomy, he may place the patient's own nipple on her inner thigh or inguinal area and salvage it later, or he may reconstruct a nipple from labial tissue. A dressing will be applied or a surgical bra may be fitted.

Complications

Breast reduction causes scars on the breast. Decreased sensitivity of the breast and nipple does occur, and sensitivity may not return for as long as 6 months. A hematoma formation or tissue ischemia may occur in the nipple and areola.

Complications of breast augmentation depend on the type of implant. Recent studies have shown that silicone implants may leak and can possibly burst, causing the release of silicone into the surrounding breast tissue (resulting in pain and hardness in the tissue).

Care considerations
Before surgery
• Inform the patient that blood transfusions may be necessary during surgery so that she can bank autologous blood before surgery.
• Instruct the patient to stop taking aspirin or any medication containing aspirin 1 week before surgery.
• Describe the procedure to the patient and explain that she may have drains inserted after surgery. Explain their purpose and reassure her that they will be removed.
• Reinforce the purpose of the procedure. Remind the patient that it will relieve physical discomfort and alter the size of the breast but will not solve her sexual or social problems.
After surgery
• Administer analgesics, as ordered, for pain control.
• Encourage ambulation and mobility of extremities.
• Monitor vital signs closely.
• Observe dressings for any bleeding; drains will be removed on the 2nd or 3rd postoperative day.

Home care instructions
• Teach the patient the importance of taking analgesics so that mobility of upper extremities will be achieved.
• After 1 week, surgical dressings will be removed; a soft bra should be worn at all times for several weeks.
• Tell the patient to expect swelling and skin discoloration of the breast, but that it will subside in several days.
• Tell the patient that the sutures will be removed in 2 to 3 weeks.
• Instruct the patient to avoid excessive movement and all overhead lifting for 3 to 4 weeks or as advised by the doctor. Advise her that she may return to work 2 weeks after surgery.
• Inform the patient that she should wear a support bra for the first month after surgery.
• Advise the patient that scars will remain visible up to 1 year and then will gradually fade.

MARSHALL-MARCHETTI-KRANTZ PROCEDURE

The Marshall-Marchetti-Krantz procedure, the most common surgery for stress incontinence, involves the creation of a bladder and urethral suspension by elevating the anterior vaginal wall. When stress incontinence in women doesn't respond to pubococcygeus (Kegel) muscle exercises or sympathomimetic drugs, surgery may help restore urinary sphincter competence. This relatively simple surgery eliminates stress incontinence in most patients, with minimal chance of recurrence.

A newer, less invasive procedure that elevates the urethra anteriorly is now being performed with similar results. This procedure uses a "needle-and-thread" method through the vagina and suprapubic area instead of a lower abdominal incision. The hospital stay is typically 24 to 72 hours, and the patient is sent home with a suprapubic catheter to use if she is unable to void. It remains in place until the follow-up visit with the doctor.

Purpose

• To eliminate stress incontinence by restoring the normal posterior vesicourethral angle.

Indications

The Marshall-Marchetti-Krantz procedure is recommended for stress incontinence when medical treatment and exercises fail.

Procedure

With the patient under general anesthesia, the surgeon makes a transverse suprapubic incision and frees the bladder neck, urethra, and anterior vaginal wall. He then suspends the urethra and bladder neck by suturing both sides of the anterior vaginal wall to the periosteum of the pubic bones and to the lower rectal fascia. (If the periosteum is in poor condition, as it is in many elderly patients, he may use Cooper's ligament in the bladder neck region.) Typically, the surgeon completes the procedure by inserting a drain in the retropubic space and an indwelling urinary catheter or cystostomy tube (suprapubic catheter) and then closing the incision and applying a sterile dressing.

Complications

This procedure is associated with the risk of urethral obstruction, with resultant urine retention, and with infection caused by leakage of urine into the vagina. These complications are rare and can usually be prevented or corrected by careful postoperative monitoring, prompt intervention, and comprehensive patient teaching.

Care considerations

Before surgery

• Review the procedure with the patient.
• Ensure that the patient has signed a consent form.
• Advise the patient that a suprapubic catheter or an indwelling urinary catheter may be inserted during surgery.

After surgery

• Check the incisional drain and dressing every 4 hours for the first 24 hours and then once every shift. A small amount of serosanguineous drainage is normal. Change the dressing when it becomes wet or as ordered, remembering to use sterile technique and taking care not to dislodge an incisional drain or cystostomy tube.
• Monitor the amount and color of urine drainage from the indwelling urinary catheter or cystostomy tube. Blood-tinged urine normally occurs for 24 to 48 hours after surgery.
• Notify the doctor if urine appears bright red or if hematuria persists for longer than 48 hours.
• The patient may experience bladder spasms due to the catheter or manipulation during surgery. Notify the doctor if this occurs, and administer ordered medications.
• Report signs of urine retention, and be prepared to institute intermittent catheterization, as ordered, to drain the bladder and prevent complications.
• Teach intermittent self-catheterization if the patient continues to experience difficulty voiding. (See *Self-catheterization*, pages 155 and 156.) Intermittent catheterization isn't usually necessary after healing is complete and edema subsides.

Home care instructions

• Explain that weakness, fatigue, and incisional pain may persist for several weeks. Advise the patient to get plenty of rest and to avoid strenuous activity during the recovery period.

• If the patient requires intermittent catheterization after discharge, provide her with written instructions on self-catheterization technique.

• Instruct the patient to report signs of urinary tract infection, such as fever, chills, flank pain, and hematuria. Also tell her to report signs of wound infection, such as severe pain, redness, and swelling at the incision site.

• Encourage the patient to try to void before each catheterization and record both amounts (for example, void _____ ml; catheter _____ ml; time _____) for follow-up appointments.

MASTECTOMY

Mastectomy is the surgical removal of all or part of one or both breasts. Primarily performed to remove malignant breast tissue and any regional lymphatic metastases, mastectomy is commonly combined with radiation therapy and chemotherapy. Until recently, radical mastectomy was the treatment of choice for breast cancer. Now, different types of mastectomy can be performed depending on the size of the tumor and the presence of metastasis.

A *partial mastectomy*, also called a lumpectomy, tylectomy, or segmental resection, is indicated for stage I lesions, which are small and peripherally located. This approach leaves a cosmetically satisfactory breast but may fail to remove all malignant tissue or to detect metastasis to axillary lymph nodes.

Subcutaneous mastectomy may be used in the patient with a central, noninvasive tumor. It's also used for chronic cystic mastitis, multiple fibroadenomas, or hyperplastic duct changes.

Simple mastectomy may be performed if a tumor is confined to breast tissue. It's also used palliatively for advanced, ulcerative stages of breast cancer and as treatment for extensive benign disease.

A *modified radical mastectomy*, the standard surgery for stage I and II lesions, removes small, localized tumors. Causing less disfigurement and disability than radical mastectomy, this procedure reduces postoperative arm edema and shoulder problems.

A *radical mastectomy* is indicated to treat large primary lesions with deep extension to the pectoral fascia and metastasis to the axillary lymph nodes. Later, breast reconstruction may be performed using a portion of the latissimus dorsi. Rarely, an *extended radical mastectomy* may be used to treat cancer in the medial quadrant of the breast or in subareolar tissue. The procedure is used to remove possible metastasis to the internal mammary lymph nodes.

Purpose

• To remove a malignant breast tumor.

Indications

Mastectomy is indicated for operable breast cancer and any regional metastasis. It is also indicated in the treatment of chronic cystic mastitis, multiple fibroadenomas, hyperplastic duct changes, and fibrocystic disease.

Procedure

The patient receives general anesthesia. (See *Types of breast surgery*, pages 434 and 435.) In a partial mastectomy, the surgeon removes the entire tumor mass along with at least 2.5 cm of the surrounding healthy tissue. In subcutaneous mastectomy, the surgeon removes all breast tissue but preserves the overlying skin and nipple and may also insert a prosthesis. In a simple mastectomy, the surgeon removes the entire breast and may apply a skin graft if necessary. Axillary lymph nodes closest to the breast may be removed.

To perform a modified radical mastectomy, the surgeon will use one of several techniques to remove the entire breast. He also resects all axillary lymph nodes while leaving the pector-

Types of breast surgery

The type of procedure the surgeon chooses depends on the size and location of the tumor and the presence of metastasis.

Partial (segmental) excision
In this procedure, the surgeon removes the lump, 2 to 3 cm of healthy tissue surrounding it, and the fascia over the chest muscles directly behind the lump. The axillary lymph nodes also may be removed. Some breast tissue remains. Radiation therapy may follow surgery.

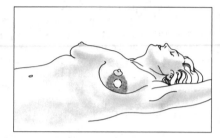

Subcutaneous mastectomy
The surgeon removes breast tissue while retaining breast skin in this procedure. The tissue is examined histologically for invasive cancer. If cancer is found, more extensive surgery is scheduled. If staging was performed during an earlier biopsy, the subcutaneous mastectomy and breast implant insertion may take place at the same time.

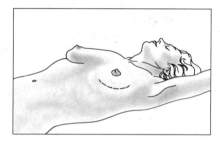

alis major muscle intact. He may or may not remove the pectoralis minor. If the patient has small lesions and no metastasis, the surgeon may perform breast reconstruction immediately or a few days or months later.

In a radical mastectomy, the surgeon removes the entire breast, the axillary lymph nodes, the underlying pectoral muscles, and adjacent tissues. During the operation, he covers skin flaps and exposed tissue with moist packs for protection and, before closure, irrigates the chest wall and axilla.

In an extended radical mastectomy, the surgeon removes the breast, underlying pectoral muscles, axillary contents, and the upper internal mammary (mediastinal) lymph node chain.

After closing the mastectomy site, the surgeon may make a stab wound and insert a catheter. The catheter removes blood that may collect under the skin flaps, prevent healing, and predispose the patient to infection. Less commonly, large pressure dressings are applied instead. If a graft was needed

Simple (total) mastectomy
In this procedure, the surgeon removes the breast tissue and the axillary lymph nodes closest to the breast. Radiation therapy commonly follows.

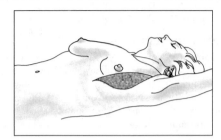

Modified radical mastectomy
In this procedure, the surgeon removes the breast, axillary lymph nodes, and chest muscle, but preserves the pectoralis major muscle. It is the most common surgery for breast cancer.

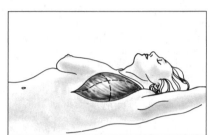

Radical mastectomy
In this procedure, the surgeon removes the breast, all the axillary lymph nodes, chest muscle, pectoralis major and pectoralis minor muscles, and surrounding fat, tissue, and skin.

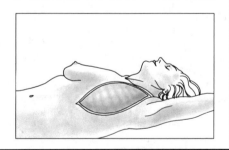

to close the wound, a pressure dressing will be placed over the donor site.

A new technique called outpatient carbon dioxide laser mastectomy is currently gaining attention. Candidates for this procedure have a diagnosis of invasive breast cancer and must have one or more supportive family members living with them at home. The patient receives preoperative sedation in the form of a scopolamine patch or sublingual haloperidol and then general anesthesia during the procedure. Excision of the breast is accomplished using a carbon dioxide laser. Silastic drains are inserted and local anesthetics are injected into the wound before closing to reduce postoperative pain. This procedure requires extreme compliance on the part of both patient and caregiver.

Complications

After any type of mastectomy, infection and delayed healing are possible. However, the major complication of radical mastectomy and axillary dissection is lymphedema, which typically occurs soon after surgery and persists for years. Dissection of the lymph nodes draining the axilla may interfere with lymphatic drainage of the arm on the affected side.

Care considerations
Before surgery
• Explore the patient's feelings about mastectomy. Listen supportively, and help the patient express her concerns.
• Review the surgeon's explanation of the procedure and all treatment options.
• Prepare the patient for her postoperative care. Inform her that she may have a drain in place. Explain the reason for it and when it may be removed.
• Provide information about the types of breast prostheses available.
• Measure the circumference of the patient's upper arms to provide baseline data.
• Ensure that the patient has signed a consent form.
After surgery
• Postoperatively elevate the patient's arm on a pillow to enhance circulation and prevent edema.
• Monitor the suction tubing to ensure proper function, and observe the drainage site for erythema, induration, and drainage.
• Record drainage every 8 hours. Drainage should change from sanguineous to serosanguineous fluid.
• Depending on the policy of the health care facility, milk the drain periodically to prevent clots from occluding the tubing.
• Teach the patient arm exercises to prevent muscle shortening and contracture of the shoulder joint and to facilitate lymph drainage. Arm extension and flexion can usually begin on the first postoperative day, and other exercises can be added each day depending on the procedure and patient's needs.
• To prevent lymphedema, make sure that no blood pressure readings, injections, or venipunctures are performed on the affected arm. Place a sign with this reminder at the head of the patient's bed.
• Because mastectomy causes emotional distress, you'll need to teach the patient to conserve her energy and to recognize the early signs of fatigue. Encourage her to view the operative site by describing its appearance and allowing her to express her feelings. Be sure to be present to offer support when she looks at the wound for the first time.
• Arrange for a volunteer who's had a mastectomy to talk with the patient. Contact the American Cancer Society's "Reach to Recovery" rehabilitation program.
• After 2 to 3 days, initiate a fitting for a temporary breast pad. Soft and lightweight, the pad may be inserted into a bra without stays or under wires.
• If appropriate, explain breast reconstruction (see the entry "Mammoplasty").

Home care instructions
• Inform the patient that prevention of lymphedema is critical. Explain that swelling may follow even minor trauma to the arm on her affected side. Tell her to wash cuts and scrapes on the affected side promptly and to contact the doctor immediately if erythema, edema, or induration occurs.
• Advise the patient to use the arm on the affected side as much as possible and to avoid keeping it in a dependent position for a prolonged period.
• Reinforce the importance of performing daily range-of-motion exercises. The patient must do them with both arms to maintain symmetry and prevent additional deformities.
• Emphasize the importance of not allowing any blood pressure readings, injections, or venipunctures on the affected arm.
• Advise the patient to wear a medical identification bracelet that reads NO

VENIPUNCTURES, BLOOD PRESSURES, OR INJECTIONS on the affected arm.

• Remind the patient that her energy level will wax and wane. Instruct her to be alert for signs of fatigue and to rest frequently during the day for the first few weeks after discharge.

• Stress the importance of monthly self-examination of the remaining breast and the mastectomy site. Demonstrate the correct technique, and have the patient repeat it.

• Explain to the patient that it is important for her to keep scheduled postoperative appointments.

• If necessary, provide information regarding a permanent prosthesis. This can be fitted 3 to 4 weeks after surgery. Prostheses are available in a wide range of styles, skin tones, and weights from lingerie shops, medical supply stores, and department stores.

• Reassure the patient that she can wear the same type of clothing she wore before her surgery.

MASTOIDECTOMY

Mastoidectomy is a surgical procedure used to excise the mastoid process or the mastoid cells of the temporal bone. There are four types of mastoidectomies: mastoidectomy, radical mastoidectomy, modified-radical mastoidectomy, and mastoid tympanoplasty.

The extent of mastoid involvement, the condition of the ossicular chain, the tympanic membrane, and the presence of cholesteatoma (a mass of dead tissue in the middle ear) will determine which procedure will be performed.

Purpose

• To remove parts of the mastoid air cells that are invaded by infection or cholesteatoma and to clean the remaining bone.

Indications

Mastoidectomy is indicated in the presence of acute mastoiditis (although rare, it occurs in children), chronic otitis media that is unresponsive to medical therapy and is associated with a perforated tympanic membrane and granulation infection, or a cholesteatoma.

Procedure

After the patient receives general anesthesia, the surgeon will select either a curved incision made behind the ear (postauricular approach) or an incision made through the ear canal (endaural approach). This exposes the bone and the mastoid.

When an acute infection is limited to the mastoid cells, a mastoidectomy is performed. All infected cells are removed and the remaining area is cleaned. Special care is taken not to injure the facial nerve that passes through the temporal bone. Radical mastoidectomy is indicated when disease has spread to the middle ear as well. If the tympanic membrane is perforated as a result of increased pressure in the middle ear, a combined mastoidectomy and tympanoplasty is performed. A modified-radical mastoidectomy may be performed to remove a cholesteatoma. This procedure leaves the tympanic membrane and the middle ear structures intact. The surgeon may insert some packing and possibly a drain, close the incision, and apply a dressing.

Complications

Facial nerve paralysis is a serious complication after mastoidectomy. It is due to possible erosion of the bone that protects the nerve. Other complications include infection, vertigo, meningitis, or brain abscess. The use of antibiotics greatly reduces the risk of postoperative infection.

Care considerations

Before surgery

• Explain to the patient that he will have a bulky dressing as well as a drain in place.

• Inform the patient that the surgeon may order the hair around the ear shaved up to 1″ (2.5 cm).

• Instruct the patient to lie on the affected side to promote postoperative drainage.

After surgery

• Administer analgesics and sedatives, as ordered, to control pain and restlessness.

• Assess for facial nerve damage. Ask the patient to smile or wink. If the patient shows signs of inability to move the affected side, such as a drooping eye, inability to smile, or inability to drink water, the surgeon must be notified immediately.

• Check the dressing frequently. A Teflon drain allows drainage of the mastoid cavity; reinforcement may be necessary. Bright red drainage should be reported to the surgeon promptly. The dressing stays in place for 4 to 5 days.

• Instruct the patient to ask for assistance when getting out of bed and to move slowly to minimize vertigo.

Home care instructions

• Tell the patient to avoid driving, blowing his nose, and heavy lifting for 1 week after surgery.

• Stress the importance of complying with the recommended drug therapy and with wound care and ear care regimens. He should keep the ear dry, using a cotton ball with mineral oil or petroleum jelly on the visible portion of the cotton ball.

• Emphasize the importance of sneezing with the mouth open, which will prevent unnecessary pressure buildup.

• Inform the patient that follow-up medical care is necessary.

• If a mastoidectomy was performed, the donor site of the graft should be checked for indications of infection. Change the dressing as necessary.

• Remind the patient that ear packing, if present, will be removed by the surgeon in 3 to 5 days.

MECHANICAL VENTILATION

Mechanical ventilation therapy, which artificially controls or supports the patient's breathing, can supply oxygen, reduce dyspnea, and allow fatigued ventilatory muscles to rest and become reconditioned. Because it also supports spontaneous breathing, mechanical ventilation allows healing to take place until normal respiratory function can resume. The ventilator delivers air to the patient's lungs through an endotracheal (ET) or tracheostomy tube.

Ventilators are available in four types: negative-pressure, pressure-cycled, volume-cycled, and high-frequency. Each type is classified according to the mechanism that cycles the ventilator.

Negative-pressure ventilators work by alternately removing and replacing air from a container that either encloses the entire body (except for the head) or just the front and sides of the chest and upper abdomen. Removing air creates a negative pressure in the chamber that forces the chest wall to expand, pulling air into the lungs. As the device's diaphragm returns to normal position, it allows the chest wall to fall, causing exhalation.

Pressure-cycled ventilators stop inspiration when they reach a preset pressure and then allow passive expiration.

Volume-cycled ventilators, the most commonly used type, stop inspiration when they've delivered a preset volume of gas, regardless of the pressure needed to deliver it, and then allow passive expiration.

High-frequency ventilators use high respiratory rates (usually four times the normal rate) and small tidal volumes (less than or equal to the patient's dead-space volume) to keep alveoli ventilated.

Purpose

• To provide oxygenation in respiratory failure
• To help control or support respiratory mechanics
• To support ventilation during neuromuscular blockade.

Indications

Mechanical ventilation is indicated when a patient cannot generate spontaneous respirations or when his respirations aren't sufficient to expand his chest and deliver enough oxygenated air to his lungs.

Two types of disorders – impaired gas exchange and extrapulmonary – require mechanical ventilation. Disorders that impair gas exchange include respiratory infections, which fill the alveoli with secretions and interfere with ventilation; pulmonary emboli; and adult respiratory distress syndrome (ARDS). In these conditions, mechanical ventilation increases the oxygen available (especially to areas least affected by infection) while the patient receives treatment for the underlying problem.

Extrapulmonary disorders include central nervous system disorders such as brain stem injury, neuromuscular diseases such as Guillain-Barré syndrome, and flail chest and other musculoskeletal disorders that lower tidal volume by keeping the chest from expanding adequately. In these situations, mechanical ventilation controls or supports respiratory mechanics.

Procedure

Mechanical ventilation often requires emergency intubation. Placement of the ET tube can be done in almost every unit in a medical facility. The most common setting for intubation and mechanical ventilation is an intensive care unit, operating room, or emergency department.

For long-term ventilator-dependent patients, mechanical ventilation therapy may be delivered in a general hospital unit, in a long-term care facility, or in the home.

The ventilator must be correctly set up according to the manufacturer's instructions, usually by a respiratory therapist. The doctor chooses specific modes based on each patient's condition and ventilatory needs. Each type of mode chosen ends expiration and signals the machine when to initiate inspiration. (See *Mechanical ventilation modes and adjuncts,* pages 440 to 442.) In addition, certain adjuncts, such as continuous positive airway pressure (CPAP) and positive end-expiratory pressure (PEEP), may be used during mechanical ventilation to help keep the patient's alveoli expanded and aid in oxygenation. CPAP, which is appropriate only for patients who can breathe spontaneously, oxygenates by increasing the patient's functional residual capacity – the amount of air remaining in the lungs after normal expiration. PEEP lets the patient exhale while maintaining a preset positive pressure at the end of expiration.

Positive-pressure levels, respiratory rate, tidal volume, flow rate, and oxygen concentration are set and then adjusted as ordered by the doctor. After the machine's settings are adjusted and all alarms are set, the patient's ET or tracheostomy tube is connected to the large-bore tubing of the ventilator, maintaining tube sterility.

Arterial blood gas (ABG) levels are checked after the patient has been ventilated for 20 minutes without interruption. This allows enough time for equilibrium of gas exchange to be established at the recommended settings. Then, based on ABG results, the ventilator settings are readjusted as needed.

(Text continues on page 442.)

Mechanical ventilation modes and adjuncts

The use of mechanical ventilation modes or adjuncts will be determined by the patient's condition and ventilatory needs. Adjuncts to mechanical ventilation, such as positive end-expiratory pressure (PEEP) and continuous positive airway pressure (CPAP), help to keep the alveoli expanded.

MODE OR ADJUNCT	INDICATION
CMV With continuous mandatory ventilation (CMV), a preset tidal volume is delivered at a preset rate regardless of the patient's inspiratory effort. The patient cannot take a spontaneous breath.	This mode is rarely used because the machine—not the patient—does the breathing, causing respiratory muscles to atrophy and making it harder to wean the patient from the machine. CMV is typically used with an unconscious patient.
ACV With assist control ventilation (ACV), the patient initiates the breath. Any decrease in pressure triggers the ventilator to deliver a breath at a preset rate. If the patient doesn't initiate a breath, the ventilator will provide full ventilation at a preset rate.	Doctors often select ACV for patients who are unable to breathe spontaneously.
IMV In intermittent mandatory ventilation (IMV), the ventilator delivers a set number of breaths at a specific volume. The patient may breathe spontaneously between the IMV breaths.	In addition to providing ventilation, IMV is used as a weaning tool and as a way to decrease mean intrathoracic pressure.
SIMV Synchronized intermittent mandatory ventilation (SIMV) is similar to IMV, with the addition of synchronization with the patient's spontaneous breathing. If the patient does not breathe within a preset time, the ventilator will deliver a mandatory breath and reset itself to respond to the patient's respiratory rate.	In addition to providing ventilation, SIMV is used as a weaning tool. Unlike IMV, SIMV prevents stacking of breaths.
PSV Pressure support ventilation (PSV) supports a spontaneous breath with positive pressure. The patient controls the length of inspiration as well as the volume. Pressure support can be delivered along with SIMV, CPAP, or PEEP.	PSV is primarily used during weaning. It functions like intermittent positive-pressure breathing.

Mechanical ventilation modes and adjuncts *(continued)*

MODE OR ADJUNCT	INDICATION
HFPPV High-frequency positive-pressure ventilation (HFPPV) is a mode of respiratory support in which small tidal volumes (as low as 100 cc) are delivered at high respiratory rates (as high as 200 breaths/minute). The smaller tidal volumes produce lower airway pressures, reducing the chance of barotrauma and circulatory impairment.	Although it is still used infrequently and under research, HFPPV is useful on patients with bronchopleural fistulas. It is also useful during bronchoscopy, laryngoscopy, and in anesthesia during lithotripsy.
HFJV During high-frequency jet ventilation (HFJV), small jets of gas are delivered to the patient at a rate of 100 to 140 times per minute. HFJV requires the use of a high-frequency jet ventilator.	HFJV is still used infrequently and under research; however, it's indicated in reconstructive surgery of the upper airways. HFJV is also appropriate for patients who require mechanical ventilation for management of bronchopleural fistulas.
High-frequency oscillation High-frequency oscillation is produced by a piston pump through a low-compliance tubing connected to the endotracheal (ET) tube. The piston pump delivers a column of gas. The frequency of piston movement determines the respiratory rate. The stroke volume of the piston determines the tidal volume. The use of high-frequency oscillation reduces the incidence of barotrauma and respiratory-induced oxygen injury in the neonate.	This mode is frequently used by pediatricians in the treatment of respiratory distress syndrome in neonates, but the procedure is still investigational.
PCIRV Pressure-controlled inverse ratio ventilation (PCIRV) increases inspiratory time by inverting the conventional inspiratory-expiratory ratio.	PCIRV is useful in patients with diffuse lung disease and oxygen desaturation who do not respond to high levels of PEEP treatment. Indications for PCIRV that have not been proven include adult respiratory distress syndrome (ARDS) and infants with respiratory distress syndrome.

(continued)

Mechanical ventilation modes and adjuncts *(continued)*

MODE OR ADJUNCT	INDICATION
DLV Differential lung ventilation (DLV), a nontraditional form of ventilatory support, permits selective ventilation of the left lung, the right lung, or both. The use of double ET tubing makes selective ventilation possible.	Indications for DLV include differential bronchospirometry, anesthesia during lung resection or pulmonary lavage, and unilateral lung disease in critically ill patients. Other applications include treatment of bronchopleural fistulas, atelectasis, lobar pneumonia, unilateral lung contusion, pulmonary hemorrhage, bilateral lung disorders, and aspiration.
PEEP When PEEP supplements mechanical ventilation, a constant pressure is exerted across the alveoli.	PEEP works to improve oxygenation by increasing the patient's functional residual capacity. PEEP is also indicated for patients with ARDS.
CPAP Based on the same principles as PEEP, CPAP provides continuous positive airway pressure in a patient breathing spontaneously.	CPAP may be considered for hypoxemic patients who can breathe on their own; CPAP is often used with neonates.

Complications

Mechanical ventilation affects many body systems. Potential complications include acid-base balance alterations, arrhythmias, asynchronous breathing, atelectasis, tension pneumothorax, decreased cardiac output, fluid volume excess caused by humidification, barotrauma, decreased venous return, GI alterations, infection, and oxygen toxicity. The patient may experience psychological reactions, including anxiety, fear, and loss of control.

Care considerations

Before therapy
• Explain to the patient the type of ventilator system being used, describing its benefits and the sensations he'll experience.

• Keep in mind that the patient's anxiety may make him fight the machine, defeating its purpose.
• Position the patient in semi-Fowler's position if possible to promote lung expansion, but be sure to change his position every 2 hours.
• Obtain baseline vital signs and ABG readings.
• A bite block may be used with an oral ET tube to prevent the patient from biting the tube and obstructing gas flow. Do not use an oral airway for this.
• As the ET tube passes through the larynx, the patient will be unable to speak. Be sure to establish a communication system with the patient. Provide reassurance that a nurse will be nearby at all times. Make sure that a call bell or communication device is within reach.

During therapy

• If necessary, use soft restraints to prevent the patient from extubating himself.

• Make sure that the patient can reach his call bell.

• Monitor respiratory status every hour in an acutely ill patient and every 2 to 4 hours in a stable, chronically ill patient to detect the need for suctioning and evaluate response to treatment.

• If the patient is receiving high-pressure ventilation, assess for pneumothorax, signaled by absent, diminished, or distant breath sounds on the affected side; acute chest pain; and possible tracheal deviation or subcutaneous or mediastinal emphysema.

• If the patient is receiving a high oxygen concentration (more than 50%), watch for signs of toxicity: substernal chest pain, increased coughing, tachypnea, decreased lung compliance and vital capacity, and decreased partial pressure of oxygen in arterial blood without a corresponding change in oxygen concentration.

• If the patient is fighting the ventilator and ineffective ventilation results, administer a sedative and neuromuscular blocking agent, as ordered. Observe the patient closely.

• Auscultate the lungs to check for decreased breath sounds on the left side — an indication of tube slippage into the right mainstem bronchus.

• Monitor fluid and electrolyte status. Check weight daily in critically ill patients.

• Check ABG levels or pulse oximetry whenever a change is made on the ventilator setting, when the patient appears to be in respiratory distress, and routinely as ordered.

• Change the patient's position frequently, and perform chest physiotherapy as necessary.

• Suction the patient as indicated by breath sounds, noting the amount, color, consistency, and odor of secretions.

• Provide emotional support to reduce stress, and give antacids, histamine-2 (H_2) receptor blockers, and other medications, as ordered, to reduce gastric acid production and help prevent GI complications.

• Attempt to wean the patient, as ordered, based on his respiratory status.

• If the patient can't be weaned and requires long-term ventilatory support, begin to provide instructions on home care.

• Mechanical ventilation requires close monitoring to avoid potential complications. Perform the following steps every 1 to 2 hours:

—Check all connections between ventilator and patient.

—Make sure that critical alarms are turned on and set properly. This includes a low-pressure alarm that indicates a disconnection in the system and a high-pressure alarm (set at 20 cm H_2O greater than the patient's peak airway pressure) to prevent excessive airway pressures. Volume alarms, if available, should also be used.

—Verify that ventilator settings are correct and that the ventilator is operating on those settings by comparing the patient's respiratory rate with the setting of the volume-cycled machine; watch that the spirometer reaches the correct volume. For a pressure-cycled machine, use a respirometer (one that is part of the ventilator or a hand-held model) to check exhaled tidal volume and check the pressure manometer to ensure that the pressure is correct.

—Check the humidifier and refill it as necessary. Check the corrugated tubing for condensation; drain any condensed liquid into another container and discard. (Do not drain condensation into the humidifier because it may be contaminated with bacteria.) Also check the temperature of inspired air from heated humidifier.

• Use aseptic technique to change the humidifier, nebulizer, and ventilator tubing every 24 to 48 hours if the res-

Managing ventilator problems at home

A patient's home caregiver must know how to handle certain common ventilator problems and when to call for emergency help. Emphasize to the caregiver the importance of remaining calm when a ventilator problem develops. And teach management of the following common problems.

Obstructed tracheostomy tube
• Disconnect the patient from the ventilator.
• Provide oxygen, using a hand-held resuscitation bag.
• Suction the patient.
• Irrigate with 0.9% sodium chloride solution, if necessary.
• Reconnect the patient to the ventilator, and assess respiratory status.
• If respiratory distress persists, call for an ambulance.

Water in the tubing
• Disconnect the tubing from the ventilator.
• Empty the water from the tubing, and reconnect the tubing to the ventilator.

Incorrect cuff pressure
• Inflate or deflate the cuff to the correct pressure.

---

piratory therapist has not done so. Ventilate the patient manually during this time.
• Check the temperature gauges, which should be set between 89.6° F (32° C) and 98.6° F (37° C). Also check that the gas is being delivered at the correct temperature.
• Subsequently, check oxygen concentrations every 8 hours and overall ABG or pulse values whenever ventilator settings are changed.

Home care instructions

• If the patient will use a ventilator at home, teach him and a family member to check the device and its settings, the nebulizer, and the oxygen equipment at least once a day.
• Tell the patient to inform the fire department and electric and phone companies that he has a ventilator and oxygen in the home. (See *Managing ventilator problems at home*.)
• Arrange for a visiting nurse and respiratory therapist, at least for the initial discharge period.
• Instruct the patient to refill the humidifier as necessary.

• Advise the patient to call the doctor if he experiences chest pain, fever, dyspnea, or swollen extremities.
• Teach the patient how to count his pulse rate, and urge him to report any changes in rate or rhythm.
• If the patient is able to be weighed at home, instruct him to report a weight gain of 5 lb (2.3 kg) or more within a week.
• Explain the importance of daily tracheostomy care using the technique taught by the nurse or respiratory therapist. If the patient is using nondisposable items, tell him to keep them clean.
• Instruct the patient to try to bring his ventilator along if he needs hospital treatment for an acute problem. It may be possible to stabilize him without hospital admission.
• Provide the patient with emergency numbers, and tell him to call his doctor or respiratory therapist if he has any questions or problems.

MILIEU THERAPY

Milieu therapy refers to the use of the patient's environment as a tool for overcoming mental and emotional disorders. It can be used in the hospital or in a community setting. Specifically, the patient's surroundings become a therapeutic community, with the patient himself involved in goal setting, which includes planning, implementing, and evaluating his treatment, as well as in sharing with staff and other patients the responsibility for establishing group rules and policies. The patient may then progress to a transitional or halfway house. Then, if the patient continues to improve in this less structured environment, he may return to the outside community ready to apply the positive behaviors and skills he has learned. Or he may be discharged directly to his home with psychiatric aftercare plans.

The candidate for milieu therapy must be able to participate in group activities and must show a willingness to accept responsibility for daily activities.

In milieu therapy, the staff will usually wear street clothes instead of uniforms. They typically keep units unlocked and supervise activities in a community room that is the center for meetings, recreation, and meals. They also provide individual, group, art, music, recreation, psychodrama, and occupational therapy.

Nurses play a key role in milieu therapy. They work closely with psychiatrists and social workers, planning programs, assisting with therapy, and sharing observations and suggestions for modifying treatment plans to reach realistic, therapeutic goals.

Purpose
• To promote behavioral change and personal growth in a controlled therapeutic community.

Indications
Milieu therapy is indicated when a patient needs to learn or relearn how to function in a socially and emotionally appropriate way.

Procedure
The patient follows a schedule of therapeutic programming that includes individual and group therapy sessions as well as group meetings. The patient learns to interact appropriately with staff and other patients. He also participates in other forms of therapy such as art, music, and occupational therapy.

In many cases, milieu therapy allows exploration of the aspects of the patient's environment that seem to contribute to the patient's behavior either by their presence or absence. New strategies may help the patient develop healthy coping behaviors.

Complications
As the type of milieu or environment can vary, so can the complications. In a restricted environment, patients may lose some autonomy and decision-making abilities. If the inpatient therapy is prolonged, patients may become apathetic about discharge and become more dependent on the setting for their care.

Care considerations
Before therapy
• Explain the purpose of milieu therapy to the patient, stating what you expect of him and how he can participate in the therapeutic community.
• Orient him to the community's routines, such as the schedule for various activities.
• Introduce him to other patients and staff.
During therapy
• Regularly evaluate the patient's symptoms and therapeutic needs as he responds to treatment. Oversee activities.
• Encourage interaction with others to avoid withdrawal or isolation. Point out

the importance of respect for others and for his environment.
• Encourage and support healthy coping behaviors.

Home care instructions
• When the patient returns to the outside community, encourage him to keep follow-up appointments with his therapist.
• Help the patient to develop a strong support network, if possible.

MINERAL SUPPLEMENTS

Supplements correct mineral deficiency caused by inadequate dietary intake, increased metabolic demands, or disease.

Minerals help build bone and soft tissue and form hair, nails, and skin. They also serve other physiologic purposes. Iron and copper, for instance, promote synthesis of hemoglobin and red blood cells. Other minerals help regulate muscle contraction and relaxation, blood clotting, and acid-base balance.

Purpose
• To correct mineral deficiencies or to help meet increased metabolic demands
• To offset poor mineral absorption.

Indications
Mineral supplements are most commonly prescribed for children, pregnant patients, elderly patients, and patients with burns or other severe injuries. Mineral supplements are also given to patients receiving total parenteral nutrition.

Calcium should be given cautiously if the patient has a history of renal calculi because calcium can precipitate into the urine. Insufficient calcium or excessive phosphorus may cause tetany.

Administer sodium cautiously in patients with congestive heart failure, impaired renal function, or edema.

Potassium is contraindicated in patients with severe renal impairment or heart block, acute dehydration, excessive tissue damage (from surgery, for example), or in those receiving therapy with captopril or digitalis glycosides because hyperkalemia may occur. Also use potassium supplements cautiously with potassium-sparing diuretics, salt substitutes, low-salt milk, or other potassium-containing drugs. Use oral potassium supplements cautiously if the patient is taking atropine or related compounds because GI lesions can result.

Magnesium is contraindicated in patients with impaired renal function, myocardial damage, or heart block, and in those patients in active labor.

Oral and parenteral iron supplements are contraindicated in hemosiderosis, hemochromatosis, and all forms of anemia other than iron deficiency anemia. Oral iron should be used cautiously in patients with peptic ulcer, regional enteritis, and ulcerative colitis. Parenteral iron should be used with extreme caution in impaired hepatic function and rheumatoid arthritis.

Adverse reactions
Adverse reactions to calcium may include muscle spasms, oral and peripheral paresthesia, abdominal pain, hair loss, and arrhythmias. Potassium supplements may cause impaired kidney function and arrhythmias. Excessive amounts of phosphorus may cause fluid retention. Sodium administration can cause electrolyte imbalances. Reactions to oral iron supplements may include constipation, staining of teeth, and GI upset, and reactions to parenteral iron may range from pain, inflammation, and myalgia to hypotension, shock, and even death.

Care considerations

For calcium

• If the patient is taking a digitalis glycoside, monitor serum drug levels. Increased calcium levels can increase the risk of digitalis toxicity.

• To prevent impaired absorption, don't give with dairy products, bran cereal, spinach, rhubarb, or corticosteroids.

• Monitor serum and urine calcium levels, and report excessive increases, which could indicate hypercalcemia.

• When administering calcium, be alert for muscle spasms, paresthesia around the mouth and in the extremities, abdominal pain, hair loss, and arrhythmias.

For potassium

• Keep in mind that the parenteral form of potassium must be diluted in large amounts of fluid and given slowly. *Note:* Direct injection of undiluted potassium can cause death.

• Monitor intake and output to check kidney function. Check the patient's electrocardiogram for possible arrhythmias; report them to the doctor.

• Don't give potassium supplements postoperatively until urine flow is established.

For phosphorus

• Dilute phosphorus in a large amount of fluid, and infuse slowly to prevent vessel irritation.

For sodium

• Monitor sodium or potassium levels, depending on which salt is used. Report elevations.

• Monitor serum electrolyte levels frequently because imbalances can occur during sodium therapy.

• Check intake and output daily; excessive sodium levels can cause fluid retention. Weigh the patient daily.

For oral iron

• Iron supplements should be taken with food to prevent GI upset but not for at least 2 hours after eating dairy products, eggs, coffee, tea, or whole grain bread or cereals because these foods interfere with absorption. Liquid iron preparations may be diluted with orange juice or water but not with antacids.

• During oral iron supplement administration, check for constipation and record the color and amount of stools.

• To avoid staining the teeth, administer iron elixir through a glass straw.

• Monitor hemoglobin and reticulocyte counts during iron supplement therapy.

For parenteral iron

• Check hospital policy before giving I.V. iron dextran.

• Give iron injections deeply, using the Z-track method, into the upper outer quadrant of buttock – never into an arm or other exposed area.

• Monitor the patient's vital signs during I.V. administration.

• Monitor hemoglobin and hematocrit levels and reticulocyte count.

For magnesium

• Use parenteral administration with extreme caution in patients receiving digitalis glycosides. Treating magnesium toxicity with calcium in such patients could cause serious alterations in cardiac conduction and lead to heart block.

• An I.V. bolus dose must be injected slowly to avoid respiratory or cardiac arrest.

• If available, use an infusion pump for I.V. administration. The maximum flow rate is 150 ml/minute. A rapid drip rate causes a feeling of heat.

• Monitor vital signs every 15 minutes when giving I.V. for severe hypomagnesemia. Watch for respiratory depression and signs of heart block. The respiratory rate should exceed 16 breaths/minute before the dose is given because magnesium can cause respiratory depression.

• Monitor intake and output. Output should be 100 ml or more during the 4-hour period before dose.

• Test patellar reflexes before each additional dose. If absent, give no more magnesium until reflexes return.

• Keep I.V. calcium available to reverse magnesium intoxication.

For copper and zinc
• Monitor serum levels during therapy.

Home care instructions

• Inform the patient that many mineral supplements are sold in combination with vitamin preparations.
• Teach dietary measures for preventing constipation to the patient receiving iron supplements.
• Inform the patient receiving iron that stools may turn black because of unabsorbed iron. Reassure him that this effect is harmless.
• To prevent iron toxicity, tell the patient who misses a dose to continue the regular dosage schedule and never to double-dose.
• Tell the patient to take potassium supplements immediately after meals to help prevent GI upset.
• Warn the patient that oral iron is toxic and that such symptoms as vomiting, upper abdominal pain, pallor, cyanosis, diarrhea, and drowsiness indicate toxicity. Provide the phone number of the local poison control center, and suggest keeping ipecac syrup available.
• Tell the patient to take zinc with meals but not with dairy products, which can decrease absorption.
• Remind the patient that many drugs can interact with oral mineral supplements. For example, advise him not to take tetracyclines or quinolones at the same time he is taking oral calcium, magnesium, or iron supplements. Tell the patient to check with the doctor or pharmacist if he is taking other drugs with mineral supplements.

MIOTICS

Miotics include cholinergics, which directly stimulate parasympathetic cells, and cholinesterase inhibitors, which inhibit cholinesterase. Cholinergics, which include *acetylcholine, carbachol,* and *pilocarpine,* cause the sphincter muscle of the iris to contract, resulting in miosis. Cholinesterase inhibitors, which include *demecarium, echothiophate, isoflurophate,* and *physostigmine,* inhibit the enzymatic destruction of acetylcholine by inactivating cholinesterase. This leaves acetylcholine free to act on the iridic sphincter, thereby causing pupillary constriction.

Purpose

• To reduce intraocular pressure.

Indications

Miotics (especially pilocarpine) are used in the treatment of acute angle-closure glaucoma, but they have been largely replaced by beta-adrenergic blockers in the initial treatment of chronic open-angle glaucoma. Miotics are also therapeutic in iridectomy, anterior segment surgery, and other eye surgeries. When used with mydriatics, they prevent adhesions after ocular surgery.

Because miotics worsen inflammation, they're contraindicated in iritis and corneal abrasions. They should be used cautiously in acute heart failure, bronchial asthma, peptic ulcer, hyperthyroidism, and Parkinson's disease.

Adverse reactions

The most common reactions to miotics are painful ciliary spasm, blurred vision, and poor vision in low light. Other adverse ocular reactions may include burning, lacrimation, pain, headache, photophobia, twitching of the eyelids, conjunctival congestion, and lacrimal passage stenosis. Miotics can also cause iris cysts, anterior chamber hyperemia, and activation of iritis or uveitis, but these reactions are more common with long-acting cholinesterase inhibitors.

Systemic effects of miotics may follow frequent or prolonged topical use, especially with long-acting miotics. Such effects may include nausea, vomiting, diarrhea and cramps, frequent urination, excessive salivation, sweating, pallor, cyanosis, and bronchoconstriction. Systemically absorbed miotics have precipitated asthmatic attacks and cardiac arrest after vagal stimulation during surgery. Severe miotic toxicity may cause tremor, muscle weakness, cardiac arrhythmias, hypotension, central nervous system excitation and depression, confusion, ataxia, seizures, and coma.

Care considerations

• Before giving miotics, check the patient's drug history for possible interactions. Concurrent use of anticholinergics may have additive effects.
• After administration, observe for signs of local allergy, such as redness or itching. Don't use echothiophate or isoflurophate in patients who are exposed to organophosphate insecticides.
• Watch for retinal detachment, which can occur from 1 hour to several weeks after therapy begins. Also pay special attention to any complaints of acute, severe eye pain; headache; and visual problems.
• Evaluate the patient's vision in dim light. If his night vision is poor, make sure he can ambulate safely.
• Monitor the patient taking cholinesterase inhibitors for signs of an overdose: weakness, hypersalivation, sweating, nausea, vomiting, abdominal pain, urine incontinence, diarrhea, bradycardia, severe hypotension, and bronchospasm. If any of these signs occur, discontinue the drug and notify the doctor.
• Observe for signs of systemic reactions. Miotics should be discontinued, at least temporarily, if they cause systemic reactions.

Home care instructions

• Teach the patient how to instill the eyedrops. Warn him not to touch the tip of the dropper to the eye or surrounding tissue. Instruct him to apply light finger pressure to the lacrimal sac for 1 minute after instillation to reduce systemic absorption.
• Instruct the patient to stop the drug immediately and contact the doctor if he develops excessive salivation, diarrhea, weakness, or other signs of toxicity.
• Reassure the patient that the blurred vision caused by these drugs usually diminishes with continued use. However, if these drugs cause poor night vision, caution him against driving or operating machinery after dark.
• Explain that close medical supervision is vital during miotic therapy to monitor intraocular pressure.

MONOAMINE OXIDASE INHIBITORS

Three monoamine oxidase (MAO) inhibitors—*isocarboxazid, phenelzine,* and *tranylcypromine*—are used to treat depression. Although some clinicians only prescribe them when tricyclic antidepressants and electroconvulsive therapy are ineffective or contraindicated, others may use them as first-line agents.

Both isocarboxazid and phenelzine produce a delayed therapeutic effect; overt improvement begins roughly 4 weeks after the start of therapy. Tranylcypromine usually produces therapeutic effects within a few days but is associated with a higher incidence of central nervous system (CNS) stimulation than other MAO inhibitors.

The key responsibility during care of the patient receiving an MAO inhibitor is the prevention or monitoring of adverse reactions.

Purpose

• To relieve depression by increasing CNS levels of catecholamines (dopamine, norepinephrine, and epinephrine).

Indications

Isocarboxazid, phenelzine, and tranyl-cypromine are used to treat depression in adults. Their use is contraindicated in children because of potential growth retardation and in elderly patients because of the increased risk of cerebrovascular accident. They're also contraindicated in patients with cardiovascular disease or impaired renal or hepatic function.

MAO inhibitors are contraindicated for combined use with agents such as analgesics, anesthetics, anticoagulants, anticonvulsants, tricyclic antidepressants, antihistamines, antiparkinsonian drugs, antihypertensives with CNS depressant effects, anxiolytics, caffeine-containing preparations, diuretics, other MAO inhibitors, and tyramine-containing foods and beverages.

Adverse reactions

The most serious adverse reaction to MAO inhibitors is hypertensive crisis, characterized by increased blood pressure, severe headache, palpitations, nausea, vomiting, neck stiffness or soreness, fever, clammy skin, and mydriasis, photosensitivity, or other visual disturbances. In extreme cases, intracranial hemorrhage may occur. The most common reactions to MAO inhibitors include restlessness, drowsiness, dizziness, headache, insomnia, constipation, nausea, vomiting, anorexia, weakness, arthralgia, dry mouth, blurred vision, peripheral edema, urine retention, transient impotence, rash, and purpura. MAO inhibitors may also cause hypotension, hypertension, and hepatitis.

Care considerations

• Ensure that the patient's diet doesn't include caffeine- or tyramine-containing foods and that the drug regimen doesn't include drugs that interact with MAO inhibitors.
• Warn visitors not to give the patient coffee, chocolate, cheese, alcohol, or any over-the-counter drugs. Ingestion of any of these can cause hypertensive crisis. If hypertensive crisis occurs, discontinue the MAO inhibitor immediately and slowly give 5 mg of phentolamine I.V., as ordered. Reduce fever by external cooling.
• Regularly monitor the patient's blood pressure and liver function tests because long-term use of MAO inhibitors can cause hypotension, and hepatitis.
• Observe for unusual sweating; fever; cold, clammy skin; enlarged pupils; increased sensitivity to light; and an unusually rapid or slow heart rate. Tell the patient to report severe dizziness or chest pain, nausea, vomiting, a stiff or sore neck, persistent constipation, urine retention, or light-headedness, drowsiness, or dry mouth.
• If the patient becomes constipated, increase his fluid intake and provide a stool softener, as ordered. Give throat lozenges to help relieve dry mouth. To prevent dizziness resulting from orthostatic hypotension, instruct the patient to rise slowly and sit on the bed or in a chair before standing.

Home care instructions

• Instruct the patient not to change the dosage or discontinue taking the drug. Remind him that therapeutic effects may take several weeks to develop.
• Tell him to take a missed dose if he remembers it within 2 hours of the scheduled administration time; otherwise, he should skip the missed dose. Recommend not taking the drug close to bedtime because it may cause insomnia.
• Teach the patient and his family what foods to avoid, even when dining out. Emphasize that the restricted diet must be maintained for at least 2 weeks after MAO drug therapy ends to allow for regeneration of monoamine oxidase. Describe the signs of hypertensive crisis, and tell the patient to go to a hospital emergency department immediately if such signs occur.

• Emphasize the need to avoid non-prescription drugs to prevent a possible dangerous drug interaction.
• Warn the patient not to get up suddenly from a kneeling, sitting, or lying position.
• Advise the patient to delay elective surgery or dental work until 2 weeks after discontinuing the drug. Suggest that he carry a medical identification card in case of an emergency.
• Refer the patient to an outpatient treatment center for continued support.

MYDRIATICS

Topical mydriatics include a group of anticholinergic drugs: *atropine, cyclopentolate, homatropine, scopolamine,* and *tropicamide.* They also include a group of adrenergic drugs: *epinephrine, dipivefrin, apraclonidine,* and *phenylephrine.*

Purpose
• To dilate the pupil and paralyze accommodation by blocking the action of acetylcholine
• To constrict the dilator muscle of the pupil.

Indications
Atropine, homatropine, and scopolamine help relieve acute inflammation of the iris (iritis), ciliary body, or choroid (uveitis). Cyclopentolate, phenylephrine, and tropicamide are used in diagnostic procedures; the adrenergic drugs help treat chronic open-angle glaucoma.

Because mydriatics increase intraocular pressure, they're contraindicated in acute angle-closure glaucoma.

Adverse reactions
Mydriatics may cause blurred vision, eye dryness, photophobia, contact dermatitis, and ocular congestion. Systemic reactions may include flushing, tachycardia, fever, ataxia, irritability, confusion, somnolence, hallucinations, seizures, and behavorial changes in children. Epinephrine preparations frequently cause local reactions: burning, stinging, lacrimation, pain, and rebound conjunctival hyperemia. Systemic reactions to epinephrine may include palpitations, tachycardia, cardiac arrhythmias, hypertension, headache, trembling, pallor, and faintness. Phenylephrine also causes frequent ocular reactions, such as burning, stinging, blurred vision, reactive hyperemia, dermatitis, brow pain, and iris floaters. Systemic reactions to phenylephrine include tachycardia, cardiac arrhythmias, hypertension, pallor, sweating, and trembling.

Care considerations
• In a patient with anatomically narrow ocular angles, be alert for symptoms of acute angle-closure glaucoma: pain, blurred vision, and headache when the drug dilates the pupil.
• In children and especially in elderly patients, check for systemic effects, including tachycardia, flushing, and dry skin. Also ask about photophobia and blurred vision.
• If the patient is taking an adrenergic mydriatic, tell him to report brow pain, headache, blurred vision, or tearing. Also observe for pigment granules (aqueous floaters) in the anterior chamber. These should disappear 12 to 24 hours after instillation of the drug.

Home care instructions
• Teach the patient the correct way to instill the drug. Warn him not to touch the tip of the dropper or tube to the eye or the surrounding tissue.
• Show the patient how to reduce systemic effects by applying light finger pressure on the lacrimal sac for 1 minute after instillation.
• Stress the importance of immediately reporting signs of increasing intraocu-

lar pressure, such as pain and persistent blurred vision.

• Because mydriatics will temporarily blur vision, warn the patient to avoid driving or operating machinery until his vision clears.

• If photophobia occurs, suggest that the patient wear dark glasses when outdoors in the daytime.

• Instruct the patient to keep the medication container tightly sealed and to store it away from heat and light. Tell the patient not to use the mydriatic if it becomes discolored or cloudy.

MYELOMENINGOCELE REPAIR

Myelomeningocele (meningomylocele) is a congenital spinal defect resulting from defective neural tube closure during the first trimester of pregnancy. This defect consists of a fragile saclike structure that protrudes over the spinal column and contains meninges, cerebrospinal fluid (CSF), and a portion of the spinal cord. CSF leakage from this sac can cause infection and can leave the infant with permanent neurologic deficits below the level of the lesion. For these reasons, most surgeons recommend prompt repair of this defect.

Repair is ideally performed within the first 24 to 48 hours after birth. The advantage of early surgical intervention is the prevention of infection and injury to the sac and further deterioration of neural tissue due to enlargement of the sac. Some surgeons delay closure to evaluate the infant's neurologic function. However, surgery is usually delayed only when the infant is seriously debilitated or has associated defects that could complicate surgery.

Unfortunately, surgery can't reverse any existing neurologic deficits. It may, however, preserve existing function in the infant and prevent further deterioration.

Purpose

• To repair the congenital defect and prevent further neurologic compromise of the legs, bowel, and bladder.

Indications

Myelomeningocele repair is the treatment of choice for this defect.

Procedure

With the infant in a prone position and under general anesthesia, the surgeon isolates the neural tissue from the rest of the sac. After establishing this tissue's point of continuity with the spinal cord and nerve roots, he fashions a flap from the tissue. This flap protects the nerve junctions and eventually will become contiguous with the dura surrounding the spinal cord. He then sutures the skin closed over the defect and covers the wound with a sterile gauze dressing and then a waterproof covering to protect the dressing from contamination by feces or urine. Because the defect is usually relatively small, he rarely orders skin grafts for cosmetic repair.

Complications

Complications associated with myelomeningocele repair include infection (meningitis or ventriculitis), hydrocephalus, delayed wound healing, and increased intracranial pressure (ICP).

Care considerations

Before surgery

• Protect the fragile defect from infection and damage while the infant awaits surgery. Keep the site covered with sterile dressings moistened with 0.9% sodium chloride solution; clean it gently with sterile 0.9% sodium chloride solution or a bactericidal solution, as ordered; and inspect it for signs of infection.

• To prevent irritation of the sac, don't dress the infant in clothing or a diaper; instead, keep him warm in an incubator.

• Position the infant on his side or abdomen, never on his back, to protect the fragile sac from rupture and to minimize the risk of contamination from urine or feces. Put a diaper under him and change it often, and keep the anal and genital areas clean. Protect against skin breakdown by placing him on a sheepskin or foam pad and applying lotion to his knees, elbows, chin, and other pressure points.

• Encourage the parents to hold their infant as often as possible to promote bonding. Teach them to place the infant, lying on his abdomen, across the lap.

• Measure the child's head circumference, and perform a baseline assessment of the neuromuscular and sensory function below the defect.

• Explain the surgical procedure to the parents and answer any questions. Prepare them for the possibility of some permanent physical and mental impairment. Make sure they understand that surgery cannot reverse existing neurologic damage.

After surgery

• After surgery, carefully monitor the infant's vital signs and observe for signs of hydrocephalus and meningitis, which commonly follow such surgery.

• Measure head circumference regularly, and notify the doctor of any increase.

• Look for signs of ICP, especially bulging fontanels and projectile vomiting. (Remember that excessive vomiting can lead to dehydration, which can prevent bulging fontanels and thus mask this classic sign of increased ICP.)

• Also watch for fever, nuchal rigidity, opisthotonos, and more subtle signs of infection, such as irritability and refusal to eat.

• Change the surgical dressing regularly, and check for drainage and wound infection.

• As before surgery, keep the infant positioned on his abdomen and protect his skin from breakdown. Place his hips in abduction and his feet in a neutral position. Reposition his arms, legs, and head frequently.

• If ordered, provide passive range-of-motion exercises, handling the infant very gently.

• Monitor intake and output, and watch for decreased skin turgor, skin dryness, and other signs of dehydration.

• Check for urine retention and constipation resulting from decreased nerve function. If necessary, express urine manually to prevent urinary tract infection. Intermittent catheterization may be necessary.

• Administer a mild laxative, as ordered, to prevent constipation.

• As the infant recovers from surgery, periodically assess neurologic function. Compare the findings to your preoperative baseline assessment.

• Before discharge, prepare the infant's parents for their child's continuing care needs. Develop a patient-teaching plan for the parents; if possible, coordinate this plan with the home health care nurse who will be providing care after discharge. Begin parent teaching early to give them time to gain confidence in their ability to cope with their child's problems and meet long-range treatment goals. Throughout teaching, provide support and encourage a positive attitude.

Home care instructions

• Teach the parents proper wound care techniques. Make sure they know how to recognize early signs of infection, such as redness or swelling. Tell them to keep the incision clean and dry and to provide frequent diaper changes and cleanings. Explain that the doctor will probably remove the sutures on the 10th day after surgery.

• Explain skin care measures to prevent breakdown, such as frequent repositioning, massage, and application of lotion to pressure areas.

• If necessary, teach the parents how to express urine manually from the child's

bladder; instruct them to do this regularly. Encourage them to begin bladder training when their child reaches age 3.
• If the doctor has prescribed an antibiotic, teach the parents how to administer the drug and explain the need to follow the dosing schedule.
• Discuss the possibility of arranging for a visiting nurse to provide periodic in-home care.
• Emphasize the importance of regular neurologic assessments and physical examinations to evaluate development.
• If appropriate, refer the parents to genetic counseling and a local support group.

MYRINGOTOMY

Myringotomy is a surgical incision in the tympanic membrane performed to relieve pain and prevent membrane rupture by allowing drainage of pus or fluid from the middle ear. It's most commonly performed on children with acute otitis media.

Myringotomy may be performed on one or both ears. After myringotomy, a pressure-equalizing tube may be inserted through the incision to allow fluid drainage. Myringotomy usually provides almost instant symptomatic relief, and the incision typically heals in 2 to 3 weeks. (If tubes have been inserted, they remain in place for about 6 months or until they spontaneously fall out.)

Purpose
• To relieve pain and drain fluid from the middle ear
• To aerate the middle ear when eustachian tube dysfunction prevents it
• To obtain material for culture and sensitivity tests.

Indications
Myringotomy is typically performed to treat otitis media when antibiotics and decongestants or antihistamines fail to correct the causative infection or when the infection damages the middle ear mucosa or causes such severe pressure that the tympanic membrane may rupture. If the tympanic membrane does rupture and does not heal spontaneously, the surgeon may perform a myringoplasty to close the perforation.

Procedure
First, a local anesthetic is administered to an adult or older child. However, if the patient is a young child, is uncooperative, or has severe otitis media, he may receive a light general anesthetic. (An infant may receive no anesthetic.)

After the anesthetic takes effect, the doctor visualizes the tympanic membrane and makes a radial or circumferential incision. A radial incision, used when serous fluid is present, involves a small slit in the membrane. Afterward, the doctor may insert a tube (pressure-equilizer tubes, ventilation tubes, or Teflon grommets) to facilitate continuous drainage, equalize pressure within the middle ear, and allow the eustachian tube to recover.

A larger U-shaped incision, used when pus or thick drainage is present, permits more drainage. The surgeon may then irrigate the middle ear or apply gentle suction to remove tenacious drainage. If drainage is copious, the doctor may apply a small piece of sterile cotton loosely in the external ear canal. If the patient requires a bilateral myringotomy, the procedure is repeated on the other ear.

Complications
Myringotomy can cause minor complications, such as bleeding during tube insertion if the ear canal is inadvertently scratched, and scars or sclerotic patches on the tympanic membrane. When tubes are inserted, ear discharge can become chronic. The tubes may become occluded and need to be reinserted. Another complication associ-

ated with tube insertion is contamination by entrance of water into the middle ear under pressure.

Care considerations

Before surgery

• Explain to the patient or parents that myringotomy removes fluid or pus from the middle ear and relieves ear pain.

• Inform the patient or parents whether the surgery will be performed on one or both ears and whether a local or general anesthetic will be used.

• Mention that the surgeon may insert a tube through the incision to allow drainage until the inflammation subsides. Then the surgeon may either remove the tube or leave it in place to drop out naturally.

• Before the procedure, make sure the patient or a responsible family member has signed a consent form.

After surgery

• Assess the condition of the patient's ear. Note if there is drainage and, if so, the amount, type, color, and odor. If bright red blood is present, notify the doctor immediately; this may indicate injury to the ear canal.

• Notify the doctor if the patient continues to complain of ear pain, if pain reoccurs, if he develops a headache or becomes disoriented, or if his temperature is elevated.

• If necessary, insert a cotton ball gently into the ear's orifice to absorb drainage. Apply petroleum jelly or zinc oxide to the external ear to protect it from excoriation by drainage, and change the cotton as needed. If exudate cakes on the outer ear, remove it by gently swabbing with a cotton-tipped applicator dipped in hydrogen peroxide. Don't attempt to clean the ear canal or allow peroxide to run into the ear.

• If the doctor has placed sterile cotton in the external ear canal, this should be changed when it becomes moist to prevent a secondary infection. The ear may drain for 2 to 3 days after the procedure.

Home care instructions

• If the patient has a cotton ball in place to absorb ear drainage, tell him or his parents to wash their hands before and after changing it and to dispose of old cotton by placing it in a small paper or plastic bag before throwing it in the trash. Emphasize the need to notify the doctor if drainage lasts more than 1 week or changes color or character (for example, from serous to purulent). Advise them to report any ear pain or fever, which may signal blocked tubing or reinfection.

• Emphasize the importance of keeping water out of the ear canal until the tympanic membrane is intact. Show the patient or his parents how to roll absorbent cotton in petroleum jelly to form a plug and then how to insert the plug in the outer part of the ear before showering or washing hair. If the doctor permits swimming, advise the patient to insert ear plugs first and to avoid immersing his head. Diving is prohibited. Advise the patient that getting small amounts of clean water into the ear is usually not a problem. Custom-made earplugs are available but are very expensive.

• Tell the patient or parents to expect considerable drainage through the tubes.

• Tell the parents what to look for if the child's tubes fall out. Tell them that the tubes are small, white, spool-shaped, and plastic.

• Emphasize the need to return for follow-up examinations and to notify the doctor if the tubes fall out prematurely.

• If the doctor has ordered antibiotic eardrops, the patient or parents should instill the drops as prescribed and continue them for several days after the drainage stops.

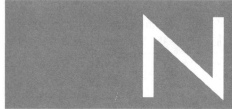

NASAL IRRIGATION

Nasal irrigation is the instillation of water or 0.9% sodium chloride solution into the nasal cavity to facilitate the drainage of mucus or debris.

A layer of mucus is formed by the mucous membrane that lines the nasal cavity and acts as a filter to remove bacteria, viruses, and particles from the air when it enters the nose. Cilia (hairlike projections) continually vibrate and assist with filtering by direct contact with the mucous layer. Continuous ciliary propulsion pushes the mucus toward the sinus opening and down into the posterior pharyngeal area. When normal ciliary function fails, nasal deposits may impede sinus drainage and air flow and cause headaches, infections, and unpleasant odors.

Nasal irrigations may be performed manually with a bulb syringe or oral irrigating device. Irrigating solutions should always be tepid; solutions that are too hot or cold may irritate the nasal mucosa.

Purpose
• To facilitate the cleaning of the mucous membranes of the nasal cavity and paranasal sinuses
• To soothe irritated mucous membranes
• To aid breathing.

Indications
Nasal irrigation is indicated when a patient's ciliary function is inadequate. Factors that interfere with natural cil-iary flow are nasal polyps, nasal septal deviation, cystic fibrosis, allergic rhinitis, nasal trauma, chronic sinusitis, mucosal edema, and granulomatous diseases. Patients who have been long-term users of inhalants (such as cocaine or nose drops containing phenylephrine chloride) and those who regularly inhale occupational toxins or allergens (paint fumes, sawdust, pesticides, or coal dust) may also benefit from this procedure.

Nasal irrigation should not be performed on patients with an absent gag reflex because aspiration can occur. Nasal irrigation may be contraindicated in patients who have had recent sinus surgery, severe destruction of the sinuses, or a history of frequent epistaxis.

Procedure
This procedure may be performed by the nurse or the patient. The patient sits upright with his head bent forward over a basin or sink and well flexed on his chest. A warmed solution is introduced into the nostril by either a bulb syringe or an oral irrigating device (such as the Water-Pik). Both types of devices facilitate the drainage of mucoid debris and loosen nasal crusting. Each nostril is irrigated alternately until the return irrigant runs clear. Nasal irrigation can safely be performed twice daily unless it causes excessive irritation; if so, one irrigation daily is adequate. (See *Nasal irrigation: Guide to self-care.*)

Nasal irrigation is usually performed with 0.9% sodium chloride solution, which mimics the body's own fluid. The patient may use a commer-

Nasal irrigation: Guide to self-care

Thorough teaching will help the patient perform nasal irrigation at home.

Equipment

The patient needs a bulb syringe or an oral irrigating device (such as the Water-Pik), rigid or flexible disposable irrigation tips, 0.9% sodium chloride solution, plastic sheet, apron or towels, facial tissues, bath basin, and gloves. She should warm the solution to about 105° F (40.5° C) and then warm the bulb by drawing up and expelling some irrigating solution. If she's using an oral irrigating device, she plugs it into an electrical outlet and runs 8 oz (240 ml) of solution through the tubing to clear previous solutions and warm the tubing. Then, she fills the reservoir of the device with warm 0.9% sodium chloride solution.

Procedure

The patient begins by assuming a comfortable upright position with head bent over the basin and well flexed on the chest.

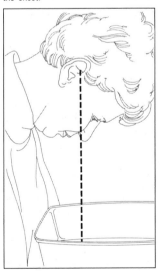

The nose and ear should be on the same vertical plane. The patient is less likely to breathe in the irrigating solution when holding the head in this position. Moreover, this position should keep the irrigant from entering the eustachian tubes. The patient should also keep the mouth open and breathe rhythmically during the irrigation.

To use a *bulb syringe*, the patient fills the bulb syringe with irrigating solution, inserts the tip about ½" (1.3 cm) into the nostril, and then squeezes the bulb until a gentle stream of warm irrigant washes through the nose. Forceful squeezing should be avoided to prevent driving debris from the nasal passages into the sinuses or eustachian tubes.

To use an *oral irrigating device*, the patient inserts the catheter tip into the nostril about ½" to 1" (1.3 to 2.5 cm) and then turns on the irrigating device. The patient should start with a low-pressure setting and then increase the pressure as needed to obtain a gentle stream of irrigating solution.

Care considerations

With either type of irrigating device, both nostrils should be irrigated and the returning irrigant should be inspected.

Changes in color, viscosity, or volume or the presence of blood or necrotic tissue should be reported to the doctor.

The patient should wait for a few minutes after the irrigation and then blow excess fluid from both nostrils at once. The device is then cleaned with disinfectant.

cially prepared isotonic solution (such as Ocean, Ayr, or NaSal) or may prepare his own solution by adding ½ tsp of salt for every 8 oz (240 ml) of warm water. The amount of solution used for irrigation varies depending on the amount of crusted mucus. A typical irrigation requires 17 to 34 oz (500 to 1,000 ml).

Complications

Complications associated with nasal irrigation include irritation of the nasal mucosa resulting from too-frequent irrigation or extreme temperatures of the solution. Aspiration is rare but can occur in patients with an absent gag reflex.

Care considerations

Before the procedure

• Thoroughly explain the procedure to the patient.
• Remind the patient to keep his mouth open and not to speak or swallow during the irrigation to avoid forcing infectious material into the sinuses or eustachian tubes.

During the procedure

• Be sure to insert the irrigating tip far enough to ensure that the irrigant cleans the nasal membranes before draining out.
• Avoid forceful squeezing of the bulb syringe, which may drive debris from the nasal passages into the sinuses or the eustachian tubes.
• When using an oral irrigating device, be sure to run a small amount of solution through the tubing before inserting it into the nose to clear any debris and to warm the tubing. Turn the device off until the irrigating tip is inside the nose; then begin irrigating with a low-pressure setting (adjusting it higher, as needed). If using a bulb syringe, first draw some irrigant into the bulb and expel it to clear the bulb of any debris.
• Inspect the returning irrigant. Watch for an increased amount of or change in

consistency or color of irrigant. Yellow or green mucus may signal an infection and should be reported to the doctor. Also report the presence of blood or necrotic tissue.

After the procedure

• Expect fluid to flow from the patient's nose for a brief time after the irrigation and before he blows his nose.
• Have the patient wait a few minutes and then clear excess fluid from both nostrils at once. This will help prevent fluid or pressure from building up in the sinuses and also help loosen and expel crusted secretions and mucus.
• To clean the electronic device, run about 8 oz (240 ml) of 0.25% acetic acid solution through the irrigating tip and tubing. Shake the excess moisture from the parts and allow them to dry thoroughly. If using a bulb syringe, draw the acetic acid solution into the bulb and swirl and expel the solution. Repeat two or three times.

Home care instructions

• Teach the patient to prepare a 0.9% sodium chloride solution and 0.25% acetic acid solution using the following methods:
– For a 0.9% sodium chloride solution, tell the patient to fill a clean 1-liter plastic bottle with 1,000 ml (34 oz) tap water or distilled water, add 1½ tsp of table salt, and then shake the solution until the salt dissolves.
– For a 0.25% acetic acid solution, tell the patient to add 50 ml (1¾ oz) of plain white vinegar to a clean 1-liter plastic bottle with a tight-fitting cap, fill it with tap water to the 1,000-ml level, and shake well to mix the solution.
• Teach the patient how to clean the irrigating devices.
• Instruct the patient to notify his doctor of any changes in the color, amount, or consistency of the mucus or of any blood or necrotic tissue in the return irrigation.

NASAL PACKING

Nasal packing, which consists of gauze or other material, is inserted into the nasal cavity to control severe epistaxis.

Depending on the bleeding site, nasal packing can be either anterior or posterior. An anterior pack may be an absorbable gauzelike material that can remain in place for 3 to 5 days. If this type of anterior packing fails to control the bleeding, the doctor may use antibiotic-impregnated petroleum gauze strips that are layered in tiers in the nasal cavity. This type of packing is typically removed after 48 hours.

Posterior packing is commonly inserted when anterior packing does not stop the bleeding or when the doctor can't identify the bleeding vessel in the posterior portion of the nasal passage. Many times, posterior bleeding can't be seen due to the location, especially if the nasal septum is deviated. Posterior packing typically remains in place for 4 days.

The doctor will first try to control the bleeding by cautery with silver nitrate pledgets, by using electrocautery, or by applying an anesthetic that acts as a temporary vasoconstrictor. If these methods fail to control the bleeding, nasal packing is used.

An alternative to nasal packing is the use of a nasal balloon catheter. Once inflated, the balloon exerts pressure on the posterior bleeding site. Single-balloon or double-balloon catheters may be used.

Purpose

• To control severe epistaxis that's uncontrollable by other treatments.

Indications

Nasal packing is indicated for severe epistaxis that cannot be controlled by other methods. Severe epistaxis may result from nasal or facial fractures; septal deviation or perforation; cancer of the sinuses; or more obscure causes, such as hypertension, leukemia, purpura, acute rheumatic fever, and anticoagulant therapy.

Procedure

To insert anterior nasal packing, a doctor may place an absorbable packing moistened with a vasoconstrictor into the nasal cavity. If this does not control the bleeding, he then places antibiotic-impregnated petroleum gauze strips horizontally in the anterior nostrils, typically near the turbinates, until the nasal passage is completely packed.

To insert posterior nasal packing, a doctor first anesthetizes the nose. He then passes a small catheter through the nose into the nasopharynx, where it is grasped by forceps and pulled out through the mouth. The pack is usually a roll of gauze or a tampon that has three black silk sutures tied around it, each about 15″ to 18″ (37.5 to 45 cm) long. One string is tied to the catheter tip that is coming out of the mouth; then the catheter and string are pulled out through one side of the nose. This is repeated through the other side of the nose. When the pack is in position, the two strings coming out of the anterior nose are tied around a roll of gauze placed at the anterior nares; the third string, which is left hanging from the mouth, is taped to the cheek.

Alternative methods to control posterior epistaxis include insertion of an indwelling urinary catheter or a nasal balloon catheter. (See *Understanding nasal balloon catheters,* page 460.)

Complications

Possible complications of nasal packing include hypoxia and shock from blood loss and respiratory compromise. In the patient who is sedated for posterior packing, aspiration and airway obstruction may also occur. Less frequent complications include sinusitis, otitis media, and pressure necrosis. Nasal balloon

Understanding nasal balloon catheters

To control posterior epistaxis, the doctor may insert a nasal balloon catheter instead of posterior nasal packing. These catheters are self-retaining and disposable and include either a single balloon or double balloon. These balloons are inflated with 0.9% sodium chloride solution, not air, because air will leak slowly.

Single-balloon catheter

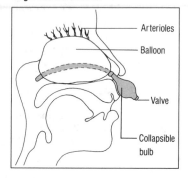

The single-balloon catheter includes a balloon that, when inflated, compresses the blood vessels and a soft, collapsible outside bulb that prevents the catheter from slipping out of place posteriorly.

Double-balloon catheter

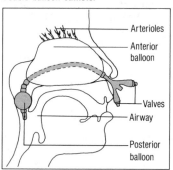

The double-balloon catheter includes a posterior balloon that, when inflated, secures the catheter in the nasopharynx; an anterior balloon that, when inflated, compresses the blood vessels; and a central airway that helps the patient breathe more comfortably. Each balloon is inflated independently.

To use either type of balloon catheter, the doctor lubricates the catheter with an antibiotic ointment and then inserts it through the patient's nostril. He then inflates the balloon by instilling 0.9% sodium chloride solution into the appropriate valve. (If a double-balloon catheter is used, the doctor will inflate the posterior balloon first.) He may secure the catheter by taping its anterior tip to the outside of the patient's nose.

catheters have similar complications. In addition, balloon deflation may dislodge clots and nasal debris into the oropharynx, which could prompt coughing, gagging, or vomiting.

Care considerations
Before the procedure
• Explain the procedure to the patient, and inform him that the pack will be in place for several days. Before posterior nasal packing is done, explain that he'll

have to cooperate with the doctor to ease the passage of the catheter.

• Also explain to the patient that he'll have to breathe through his mouth, which will make it dry, but that mouthwash may relieve this. Mention that pain medication will be available to relieve the headache that often accompanies nasal packing.

• If the patient will be sedated, explain the routine preoperative and postoperative procedures.

• Administer the prescribed sedative or tranquilizer.

During the procedure

• Have the patient lean forward to prevent blood from draining into his throat.

• Monitor the patient's vital signs, and watch for impending hypovolemic shock from blood loss.

• Offer support and reassurance during the procedure to ease fears and anxiety.

After the procedure

• After nasal packing, watch for signs and symptoms of hypoxia, such as tachycardia, confusion, and restlessness. Check arterial blood gases, as ordered, and monitor the patient's pulse and blood pressure.

• Keep emergency equipment (flashlight, scissors, and hemostat) at the patient's bedside, and place a call bell within his reach.

• If the patient has posterior nasal packing, check it frequently and remove it immediately if it's visible at the back of his throat and he appears to be choking. Avoid any tension on the sutures taped in place because this may dislodge posterior packing.

• Monitor blood loss to help detect impending hypovolemia. Note the amount of bleeding on the dental rolls, and have the patient report any fresh blood in the back of his throat or blood he expectorates.

• Also monitor fluid status. Note the patient's intake and output, and maintain the I.V. line if one is in place. Check the oral mucosa and skin turgor for signs of dehydration, and instruct the patient to report any nausea and vomiting.

• Offer mouthwashes or ice chips to moisten the patient's mouth, and provide sedation and analgesics, as ordered. Also monitor temperature; fever may indicate infection.

• If a nasal balloon catheter is in place, the doctor may order the balloon deflated for 10 minutes every 24 hours to prevent damage to nasal tissue. If bleeding persists or recurs, reinflate the balloon and notify the doctor.

• While the nasal packing is in place, the patient is usually maintained on a liquid diet. The nasal packing causes a partial vacuum of the nasal passage, which makes swallowing difficult.

• Monitor the skin under the gauze roll at the anterior nares. Observe for any necrosis of the nasal tip or septum. Any sign of necrosis should be reported to the doctor immediately.

Home care instructions

• When the nasal packs have been removed and the patient is ready for discharge, instruct him to avoid blowing his nose for 2 to 3 days because this may precipitate bleeding. Tell the patient to expect slight oozing of blood-stained fluid from his nose for the next few days but to report any frank bleeding.

• Instruct the patient to use a humidifier (cool mist) at home to help prevent crusting inside the nose.

• Teach the patient ways to avoid activities that may promote nosebleeds.

NASAL POLYPECTOMY

Nasal polypectomy is the surgical removal of a nasal polyp. Nasal polyps are localized areas of swelling (fluid-filled sacs) originating from the sinus mucosa. They occur in individuals who have allergic or chronic rhinitis. Multiple polyps are common; they can occur bilaterally.

Removal of nasal polyps eliminates obstruction of the sinus openings. However, because polyps have a strong tendency to recur after surgical removal, more extensive sinus surgery may later be required.

Laser polypectomy is another technique used to remove polyps within the nasal cavity. This method is less invasive and reduces patient discomfort.

Purpose
• To reestablish the normal flow of mucus from the sinuses
• To prevent recurrent or chronic infection
• To eliminate airway obstruction.

Indications
Nasal polypectomy combined with topical and systemic corticosteroids is the optimal therapy for nasal polyposis.

Procedure
The surgeon administers a local or a general anesthetic, depending on the extent of polyposis; then, placing a wire snare around the base of the polyp, he removes it. If laser polypectomy is the chosen technique, the surgeon uses a laser beam to cut, coagulate, and vaporize tissue.

Complications
Complications are rare but may include bleeding and infection.

Care considerations
Before surgery
• Administer topical and systemic corticosteroids, as ordered, to decrease mucosal inflammations and polyp size.
• Give the patient appropriate preoperative and postoperative instructions.

After surgery
• Monitor vital signs carefully.
• Elevate the head of the bed to reduce edema.
• Check the nasal dressing frequently, and report bright red drainage to the doctor.
• Nasal packing, if inserted at the end of surgery, will be removed at the surgeon's discretion.
• Administer analgesics, as ordered, to control pain.

Home care instructions
• The doctor may advise the patient not to return to work for up to 10 days if his work is physically strenuous.
• Advise the patient to avoid heavy lifting or straining, not to blow his nose, and to sneeze with his mouth open. This will prevent unnecessary pressure and reduce the chance of bleeding.
• Instruct the patient to wear the nasal dressing until drainage subsides, possibly as long as 10 days.
• Teach the patient how to use sodium chloride solution nasal spray and how to provide nares care. Removal of crusting prevents scarring.
• Emphasize the importance of follow-up care.
• Advise the patient to call the doctor if bleeding or other complications occur.

NASOENTERIC DECOMPRESSION

Nasoenteric decompression is a procedure for removing intestinal contents to relieve intestinal obstruction. It involves passing a long, weighted tube through the nose and then advancing the tube beyond the stomach into the intestines.

Various types of tubes may be used for this procedure. All of these tubes have a balloon that may be weighted with mercury, air, or water to stimulate peristalsis and facilitate the tube's passage through the pylorus into the intestinal tract. Some of the tubes have double and triple lumens, allowing for irrigation, aspiration, and balloon inflation.

Purpose

• To relieve acute intestinal obstruction
• To aspirate gastric contents for examination
• To prevent nausea, vomiting, and abdominal distention after GI surgery.

Indications

Nasoenteric decompression is the initial treatment for acute intestinal obstruction, along with fluid and electrolyte replacement. Obstruction may result from polyps, adhesions, fecal impaction, volvulus, or localized cancer. Decompression usually relieves the obstruction, especially in the small intestine. However, if decompression fails to relieve the obstruction or if the patient's condition deteriorates, bowel resection may be necessary.

Nasoenteric decompression may also be performed to aspirate gastric contents for testing purposes or to prevent GI upset after abdominal surgery.

Procedure

A doctor or specially skilled nurse may perform decompression. The doctor chooses the appropriate nasoenteric decompression tube, basing the choice on the size of the patient and of his nares, the estimated duration of the intubation, and the reason for the procedure. The tube is passed through the nares and advanced into the nasopharynx and into the stomach. The patient is then positioned on his right side until the tube clears the pylorus, which usually takes up to 2 hours. Passage into the stomach will be confirmed by X-ray. After the tube clears the pylorus, the doctor may order that the tube be advanced 2″ to 3″ (5 to 7.5 cm)

every hour until a premeasured mark on the tube meets the patient's nostril. After the tube progresses the necessary distance and X-ray confirms correct placement, the tube is connected to intermittent suction.

When the tube is no longer necessary, it is removed.

Complications

Common complications include esophagitis, nasal or oral inflammation, and nasal or laryngeal ulcers. Rarely, atelectasis and pneumonia may result from the presence of the tube in the esophagus and its interference with normal coughing. Excessive intestinal drainage can produce acid-base imbalance or malposition of the tube within the intestine.

Care considerations

Before the procedure

• Briefly explain the procedure. Tell the patient to expect mild discomfort as the doctor inserts and advances the tube. Reassure him that a sedative will be given if intubation proves difficult or painful.
• Gather and prepare the equipment as indicated for the type of tube.
• Place the patient in semi-Fowler's position.
• Help the patient to relax.
• It may be necessary for you to stiffen a flaccid tube by placing it in a basin of ice or to soften a stiff tube in warm water.
• Check the tubing for leaks and then add mercury, air, or water to the tube as appropriate for the type of tubing.

During the procedure

• Apply a water-soluble lubricant to the tube to reduce friction and ease insertion.
• Insert the tube into the selected nostril.
• Instruct the patient to repeatedly swallow to advance the tube when the tube reaches the nasopharynx.

- Offer small sips of water or ice chips, as allowed by the doctor, to facilitate swallowing when the tube passes the trachea.
- Administer a sedative, as ordered, for difficult intubation.
- Advance the tube slowly until it reaches the stomach.
- Confirm correct placement.
- Position the patient (usually on his right side until the tube passes through the pylorus, then in Fowler's position).
- If ordered, test the pH of the intestinal aspirate (normal intestinal pH is greater than 7.0).

After the procedure
- Confirm tube placement through abdominal X-rays.
- Secure the tube to prevent further advancement and to prevent its dislodgment. (Never tape the tube directly to the patient's skin; instead wrap it with gauze and then tape the gauze to the cheek.)
- As ordered, connect the tube to intermittent suction.
- Frequently check the tube's patency and the effectiveness of intestinal suction and decompression.
- Note and record the amount and nature of drainage.
- As ordered, irrigate the tube with 0.9% sodium chloride solution.
- Regularly check the patient's vital signs, and assess fluid and electrolyte status.
- Record intake and output, and be sure to watch for signs of fluid imbalance, such as decreased urine output, poor skin turgor, dry skin and mucous membranes, lethargy, and fever.
- Monitor for acid-base imbalance.
- Watch for signs of metabolic alkalosis (altered level of consciousness, slow and shallow respirations, hypertonic muscles, and tetany) or acidosis (dyspnea, disorientation and, later, weakness, malaise, and deep, rapid respirations).
- Also watch for signs of secondary infection, such as fever and chills.
- Provide mouth care and apply petroleum jelly to the nares at least every 4 hours.
- Check for signs that indicate the return of peristalsis. These include the presence of bowel sounds, decreased abdominal distention, passage of flatus, or a spontaneous bowel movement.
- Record and notify the doctor of patient's progress.

Home care instructions
- The nasoenteric tube is removed before discharge. As a result, the patient doesn't require treatment-related directions for home care. However, instruct the patient about proper nutrition, the addition of dietary fiber, and adequate fluid intake to promote normal bowel function.

NEPHRECTOMY

Nephrectomy is the surgical removal of a kidney. Nephrectomy may be unilateral or bilateral. Unilateral nephrectomy (removal of one kidney), the more commonly performed procedure, usually doesn't interfere with renal function as long as the kidney that remains is healthy. Bilateral nephrectomy (removal of both kidneys) requires lifelong dialysis or transplantation to support renal function.

Three major types of nephrectomy are performed: partial nephrectomy, involving resection of only a portion of the kidney; simple nephrectomy, removal of the entire kidney; and radical nephrectomy, resection of the entire kidney, the perinephric fat, and the entire ureter. Complete ureteral removal is advocated only for transitional cell carcinoma of the upper collecting system (for example, of the renal pelvis). Except for variations in the extent of tissue resection, the surgical approach remains basically the same for all types of nephrectomy.

Purpose

• To remove one or both kidneys to help treat renal cancer or other renal disease
• To obtain a healthy organ for transplantation.

Indications

Nephrectomy is the treatment of choice for advanced transitional or renal cell cancer that's refractory to chemotherapy and radiation; it's also indicated as the primary treatment for resectable, nonmetastatic renal lesions. Nephrectomy is also used to harvest a healthy kidney for transplantation. When conservative treatments fail, nephrectomy may be used to treat renal trauma, infection, hypertension, hydronephrosis, and other lesions.

Procedure

The surgeon performs the surgery with the patient under general anesthesia. A thoracoabdominal or transthoracic incision may be used if extensive renovascular repair or radical excision of the kidney and surrounding structures is necessary or if the patient has respiratory or cardiac dysfunction. Some alternative routes are the anterior transperitoneal approach, which permits primary pedicle control for trauma or tumors; the anterior extraperitoneal approach; the open flank approach for simple nephrectomy in selected cases; and the percutaneous endosurgical flank approach, also done in selected cases. Once the kidney is exposed, the surgeon frees it from the surrounding fat and adhesions and from the ureter, removes the kidney, and ligates the ureter. If necessary, he then inserts a Penrose drain and closes the wound.

Complications

Nephrectomy can cause serious complications. Rare complications include infection, hemorrhage, atelectasis, pneumonia, venous thrombosis, and pulmonary embolism.

Care considerations
Before surgery

• Reinforce the surgeon's explanation of the surgery, and describe the preoperative and postoperative care.
• Ensure that the patient or a responsible family member has signed a consent form.
• Tell the patient that an indwelling urinary catheter will be in place after surgery to allow precise measurement of urine output and that a nasogastric tube will be in place to prevent abdominal pain, distention, and vomiting. He'll also have a dressing and possibly a drain at the incision site. Prepare him for frequent dressing changes.
• Explain to the patient that he won't receive food or fluids by mouth after surgery until bowel sounds have returned, but that he'll receive I.V. fluids to maintain hydration.
• Reassure the patient who's having a unilateral nephrectomy that one healthy kidney provides adequate function. The kidney increases its function so that it assumes 70%, rather than 50%, of the original kidney's workload. Prepare the patient who's scheduled for bilateral nephrectomy or the removal of his only kidney for radical life-style changes, notably the need for regular dialysis. If appropriate, reinforce the doctor's explanation of the possibility of a future kidney transplantation to restore normal function.
• Stress the need for postoperative deep-breathing and coughing to prevent pulmonary complications.

After surgery

• If the patient has a remaining kidney, measure intake and output meticulously every hour to monitor kidney function. Weigh the patient daily. Note the appearance of the urine, and check for blood clots in the urine.
• Maintain fluid and electrolyte balance. Administer I.V. fluids, as ordered. Note serum electrolyte levels.
• Monitor the patient's heart and lung sounds, checking for signs of fluid

overload: tachycardia, tachypnea, crackles, and wheezes. Notify the doctor of problems.

• Encourage coughing, deep-breathing, incentive spirometry, and position changes. Regularly assess respiratory status. Be alert for signs of pulmonary embolism, especially 5 to 10 days after surgery. Watch for dyspnea, tachypnea, pleuritic chest pain, and hemoptysis; if these develop, immediately notify the doctor, raise the head of the patient's bed at least 30 degrees, and administer oxygen.

• Check the patient's dressing and drain every 4 hours for the first 24 to 48 hours and then once every shift to assess the amount and nature of drainage. Maintain patency of the drain if one is in place. Change dressings as ordered, checking the incision for signs of infection and inflammation.

• Maintain food and fluid restrictions, as ordered. Periodically auscultate for bowel sounds; when they return and the patient is able to pass flatus, typically by the 4th postoperative day, notify the doctor and prepare to resume oral feedings. When oral intake is permitted, encourage fluids – up to 3 liters a day.

• To reduce the risk of venous thrombosis, encourage early and regular ambulation, apply antiembolism stockings, and encourage leg exercises (calf-pumping and ankle circles, as ordered). Assess for signs and symptoms of venous thrombosis, such as leg pain, edema, and erythema.

• Monitor for signs of hemorrhage and shock. Keep in mind that bleeding is most likely to occur during the first 24 to 48 hours after surgery.

• After nephrectomy to treat renal cell cancer, most recurrences are pulmonary.

Home care instructions

• Teach the patient how to monitor intake and output at home, and explain how this helps assess renal function.

Instruct him to call the doctor immediately if he detects any significant decrease in urine output, a reliable sign of renal failure.

• Tell the patient to notify the doctor if fever, chills, hematuria, or flank pain occur. Explain that these signs and symptoms may indicate urinary tract infection, a common response to indwelling urinary catheter insertion.

• Tell the patient to notify his doctor if he has weight loss, bone pain, altered mental status, and numbness in the extremities – signs of tumor metastasis.

• Emphasize the importance of following the doctor's guidelines on fluid intake and diet restrictions.

• Explain that the patient may experience incisional pain and fatigue for several weeks after discharge; reassure him that these are normal postoperative effects. Advise him to avoid strenuous exercise or heavy lifting and to refrain from sexual relations until the doctor recommends resuming them (usually after at least 6 weeks).

• Stress the need for regular follow-up examinations to evaluate kidney function and to assess for possible complications.

NERVE BLOCKS

Nerve blocks control moderate to severe pain by anesthetizing specific nerves to block the conduction of pain impulses to the central nervous system. The most common agents used are local anesthetics, such as *bupivacaine, etidocaine, lidocaine, procaine,* and *tetracaine.* (If inflammation is present, a corticosteroid may be added.) These nerve-blocking agents may be injected into the subarachnoid or epidural space, the paravertebral somatic nerve, sympathetic ganglion nerve, a peripheral nerve, or nerve endings. (See *Comparing nerve blocks,* pages 468 and 469.)

Purpose
• To provide analgesia or anesthesia by interrupting pain pathways.

Indications
Nerve blocks may be the treatment of choice for pain relief in some disorders, such as reflex sympathetic dystrophy; for symptomatic pain relief, such as for the pain of certain cancers; or to provide anesthesia during surgery to a specific area.

Nerve blocks are contraindicated in local infection, bleeding disorders, history of allergic reaction to the drug or another similar drug, concurrent anticoagulant therapy, and deafferentation syndromes (which eliminate or interrupt afferent nerve impulses).

Procedure
After the patient has been prepared, the doctor inserts the needle into the appropriate area and may use fluoroscopy to verify proper placement. Before injection of the anesthetic agent, the doctor attempts aspiration to prevent inadvertent intravascular or intrathecal injection, thus further verifying proper needle placement. Once proper needle placement has been verified, the doctor injects a test dose. If no adverse reactions occur, the remainder of the anesthetic is injected, usually in small increments. After completing the injection, the doctor removes the needle and applies pressure over the site. The patient remains recumbent for the specified time and is then returned to his room.

Complications
Nerve blocks can cause puncture of the dura, subarachnoid space, or a blood vessel during injection. Dural puncture can lead to headache, whereas subarachnoid puncture can cause severe cardiovascular complications and respiratory failure. Puncture of a blood vessel can cause hemorrhage.

Absorption of a sufficient amount of anesthetic into the bloodstream may produce systemic effects, including changes in heart rate or blood pressure, alterations in taste, altered mental status, excitation, and seizures. Absorption increases in vascular areas, such as the upper respiratory passages, the urethra, and the large venous plexus of the caudal canal. Most such reactions occur within 10 minutes of injection. Rarely, injection causes anaphylaxis.

Care considerations
Before the procedure
• Reinforce the doctor's explanation of the procedure, and answer the patient's questions. Also ask if he's ever experienced an adverse reaction to local anesthetic.
• Be sure preliminary testing has been performed before the procedure as appropriate. Some clinicians may require bleeding times or coagulation studies before epidural or intraspinal injections.
• Obtain the patient's drug history. Check for the use of oral anticoagulants or aspirin.
• Inform the patient that the duration of the procedure depends on the type of nerve block used and that he'll be awake and alert during the injection. If he's anxious, a sedative may be given to help him relax.
• Instruct the patient not to move during the injection to confine the local anesthetic and avoid injury. Tell him to report any pain to the doctor.
• Make sure the patient has signed a consent form.
• Establish a baseline for pain. Using a scale of 0 (for no pain) to 10 (for the worst pain imaginable), ask the patient to estimate the pain's severity. Also record any evidence of hypalgesia or other sensory changes, motor dysfunction, or reflex abnormalities.
• Ensure that monitoring and resuscitation equipment are nearby and that

Comparing nerve blocks

NERVE BLOCK	INDICATIONS
Subarachnoid Most commonly given in the lumbar region to interrupt sensory motor and autonomic components of nerves	• Diagnostic before surgery or a neurolytic block • Postamputation pain • Visceral pain • Cancer pain
Epidural Most commonly given in the lumbar region to interrupt sensory motor and autonomic components of nerves; onset is slower than with subarachnoid block	• Radicular or visceral pain • Postoperative pain • Causalgia • Reflex sympathetic dystrophy • Anesthesia during cesarean section or pain relief during vaginal delivery
Paravertebral somatic nerve May be given in the cervical, thoracic, or lumbar region to interrupt sensory and pain pathways	• Prognostic before surgery or a neurolytic block • Neuralgia • Cancer pain • Causalgia • Vertebral fracture pain
Sympathetic ganglion nerve Most commonly given in the stellate ganglion, celiac plexus, or lumbar sympathetic nerves to eliminate vasomotor, sudomotor, and visceromotor hyperactivity and to inhibit activity of the neuroaxis responsible for some chronic pain	• Causalgia • Postherpetic neuralgia • Visceral pain • Phantom pain • Acute herpes zoster
Peripheral nerve Most commonly given at the intercostal nerves, the lateral femoral cutaneous nerve, or the sciatic nerve to interrupt sensory and pain pathways	• Rib fracture or hip pain • Postherpetic neuralgia • Postoperative pain • Meralgia paresthetica
Local infiltration (trigger point injection) Given to interrupt sensory and pain pathways in a muscle in which palpation produces pain	• Costal chondritis • Myofascial pain • Pyriformis syndrome

SPECIAL CONSIDERATIONS

- May block more segments than necessary; may preview effects of neurolytic injection.
- Complications include motor weakness, paralysis, meningitis, dysesthesias, neuropathies, arachnoiditis, and myelopathy.

- Appropriate concentration of local anesthetic can produce sensory and vasomotor block without involving skeletal muscles.
- Complications include hypotension and headache.

- Sensory and motor functions are affected similarly.
- Muscle weakness or paralysis and loss of proprioception and touch sensation may result in a useless limb.
- Cervical injection may cause vertebral artery puncture and phrenic and vagus nerve block. Thoracic injection may cause pneumothorax.

- A successful block causes vasodilation and suppresses the galvanic skin response.
- Complications of stellate ganglion block include phrenic or laryngeal nerve paralysis and pneumothorax.
- Complications of celiac plexus block include hypotension.
- Complications of lumbar sympathetic block include hemorrhage, hypotension, sexual impotence, and block of lumbar somatic nerves.

- Appropriate concentration of local anesthetic affects sensory fibers but not motor conduction.
- Can cause pneumothorax and hemorrhage.

- Is useful for localized pain.

epinephrine, bronchodilators, and antihistamines are readily available. Prepare the nerve block tray with a variety of needle sizes. Also prepare the injection site, and insert an I.V. line, as ordered. Then position the patient (usually lying down) to reduce the risk of syncope.

- If the patient will be receiving a neurolytic block, position him as ordered. If he'll be receiving an alcohol injection, warn that painful paresthesia may occur during the injection. If he'll be receiving phenol, tell him to expect a warm, tingling sensation in the involved dermatomes.

During the procedure

- Assist with the procedure as necessary.
- Maintain the patient in proper body position, as ordered.
- Observe the patient continuously for adverse reactions, such as tinnitus, headache, tachycardia or tachypnea, confusion, muscle twitching, taste alteration, seizures, and hypertension. If any reactions occur, the doctor will stop the injection and begin emergency treatment, such as administration of oxygen and appropriate drugs.

After the procedure

- After a nerve block, closely observe the needle insertion site for bleeding or hematoma formation every 30 minutes for 4 hours. Immediately notify the doctor if either occurs.
- Monitor the patient's vital signs; report hypotension, dyspnea, or a change in pulse rate.
- After an epidural nerve block, have the patient maintain the side-lying position for 30 minutes so that decreased sensitivity to pain is confined mostly to the dependent side. After an intrathecal block, reevaluate motor function and bowel and bladder function for 24 to 48 hours. After stellate ganglion and intercostal nerve blocks, auscultate the lungs to rule out pneumothorax.

• If the patient has had a cervical plexus block, caution him to lift his head and body slowly when rising because extensive vasodilation commonly causes severe orthostatic hypotension. If the patient experiences severe orthostatic hypotension after a neurolytic block, apply an abdominal binder and administer an oral vasopressor, as ordered.

• Evaluate the effects of the nerve block by comparing current pain levels to the recorded baseline. Also, review the patient's analgesic requirements. If appropriate, the opioid dosage should be reduced gradually to avoid withdrawal symptoms. Be aware that patients with cancer may have pain in areas that haven't been blocked and may continue to need analgesics.

Home care instructions

• If the patient is discharged with an anesthetized extremity, advise him to change his position every 30 minutes to prevent skin breakdown. Tell him to avoid falls by moving cautiously.

• Instruct the patient to immediately report any bleeding, fainting, difficulty breathing, or decreased motor function.

• If a neurolytic block causes sexual impotence or bladder or bowel dysfunction, refer the patient for appropriate intervention and counseling.

NITRATES

The oldest and most commonly used vasodilators, nitrates help treat and prevent acute angina. Available in various forms, the nitrates include *isosorbide dinitrate, nitroglycerin,* and *pentaerythritol tetranitrate.* Choice of drug and form depends on the type of angina. For example, sublingual nitroglycerin and sublingual or chewable isosorbide dinitrate provide relief of acute angina pectoris. The long-acting nitrates and topical, transdermal, transmucosal, and extended-release oral nitroglycerin provide prophylaxis and long-term management of recurrent angina. I.V. nitroglycerin is used during the critical phase of unstable angina or in preinfarction angina.

Purpose

• To relieve or prevent angina by reducing cardiac oxygen demands through relaxation of all smooth muscle

• To increase blood flow through collateral coronary vessels.

Indications

Nitrates are indicated in the treatment of both angina pectoris and Prinzmetal's angina. They're also used to reduce cardiac work load in congestive heart failure and acute myocardial infarction (MI).

Nitrates are contraindicated in patients with hypersensitivity to one of the drugs, severe anemia, profound hypotension, increased intracranial pressure, glaucoma, head trauma, or cerebral hemorrhage. They should be used cautiously during early MI and in hepatic or renal insufficiency and hyperthyroidism.

Adverse reactions

Adverse reactions associated with nitrates include circulatory collapse, seizures, coma, and respiratory failure. Additional adverse reactions include headache (sometimes with throbbing), dizziness, weakness, tachycardia, sublingual burning, flushing, blurred vision, dry mouth, postural hypotension, palpitations, and syncope.

Care considerations

• At the beginning of therapy, monitor the patient's blood pressure and the intensity and duration of his response to the medication. Note the relief of anginal pain and reduction in the frequency of attacks.

• Be alert for serious adverse effects. Notify the doctor immediately of such effects, and begin emergency treatment.

• Check the patient's drug regimen for possible interactions. For example, taking nitroglycerin with an antihypertensive may potentiate orthostatic hypotension. Combining nitroglycerin and tricyclic antidepressants may cause hypotension.

• I.V. nitroglycerin must be prepared only in glass containers and delivered through special nonabsorbent tubing because regular plastic I.V. containers or tubing can absorb up to 80% of the drug.

Home care instructions

• Tell the patient to take the drug as prescribed, even if he isn't experiencing anginal pain. Explain that taking the drug on schedule will help prevent this pain. Reassure the patient that the drug isn't habit-forming.

• Tell the patient to call the doctor immediately if he develops symptoms of possible toxicity: blue lips, palms, or fingernails; syncope or extreme dizziness; a feeling of pressure in the head; dyspnea; weakness or fatigue; weak, rapid heartbeat; fever; or seizures.

• Advise the patient to store the drug in a cool, dark place in a tightly closed container and to replace the supply every 3 months.

• Warn the patient to avoid alcohol, which may lower blood pressure when taken with nitrates.

• Instruct the patient to take oral tablets on an empty stomach, 30 minutes before or 1 to 2 hours after meals. Unless they're chewable tablets, the patient should swallow them whole.

• Tell the patient who is taking sublingual tablets to take a tablet as soon as he feels anginal pain; to wet the tablet with saliva, place it under his tongue, and then sit or lie down and relax; to allow the tablet to dissolve naturally and not swallow until it has done so; then to relax for 15 minutes after the pain subsides to prevent dizziness.

• Explain that if one tablet doesn't relieve the pain within 5 minutes, he should take a second one; and if there's no relief within another 5 minutes, to take a third tablet. If pain persists after another 5 minutes, the patient should notify the doctor immediately. Warn the patient never to take more than three tablets.

• Tell the patient to take an additional dose of the short-acting oral or sublingual form 5 to 10 minutes before a stressful situation or strenuous exercise; the drug's effect will last up to 30 minutes.

• If the doctor has prescribed topical nitroglycerin ointment, show the patient how to apply it: he should spread it in a uniform, thin layer on any hairless area (without rubbing it in) and then cover it with plastic film to aid absorption and protect clothing. If he's using ointment applied to a strip of ruled paper, tell him to keep the paper on the skin to protect his clothing and ensure that the ointment remains in place.

• If the patient is using the transdermal patch, show him how to apply it. Explain that he can apply it to any hairless area except the distal parts of his arms or legs (absorption is poorer at these sites). Also, warn him to avoid prolonged proximity to microwave ovens. Explain that a radiation leak may heat the patch's aluminum backing, causing burns.

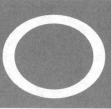

OBESITY, SURGICAL TREATMENT

Surgical treatment of morbid obesity helps patients lose weight and avoid life-threatening weight-related complications. Three commonly performed procedures are jejunoileal bypass, gastric bypass, and vertical banded gastroplasty. However, none of these procedures is totally effective or safe.

Jejunoileal bypass allows weight reduction by shortening the small intestine. Performed frequently in the 1970s, this procedure is now used less often because of the incidence of postoperative complications. Gastric bypass and vertical banded gastroplasty are thought to produce weight loss by limiting the amount of food that can be ingested. These procedures are less likely than jejunoileal bypass to cause complications; however, their long-term effects are unknown.

Surgical treatments are contraindicated in patients who do not meet strict selection criteria.

Purpose

• To provide permanent weight loss in morbidly obese patients who do not respond to traditional treatment.
• To decrease the incidence of hypertension, degenerative arthritis, cardiac dysfunction, cholelithiasis, diabetes mellitus type II, and other disorders associated with morbid obesity.

Indications

Only patients who are morbidly obese (weighing at least two times the ideal weight) should be considered for weight-reduction surgery. Candidates for surgery include patients who have tried conventional methods of weight reduction and have been approved for the procedure after a psychological consultation (which includes examination of emotional stability and addictive behaviors). Patients must be free of endocrine or metabolic disorders that can be treated effectively without surgery and free of liver, cardiac, inflammatory bowel, and kidney disease. Patients must also comply with postoperative care (follow-up appointment schedule and diet restrictions).

Patients with hypertension, diabetes mellitus, disabling bone disease, or extreme endocrine dysfunction may be considered for weight-reduction surgery without meeting the above criteria if the perceived benefits of surgery outweigh the risks.

Procedure

Jejunoileal bypass involves shortening the small bowel, thereby causing weight loss by decreasing the absorption of nutrients ingested. The gastric bypass procedure uses a constructed pouch that is drained into a loop of the jejunum; bypassing the lower stomach and small intestine limits the amount of food ingested as well as the absorption of ingested nutrients. Vertical banded gastroplasty is performed by creating a pouch in the upper stomach using vertically placed staples. This pouch communicates with the lower stomach via a small (1-cm) conduit encircled by a Teflon ring. Vertical banded gastroplasty drastically reduces the amount the stomach can hold.

Complications

Postoperative complications of these procedures include atelectasis, deep vein thrombosis, vomiting, dehydration, bleeding, superficial and deep wound infection, pneumonia, and pulmonary embolus.

Surgery-specific complications can include vitamin B_{12}, iron, calcium, and potassium deficiencies; other fluid and electrolyte imbalances; and malnutrition. (These deficiencies are correctable with administration of oral and I.V. supplements.) Foul breath, body odor, flatulence, bloating, cramping abdominal pain, and diarrhea are common in malabsorptive conditions. Psychological problems that require inpatient or outpatient treatment often develop postoperatively. Intra-abdominal abscess, bypass enteritis, perforation at the surgical site, intestinal obstruction, and symptomatic duodenal ulcers in the bypassed segment are sometimes noted. After jejunoileal bypass, diarrhea occurs in all patients; migratory polyarthritis and liver and kidney dysfunction may also occur.

Care considerations

Before surgery

• Review the purpose and procedure with the patient and family, and answer any questions.
• Ensure that the consent form has been signed.
• Administer prophylactic antibiotics.

After surgery

• Administer antibiotics.
• Administer prophylactic thromboembolytic therapy.
• Administer antidiarrheal medication (diphenoxylate atropine or loperamide) as appropriate.

• Monitor the patient's bowel sounds and bowel movements; assess for signs of complications.
• Ensure patency of the nasogastric tube. (Do not reposition the tube after gastric-reduction surgery; this may disrupt the suture line.)
• Progress diet from clear liquids to pureed foods, and advance as tolerated. (Some patients may continue a liquid diet for 8 to 12 weeks.) Also cautiously progress volume of fluid ingested, as ordered.
• Monitor for nausea, vomiting, and abdominal discomfort. These symptoms may indicate excessive ingestion of fluid or food.

Home care instructions

• Provide the patient and family with information on obesity, the surgical procedure, and postoperative care.
• Tell the patient and family to report any of the following signs and symptoms to the doctor: persistent nausea and vomiting, diarrhea, and temperature above 101° F (38.3 C).
• Schedule follow-up appointments, and emphasize their importance.
• Encourage social rehabilitation and participation in a support group.
• Provide dietary counseling. Advise the patient to adhere to a daily multivitamin schedule and to drink high-protein liquids. Also provide exercise instructions.
• Instruct the patient to eat slowly and to chew food completely before swallowing. Tell the patient to stop eating if he senses fullness because overeating will cause vomiting.
• Provide referrals for motivational support and counseling (stress reduction, self-esteem, communication, and assertiveness classes).

OOPHORECTOMY AND SALPINGECTOMY

Oophorectomy is the surgical removal of one (unilateral) or both (bilateral) ovaries. Salpingectomy is the surgical removal of one or both fallopian tubes. When the procedures are done together, it may be referred to as a salpingo-oophorectomy.

A bilateral oophorectomy eliminates much of the patient's production of estrogen and progesterone, and the loss of estrogen may result in a variety of signs and symptoms. This procedure, therefore, must be considered carefully before use in the young woman who still requires the benefits of circulating estrogen.

Purpose
• To remove one or both ovaries
• To remove one or both fallopian tubes.

Indications

Oophorectomy is indicated to treat ovarian cysts, ovarian cancer, an estrogen-dependent tumor, or an ectopic pregnancy. Bilateral oophorectomy may be performed during a hysterectomy if uterine disease has spread to the ovaries.

Salpingectomy may be performed to treat salpingitis (infection of the fallopian tubes), severe pelvic inflammatory disease, endometriosis, or an ectopic pregnancy or to provide permanent contraception.

Salpingectomy almost always accompanies routine hysterectomy because the fallopian tubes offer no benefit if the patient will never again be pregnant. Many experts debate whether one or both ovaries should also be removed routinely. The removal of only one ovary ensures that the patient will continue to have the benefit of estrogen production. If both ovaries are removed, the patient will probably require estrogen replacement therapy, which carries risks of its own.

Procedure

With the patient under general anesthesia, the surgeon, using either a transverse or vertical incision, will locate and remove one or both ovaries or fallopian tubes. If a hysterectomy is indicated, the uterus will also be removed. If the ovary is being removed because of cancer, the surgeon will also remove adjacent lymph nodes for biopsy.

Complications

Complications are rare but include hemorrhage, infection, atelectasis, pulmonary embolism, psychological problems resulting from changes in self-concept, and physical (menopausal) changes resulting from loss of estrogen. Menopausal symptoms are usually delayed for several days or weeks after surgery unless both ovaries were removed.

Care considerations
Before surgery
• Careful preoperative education will help prevent potential problems with self-concept. Encourage the patient to discuss her feelings related to the loss of reproductive abilities if both ovaries are to be removed.
• Instruct the patient to douche with povidone-iodine preoperatively, if ordered, to clean the vagina and prevent the ascent of microorganisms into the reproductive tract.
• Insert an indwelling urinary catheter so that gravity drainage will prevent the accidental perforation of the bladder during surgery. Tell the patient that this catheter will be in place for 24 hours postoperatively.
After surgery
• Monitor vital signs every 15 minutes for at least the 1st hour.
• Observe the dressings frequently for signs of hemorrhage.

- Teach the importance of coughing and deep-breathing every hour.
- Encourage early and frequent ambulation to prevent phlebitis and atelectasis.
- Maintain and administer I.V. therapy to ensure adequate hydration and prevent hypotension.
- Administer analgesics as needed to control pain.
- Administer any estrogen replacement (usually prescribed when the patient is ambulatory).

Home care instructions

- Teach the patient the importance of taking any ordered medication as directed. Make sure the patient understands why estrogen replacement is given and its risks and benefits.
- If the uterus was also removed, make sure the patient understands that her menses will no longer occur.
- Tell the patient that it is important she return for a follow-up pelvic examination in 6 to 8 weeks to check healing of the internal incisions.
- Make sure the patient understands that even if she has had a hysterectomy, she will require annual Papanicolaou tests to screen for cervical cancer.
- Teach the patient to immediately report any abnormal bleeding, pain, fever, or problems with voiding.

ORCHIOPEXY

Orchiopexy is a surgical procedure that secures the proper position of a testicle in the scrotum. When successful, orchiopexy decreases the risk of sterility, testicular cancer, and testicular trauma from abnormal positioning. If a testicle is missing or must be removed, a Silastic prosthesis is inserted to achieve a normal appearance and foster the patient's positive body image. Orchiopexy for correction of cryptorchidism is usually performed in children ages 1 to 6.

Purpose

- To correct cryptorchidism (undescended testicle) or testicular torsion by securing the testicle within the scrotal sac.

Indications

Orchiopexy is indicated in cryptorchidism when other treatments, such as hormonal therapy with human chorionic gonadotropin, fail. It is indicated in testicular torsion when the testicle remains viable.

Procedure

Orchiopexy is performed under general anesthesia. If the patient has testicular torsion, the surgeon makes an incision in the scrotal skin and attempts to untwist and stabilize the spermatic cord. He may remove a hydrocele, if present. For a necrotic testicle, he performs an orchiectomy (removal of testicle).

If the patient has an undescended testicle, the surgeon makes an inguinal or lower abdominal incision to expose the testicle and a small incision to open the scrotum. He then frees the testicle, lowers it into the scrotal sac, and secures it with sutures. If cryptorchidism is bilateral, he repeats this procedure for the other testicle.

In two-stage orchiopexy, an alternative procedure, the surgeon brings the testicle down into the scrotal sac and sutures it to the thigh; then, 2 to 3 months later, he imbeds it in the scrotal sac. If the spermatic cord is too short to accommodate repositioning of the testicle, the surgeon may perform the Fowler-Stephens procedure, in which he severs the spermatic cord before placing the testicle in the scrotal sac. After completing the procedure, the surgeon sutures the incision and applies a dressing.

Complications

Complications of this procedure are uncommon but include hemorrhage, infection, and dysuria.

Care considerations

Before surgery

• Explain the surgery to the patient and, if appropriate, to the patient's parents.
• Provide emotional support. Encourage the patient and parents to verbalize their concerns about possible infertility, impaired sexual performance, and altered body image.

After surgery

• Monitor the patient's vital signs. Check the dressing frequently for signs of hemorrhage, and change it as necessary. Inspect the suture line for redness, inflammation, separation, and bleeding.
• If the surgeon has used a traction attachment that retains the testicle in the scrotum, it will typically be removed 5 to 7 days after surgery.
• Monitor and record the patient's intake and output. Be alert for urine retention or dysuria due to postoperative edema or the effects of anesthesia.
• Provide ice packs or a scrotal support to relieve the patient's discomfort. Administer analgesics, as ordered.
• Provide meticulous skin care, and encourage good personal hygiene to prevent contamination of the operative site with stool or urine.

Home care instructions

• Instruct the patient or parents to promptly report increased scrotal pain or swelling or other changes in the testicle.
• Advise the patient to gradually resume normal activities, beginning about 1 week after surgery, but to avoid heavy lifting and other strenuous activities until the doctor advises otherwise.
• Encourage the patient to wear a scrotal support to enhance comfort and control edema for the first few weeks after surgery.

• Advise the sexually active patient to avoid sexual activity for 6 weeks after surgery or for the duration recommended by the doctor.
• Teach the patient how to perform testicular self-examination. Advise him to examine both testicles regularly and to report any lumps or unusual findings. For as yet unclear reasons, patients with cryptorchidism are at increased risk for testicular cancer.

OXYGEN THERAPY

Oxygen therapy, delivered by nasal cannula, mask, or transtracheal catheter, prevents or reverses hypoxemia and reduces the work of breathing.

The type of equipment used depends on the patient's condition and on the required concentration of the fraction of inspired oxygen (FIO_2). High-flow systems, such as the Venturi mask, deliver a precisely controlled air-oxygen mixture that provides a precise oxygen concentration. Low-flow systems, such as a nasal cannula, simple mask, partial rebreather mask, and nonrebreather mask, allow variation of the percentage of oxygen delivered, depending on the patient's respiratory pattern. The FIO_2 provided by the device is determined by the device itself and by the patient's minute volume. The higher the minute volume, the lower the FIO_2; the lower the minute volume, the higher the FIO_2, except with the Venturi mask.

Nasal cannulas deliver oxygen at flow rates from 0.5 to 6 liters/minute. Inexpensive, disposable, and easy to use, nasal cannulas permit talking, eating, and easy movement. However, they can cause nasal drying, can dislodge easily, and can't deliver high oxygen concentrations.

A nonrebreather mask can theoretically deliver oxygen concentrations of near 100%, but only if the mask is tight-fitting. Partial rebreather masks allow the patient to rebreathe the first one-third of exhaled air, which contains oxygen, not carbon dioxide; they provide higher oxygen concentrations than a simple mask and lower concentrations than a nonrebreather mask. Masks may be confining, however, and may interfere with eating and talking; these problems may affect patient compliance and make masks impractical for long-term oxygen therapy.

Transtracheal catheters permit highly efficient, continuous delivery of oxygen without hindering the patient's mobility. They don't interfere with eating or talking and can be concealed by a shirt or scarf. They also avoid the adverse effects of nasal delivery systems, such as drying mucous membranes.

Purpose

• To prevent or treat hypoxemia, thereby decreasing myocardial work load and respiratory effort.

Indications

Oxygen therapy is indicated for hypoxemia resulting from many causes, including respiratory disease, cardiovascular disease, and neuromuscular disorders. It may also be indicated for conditions associated with high metabolic demands, such as massive trauma or severe burns.

Procedure

The procedure varies according to the type of delivery device.

Nasal cannula: To insert a nasal cannula, direct the curved prongs inward, following the nostrils' natural curvature. Hook the tubing behind the patient's ears and under the chin. Set the flow rate, as ordered.

Simple mask: Oxygen flows through an entry port at the bottom of the mask and exits through large holes on the sides of the mask. Select the mask size that offers the best fit. Place the mask over the patient's nose, mouth, and chin,

and press the flexible metal edge to fit the bridge of the patient's nose. Adjust the elastic band around the head to hold the mask firmly but comfortably over the cheeks, chin, and bridge of the nose. Use gauze padding as necessary to ensure comfort and a proper fit. Make sure the flow rate is at least 5 liters/minute. Lower flow rates won't flush carbon dioxide from any mask but the Venturi model.

Partial rebreather mask: This mask has an attached reservoir bag that conserves the first third of the patient's exhalation and also fills with oxygen before the next breath, delivering average estimated oxygen concentrations ranging from 40% at a flow rate of 8 liters/minute to 60% at a flow rate of 15 liters/minute, depending on the patient's breathing pattern and rate. To apply this mask, use the procedure described for the simple mask.

Nonrebreather mask: This mask has an attached reservoir bag and three one-way valves: one located between the reservoir bag and the mask and two others located on the mask itself. These valves prevent entrance of room air and allow the patient to breathe only the source gas from the bag. This mask can deliver average estimated oxygen concentrations ranging from 60% at a flow rate of 8 liters/minute to 90% at a flow rate of 15 liters/minute, depending on the patient's breathing and respiratory rate and the tightness of the mask's fit. To apply this mask, use the procedure described for the simple mask.

Venturi mask: This mask is connected to a Venturi device that mixes a specific volume of air and oxygen. Therefore, this mask delivers the most precise oxygen concentrations—to within 1% of the setting. If you use this mask, make sure its air entrainment ports don't become blocked. Otherwise, the patient's FIO_2 level could rise dangerously.

Transtracheal catheter: The patient receives oxygen through a catheter that the doctor inserts into the trachea.

Complications

High oxygen concentrations continued for 24 or more hours can lead to oxygen toxicity, which can cause cellular damage to the lungs and can result in permanent disability. Also, high concentrations in a patient with chronic hypercapnia can eliminate the patient's stimulus to breathe, deepening respiratory failure. Pressure applied by the oxygen delivery device can cause skin irritation and necrosis. Aspiration can occur if a patient, especially one who is comatose, vomits within a mask.

Care considerations

Before therapy

• Explain the treatment to the patient, and gather the necessary equipment. Instruct the patient and any roommate or visitors not to smoke. Post a NO SMOKING sign.

• Perform a cardiopulmonary assessment, and check that ordered baseline arterial blood gas (ABG) or pulse oximetry values have been obtained.

• Assemble the equipment, check all the connections, and turn on the oxygen source. Make sure that oxygen is flowing through the nasal cannula, transtracheal catheter, or mask. Set the flow rate, as ordered. Have the respiratory therapist check the flowmeter for accuracy, as needed.

During therapy

• Periodically perform a cardiopulmonary assessment. Check the patient frequently for signs of hypoxemia, including decreased level of consciousness, tachycardia, arrhythmias, diaphoresis, restlessness, altered blood pressure or respiratory rate, clammy skin, and cyanosis. Notify the doctor if any of these occur, and check the oxygen equipment for malfunction.

• Check pulse oximetry levels or measure ABG values 20 to 30 minutes after adjusting oxygen flow. Monitor the patient for any adverse reactions.

• If the patient is restricted to bed rest, change his position frequently to ensure adequate ventilation and circulation.

• Provide good skin care to prevent irritation and breakdown caused by the tubing, prongs, or mask.

• If the patient is using a nonrebreather mask, periodically check the one-way valve between the reservoir and the mask as well as the valves on the mask to see if they are functioning properly. If the valves stick closed, the patient can rebreathe carbon dioxide and not get adequate oxygen. Replace a malfunctioning mask.

• If the patient is using a nonrebreather or a partial rebreather mask, observe the reservoir bag as the patient breathes. If it collapses more than slightly during inspiration, increase the flow rate until you see only a slight deflation. Marked or complete deflation means the flow rate is too slow. Also, keep the reservoir bag from twisting or kinking and make sure it lies outside the patient's gown, sheet, and blankets so it's free to expand.

• If the patient is receiving high oxygen concentrations for more than 24 hours, ask about symptoms of oxygen toxicity, such as burning, substernal chest pain, dyspnea, and dry cough. Atelectasis and pulmonary edema may also occur. (Encourage coughing and deep-breathing to help prevent atelectasis.) Reduce oxygen concentrations as soon as ABG results support the change.

After therapy

• Monitor for signs of hypoxia.

• Discard disposasble equipment properly or send reusable equipment to the appropriate department for sterilization.

Home care instructions

• If the patient will continue to receive oxygen at home, the doctor will order the flow rate of oxygen and the hours per day to be used. With the doctor and the patient, select the oxygen device best suited to the patient. The choice of system will depend on the patient's needs and on the availability and cost of each system.

• Teach the patient how to use the ordered oxygen equipment safely and effectively. Teach the patient who will be receiving transtracheal oxygen therapy how to clean and care for the catheter. Tell the patient to keep the skin surrounding the catheter insertion site clean and dry to prevent infection.

• Emphasize the need for regular follow-up care to evaluate the patient's response to oxygen therapy.

• Warn the patient never to increase the flow rate without checking with the doctor first.

OXYTOCICS

Oxytocics are synthetic agents that mimic the effects of the endogenous hormone oxytocin, which stimulates the uterus and induces contraction of the myoepithelium of the lacteal glands. Oxytocin also exerts vasopressive and antidiuretic effects, as well as a transient relaxing effect on vascular smooth muscle. Uterine sensitivity to it increases gradually during gestation.

Purpose
• To stimulate the contraction of uterine smooth muscle
• To stimulate lactation by inducing contraction of the myoepithelium of the lacteal glands.

Indications
Oxytocics are primarily given by I.V. infusion to induce or stimulate labor. They're given I.V., I.M., or by mouth to control postpartum bleeding. The nasal form of oxytocin can be given to stimulate lactation and thus relieve breast engorgement.

To initiate or improve uterine contractions and achieve early vaginal delivery, the doctor may infuse *oxytocin* in patients with pregnancy complications resulting from Rh incompatibility, maternal diabetes, pregnancy-induced hypertension, or premature membrane rupture or in patients who are experiencing inevitable or incomplete abortion. It may also be used in some patients with uterine inactivity.

Ergonovine and *methylergonovine* are given after placental delivery to increase the frequency, strength, and duration of uterine contractions and thereby decrease uterine bleeding.

Oxytocin is contraindicated in the presence of significant cephalopelvic disproportion, unfavorable fetal position or presentation, obstetric emergencies requiring intervention, fetal distress when delivery isn't imminent, prolonged uterine inertia, severe toxemia, or hypertonic uterine patterns.

Ergonovine and methylergonovine are contraindicated during pregnancy and in patients who have shown sensitivity to these drugs. They should never be used to induce labor.

Oxytocics shouldn't be given to a patient who has received a sympathomimetic, such as epinephrine or phenylephrine, because severe hypertension or intracranial hemorrhage could occur.

Oxytocin must be used cautiously if the patient has a history of cervical or uterine surgery, grand multiparity, uterine sepsis, or traumatic delivery; if the uterus is overdistended; or if the patient is over age 35 and in her first pregnancy. This drug must be used with extreme caution during the first and second stages of labor because cervical laceration, uterine rupture, and maternal and fetal death can occur.

Ergonovine and methylergonovine must be used cautiously in patients with hypertension.

Adverse reactions
Adverse maternal reactions to oxytocin include fluid overload, hypertension or hypotension, postpartum hemorrhage,

Preventing the perils of oxytocin administration

Oxytocin infusion can cause excessive uterine stimulation and fluid overload. To help forestall these complications, follow these guidelines.

Excessive uterine stimulation

Drug overdose or hypersensitivity may cause excessive uterine stimulation, leading to hypertonicity, tetany, rupture, cervical and perineal laceration, fetal hypoxia, or rapid forceful delivery.

To prevent these complications, always administer oxytocin by piggyback infusion so that the drug may be discontinued, if necessary, without interrupting the main I.V. line. Every 15 minutes, monitor uterine contractions, intrauterine pressure, fetal heart rate, and the character of blood loss.

If uterine contractions occur less than 2 minutes apart, last 90 seconds or longer, or exceed 50 mm Hg, stop the infusion, turn the patient on her side (preferably the left side), and notify the doctor. Contractions should occur every 2½ to 3 minutes, followed by a period of relaxation.

Keep magnesium sulfate (20% solution) available to relax the myometrium.

Fluid overload

Oxytocin's antidiuretic effect increases renal reabsorption of water. This can cause fluid overload, leading to seizures and coma.

To identify fluid overload, monitor the patient's intake and output, especially during prolonged infusion and administration of doses above 20 milliunits/minute. The risk of fluid overload also increases when oxytocin is given after abortion induced by hypertonic sodium chloride solution.

Fetal adverse reactions include bradycardia, neonatal jaundice, arrhythmias, and anaphylactic reactions.

Ergonovine and methylergonovine may cause uterine hyperstimulation or hypertension. Ergonovine may lower prolactin levels, which can interfere with breast-feeding.

Care considerations

• Monitor the patient continuously during oxytocin infusion. Check her blood pressure and pulse every 15 minutes; high doses may cause an initial drop in blood pressure followed by a sustained elevation.
• If the patient is receiving cyclopropane anesthesia, concurrent administration of oxytocin may produce severe hypotension and cardiac arrhythmias.
• Monitor uterine contractions, and watch closely for signs of fluid overload. (See *Preventing the perils of oxytocin administration.*)

Home care instructions

• Advise the patient to contact the doctor immediately if she has any abnormal vaginal bleeding.
• If the patient is using oxytocin nasal spray to promote lactation, instruct her to clear her nasal passages before administering the solution.

arrhythmias, premature ventricular contractions, afibrinogenemia, nausea and vomiting, and pelvic hematoma. An overdose or hypersensitivity to the drug may lead to uterine hypertonicity, tetanic contractions, or uterine rupture.

PACEMAKERS, PERMANENT

Permanent cardiac pacemakers may be required to maintain an effective heart rate after conduction disturbances have been stabilized and adequate pumping function has been established. Technologic improvements—for example, advances that make pacemakers more effective and small, lightweight pulse generators that contain batteries that last 7 to 10 years—have greatly extended the clinical applications of permanent pacemakers.

Permanent pacemakers consist of a subcutaneously implanted pulse generator that contains the battery and the electronic circuitry and a pacemaker catheter with a lead on the end. The catheter carries the impulses from the pulse generator to the heart and returns messages from the heart to the pulse generator. The lead with an electrode on its tip is in contact with heart tissue; it delivers the impulse and senses the activity of the heart. Pacemaker leads can be placed in the atria, ventricles, or both chambers. Having leads in contact with the atria and ventricle provides the closest simulation of normal cardiac output.

Permanent pacemakers can function in either a fixed (asynchronous) or a demand (synchronous) mode. A fixed mode releases the impulse at the preset rate and milliamperage regardless of the intrinsic activity of the heart. A demand mode senses the intrinsic activity of the heart and inhibits firing of the pulse generator as long as the cardiac rate exceeds a rate programmed in the permanent pacemaker. Most pacemakers are programmed in the demand mode to avoid interference with the intrinsic activity of the heart.

Pacemakers vary in their capabilities; a coding system has been devised to clearly identify pacemaker capabilities. (For more information, see *Guide to pacemaker codes*, page 482.) One of the newest advances in permanent pacemaker design is the ability to adjust the rate in response to the patient's activity unlike conventional pacemakers, which pace at a preset rate regardless of the patient's activity. This function more closely simulates the normal function of the heart. For example, the heart rate accelerates with activity to meet the body's increased need for oxygen; a greater cardiac output is needed at such times. Likewise, during sleep the heart rate is slower.

Early pacemakers required avoidance of exposure to microwave ovens, which interfered with pacemaker function. Now, a metal covering protects the circuitry in the permanent pacemaker pulse generator so exposure to microwaves is no longer hazardous. However, some hazards remain. For example, magnetic resonance imaging is contraindicated in patients with permanent pacemakers. During surgery, patients must be closely monitored if electrocautery will be used. Radiation therapy can have a cumulative effect on the pulse generator's circuitry, changing the molecular structure of the silicone chip and causing pacemaker failure. The pacemaker should be covered with a lead shield

Guide to pacemaker codes

A permanent pacemaker's code refers to its capabilities.

I Chamber paced	II Chamber sensed	III Response to sensing	IV Programmable functions: Rate modulation	V Antiarrhythmia functions
V — ventricle **A** — atrium **D** — dual (A + V) **O** — none **S** — A or V	**V** — ventricle **A** — atrium **D** — dual (A + V) **O** — none **S** — A or V	**T** — triggers pacing **I** — inhibits pacing **D** — dual (T + I) **O** — none	**P** — simple programmable rate or output **M** — multiprogrammability of rate, output, sensitivity **C** — communicating functions (telemetry) **R** — rate modulation **O** — none	**P** — pacing (antitachyarrhythmia) **S** — shock **D** — dual (P + S) **O** — none

during radiation therapy and checked for proper function afterward.

A permanent pacemaker will last several years, depending on how it is programmed and how often the heart paces on its own. The more often the pacemaker must initiate an impulse, the sooner the battery will be depleted of its charge. The usual life expectancy of a lithium battery is 7 to 10 years.

Most permanent pacemakers can now be reprogrammed by a doctor or other specially trained person if pacemaker problems arise after implantation. A magnetic device supplied by the manufacturer is placed on the skin over the location of the pulse generator; using certain commands, the device can reprogram the pacemaker mode, the rate, the sensitivity, the amount of energy delivered for each stimulus, and other variables.

Purpose

• To provide electrical impulses to the heart at a rate adequate to maintain the patient's cardiac output.

Indications

Candidates for permanent pacemakers include patients with persistent symptomatic bradyarrhythmia, complete heart block, and slow ventricular rates resulting from congenital or degenerative heart disease or cardiac surgery. Patients with Stokes-Adams syndrome, Wolff-Parkinson-White syndrome, or sick sinus syndrome may also benefit from permanent pacemaker implantation.

Procedure

Permanent pacemakers are inserted by a surgeon or cardiologist in an operating room. Local anesthesia is generally used, but other forms of anesthesia may be used depending on the patient and route of pacemaker insertion.

The surgeon may implant the leads epicardially, using a transthoracic approach with direct penetration of the chest wall and attachment of the lead to the external surface of the heart. The epicardial approach provides stability for the leads, but implantation of the leads requires surgery under general anesthesia; therefore, this approach is used during open-heart surgery. More commonly, the surgeon inserts the leads endocardially, using a transvenous approach. He threads the leads through a vein into the right atrium, right ventricle, or both. The transvenous approach uses the subclavian vein (most common), the cephalic vein, or the external or internal jugular vein. The surgeon attaches the lead wire(s) to the pulse generator, which he implants in a subcutaneous subclavicular pocket (most common) or in a subcutaneous abdominal pocket. He programs and tests the pulse generator and closes the incision.

Complications

Complications of permanent pacemakers include infection, arrhythmia, or displacement of the lead wires. After epicardial placement, the patient is at risk for complications associated with thoracotomy and general anesthesia (such as pneumonia). If the transvenous approach is used, the patient is at risk for thrombus and embolus formation.

Other complications are related to the pacemaker (for example, battery failure, a displaced electrode, or pacemaker-mediated arrhythmias) For more details on complications, see the entry "Pacemakers, Temporary."

Care considerations
Before the procedure
• Teach the patient about pacemaker insertion. Include the reason for the pacemaker and what the pacemaker does; show a sample pacemaker unit; discuss the type of anesthesia to be used; and explain what to expect in the operating room, in the recovery area, and on return to the unit after the pacemaker has been inserted.
• Obtain electrocardiogram (ECG) baseline.
• Obtain baseline vital signs.
• Make sure that the patient has signed a consent form.
• Prepare the surgical site, as ordered, or according to the policy of the health care facility.
• Establish I.V. access in case emergency medications are needed.
• Provide sedation, as ordered.

After the procedure
• Monitor ECG, vital signs, and level of consciousness for at least the first 24 hours after insertion of the pacemaker.
• Check the dressing for bleeding, and change it according to the policy of the health care facility.
• Assess the patient for pain; administer analgesics, as prescribed.
• Remind the patient of any ordered limitations of activities. Such restrictions typically include limited use of the involved extremity for the first 24 to 72 hours. Assist with activities of daily living, as needed.
• Document the type of pacemaker that was inserted, and note the programmed settings (such as rate, intervals, and mode).
• To ensure that the pacemaker is functioning, evaluate the patient's ECG and assess the patient for signs of pacemaker malfunction or failure.
• Administer antibiotics for 24 to 48 hours, as prescribed.

Home care instructions
• Teach the patient how to recognize the signs and symptoms of infection at the incision or insertion site.
• Tell the patient to inform any dentists or doctors that he has a permanent pacemaker.
• Advise the patient to take his resting pulse daily; tell him what constitutes an acceptable and unacceptable dis-

crepancy between pulse readings and whom to notify about an unacceptable discrepancy.
• Tell the patient when or how to schedule a follow-up visit with the doctor.
• Tell the patient what to do in case of pacemaker malfunction or failure.
• Show the patient how to use the telephone to monitor pacemaker function.
• Provide the patient with an identification card that lists pacemaker data as well as the date of implantation and the doctor's name.

PACEMAKERS, TEMPORARY

A temporary pacemaker is an electrical device that provides short-term artificial stimulation to the heart. It is frequently used during emergency situations that require immediate cardiac pacing; it can be a lifesaving intervention for a patient with a hemodynamically unstable cardiac rhythm.

A temporary pacemaker has three components: the pulse generator, the catheter or lead wire, and the lead(s). Unlike permanently implanted pacemakers, the temporary pacemaker has an external pulse generator that the patient may wear on his chest, waist, or upper arm or that may be hung at the bedside. The pulse generator produces the electrical impulses and contains the power source (a lithium or alkaline battery) and the electronic circuitry. The catheter or lead wire is the avenue by which the electrical impulse initiated by the pulse generator travels to the heart and is the pathway or mechanism by which the activity of the heart is communicated back to the pulse generator. The catheter or lead wire is contained in insulated materials.

Electrodes at the tip of the pacemaker leads create positive or negative poles that allow the electrical impulse to travel in an electrical field. The electrodes of a temporary pacemaker are

either unipolar (negative electrode only at the tip of the catheter) or bipolar (negative electrode at the tip of the catheter and positive electrode proximal to the tip of the catheter).

Temporary pacemakers can function in either a fixed (asynchronous) or demand (synchronous) mode. A fixed mode releases the impulse at a preset rate and milliamperage regardless of the intrinsic activity of the heart. A demand mode senses the intrinsic activity of the heart and inhibits firing of the pulse generator as long as the cardiac rate exceeds the rate set on the temporary pacemaker. (For more information on types of pacemakers and their capabilities, see *Guide to pacemaker codes,* page 482.)

Electrical safety precautions must be observed when a patient has a temporary pacemaker because the pacing wire provides a direct route to the heart for stray electrical current. Electrical equipment must be kept to a minimum and must be properly grounded. Caregivers must avoid simultaneous contact with the patient and electrical equipment.

Do not hesitate to defibrillate a patient when necessary; to do so, turn the pulse generator off before defibrillation, if possible, to avoid its potential malfunction.

Purpose
• To initiate an artificial electrical impulse to the heart when the intrinsic rate is too slow or when the normal impulse encounters a conduction disturbance that does not allow an adequately pumping heart to meet the body's requirements
• To act as prophylaxis when abnormal impulse formation or conduction disturbances may lead to myocardial infarction, cardiac surgery, drug toxicity, or metabolic abnormalities
• To interrupt tachyarrhythmias that are unresponsive to drug intervention (less common use).

Indications

Temporary pacing is indicated for certain arrhythmias that may result in symptomatic bradycardia and are unresponsive to drug therapy—for example, sinus bradycardia, sinus arrest, and sick sinus syndrome. Temporary pacing is generally required for a second-degree type II heart block (Mobitz II) and for a third-degree heart block (complete heart block).

Ventricular tachycardia or supraventricular tachycardias that are unresponsive to drug therapy or cardioversion may respond to rapid overdrive pacing with a temporary pacemaker.

Procedure

Temporary pacemakers are usually inserted by a cardiologist. A nurse customarily will assist during the procedure; additional staff may be present, as needed.

Temporary pacing can be accomplished using several methods. Endocardial or transvenous pacing is the most common type of temporary pacing. A transvenous pacing catheter is inserted through a vein (femoral, brachial, external jugular, or subclavian) to the apex of the right ventricle of the heart. The tip of the transvenous pacing catheter is put in contact with the endocardial or inner layer of the heart. A temporary atrioventricular pacemaker may be inserted if the patient needs the atrial kick from atrial contractions. In this case, one catheter tip is inserted in the right atrium and another in the right ventricle.

Temporary epicardial pacing is commonly accomplished through a thoracotomy, but it can be done through a subxiphoid incision. The pacing electrodes are placed on the epicardial or outer layer of the heart. This type of pacemaker is commonly used during and for the first few days after open-heart surgery. Typically, the pacing electrodes are sutured to the epicardium, brought out through the chest wall incision, and attached to a pulse generator or capped until they are needed.

External pacing is noninvasive. Pacing electrodes are placed on the patient's chest and back. From an external power source, small amounts of electricity are delivered through the pacing electrodes to the heart. External pacing is used for emergency situations (while the patient awaits insertion of a transvenous temporary pacemaker) or as backup for a permanent pacemaker during battery replacement. It is commonly used for reperfusion arrhythmias associated with thrombolytic therapy that results in symptomatic bradyarrhythmias with decreased cardiac output. Often, inserting a central venous catheter that would be used to insert a transvenous pacing lead is contraindicated during and for several hours after thrombolytic therapy; therefore, an external device may be used.

Following lead placement, the temporary leads are connected to the external pulse generator. The catheter may be sutured in place, and a dressing is applied to the insertion site.

Complications

Various types of arrhythmias may result as a complication of temporary pacing. For example, asystole can follow abrupt cessation of pacing; ventricular tachycardia or ventricular fibrillation can result from the ventricular irritability caused by the catheter tip touching the ventricle.

Thrombus or embolus formation can result from the presence of the catheter or from inactivity. Rarely, ventricular perforation or cardiac tamponade related to insertion or migration of the catheter may occur. Pericarditis may also result from the use of temporary pacing. Hiccoughs or abdominal twitching can result from placement of the pacing catheter against a thin-walled right ventricle or from ventricular rupture, which leads to electrical stimulation of the diaphragm. Retrograde migration of the pacing catheter into the right atrium results in atrial pacing or inhibition of the pacing impulses through sensing of the atrial impulses.

Complications at the insertion site include infection, phlebitis, blood vessel occlusion, hemorrhage, and allergic reactions to the local anesthetic.

A temporary pacemaker system can malfunction because of failure of discharge of the electrical stimulus, failure to capture in the chambers involved, or failure to sense the intrinsic activity of the involved chambers. These problems are usually the result of malpositioning of the pacing electrode tip.

Care considerations
Before the procedure
• Review the procedure with the patient and family.
• Ensure that the patient or a family member has signed a consent form.
• Provide sedation, as ordered.
• Establish an I.V. line in case emergency medications are necessary to control arrhythmia.
• Establish baseline vital signs and a baseline electrocardiograph (ECG) tracing.
• Ensure that all the necessary supplies have been gathered.
• Ensure that the pulse generator has a battery or that the lithium battery has an adequate charge.
• Ensure that all electrical equipment is properly grounded to prevent accidental shocks to the heart that could lead to ventricular fibrillation. Keep electrical equipment use to a minimum to decrease this risk.
• Alert additional personnel who may be needed during the procedure (such as an X-ray technician and a respiratory therapist).

During the procedure
• Have emergency equipment at the bedside in case of ventricular arrhythmias or cardiac arrest.
• Monitor the patient's cardiac status continuously during insertion of the pacing catheter. Assist with the procedure, as needed.
• When the catheter is correctly positioned, don rubber gloves and attach the pacemaker leads tightly into their respective slots in the pulse generator (place the positive lead [proximal] in the positive slot, and the negative lead [distal] in the negative slot).
• Check the stimulation threshold so that adequate stimulus is delivered to the heart. To determine the stimulation threshold, increase the pacemaker rate above the patient's heart rate, as ordered. Increase the milliamperage, as ordered, and watch the ECG for capture – a pacemaker spike followed by a QRS complex. Stop increasing the milliamperage when 100% capture is achieved. Slowly decrease the milliamperage until you lose capture. Record the threshold as the lowest milliamperage that achieves capture.
• Set the milliamperage and rate, as ordered. Usually the milliamperage is set 5% to 10% greater than the stimulation threshold to allow for the resistance that results with prolonged pacing. Also set the pacemaker to demand (synchronous) or asynchronous mode, as ordered.
• Secure the pulse generator to the patient's chest, waist, or upper arm or to an I.V. pole at the bedside.
• Ensure that the protective plastic cover is over the controls on the pulse generator to avoid moisture and accidental changes of the settings.
After the procedure
• Cover all exposed metal parts of the pacemaker setup (such as electrode connections) with nonconductive tape, or place a rubber surgical glove over each electrode to insulate them. If possible, a pulse generator should be at-

tached to the electrodes so that they are not exposed, even if the pulse generator is turned off. Ensure that the electrodes are securely placed in the terminal slots so that no metal is exposed.

• Make the patient comfortable.

• Administer pain medication, as prescribed.

• Immobilize the extremity if a femoral or brachial approach was used, to avoid stressing the pacing wires.

• Monitor the patient's heart rhythm continuously, and obtain ECG tracings for documentation and comparison purposes.

• Document the pacemaker settings to include the rate, mode (demand or fixed), output in milliamperage, and sensitivity.

• Check or change the battery. Alkaline batteries should be changed every 300 hours or according to the policy of the health care facility. Lithium batteries are good for 7 to 10 years.

• Check the patient's stimulation threshold, usually daily, because drugs, electrolyte changes, or ischemia can alter the threshold.

• Observe the patient for signs and symptoms of pacemaker malfunction—for example, a change in pulse rate, dyspnea, fatigue, chest pain, vertigo, distended neck veins, and crepitant crackles at the base of the lungs. Notify the doctor if these occur.

• Assess the insertion site daily for indications of infection, and re-dress it using aseptic technique, as ordered.

• Tape the catheter securely if it was not sutured, to avoid dislodgment.

• Assess circulation in the extremity below the site of insertion by evaluating the distal pulse and the color, temperature, and sensation of the extremity.

• Assess for thrombosis in the calf veins if the femoral approach was used.

• After the catheter is withdrawn, apply pressure to the insertion site.

Home care instructions

• Patients are not discharged with a temporary pacemaker. Advise the patient, however, to keep follow-up appointments, as scheduled.

PAIN CONTROL, COGNITIVE TECHNIQUES

Cognitive pain control refers to "mind over pain" methods, including *relaxation, biofeedback, distraction, guided imagery, hypnosis, meditation,* and *behavior modification,* that help the patient reduce the suffering associated with pain. The patient participates in treatment by using his cognitive abilities to achieve a degree of control over his pain.

These techniques are virtually risk-free and have few contraindications. However, if the patient has a significant psychiatric problem, relaxation techniques should be taught by a psychotherapist.

Purpose

• To reduce pain by promoting relaxation or a behavioral change.

Indications

Pain-control techniques are indicated for acute and chronic pain and may be used with analgesics for control of intense pain.

Procedure

The nurse can teach cognitive pain-control techniques. Teaching should begin when the patient's pain is absent or mild because the techniques require concentration.

Relaxation involves using rhythmic, slow abdominal breathing to achieve skeletal muscle relaxation and to ward off fatigue, which lowers pain tolerance and increases intensity of pain. The rate of breathing is about 6 to 9 breaths per minute and the rhythm is slow (in, 2-3, out, 2-3). The nurse may count for the patient or breathe with him when teaching this technique.

In biofeedback, the patient uses a relaxation technique (the one he finds most helpful) while he is connected to a biofeedback machine. The patient recognizes and controls the relaxation process, taking his cues from the device's audible tones, flashing lights, or digital readouts of changes in blood pressure, pulse, or skin temperature. These indicate whether the patient is becoming more relaxed.

Distraction involves having the patient shift his attention away from the pain. The patient focuses his attention on a sensory stimulus such as music, television, humming, singing, or reading and concentrates on the images these things evoke. The patient may also visually focus on a specific object, keep time to music, or use rhythmic breathing at this time. The patient may use a headset when listening to music, increasing the volume when the pain worsens. This method is easily taught; it is most effective when multiple senses are involved.

In guided imagery, the patient uses his imagination to achieve the specific result of pain relief and relaxation. The patient concentrates on a peaceful, soothing, vivid image while the nurse describes the sensations associated with it, such as the smell of grass or the warmth of the sun. This technique requires practice, about three times a day for 5 minutes; several days may pass before some pain relief is obtained using this method. The patient must have a vivid imagination and excellent concentration.

Hypnosis must be done by a therapist, who may employ such techniques as symptom suppression, to block awareness of pain, or symptom substitution, which allows a positive interpretation of pain. The patient may continue to see the therapist or may learn self-hypnosis techniques.

Meditation involves having the patient repeat a word or phrase or stare at an object until relaxed. This method also focuses attention away from pain and may be especially useful while waiting for the onset of analgesic effect.

In behavior modification, the patient identifies behaviors that reinforce pain, suffering, and disability, such as being too dependent on others or using a cane when it's not medically necessary. Behavior modification also helps the patient to define his goals, such as decreasing his dependence on others, and to use appropriate reinforcements to achieve desired behavior patterns. Behavior modification can improve the patient's self-esteem, activity, and productivity and reduce his preoccupation with pain, suffering, and disability.

Complications
Virtually no complications are associated with these therapies.

Care considerations
Before therapy
• Perform a thorough assessment of the patient, evaluating environmental factors, family relationships, and any psychosocial considerations that may intensify pain.
• Explain the technique to the patient, and stress the importance of his role in the process.
• Tell the patient to begin using these techniques when pain is absent or mild because they require concentration. However, if the pain is persistent, begin with short, simple exercises and build on the patient's abilities.
• The patient should remove or loosen restrictive clothing, dim the lights, and keep noise to a minimum.
During therapy
• If the patient is learning biofeedback, inform him that he'll be connected to a monitor that will measure changes in his blood pressure, pulse, and skin temperature. These readings will help the patient determine his level of re-

laxation. He should not fight the monitor because doing so will increase his tension.

• Mention to the patient who is learning distraction techniques that the more absorbed he becomes in this activity, the less pain he's likely to feel.

• Inform the patient receiving guided imagery that the more vivid the image, the better the results.

• Explain to the patient learning meditation that he may feel warmth, heaviness, lightness, or tingling while relaxed.

After therapy

• Communicate the chosen approach to all staff members, and have them reinforce it.

• Encourage the patient to practice the technique, and evaluate his ability to perform it properly.

• Encourage the patient using biofeedback to practice his relaxation technique without the machine to avoid becoming dependent on it.

• End each session on a positive note; for example, point out improvements.

• Assess the patient's pain to evaluate the effectiveness of the technique.

Home care instructions

• Advise the patient with overwhelming psychosocial problems to seek help in psychotherapy. Any gains in pain management may be quickly lost unless he deals with these factors.

• Suggest that the patient continue to use pain-control techniques after his pain has resolved because they may help relieve everyday stress.

PANCREATECTOMY

Pancreatectomy is the surgical removal of all or part of the pancreas. It may involve various resections, drainage procedures, and anastomoses, depending on the patient's condition, the extent of disease and metastasis, and the amount of endocrine and exocrine function the pancreas retains. Usually the type of procedure is determined only after surgical exploration of the abdomen.

Purpose

• To remove diseased pancreatic tissue
• To preserve functioning pancreatic tissue through adequate drainage and the prevention of metastasis
• To relieve pain when tissue function cannot be preserved.

Indications

Pancreatectomy is used when more conservative techniques for treating pancreatic diseases have failed. It is used for palliative treatment of pancreatic cancer and chronic pancreatitis related to chronic alcohol abuse. It is also used in the treatment of islet cell tumors (insulinomas).

Procedure

With the patient under general anesthesia, the surgeon makes an abdominal incision. The surgeon selects the procedure based on evaluation of the pancreas, liver, gallbladder, and common bile duct. If the disease is localized, he may resect a portion of the pancreas and the surrounding organs. If the surgeon detects either metastatic disease in the liver or lymph nodes or tumor invasion of the aorta or superior mesenteric artery, he may bypass the obstruction to relieve the patient's pain.

For further information on the various procedures, see *Understanding types of pancreatectomy,* pages 490 and 491.

Complications

Major complications of pancreatectomy include hemorrhage (during and after surgery), fistulas, abscesses (common with distal pancreatectomy), common bile duct obstruction, and pseudocysts. Subtotal resection sometimes causes insulin dependence; total pancreatec-

(Text continues on page 492.)

Understanding types of pancreatectomy

Pancreaticojejunostomy

Indications
- Chronic pancreatitis with extensive disease
- Multiple strictures
- Palpable ductal dilation
- Pancreatic ascites

Procedure
Connects the pancreatic duct, if large enough, to the jejunum, bypassing obstruction; pancreatic tissue is preserved

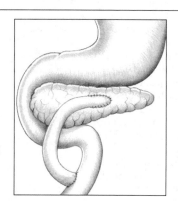

Distal pancreatectomy (subtotal)

Indications
Islet cell tumors (insulinomas) confined to tail of pancreas

Procedure
Removes the neck, body, and tail of the pancreas plus the spleen and splenic vessels; pancreatic duct may be drained into stomach or jejunum; leaves the head and uncinate process of the pancreas to the left of the mesenteric vessels

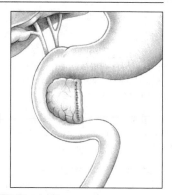

Distal pancreatectomy

Indications
- Acute pancreatitis
- Chronic pancreatitis with extensive disease and diffuse calcification
- Multiple strictures or obstructions
- Intrahepatic cyst formation
- Failure of other procedures, such as surgical repair of biliary or pancreatic ducts or the sphincter of Oddi

Procedure
Removes the neck, body, and tail of the pancreas as well as a major portion of the head and uncinate process and the entire spleen; leaves a rim of pancreatic tissue supplying blood to the duodenum and common bile duct; also includes vagotomy and gastrojejunostomy

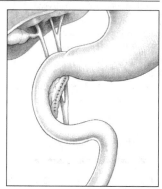

Understanding types of pancreatectomy *(continued)*

Total pancreatectomy

Indications
- Chronic pancreatitis with marked pancreatic destruction
- Multiple intraductal obstructions
- Failure of conservative measures, such as medications and diet, to control severe pain
- Cancer

Procedure
Removes the pancreas and spleen completely, leaving the hepatic duct anastomosed to the jejunum; also includes hemigastrectomy and vagotomy or 75% gastrectomy and duodenectomy

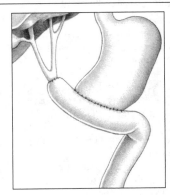

Radical pancreaticoduodenectomy (Whipple procedure)

Indications
Cancer confined to head of pancreas

Procedure
Removes the head of the pancreas with the duodenum, pylorus, and distal half of the stomach, gallbladder, and lower end of the common bile duct

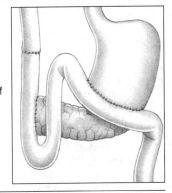

Partial pancreaticoduodenectomy (Modified Whipple procedure)

Indications
Cancer confined to head of pancreas

Procedure
Preserves the pylorus and stomach by anastomosing the pancreatic remnant to the antrum of the stomach (pancreaticogastrostomy)

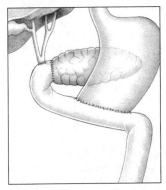

tomy always causes permanent and complete insulin dependence.

Care considerations

Before surgery

• Explain that the surgeon will select the specific procedure during abdominal exploration.

• Arrange for the necessary diagnostic studies, as ordered, to help the surgeon define the anatomic structure and evaluate endocrine and exocrine function.

• Provide enteral or parenteral nutrition for the patient with chronic pancreatitis or cancer.

• Monitor blood and urine glucose levels. Administer insulin and oral hypoglycemics, as ordered.

• Monitor the patient with a recent history of alcohol abuse for symptoms of withdrawal: agitation, tachycardia, tremors, anorexia, and hypertension.

• Advise the patient who smokes to stop smoking before surgery. Evaluate his pulmonary status to establish baseline information, and instruct him in turning, deep-breathing, and coughing techniques to be used after surgery.

• Assess the patient for jaundice and increased hematoma formation; these are signs of liver dysfunction, which commonly accompanies pancreatic disease. As ordered, arrange for liver function and coagulation studies. If the patient has a prolonged prothrombin time, expect to give vitamin K to prevent postoperative hemorrhage.

• As ordered, perform mechanical and antibiotic bowel preparation and administer prophylactic systemic antibiotics because resection of the transverse colon may be necessary.

• Insert a nasogastric (NG) tube and an indwelling urinary catheter.

• Provide emotional support and reassurance. Encourage the patient to verbalize his concerns. If necessary, obtain an order for medications to relieve pain and anxiety.

• Tell the patient what to expect immediately after surgery: the presence of tubes and drains, treatment in the intensive care unit (ICU), and invasive monitoring procedures.

After surgery

• After surgery, the patient usually spends the first 48 hours in the ICU. Monitor vital signs closely, and administer plasma expanders, as ordered. Use central, arterial, or pulmonary catheter readings to evaluate hemodynamic status; correlate these readings with urine output and wound drainage. If the patient's central venous pressure and urine output drop, give fluids to avoid hypovolemic shock.

• Provide meticulous skin care to prevent tissue breakdown that could complicate postoperative healing.

• Evaluate drainage from the NG tube, which should be green-tinged as bile drains from the stomach. A T tube may be placed in the patient's common bile duct. Notify the doctor if bile drainage doesn't decrease because this may indicate a biliary obstruction that could lead to possibly fatal peritonitis.

• Assess abdominal drainage, and inspect the dressing and drainage sites for frank bleeding. If a pancreatic drain is in place, prevent skin excoriation from highly corrosive pancreatic enzymes by changing dressings frequently or by using a wound pouching system to contain the drainage.

• Closely monitor the patient's fluid and electrolyte balance, evaluate arterial blood gases, and provide I.V. fluid replacement, as ordered. Be alert for signs of metabolic alkalosis, which may result from the constant gastric drainage, and signs of metabolic acidosis, which may be caused by loss of bile and pancreatic secretions.

• Evaluate serum calcium levels periodically because serum amylase levels commonly rise after pancreatic surgery, and amylase can bind to calcium.

• Check urine and blood glucose levels periodically. Give insulin, if prescribed.

• Monitor respiratory status. Watch closely for shallow breathing, decreased respiratory rate, and respiratory distress.

• Administer oxygen, if ordered. Reinforce deep-breathing techniques and encourage coughing.

• Be alert for absent bowel sounds, severe abdominal pain, vomiting, or fever – evidence of such complications as fistula and paralytic ileus. Also, check the wound for redness, pain, edema, unusual odor, or suture line separation. Report any of these findings to the doctor.

• If no complications develop, expect the patient's GI function to return in 24 to 48 hours. Then remove the NG tube, as ordered, and have the patient begin oral fluids.

Home care instructions

• Teach the patient to carefully clean and dress his wound each day. Tell him to report any signs of wound infection promptly.

• Teach the patient how to test his urine for glucose and ketones and how to monitor blood glucose levels. After a total pancreatectomy, provide routine diabetic teaching and instruct the patient and a responsible family member how to administer insulin.

• For a patient with chronic pancreatitis, stress the importance of regular medical follow-up and the avoidance of alcohol. As needed, provide referral to an outpatient or chemical dependency clinic.

• Because pancreatic exocrine insufficiency leads to malabsorption, provide dietary instructions. Inform the patient that he may eventually need pancreatic enzyme replacement.

PARACENTESIS

Paracentesis is the removal of ascitic fluid from the peritoneal cavity through a needle or trocar inserted in the abdominal wall.

Patients with markedly distended bowels should not be considered for this procedure because of the potential for laceration of the bowel. Rapid removal of ascitic fluid is contraindicated because hypovolemic shock may occur from fluid shifting from the intravascular compartment to the peritoneal space. Repeated paracentesis procedures should be attempted with caution because hypovolemia, electrolyte imbalances, and protein depletion may occur.

Purpose

• To obtain a specimen of ascitic fluid for diagnosis of the cause of fluid accumulation (such as malignant ascites, spontaneous peritonitis, infectious organisms, or intra-abdominal hemorrhage)

• To relieve ascitic abdominal pressure and thereby ease associated abdominal and respiratory discomfort.

Indications

Paracentesis is most commonly performed in patients with hepatic cirrhosis, suspected intra-abdominal hemorrhage from blunt trauma to the abdomen or duodenum, malignant lymphoma or other cancer, or other conditions that obstruct hepatic blood flow and cause fluid shift into the peritoneal space. Paracentesis aids diagnosis in patients with ascites of unknown etiology.

Procedure

If the clinical situation allows, fluid restriction is imposed before paracentesis to avoid hyponatremia. Local anesthesia is employed before the procedure. This procedure is typically performed under local anesthesia in the patient's hospital room or in a special procedure room.

The doctor may first make a small incision and then will insert a spinal needle or trocar to remove the ascitic fluid. Typically, the amount of fluid removed from the peritoneal space at one time is limited to 1,000 to 1,500 ml to avoid intravascular depletion and hemodynamic compromise. After removing the needle or trocar, the doctor may suture the incision. A dry sterile pressure dressing is applied.

Complications

Rapid diuresis may cause intravascular fluid to shift into the peritoneal space, resulting in electrolyte imbalances (such as hypokalemia), protein depletion, and hypovolemic shock. Other complications include perforation of abdominal organs by the needle or trocar, hepatic coma from decreased systemic circulation and reduced tissue perfusion, wound infection, and peritonitis.

Care considerations

Before the procedure

• Review the purpose of the paracentesis with the patient and family, and describe the procedure. Answer their questions.
• Ensure that the patient or a family member has signed a consent form.
• To prevent inadvertent puncture of the bladder during the procedure, encourage the patient to void beforehand.
• Assess and record the patient's baseline vital signs, abdominal girth, and weight.
• Assist the patient to a sitting position so that fluid accumulates in the lower abdominal cavity. The internal abdominal structures provide counterresistance and additional pressure to facilitate fluid flow.
• Ensure patency of the I.V. line or heparin lock, if ordered.
• Tell the patient to stay as still as possible during the procedure to prevent injury from the needle or trocar.

During the procedure

• Assist the doctor with specimen collection in the appropriate containers. Wear clean gloves to protect yourself from possible body fluid contamination.
• Monitor vital signs every 15 minutes; observe for signs of hypovolemic shock, and report such signs promptly.
• Provide emotional support to the patient.
• Document the site, amount, and character of drained fluid and the patient's response to the procedure.

After the procedure

• Monitor vital signs, and check the dressing for drainage. (Assess for signs of shock, peritoneal fluid leak, and wound infection.)
• Maintain daily records of the patient's weight and abdominal girth.
• Notify the doctor of changes in vital signs, increased abdominal girth, or scrotal edema.
• Ensure that the patient remains on bed rest until vital signs return to baseline.
• Send the labeled specimen tubes to the laboratory with the special request form.

Home care instructions

• Provide the patient and his family with appropriate information related to the diagnosis determined by the paracentesis.
• Inform the patient and family members about signs and symptoms they should report to the doctor (such as weight gain, increased abdominal girth, respiratory difficulty, scrotal edema, and abdominal discomfort).
• Remind the patient of follow-up appointment dates and times.

PARATHYROIDECTOMY

Parathyroidectomy is the surgical removal of one or more of the four parathyroid glands located at the back of the thyroid gland. It is performed to treat parathyroid cancer or primary hyperparathyroidism.

The parathyroid glands release parathyroid hormone (PTH), which contributes to calcium metabolism. In primary hyperparathyroidism and most parathyroid cancers, the glands secrete excessive PTH, causing high serum calcium and, often, low serum phosphorus levels.

How many of the glands are removed depends on the underlying cause of excessive PTH secretion. For example, if the patient has a single adenoma, excision of the affected gland corrects the problem. However, if more than one gland is enlarged, subtotal parathyroidectomy (removal of the three largest glands and part of the fourth gland) can correct the hyperparathyroidism. The surgeon usually tries to leave some glandular tissue to prevent postoperative hypocalcemia.

Purpose
• To remove diseased parathyroid tissue, decreasing circulating levels of PTH and serum calcium.

Indications
Parathyroidectomy is indicated in the treatment of primary hyperparathyroidism. Total parathyroidectomy and radical excision of all abnormal adjacent tissue is necessary in parathyroid cancer. The surgeon may also perform a subtotal thyroidectomy if he is unable to locate the abnormal tissue or adenoma and he suspects an intrathyroid lesion.

Patients who undergo total parathyroidectomy may require treatment for hypoparathyroidism.

Procedure
With the patient under general anesthesia, the surgeon makes a neck incision and exposes the thyroid gland. He then locates the four parathyroid glands, identifies and tags them, examines all four glands for hyperplasia, and removes the affected ones. The surgery may be extended to the thyroid gland, or further studies may be needed and a second surgery performed if the doctor is unable to locate the abnormal tissue or all the parathyroid glands. Some surgeons may insert a Penrose drain or a closed wound drainage device before closing the incision and applying a dressing.

Complications
Complications are rare but include hemorrhage, damage to the recurrent laryngeal nerves, respiratory problems, and hypoparathyroidism. A complication known as "hungry bone syndrome" is associated with hypocalcemia and can occur within 48 hours after surgery in patients with significant bone disease. In this complication, bone rapidly remineralizes by drawing calcium from the serum.

Care considerations
Before surgery
• Explain the surgical procedure, and tell the patient he will be intubated and will receive a general anesthetic.
• Inform the patient that a subtotal thyroidectomy or a second surgery may be necessary if the surgeon can't find the diseased parathyroid tissue or all of the glands.
• Maintain calcium restrictions, as ordered.
• Provide plenty of fluids to dilute excess calcium.
• If the patient's hypercalcemia is severe, give him 0.9% sodium chloride solution with potassium I.V., as ordered, and expect to administer a diuretic such as furosemide. If the calcium level remains elevated after diuresis has begun, expect to give plicamycin (an antihypercalcemic agent), as prescribed. As an adjunct, the doctor may also order inorganic phosphates, which appear to lower serum calcium levels by promoting calcium deposition in bone.

After surgery

• Keep the patient in high Fowler's position after surgery to promote venous return from the head and neck and to decrease oozing from the incision. Check the patient's dressing, and palpate the back of his neck, where drainage tends to flow. Expect about 50 ml of drainage in the first 24 hours. If a Penrose drain is in place but no drainage is evident, check for kinking of the drain; if a closed wound drainage device is in place, reestablish suction. Expect only scant drainage after 24 hours.

• Keep a tracheotomy tray at the patient's bedside for the first 24 hours after surgery, and assess the patient frequently for signs of respiratory distress, such as dyspnea and cyanosis, which may signal upper airway obstruction.

• Give mild analgesics, as prescribed, to relieve pain.

• Obtain serum calcium levels, as ordered. Serum calcium typically declines to slightly below normal by the 3rd day, then normalizes within 4 to 5 days.

• Watch closely for signs of increased neuromuscular excitability from hypoparathyroidism and associated hypocalcemia.

• Tell the patient to report numbness and tingling of his fingers, toes, and around his mouth (early signs of hypocalcemia) as well as muscle cramps. Check for positive Chvostek's and Trousseau's signs, which can signal tetany. Keep I.V. calcium on hand in case of tetany.

• Assess the patient for hoarseness and other voice changes, which can indicate damage to the recurrent laryngeal nerves, a rare complication.

Home care instructions

• Tell the patient to keep his incision site clean and dry, and explain that it will need to be checked in follow-up appointments.

• Explain the need for periodic serum calcium determinations to help evaluate the outcome of surgery.

• Advise the patient to avoid taking over-the-counter drugs without his doctor's approval. Tell him to avoid magnesium-containing laxatives and antacids, mineral oil, and vitamins A and D; these may affect calcium absorption or blood levels.

• Instruct the patient who has had a total parathyroidectomy to follow a high-calcium diet, as ordered, and to take calcium and other medications, as prescribed.

PARENTERAL NUTRITION

Parenteral nutrition refers to the administration of a nutrient solution containing dextrose, amino acids, fats, electrolytes, vitamins, micronutrients, and water through a catheter inserted in a central or a peripheral vein.

Total parenteral nutrition (TPN), sometimes called hyperalimentation, is administered through a central venous line. It can be used to meet nutritional needs for a prolonged period and may be used as a preventive therapeutic measure. TPN provides 2,000 to 5,000 calories daily and is used to replace nutrients in markedly malnourished and severely catabolic patients.

Direct central lines carry a risk of pneumothorax but offer several advantages over peripheral lines: they're easily dressed and don't restrict activity; they permit the administration of any type of solution, regardless of osmolarity (density); and they eliminate the need for repeated venipuncture.

Peripheral parenteral nutrition (PPN) is administered through a peripheral line and supplies 1,400 to 2,000 calories daily. It is usually used for nutritional maintenance in patients who have had nothing by mouth for more than 3 days and who are not expected to eat again for the next 10 to 14 days. PPN supplies the patient's full caloric needs without the risks associated with central venous access. Peripheral administration can be used only for isotonic or slightly hypertonic solutions. Because this limits what can be added to the solution, PPN cannot meet full nutritional needs.

The type of solution used depends on the patient's needs and clinical status. TPN solutions are hypertonic, with an osmolarity of 1,800 to 2,400 mOsm/liter. Electrolytes, vitamins, micronutrients, and water added to the base solution help satisfy daily requirements. Lipids may be given as a separate solution with dextrose and amino acids. PPN solutions have a lower tonicity than TPN solutions; therefore, the patient receiving PPN must be able to tolerate large volumes of fluid.

Purpose
• To provide essential nutrients for patients who cannot take food via the GI tract
• To provide supplemental nutrients for patients with protein-wasting conditions.

Indications
Parenteral nutrition can be used for certain patients, such as those with severe Crohn's disease, intestinal fistulas, short-bowel syndrome, or ulcerative colitis, in whom GI feeding is contraindicated or ineffective. It's also used to provide supplemental nutrition in malnourished and comatose patients and in those with burns, trauma, or cancer.

Procedure
The central venous catheter is inserted into a large vein by the doctor, either at the bedside or in the operating room. The peripheral venous catheter, which is inserted into a peripheral vein, may be inserted by a specially trained nurse.

Meticulous care of the insertion site (using sterile technique), especially of the central venous catheter, is important to prevent infection.

The solution is connected to an I.V. line and then infused using an infusion pump. The catheter may be flushed with a 0.9% sodium chloride and heparin solution before and after administration to help ensure patency. The infusion pump allows careful monitoring of the flow rate of the solution. The infusion begins at a slow rate, is gradually increased, and then is slowly tapered to discontinue. Parenteral nutrition may be given around the clock or as a nighttime feeding to allow greater freedom of movement during the day.

Complications
Parenteral nutrition can cause potentially severe complications, such as infection, hyperglycemia, and hypokalemia (see *Dealing with TPN hazards*, pages 498 and 499). Most complications can be prevented by careful monitoring of the catheter insertion site, infusion rate, and laboratory studies.

Care considerations
Before the procedure
• Explain the procedure, and give the patient an opportunity to express his concerns. Be alert for signs of depression or resistance to parenteral nutrition, especially in a patient who requires long-term therapy.
• Remove the hyperalimentation solution from the refrigerator, and allow it to stand for at least 30 minutes to reach room temperature. Compare the label with the doctor's orders. Check the container for cracks, and inspect the solution for cloudiness, turbidity, or particles.
During the procedure
• Check the infusion rate, catheter integrity, connections, and dressings. The catheter may have several connection
(Text continues on page 500.)

Dealing with TPN hazards

Complications of total parenteral nutrition (TPN) can result from catheter-related, metabolic, or mechanical problems. To help you identify and treat these common complications, use this chart.

COMPLICATION	SIGNS AND SYMPTOMS	INTERVENTIONS
Catheter-related complications		
Cracked or broken tubing	Fluid leaking out of the tubing	• Apply a padded hemostat above the break to prevent air from entering the line.
Dislodged catheter	Catheter out of the vein	• Place a sterile gauze pad on the insertion site and apply pressure.
Pneumothorax and hydrothorax	Dyspnea, chest pain, cyanosis, decreased breath sounds	• Suction patient. • Chest tube will be inserted.
Sepsis	Fever, chills, leukocytosis, erythema or pus at insertion site	• Remove catheter and culture tip. • Give appropriate antibiotics.
Metabolic complications		
Hepatic dysfunction	Increased serum transaminase, lactate dehydrogenase, and bilirubin levels	• Use special hepatic formulations. • Decrease carbohydrate and add I.V. lipids.
Hyperglycemia	Fatigue, restlessness, confusion, anxiety, weakness, and (in severe cases) delirium or coma; polyuria; dehydration; elevated blood and urine glucose levels	• Start insulin therapy or adjust TPN flow rate.
Hyperosmolar non-ketotic syndrome	Confusion, lethargy, seizures, coma, hyperglycemia, dehydration, glycosuria	• Stop dextrose. • Give insulin and 0.45% sodium chloride solution to rehydrate.
Hypocalcemia	Polyuria, dehydration, elevated blood and urine glucose levels	• Increase calcium supplementation.
Hypoglycemia	Sweating, shaking, irritability after infusion ends	• Infuse dextrose 10% solution.
Hypokalemia	Muscle weakness, paralysis, paresthesia, arrhythmias	• Increase potassium supplementation.

Dealing with TPN hazards *(continued)*

COMPLICATION	SIGNS AND SYMPTOMS	INTERVENTIONS
Metabolic complications *(continued)*		
Hypomagnesemia	Tingling around mouth, paresthesia in fingers, mental changes, hyperreflexia	• Increase magnesium supplementation.
Hypophosphatemia	Irritability, weakness, paresthesia, coma, respiratory arrest	• Increase phosphate supplementation.
Metabolic acidosis	Increased serum chloride level, decreased serum bicarbonate level	• Use acetate or lactate salts of sodium or hydrogen.
Mechanical complications		
Air embolism	Apprehension, chest pain, tachycardia, hypotension, cyanosis, seizure, loss of consciousness, cardiac arrest	• Clamp catheter. • Place patient in the Trendelenburg position on left side. • Give oxygen, as ordered. • If cardiac arrest occurs, initiate cardiopulmonary resuscitation.
Clotted catheter	Interrupted flow, hypoglycemia	• Reposition catheter. Attempt to aspirate clot. • If unsuccessful, instill urokinase to clear catheter lumen, as ordered.
Extravasation	Swelling of tissue around the insertion site, pain	• Stop I.V. infusion. • Assess patient for cardiopulmonary abnormalities. • Chest X-ray may be performed.
Phlebitis	Pain, tenderness, redness, warmth	• Apply gentle heat to the insertion site. • Elevate the insertion site.
Rapid infusion	Nausea, headache, lethargy	• Check the infusion rate. • Check the infusion pump.
Thrombosis	Erythema and edema at the insertion site; ipsilateral swelling of arm, neck, and face; pain at the insertion site and along vein; malaise; fever; tachycardia	• Remove catheter promptly. • Administer heparin, if ordered. • Venous flow studies may be done.

sites, which may need to be taped to avoid accidental disconnection.
• Carefully record the patient's intake and output.
• Monitor results of laboratory studies carefully.

After the procedure
• Weigh the patient every day at the same time, using the same scale, and with the patient wearing the same type of clothing.
• Watch for edema, and report it to the doctor promptly.
• Change the I.V. tubing and dressings every 2 to 3 days. When changing the dressing, inspect the catheter insertion site and report any redness, swelling, discharge, or drainage.
• To prevent oral lesions and parotitis, have the patient brush his teeth and tongue frequently and use mouthwash and lip balm, as necessary.

Home care instructions

• Remind the patient that the suture at the catheter site will need to be removed at a follow-up visit when the site is healed.
• If parenteral nutrition will be continued at home, observe the patient's family caregivers in the hospital as they demonstrate the procedure for administering it.
• Explain correct storage and refrigeration of the hyperalimentation solution. Point out that each bag has an expiration date. Tell the patient or caregiver to check the solution's date, composition, and appearance and then, if the solution is suitable for use, to allow it to warm to room temperature before using it. For most patients, the solution will be delivered daily or will have to be picked up from a local pharmacy.
• Tell family caregivers to change the patient's dressing whenever it becomes soiled or loose, at least once a week (for transparent polyurethane dressings) or every other day (for gauze dressings). Teach them to use aseptic technique when changing the dressing.

• Instruct the patient or family caregivers to inspect the catheter insertion site regularly for swelling, redness, or drainage. If the patient must inspect his own dressing, suggest that he use a mirror.
• Demonstrate how to irrigate the catheter. Long-term venous access devices must be heparinized to remain patent; Silastic atrial catheters may require daily irrigation with a heparin and 0.9% sodium chloride solution, depending on the hyperalimentation solution used and the frequency of administration. Implanted infusion ports must be flushed with a heparin and 0.9% sodium chloride solution every 4 weeks. In addition, the catheter should be irrigated with this solution after every infusion to clear the lumen of residual hyperalimentation solution.
• Explain to the patient and family that the patient should be weighed daily at the same time, on the same scale, and while wearing similar clothing.
• Show the patient and family how to check urine glucose levels and how to monitor intake and output. Warn them to watch for swelling of extremities, which indicates electrolyte imbalances, and to be alert for signs of infection.
• Review the potential complications of parenteral nutrition. Advise the patient to keep the telephone numbers of his local police and fire department, ambulance company, hospital, and doctor within easy reach.
• Patients infusing parenteral nutrition at home should have a home health care nurse visit for at least the 1st week to be sure that the home infusions are being administered correctly. The home environment, especially the area where the equipment is stored, should be checked for sanitary conditions.
• Provide written instructions and information about complications.

PAROTIDECTOMY

Parotidectomy is the surgical excision of the parotid gland. A parotidectomy may be total or superficial, depending on the extent of parotid involvement. Total parotidectomy is performed when infection or tumor involves the deep lobe of the parotid gland; superficial parotidectomy, when only the superficial lobe is involved. Although superficial parotidectomy is not necessary when disease is localized to the deep lobe, removal of the superficial lobe allows easier identification of the facial nerve.

Purpose

• To eliminate recurrent infection of the parotid gland
• To prevent the formation of fistulas or abscesses in chronic parotitis
• To remove tumors involving the parotid gland.

Indications

Parotidectomy is indicated in chronic parotitis unresponsive to medical therapy, when a mass or lesion is present in the parotid gland, when there is metastasis or a chance of metastasis to the parotid gland, or if a parotid duct stone is present.

Procedure

The surgeon makes an incision where the helix of the pinna attaches to the side of the face and extends the incision to the neck. A flap is carefully dissected, and the facial nerve is identified. The affected parotid gland and tissue are removed. The facial nerve and its branches are examined for integrity and are stimulated by a nerve stimulator to confirm function. A drain is inserted during surgery to remove excess fluid and prevent hematoma, and a pressure dressing is applied.

Complications

Potential postoperative complications include facial nerve paralysis, salivary fistula, hematoma, and infection. A potentially serious complication is the complete loss of function of all the branches of the facial nerve.

The most common long-term complication is gustatory sweating, known as Frey's syndrome.

Care considerations

Before surgery

• Describe the operative procedure and postoperative course, and answer the patient's questions.
• In patients with chronic parotitis, administer antibiotics, as prescribed.
• Check that the patient has signed a consent form.

After surgery

• Expect the patient to be hospitalized for 1 to 3 days after the procedure.
• Monitor vital signs for indications of hemorrhage or infection.
• Assess for facial nerve damage. Signs of damage include inability to smile, wink, or drink fluids.
• Check the pressure dressing for drainage. If it becomes saturated, reinforce the dressing and notify the doctor at once. The drain is usually removed on the 1st postoperative day, and the doctor then changes the pressure dressing. The new pressure dressing will be in place for 24 to 48 hours after the drain has been removed.
• Administer analgesics to control pain.

Home care instructions

• If appropriate, instruct the patient to remove the dressing at home (usually 24 hours after the drain has been removed).
• Instruct the patient to clean the suture line with hydrogen peroxide and cotton-tipped applicators twice a day.
• Teach the importance of taking prescribed antibiotics.

• Inform the patient that a follow-up appointment is necessary 5 to 7 days after surgery for removal of sutures.
• Instruct the patient not to wash his hair until after the sutures are removed and the doctor gives permission.
• Explain that the patient may notice some numbness in the cheek and ear (on the surgical side). The numbness may last for 3 to 6 months. Instruct the patient to cover his face and ear in frigid weather to prevent frostbite because he may not feel the cold.

PATIENT-CONTROLLED ANALGESIA

Patient-controlled analgesia (PCA) is a method of self-administering medication, commonly via the I.V. route, to provide optimal pain control. Delayed or inadequate administration of analgesics can cause unrelieved pain to escalate and become difficult to control. By allowing the patient who is experiencing pain to control administration of analgesics, PCA avoids delayed treatment and decreases the patient's anxiety.

Purpose
• To achieve satisfactory control of pain.

Indications
PCA is effective in the management of both chronic and acute pain syndromes. It is commonly used postoperatively, after trauma, and in terminal cancer. The primary consideration for PCA is the patient's ability to understand directions and learn how to use the PCA pump.

Procedure
PCA therapy is ordered by the doctor and initiated by the nurse. The nurse selects an appropriate PCA pump. (See *Types of PCA systems.*) The PCA pump is programmed to deliver a preset bolus

of analgesia when the patient presses a button. The pump can be programmed with a lock-out time (in minutes) to place a safe limit on the time between boluses and to monitor the number of times the button is pushed. Certain pumps can deliver a continuous infusion of analgesia with boluses, as required.

Complications
Complications are rare but can be related to adverse reactions to the analgesic drug, errors in programming the pump, or pump malfunction.

Care considerations
Before therapy
• Check for a history of allergy to the analgesic.
• Determine the availability of the pump and the drug, and review refill requirements.
• Instruct the patient or caregiver about pain management, use of the pump, and management of adverse reactions. Explain that the patient should take enough analgesic to relieve acute pain but not enough to induce drowsiness. Have the patient practice with a sample device.
• Check the doctor's order. It should specify a loading dose, the appropriate lock-out interval, the maintenance dose, the amount of analgesic the patient will receive when he activates the device, and the maximum amount the patient can receive within a specified time.
During therapy
• Program the pump.
• Observe the patient for changes in levels of sedation. Monitor his respirations, assess him for constipation and nausea, and check for infiltration of I.V. infusions and for catheter occlusion.
• Document accurately the number of boluses required and any attempted boluses for which no analgesia was administered. Use this information when making analgesia adjustments.

Types of PCA systems

The accompanying illustrations show commonly used patient-controlled analgesia (PCA) devices.

The first device is a reusable, battery-operated pump that delivers a drug dose when the patient presses a call button at the end of a cord.

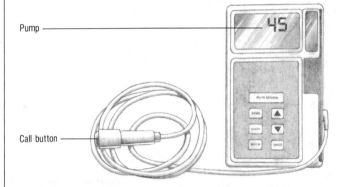

Pump ————

Call button ————

The other device is disposable and mechanically operated. It contains an infusor and a unit that's worn like a wristwatch. The patient pushes a button on the device to receive the analgesic from a collapsible chamber.

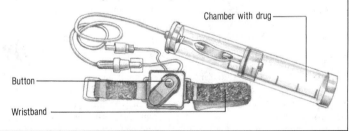

Chamber with drug ————

Button ————

Wristband ————

• Assess pain control as described by the patient, and adjust analgesia as necessary. If the patient reports insufficient relief of pain, notify the doctor.

Home care instructions

• Locate a local resource for problem solving and continuity of care.
• Make certain that patients on home PCA have caregiver and professional support available.
• Because the cost of PCA can be considerable, resolve potential financial or reimbursement problems before initiating home therapy.

• Establish I.V. access. Teach the patient and family caregiver appropriate methods to reestablish access.
• Teach the patient and family caregiver to recognize I.V. site complications and adverse effects of analgesia. Explain how to use and program the pump, as well as principles of pain management.
• Offer the patient referral to community resources, as needed.

Pediculicides

The topical drugs *lindane, crotamiton, pyrethrins,* and *permethrin* are available in various forms, including shampoos, creams, lotions, gels, and topical solutions. Typically, treatment with pediculicides requires two applications: the first eradicates adult lice; the second, given about 10 days later, kills newly hatched lice.

Purpose
• To eradicate infestations of lice.

Indications
Pediculicides are indicated in the treatment of infestations of head, body, or pubic lice.

Pediculicides are generally safe, causing only local stinging and burning. Occasionally, they cause a severe rash. However, they should be applied cautiously, especially in children, because systemic absorption can cause central nervous system (CNS) reactions.

Adverse reactions
All pediculicides may cause itching, irritation, mild erythema, rash, or hypersensitivity reactions; a local burning sensation is common.

Lindane penetrates human skin and causes systemic reactions. These include adverse CNS reactions ranging from dizziness to seizures. These neurotoxicities are more severe in young patients and after repeated use.

Pyrethrins, although poorly absorbed through the skin, can cause sneezing, sinusitis, wheezing, vomiting, respiratory distress, and paralysis if inhaled.

Care considerations
• When treating patients for lice infestation, watch for local and systemic reactions and assess the effectiveness of therapy.

• Although the patient's skin may be irritated by the lice infestation itself, be alert for any new rashes that occur after treatment, and report them to the doctor; they may require treatment with topical corticosteroids.
• Check the patient's skin and scalp for lice and nits. Also check other family members because transmission is common.
• When using preparations containing lindane, watch for signs of systemic absorption and CNS toxicity, especially in young patients. Dizziness, muscle cramps, irritability, tachycardia, vomiting, and seizures are common signs of CNS toxicity.
• When using pyrethrins, watch for signs of respiratory distress caused by inadvertent inhalation of the drug.

Home care instructions
• Because pediculicides are usually applied at home, provide thorough directions for their use. Keep in mind that the method of application depends on the product used.
• If the patient is using lindane shampoo, tell him to apply it to dry hair, rub it in thoroughly, and leave it in place for 4 minutes. Then he should apply a little water, work the shampoo into a lather, and rinse his hair thoroughly. Afterward, he should use a fine-tooth comb to remove nits and nit shells.
• Depending on the type of infestation, pyrethrins may be applied to the scalp, body, or pubic area. If using a gel or solution form, the patient should first wash the affected area with warm water and soap or regular shampoo; if using a shampoo, he should apply it to dry hair and work it into a lather using a small amount of water. The patient should leave all forms of pyrethrins on the affected area for 10 minutes and then rinse thoroughly. Afterward, he should comb his hair with a fine-tooth comb.
• No matter which pediculicide is used, instruct the patient to apply it again

after 7 to 10 days to kill any newly hatched lice.

• Warn the patient never to apply pediculicides on broken skin, the face (especially the eyes), mucous membranes, or the urethral meatus.

• Briefly describe the signs of CNS toxicity, and advise the patient to notify the doctor immediately if any occur.

• Advise the patient not to use lindane during or immediately after a bath or shower and that pyrethrins should be applied in a well-ventilated area.

• Tell the patient to wash the medication off if a rash or an irritation develops during application and to notify the doctor. Inform the patient that pruritus may persist for several weeks after successful treatment and may be treated with topical corticosteroids.

• Tell the patient how to prevent reinfestation: to clean the house thoroughly, vacuuming upholstered furniture, rugs, and floors; to wash all recently worn clothing, bed linens, and towels in hot water or have them dry-cleaned; and to wash hair brushes and combs in hot, soapy water for 5 to 10 minutes. Emphasize that hats, combs, and brushes should never be shared.

• If the patient is undergoing treatment for pubic lice, explain that the toilet seat should be scrubbed frequently and that sexual partners must receive concurrent treatment.

PENICILLINS

Because of their effectiveness, low toxicity, and minimal cost, penicillins are among the most widely used antimicrobial agents. They consist of extracts and semisynthetic derivatives of several strains of Penicillium mold. Penicillin derivatives differ in their spectrum of antimicrobial activity, gastric acid stability, degree of protein binding, and resistance to inactivation by penicillinases.

Choice of a specific penicillin can be complicated because a previously susceptible organism sometimes develops resistance. For example, staphylococci have become resistant to penicillin G even though other bacteria, such as streptococci, remain susceptible to it.

Purpose

• To combat bacterial infection by interfering with the formation of bacterial cell walls, causing lysis and cell death

• To provide prophylaxis before invasive procedures.

Indications

Penicillins effectively treat bacterial infections such as streptococcal pharyngitis, pneumococcal pneumonia, gas gangrene, gonorrhea, syphilis, tetanus, and cellulitis. (See *Comparing penicillins*, pages 506 and 507.)

Penicillins are contraindicated in any patient with a previous anaphylactic reaction to penicillin or a cephalosporin (because of possible cross-allergenicity). However, a negative history doesn't rule out the possibility of a future allergic reaction.

Adverse reactions

Hypersensitivity, the major adverse reaction, occurs with both natural extracts and semisynthetic derivatives and most commonly affects patients with asthma or a history of allergies. This reaction ranges in severity from a rash and pruritus to serum sickness and anaphylaxis.

GI reactions are more common and can follow use of oral and other routes of administration. GI reactions include sore mouth or tongue, furry tongue, vomiting, cramping, mild diarrhea, or such severe reactions as pseudomembranous colitis.

Comparing penicillins

DRUG AND ROUTE	INDICATIONS	SPECIAL CONSIDERATIONS
Natural penicillins		
penicillin G benzathine P.O. **penicillin G potassium** P.O., I.M., I.V. **penicillin G procaine** I.M. **penicillin G sodium** I.M., I.V. **penicillin V** P.O.	Infections caused by various organisms, including gram-positive, aerobic, and anaerobic bacteria	• Contraindicated in patients with a history of severe hypersensitivity reactions to penicillins or cephalosporins; use cautiously in patients with allergies, colitis (antibiotics can cause pseudomembranous colitis), or renal impairment. • Notify the doctor if a hypersensitivity reaction develops. • Expect false-positive reactions on copper sulfate urine glucose tests. • Oral form can cause nausea, vomiting, and diarrhea. • For best absorption, tell the patient to take penicillin G 1 hour before or 2 hours after meals; he should avoid taking it with fruit juice because acidic fluids inactivate the drug. • Penicillin V is better absorbed orally and is not greatly affected by food or acid. • Concurrent use of allopurinol increases the incidence of rashes; probenecid raises blood levels of penicillins.
Aminopenicillins		
amoxicillin P.O. **ampicillin** P.O., I.M., I.V. **ampicillin/ sulbactam sodium** I.M., I.V. **amoxicillin/ clavulanic acid** P.O. **bacampicillin** P.O.	Infections caused by gram-positive and gram-negative bacteria *(Haemophilus influenzae, Proteus mirabilis, Salmonella, Shigella,* and most strains of *Escherichia coli);* especially useful in treating upper respiratory tract infections	• Contraindicated in patients with a history of severe hypersensitivity reactions to penicillins or cephalosporins; use cautiously in patients with allergies, colitis, infectious mononucleosis, or renal impairment. • Notify the doctor of any hypersensitivity reaction. • For best absorption, tell the patient to take the drug on an empty stomach; amoxicillin and bacampicillin can be taken without regard to meals. • Expect false-positive reactions on copper sulfate urine glucose tests. • Concurrent use of allopurinol may cause a rash; probenecid raises blood levels of penicillins and is often used for this purpose. • A generalized maculopapular rash may occur in about 10% of patients taking ampicillin after 7 to 10 days; this occurs more frequently in patients taking allopurinol, those with infectious mononucleosis or lymphatic leukemia, and is not an allergic reaction.

Comparing penicillins *(continued)*

DRUG AND ROUTE	INDICATIONS	SPECIAL CONSIDERATIONS
Penicillinase-resistant penicillins		
cloxacillin P.O. **dicloxacillin** P.O. **methicillin** I.M., I.V. **nafcillin** P.O., I.M., I.V. **oxacillin** P.O., I.M., I.V.	Systemic infections caused by penicil-linase-producing staphylococci	• Contraindicated in patients with a history of severe hypersensitivity reactions to peni-cillins or cephalosporins; use cautiously in patients with allergies or colitis. • Notify the doctor if a hypersensitivity reac-tion develops. • For best absorption, give oral form of the drug on an empty stomach. • During therapy with oxacillin, monitor for elevated hepatic enzyme levels. • During therapy with methicillin, monitor renal function for signs of acute interstitial nephritis. • Probenecid increases penicillin blood levels and is often used for this purpose.
Extended-spectrum penicillins		
carbenicillin indanyl sodium P.O. **mezlocillin** I.M., I.V. **piperacillin** I.M., I.V. **ticarcillin disodium** I.M., I.V. **ticarcillin/ clavulanic acid** I.V.	Systemic infections caused by suscep-tible gram-positive and gram-negative organisms; carbeni-cillin indanyl so-dium is only used to treat urinary tract infections	• Contraindicated in patients with a history of severe hypersensitivity reactions; use cautiously in patients with allergies or coli-tis or in those on sodium-restricted diets. • Dosage modifications may be necessary for patients with renal impairment to prevent further nephrotoxicity. • Monitor intake and output. • Monitor complete blood count because these drugs may cause thrombocytopenia. • Contact the doctor if a hypersensitivity re-action develops. • Ticarcillin disodium contains large amounts of sodium; monitor serum potassium levels, which may fall because of increased sodium. • Give carbenicillin indanyl sodium on an empty stomach to promote absorption.

Electrolyte abnormalities can occur with high doses of either sodium or potassium salts of penicillins.

Higher doses of penicillins, espe-cially in patients with renal disease, have been associated with signs of cen-tral nervous system toxicity: lethargy, irritability, hallucinations, and sei-zures.

Care considerations

• Always keep epinephrine and other emergency resuscitation supplies available when giving penicillins.
• Watch for signs of hypersensitivity, such as rash or pruritus, which may develop within 20 minutes (or some-times after several days). Be especially alert for signs of anaphylaxis, such as

dyspnea, choking, precipitous hypotension, thready pulse, anxiety, weakness, sweating, and dizziness. Report such signs to the doctor immediately. Check the patient's blood pressure regularly, and prepare to give I.V. fluids for hypotension.

• Review the patient's medications for possible interactions. Concurrent use of antacids reduces the effectiveness of penicillin by decreasing its absorption from the GI tract. Erythromycins, tetracyclines, acidifying drugs (such as ammonium chloride), and acidic foods reduce oral penicillin's effectiveness. Aspirin and phenylbutazone raise serum levels of penicillin by reducing plasma protein binding; probenecid also raises serum penicillin levels and is commonly used for this purpose.

• If the patient receives penicillin for a prolonged period, observe for superinfection. This occurs most commonly in elderly, debilitated, or immunosuppressed patients.

Home care instructions

• Instruct the patient to call the doctor if he experiences a rash, hives, itching, or wheezing.

• If the patient has a history of severe penicillin reaction, stress the importance of wearing a medical identification bracelet or necklace. If the patient carries an anaphylaxis kit, review with him instructions for using it.

• Emphasize the importance of completing the full course of penicillin even if he feels better. Explain that residual organisms can cause a relapse.

• If the patient misses a dose, instruct him to take it as soon as possible. Then he should space the remaining daily doses closer together to make up for the missed dose. Penicillins are most effective if a constant serum concentration is maintained.

• Tell the patient to avoid orange juice, other acidic juices, and vitamin C supplements while taking oral penicillin; they reduce the drug's effectiveness.

• Tell the patient who develops diarrhea to check with his doctor or pharmacist before taking any antidiarrheal medication. Antiperistaltic antidiarrheals aren't recommended because they can delay elimination of toxins.

• Tell the patient to call his doctor if symptoms don't improve within a few days.

PENILE PROSTHESES

A penile prosthesis consists of a pair of semirigid rods or inflatable cylinders surgically implanted in the corpora cavernosa of the penis. These devices are the most common therapeutic intervention for impotence unresponsive to any other treatment.

Of the two types of penile prostheses, the semirigid device costs less, allows easier implantation, and is less likely to require additional surgery to correct mechanical problems. This device is especially beneficial for the patient with limited hand or finger function because its use doesn't demand manual dexterity. Its major disadvantage is continuous semierection, which may embarrass the patient. (More malleable models have been developed that can be bent into less conspicuous positions.) Some couples also complain that the semirigid prosthesis produces an erection that isn't sexually satisfying because penile girth does not increase.

The inflatable prosthesis more closely mimics a normal erection. The patient controls erection by squeezing a pump in the scrotum that releases radiopaque fluid from a reservoir into the implanted cylinders. He then presses the release valve to return fluid to the reservoir and thus lose the erection.

Purpose

• To correct erectile dysfunction by surgical implantation of a prosthetic device.

Indications

Penile prostheses are indicated for patients with impotence secondary to organic dysfunction. Causes of such dysfunction may include diabetes, arteriosclerosis, radical prostatectomy, spinal cord injury, or prolonged use of alcohol or drugs such as antihypertensives. Patients with impotence secondary to psychogenic dysfunction — including sexual performance anxiety, low self-esteem, and past failure at sustaining an erection — are usually referred for sexual counseling. Use of penile prostheses in such patients is controversial.

Procedure

Typically, the prosthesis is implanted in the operating room under general or spinal anesthesia. The semirigid device may also be implanted on an outpatient basis under local anesthesia.

To implant a semirigid prosthesis, the surgeon exposes the corpora cavernosum subcutaneously, opens each individually, and dilates a channel. The prostheses are then inserted into the prepared channels, and the incisions are closed.

To implant an inflatable prosthesis, the surgeon performs these same steps to position the cylinders. Then he makes an abdominal and a perineal incision and places a reservoir, filled with 60 ml of radiopaque fluid, through the external inguinal ring. Next, he places a pump in the lateral portion of the scrotum and connects the cylinders, reservoir, and pump with tubing. By squeezing the pump, he tests the function of the prosthesis. Some newer models exclude the suprapubic and scrotal extensions.

Complications

Complications following the implantation procedures include infection, erosion of the penis by the prosthesis, and persistent pain, which may necessitate removal of the implant.

Both types of prostheses place the patient at risk for infection, but the incidence is low (about 1% to 4%). The inflatable prosthesis may also leak fluid, or the tubing connecting the pump reservoir and cylinders may become kinked.

Care considerations

Before surgery

• Reinforce the surgeon's explanation of the implantation procedure, and answer any questions the patient or couple may have.

• Offer emotional support and reassurance. Encourage the patient and his partner to verbalize their feelings about how the implants may affect their relationship.

• Instruct the patient to shower the evening before and the morning of the surgery using an antimicrobial soap. Tell him that he'll be shaved in the operating room to reduce the risk of infection. If ordered, begin antibiotic therapy.

After surgery

• Monitor vital signs. Check the dressing for frank bleeding, and change it, as ordered. Inspect the suture line for redness, swelling, separation, or signs of infection. If a drain is present, record the amount and character of drainage.

• Apply ice packs to the patient's penis for 24 hours after surgery. Administer analgesics, as prescribed. Monitor urine output, and be alert for dysuria and urine retention.

• Warn the patient not to inflate the inflatable implant until his doctor tells him it is safe to do so.

Home care instructions

• Stress the importance of returning for all follow-up appointments to ensure that the incision is healing properly.

• Instruct the patient to wash the incision daily with an antimicrobial soap. Also instruct him to watch for signs of

infection and to report them immediately to his doctor.
• Tell the patient that scrotal swelling and discoloration may last up to 3 weeks.
• Remind the patient to pull the scrotal pump downward to ensure proper alignment.
• Warn the couple that they may experience dyspareunia when they're permitted to resume sexual activity — usually about 6 weeks after surgery. This may result from an inability to have intercourse for a prolonged period before surgery. Suggest use of a water-soluble jelly to minimize or avoid discomfort.

PERICARDIOCENTESIS

Pericardiocentesis is the needle aspiration of excess fluid from the pericardial sac.

Purpose
• To remove excessive pericardial fluid, thus relieving myocardial compression and increasing cardiac output
• To provide a sample of pericardial fluid for diagnosis.

Indications
Pericardiocentesis may be indicated in acute or chronic constrictive pericarditis. It may also be the treatment of choice for life-threatening cardiac tamponade (except when fluid accumulates rapidly, in which case immediate surgery is usually preferred).

Procedure
This procedure is typically performed by the doctor at the bedside in the critical care unit, with the nurse assisting. After the patient's skin at the insertion site has been shaved and cleaned with an antimicrobial soap, the doctor administers a local anesthetic at the puncture site. Next, he inserts the aspiration needle in one of three areas. Most common is the subxiphoid approach, with needle insertion in the angle between the left costal margin and the xiphoid process. This method avoids needle contact with the pleura and the coronary vessels and thus decreases the risk of damage to these structures. Alternative insertion sites include the fifth intercostal space next to the left side of the sternum, where the pericardium normally isn't covered by lung tissue, and the cardiac apex, which poses the greatest risk of complications (such as pneumothorax).

As the parietal pericardium is punctured, a gentle "pop" is usually felt. The doctor then very slowly and cautiously aspirates pericardial fluid. After the fluid has been withdrawn, the doctor removes the needle and places a dressing over the insertion site.

Complications
Pericardiocentesis carries some risk of potentially fatal complications, such as inadvertent puncture of internal organs (particularly the heart, lung, stomach, or liver), laceration of the myocardium or of a coronary artery, or initiation of ventricular arrhythmias.

Care considerations
Before the procedure
• Reinforce the doctor's explanation of the procedure. Offer emotional support and reassurance, and encourage the patient to verbalize his feelings. Administer tranquilizers or sedation, if ordered.
• Review the patient's coagulation profile to identify bleeding tendencies.
• Insert an I.V. line to provide access for medications. Have resuscitation equipment nearby in case of emergency.
• If necessary, shave the needle insertion site on the patient's chest. Clean the area with an antiseptic solution.
• Assist the patient to a supine position in bed, with his upper torso raised 45

to 60 degrees and his arms supported by pillows.

• Apply 12-lead electrocardiograph (ECG) electrodes. If ordered, assist the doctor in attaching the pericardial needle to the precordial lead (V) of the ECG and also to a three-way stopcock.

During the procedure

• Monitor the patient's blood pressure and central venous pressure (CVP), if appropriate.

• Administer oxygen, as ordered.

• Continuously observe ECG pattern for premature ventricular contractions and elevated ST segments, which may indicate that the needle has touched the ventricle; elevated PR segments, which may indicate that the needle has touched the atrium; and large, erratic QRS complexes, which may indicate that the needle has penetrated the heart.

• Monitor the patient for signs of organ puncture, such as hypotension, decreased breath sounds, chest pain, dyspnea, hematoma, and tachycardia.

• Note and record the volume and character of any aspirated fluid. Be aware that blood that has accumulated slowly in the patient's pericardial sac usually doesn't clot after it has been aspirated; blood from a sudden hemorrhage, however, will clot.

• Continue to offer emotional support and reassurance to the patient throughout the procedure.

After the procedure

• Monitor vital signs every 15 minutes for 1 hour, every 30 minutes for 2 hours, and then every 4 hours for 16 hours or until the patient is stable. Expect the patient's blood pressure to rise as tamponade is relieved. Be alert for rise in temperature, which may indicate possible infection.

• Maintain continuous ECG monitoring.

• Be alert for signs of recurring tamponade: decreased blood pressure, narrowing pulse pressure, increased CVP, tachycardia, muffled heart sounds, tachypnea, pleural friction rub, distended neck veins, anxiety, and chest pain. Notify the doctor of these signs immediately. Repeat pericardiocentesis or surgical drainage of the pericardium in the operating room may be necessary.

Home care instructions

• Tell the patient to notify the doctor immediately if chest pain, dyspnea, tachycardia, or palpitations recur.

• Stress the importance of keeping follow-up medical appointments.

PERITONEAL DIALYSIS

Peritoneal dialysis is a procedure in which a hypertonic dialysate is instilled through a catheter into the patient's peritoneal cavity. It uses the patient's peritoneal membrane as a semipermeable dialyzing membrane to filter out excess electrolytes, uremic toxins, water, and wastes from the blood. Peritoneal dialysis may be performed manually, by an automatic or semiautomatic cycler machine, or as continuous ambulatory peritoneal dialysis (CAPD). As its name implies, CAPD allows the patient to be out of bed and active during dialysis; it minimizes lifestyle disruption, as it does not require travel to a dialysis center.

Some patients use CAPD in combination with an automatic cycler, in a treatment called continuous-cycling peritoneal dialysis (CCPD). In CCPD, the cycler performs dialysis at night while the patient sleeps, and the patient performs CAPD in the daytime.

Peritoneal dialysis offers several advantages over hemodialysis, such as ease of performance, high safety margin, portability, and availability. Disadvantages may include patient immobilization, low efficiency, protein loss, and metabolic complications.

Purpose
• To remove toxic wastes from the blood.

Indications
Peritoneal dialysis may be indicated in the patient with chronic renal failure who doesn't respond to other treatments or when a less rapid treatment is needed. It is indicated for the patient with severe coagulopathy, cardiovascular disease, acute poisoning, hepatic coma, metabolic acidosis, or extensive burns with prerenal azotemia; in those with exhausted vascular access sites for hemodialysis, and in those who have religious objections to hemodialysis.

Contraindications for peritoneal dialysis include recent abdominal surgery, adhesions, scarring, infection, and the inability of the patient or his support persons to adequately perform the dialysis exchanges.

Procedure
Peritoneal dialysis may be performed in the operating room or at the bedside, with a nurse assisting. First, the surgeon administers a local anesthetic in a small area of the patient's abdomen below the umbilicus. After making a small incision, he inserts the catheter into the peritoneal cavity. The catheter is then secured in place and a dressing is applied. (See *Catheters for peritoneal dialysis*.)

In manual dialysis, the nurse, patient, or family member instills dialysate through the catheter inserted into the peritoneal cavity, allows it to dwell for a specified time, and then drains it from the peritoneal cavity. Typically, this process is repeated for 6 to 8 hours at a time, five or six times a week.

Peritoneal dialysis using a cycler machine requires sterile equipment and sterile connection technique. The nurse, patient, or family caregiver sets up and programs the machine to infuse the ordered volume of dialysate, allows the solution to dwell for the prescribed time, and then allows it to flow out. The cycle of infuse, dwell, and outflow is repeated (usually every half hour) for 8 to 10 hours per session.

CAPD can be performed by the patient himself. A special plastic bag is filled with dialysate, and then the solution is instilled through a catheter into the patient's peritoneal cavity. While the solution remains in the peritoneal cavity, the patient can roll up the empty bag, place it under his clothing, and go about his normal activities. After 6 to 8 hours of dwell time, the spent solution is drained into the bag. The full bag is removed and discarded. The patient then attaches a new bag of dialysate; he repeats the process four times a day to ensure continuous dialysis 24 hours a day, 7 days a week.

Complications
Peritoneal dialysis can cause severe complications. The most serious one, peritonitis, results from contamination of the peritoneal cavity by bacteria or fungi through the catheter or the insertion site. Other complications include catheter obstruction from proteinaceous debris, lodgment against the abdominal wall, or kinking; metabolic complications; hypotension; hypovolemia from excessive plasma fluid removal; and respiratory distress from upward pressure of the dialysate on the diaphragm.

Care considerations
Before the procedure
• For the first-time peritoneal dialysis patient, explain the purpose of the treatment and what to expect during and after the procedure. Explain that the surgeon will insert a catheter into his abdomen to allow instillation of dialysate; explain the appropriate insertion procedure.
• Before insertion of the catheter, measure and record the patient's baseline vital signs (be sure to check blood pressure in both the supine and standing positions), abdominal girth, and weight.

Catheters for peritoneal dialysis

The first step in any type of peritoneal dialysis is insertion of a catheter to allow instillation of dialysate. The surgeon may insert one of three different catheters, as described below.

Tenckhoff catheter
To implant a Tenckhoff catheter, the surgeon inserts the first 6¾" (17 cm) of the catheter into the patient's abdomen. The next 2¾" (7-cm) segment, which has a synthetic cuff at each end, is imbedded subcutaneously. Within a few days after insertion, the patient's tissues grow around these synthetic cuffs, forming a tight barrier against bacterial infiltration. The remaining 3⅞" (10 cm) of the catheter extends outside of the abdomen and is equipped with a metal adapter at the tip to allow connection to dialyzer tubing.

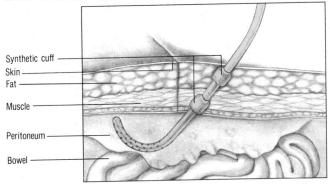

Gore-Tex catheter
To insert a Gore-Tex catheter, the surgeon positions its flanged collar just below the dermis so that the device extends through the abdominal wall. He keeps the distal end of the cuff from extending into the peritoneum, where it could cause adhesions.

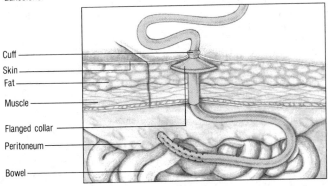

(continued)

Catheters for peritoneal dialysis *(continued)*

Column-disk peritoneal catheter

To insert a column-disk peritoneal catheter (CDPC), the surgeon rolls up the flexible disk section of the implant, inserts it into the peritoneal cavity, and retracts it against the abdominal wall. The implant's first cuff rests just outside the peritoneal membrane, and its second cuff rests just beneath the skin. Because the CDPC doesn't float freely in the peritoneal cavity, it keeps inflowing dialysate from being directed at sensitive organs; this increases patient comfort during dialysis.

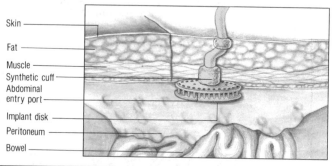

Review the patient's blood chemistry. Ask the patient to void to reduce the risk of bladder perforation and increase comfort during catheter insertion. Perform straight catheterization if necessary.

• Warm the dialysate to body temperature using a warmer, heating pad, or water bath. The dialysate may be a 1.5%, 2.5%, or 4.25% dextrose solution; heparin is often added to prevent clotting in the catheter. The bag's outer plastic wrap should be intact. Inspect the dialysate, which should be clear and colorless.

• Put on a surgical mask, and prepare the dialysis administration set. Add any prescribed medication to the dialysate at this time. Place the drainage bag below the patient to facilitate drainage by gravity, and connect the outflow tubing to it. Connect the dialysis infusion lines to the bags of dialysate, and hang the containers on a separate broad-based I.V. pole at the patient's bedside. Do not hang any other I.V. solutions on the same pole. Maintain sterile technique during preparation of the equipment to avoid introducing pathogens into the patient's peritoneal cavity.

• When the equipment and solution are ready, place the patient in a supine position and have him put on a surgical mask. Prime the tubing with solution, keeping the clamps closed, and connect one infusion line to the abdominal catheter.

• Test the catheter's patency: open the clamp on the infusion line and rapidly instill 500 ml of dialysate into the patient's peritoneal cavity. Immediately unclamp the outflow line and let fluid drain into the collection bag; outflow should be brisk.

• Warn the patient that he may feel cramping, shoulder aching, fullness in the abdomen or rectum, and aching in the penis, scrotum, or vagina during the dwell time. Encourage the patient to verbalize feelings and sensations experienced during the procedure. Offer emotional support and reassurance. If necessary, premedicate with analgesics, and make sure the patient maintains good body alignment to promote comfort.

During the procedure

• Open the clamps on the infusion lines, and infuse the prescribed amount of dialysate over 5 to 10 minutes. When the bag is empty, immediately close the clamps to prevent air from entering the tubing.

• Allow the solution to dwell in the peritoneal cavity for the ordered length of time so that excess water, electrolytes, and accumulated wastes can move from the blood through the peritoneal membrane and into the solution. At the completion of the ordered dwell time, open the outflow clamps and allow the solution to drain from the peritoneal cavity into the collection bag.

• If outflow is slow, reposition the patient and make sure that all outflow clamps are open. Check the lines to make sure that the direction of flow is with gravity. Lower the drainage bag or elevate the bed to increase the distance between the abdomen and the bag; this will increase gravitational force and enhance outflow.

• Repeat the cycle of infusion, dwell, and drainage, using new dialysate each time, until the ordered amount of solution has been instilled and the ordered number of cycles has been completed.

• Monitor blood pressure and respirations, as necessary. If respiratory distress occurs, drain the peritoneal cavity and notify the doctor.

• Observe the effluent (outflow or drainage solution), which is normally pink to bloody 24 hours after catheter insertion and then becomes progressively clear and yellow. Note the presence of fibrin, which may appear as clear or white strands in the effluent and may indicate the need for additional heparin.

• Examine the tubing and catheter dressing, noting any leakage around the insertion site.

After the procedure

• When dialysis is completed, put on sterile gloves and clamp the catheter with a small plastic clamp. Disconnect the inflow line from the catheter, taking care not to dislodge or pull on the catheter, and place a sterile protective cap over the catheter's distal end. Apply a dressing, as ordered, but do not put tape directly on the catheter. Change the dressing every 24 hours or as needed.

Home care instructions

• If the patient or a family member will perform CAPD or CCPD at home, make sure that they thoroughly understand the procedures and can perform them safely.

• Instruct the patient to wear a bracelet or carry a card that identifies him as a peritoneal dialysis patient. Instruct the patient and family to keep the phone number of the dialysis center on hand at all times in case of an emergency.

• Teach the patient to watch for and report signs of infection and fluid imbalance. Make sure he knows how to measure blood pressure, pulse, temperature, weight, and fluid intake and output to provide a record of response to treatment.

• Refer the patient and family to a dietitian to learn how to modify the patient's diet to adjust for nutritional imbalances resulting from peritoneal dialysis.

• Stress the importance of follow-up appointments with the doctor and dialysis team to evaluate the success of treatment and detect any problems.

• If possible, introduce the patient to other patients on peritoneal dialysis to help him develop a support system. As necessary, arrange for periodic visits by a home health care nurse to assess his adjustment to CAPD.

PHLEBOTOMY, THERAPEUTIC

Phlebotomy (sometimes called venesection) is the direct removal of blood from a patient's body. Historically, this therapy was known as bleeding and was among one of the earliest known medical treatments. For centuries, the widespread use of phlebotomy performed by crude blood-letting techniques was more detrimental than therapeutic. However, the removal of a safe volume (less than 15% of the total blood volume) of peripheral blood remains the treatment of choice for several clinical disorders, such as hemochromatosis.

Phlebotomy tends to be a long-term therapy. Note that one unit of whole blood or packed red blood cells (RBCs) normally contains 200 to 250 mg of iron, but patients with iron overload typically present with more than 20 g of accumulated iron. In such patients, reduction of iron stores usually requires 1 to 2 years of frequent (weekly) venesection. An initial fall in hemoglobin is usually seen, but in most cases erythropoiesis (production of erythrocytes, or RBCs) accelerates to keep pace with phlebotomy. After excess iron has been removed, a normal level is maintained with a one-unit phlebotomy every 3 to 4 months for the patient's lifetime.

Purpose

- To reduce the RBC mass and consequently reduce hematocrit levels
- To decrease blood viscosity
- To reduce circulating iron levels.

Indications

Repeated phlebotomy is the treatment of choice to reduce iron overload and maintain serum iron at a safe level. Hemochromatosis is the most common form of iron overload in the United States.

Another indication for phlebotomy is increased blood viscosity caused by the excessive production of RBCs. Polycythemia vera, a myeloproliferative stem cell disorder resulting in uncontrolled production of leukocytes, platelets, and RBCs, is the most common of these disorders. Phlebotomy may also be indicated in patients with chronic pulmonary insufficiency, cyanotic congenital heart disease, porphyria cutanea tarda, or hemoglobinopathy.

Aggressive phlebotomy is contraindicated in elderly patients and those with chronic lung disease. For these patients, cautious phlebotomies involving the removal of lesser blood volumes over a longer period of time are recommended.

Procedure

Phlebotomy is performed by qualified staff in the blood bank, on the nursing unit, or in the outpatient clinic. The procedure is performed under aseptic conditions. Skin preparation should include the use of povidone-iodine or an equally effective antiseptic.

The phlebotomist uses an integrally connected blood container and needle to reduce the risk of exposure to potentially hazardous body fluids. A polyvinyl chloride bag with a 16G needle, such as those used in allogeneic blood collection, is recommended. If venous access is poor, a smaller gauge needle can be used; however, the collection will take substantially longer and aspiration with a syringe may be required.

For small patients or those at high risk for adverse reactions, crystalloid or colloid solutions may be infused before or during phlebotomy. Use an in-line Y-connector or three-way stopcock if replacement fluids will be infused before or after the procedure. Simultaneous infusion of fluids will require a second venesection. The volume of blood being removed should be continuously monitored to ensure adequate flow and avoid hypovolemia caused by removal of an excessive volume of blood.

Complications

The most common complications of phlebotomy are vasovagal reactions (bradycardia, hypotension, fainting, seizures), local discomfort, and hematoma formation at the venesection site. Patients with active cardiopulmonary disease may have a more prolonged recovery from such reactions and therefore should be assessed and monitored closely.

Care considerations

Before the procedure

• Make sure the patient is well rested and has a clear understanding of the procedure to be performed.
• Encourage the patient to eat a balanced meal within a few hours of phlebotomy and to take additional oral fluids unless contraindicated.
• Check the medical order, which should specify the volume of blood to be removed and an acceptable hematocrit at which the procedure can be performed; it should also clearly state the type and volume of replacement solution, if any is indicated.
• Confirm that the patient has signed a consent form that includes a description of potential complications.
• Before performing the procedure, the phlebotomist should verify that the amount of blood to be removed will not exceed the patient's safe extracorporeal volume (less than 15% of total blood volume).
• Take and record vital signs, and test the hemoglobin or hematocrit immediately before each phlebotomy.

After the procedure

• Place a pressure dressing on the venesection site, and instruct the patient to leave it in place for 2 to 3 hours. Take and record vital signs before allowing the patient to rise. Liquids and a high-carbohydrate snack are recommended before the patient is released from care.
• If the patient meets all allogeneic blood donation criteria and the collection technique adheres to blood bank regulations, the unit can be used for transfusion to other patients. The bag must be labeled THERAPEUTIC PHLEBOTOMY. However, the recipient's apprehension about receiving blood from a patient rather than from a volunteer donor frequently discourages this practice.

Home care instructions

• Instruct the patient not to drink alcohol or perform prolonged or strenuous physical exercise until after eating the next balanced meal.
• Because of the potential risk of dizziness, advise the patient not to drive, operate heavy equipment, or work in other hazardous situations for several hours after phlebotomy.
• If the patient is released after phlebotomy, provide written instructions describing what to do in case of bleeding at the venesection site, dizziness, and other potential complications. Include the name and telephone number of a person who can be reached in case of emergency.
• Confirm the patient's next appointment date and time. Stress the importance of compliance and the long-term commitment required for successful phlebotomy therapy.

PLASMAPHERESIS

Plasmapheresis, also known as therapeutic plasma exchange (TPE), is the therapeutic removal of plasma from withdrawn blood and the reinfusion of formed blood elements.

Plasmapheresis techniques were first used routinely in the 1960s. Through this exchange treatment, from 50% to

90% of unwanted plasma factors can be removed. These factors may include autoantibodies, immune complexes, metabolites, or unknown mediators of disease.

The procedure can take up to 5 hours and may be performed as often as four times a week in acutely ill patients but is otherwise limited to about once every 2 weeks.

Purpose
• To remove disease mediators or toxic substances from circulating blood.

Indications
Plasmapheresis is indicated in renal disease, blood hyperviscosity, thrombotic thrombocytopenic purpura, and idiopathic thrombocytopenic purpura.

Plasmapheresis has several neurologic applications, such as in Guillain-Barré syndrome, multiple sclerosis, and especially myasthenia gravis. In myasthenia gravis, plasmapheresis removes circulating antiacetylcholine receptor antibodies. If successful, treatment may relieve symptoms for months, but results vary.

Plasmapheresis is used most commonly in patients with long-standing neuromuscular disease but may also be used to treat acute exacerbations.

Procedure
Plasmapheresis is performed under a doctor's supervision. It requires a specially trained technician or nurse to operate the cell separator and a primary nurse to monitor the patient and provide supportive care. It can be performed on an inpatient or outpatient basis.

During this treatment, blood is removed from the patient by antecubital or subclavian venous access and flows into a cell separator, where it's divided into plasma and formed elements.

The plasma is collected in a container for disposal, and the formed elements are mixed with a plasma replacement solution and returned to the patient through a vein.

In a newer method, automated pheresis, the plasma is separated out, filtered to remove a specific disease mediator, and then returned to the patient.

Whichever method is used, patients tend to do well if fluids are replaced to equal the amounts that were removed.

Complications
Plasmapheresis carries the risk of several complications. Such complications include infection around the venipuncture site, a hypersensitivity reaction to the ingredients of the replacement solution, and hypocalcemia from excessive binding of circulating calcium to the citrate solution used as an anticoagulant in the replacement solution. Hypomagnesemia can follow repeated plasmapheresis, producing severe muscle cramps, tetany, and paresthesia, plasmapheresis-induced electrolyte imbalances can cause arrhythmias. Additionally, because between 150 and 400 ml of the patient's blood is removed during treatment, the patient is at risk for hypotension and other complications of low blood volume, such as syncope. The patient with myasthenia gravis is at risk for symptoms of myasthenic crisis, such as dysphagia, ptosis, and diplopia, because of the removal of antibodies or antimyasthenic drugs from the blood. Rare life-threatening complications include hemolysis and embolism.

Care considerations
Before the procedure
• Explain the treatment and its purpose. Tell the patient that a needle will be inserted into one or both arms and that his blood will be pumped through a filtering machine, cleaned of harmful substances, and then returned to the body.
• Explain to the patient that the procedure may take up to 5 hours. Inform

him that, during treatment, frequent blood samples will be taken to monitor calcium and potassium levels and that blood pressure and heart rate will be checked regularly.

• Instruct the patient to report any paresthesia.

• Advise the patient to eat lightly before treatment and to drink milk before and during treatment to help reduce the risk of hypocalcemia.

• Tell the patient to void before the procedure because a full bladder may lead to mild hypotension as a result of fluid shift or vasovagal reaction.

• Take vital signs for a baseline. As ordered, apply electrocardiograph leads to monitor heart rate; also, obtain blood samples to determine baseline levels of hemoglobin, hematocrit, and other blood substances.

• If possible, give necessary medications after treatment to prevent their removal from the blood.

During the procedure

• If the patient doesn't have an I.V. line in place, perform one or more venipunctures in the antecubital veins, as ordered, to establish vascular access for blood withdrawal and reinfusion. Use large-bore needles to minimize resistance and prevent damage to blood cells. If venous access is not possible, the doctor may use subclavian catheters.

• Connect the patient to the cell separator, and begin treatment.

• As plasmapheresis begins, observe the patient closely for signs of a hypersensitivity reaction, such as respiratory distress, hives, diaphoresis, hypotension, or thready pulse. If any such signs occur, immediately notify the doctor, who will stop the procedure and provide emergency treatment.

• During plasmapheresis, monitor vital signs every 30 minutes. (Don't take blood pressure readings in the arm being used for blood withdrawal and reinfusion, however.) Pay particular attention to temperature; reinfusion of blood that

has cooled while in the cell separator can produce hypothermia.

• Report any serious arrhythmias, which can result from electrolyte imbalance or volume depletion.

• If the patient is undergoing plasmapheresis for unstable myasthenia gravis, keep emergency equipment on hand and monitor blood pressure and pulse. Observe for symptoms of myasthenic crisis (dysphagia, ptosis, and diplopia), which can be precipitated by this procedure.

• Monitor blood levels of calcium and potassium, and replace electrolytes, as ordered.

• Monitor intake and output to ensure adequate hydration.

• Watch for signs of circulatory compromise.

• Compare levels of hematocrit, hemoglobin, electrolytes, antibody titers, and immune complexes with pretreatment levels.

After the procedure

• Periodically assess the dressings for drainage and the puncture sites for signs of extravasation.

Home care instructions

• Tell the patient that he may feel tired for a day or two after plasmapheresis. (During repeated treatments, he may develop chronic fatigue.) Advise him to rest frequently and to avoid strenuous activities during this period. Unless contraindicated, instruct the patient to maintain a high-protein diet and to take a multivitamin with iron daily.

• Inform the patient who is undergoing repeated plasmapheresis that he may require transfusions of fresh-frozen plasma to replace the normal clotting factors lost in his removed plasma.

• Because plasmapheresis can cause immunosuppression, warn the patient to avoid contact with persons with colds or other contagious viruses.

• Instruct the patient to watch for and report any signs of hepatitis, such as fever, yellowing of the skin and whites of the eyes, and itching skin.

PNEUMATIC COMPRESSION, INTERMITTENT

Intermittent pneumatic compression (IPC) devices consist of cuffs that wrap around each leg and extend to the knee or thigh. Connected to a pump, the cuffs intermittently inflate and deflate, applying gentle compression to the leg. The inflation and deflation of the cuffs mimics the normal pumping action, thus reducing pooling of venous blood and enhancing the return of venous blood to the heart.

Purpose
- To prevent venous thrombosis
- To enhance venous blood flow
- To decrease lymphedema.

Indications
IPC is indicated for any patient at risk for deep vein thrombosis (DVT), especially immobile patients and surgical patients. Clots are more likely to form within the veins of these patients. In addition, if the veins become overdistended from pooling, small tears can develop in the inner walls of the veins, providing a site for clot formation.

IPC enhances fibrinolytic activity; in postoperative patients, it returns this activity, which usually drops for 72 hours postoperatively, to preoperative levels.

Pneumatic compression boot devices are used by professional sports teams to decrease swelling after acute musculoskeletal injury. The compression reduces the buildup of interstitial fluid and decreases pain. Within 24 hours, mobility is enhanced due to the decreased swelling. Boot devices can also be used in the treatment of lymphedema; however, different compression times and pressures are used.

IPC should not be used in patients with overt evidence of leg ischemia caused by peripheral vascular disease or in patients with venous thrombosis or thrombophlebitis. It is contraindicated in patients who have been on prolonged bed rest without prophylactic therapy for thrombosis unless impedance plethysmography (IPG) studies have ruled out thrombosis. IPC is also contraindicated in patients with congestive heart failure because it can produce fluid overload in sensitive patients.

If the cuffs cannot be placed on the legs, they may be applied to the arms; such use will not relieve venous pressure in the legs but will produce a fibrinolytic effect.

Procedure
IPC cuffs are applied to the patient by the nurse. The knee- or thigh-high cuffs are wrapped from the ankle to the knee or thigh on each leg and are then connected to a pump. One cuff inflates fully and then deflates. Then the second cuff inflates and deflates.

To prevent DVT, cuffs should be applied to the legs as soon as the immobility risk factor becomes evident. For surgical patients, the cuffs should be applied *before* anesthesia.

The cuffs should remain in place and therapy continued until the patient is fully ambulatory and the risk of DVT has diminished.

Complications
During this therapy, some patients find the cuffs hot and uncomfortable, but the use of fabric cuffs and cuffs that wrap around the calves alone now minimizes such discomfort.

Care considerations

Before therapy
• Identify patients at risk for DVT.
• Explain the use of IPC cuffs, describing their purpose and the sensations the patient should expect.

During therapy
• Observe cuff filling for at least the first two cycles (approximately 3 to 4 minutes) to ensure correct operation.
• Assess the patient's skin color, temperature, sensation, and ability to move the extremity.
• Maintain therapy for DVT prevention until the patient is no longer at risk, usually until he is fully ambulatory.
• Check pressures and time intervals regularly, according to the policy of the health care facility.
• When a patient must leave the nursing unit for diagnostic or therapeutic procedures, the IPC unit should travel with the patient and therapy should be maintained in the new location.
• If a patient's therapy is interrupted for more than 1 hour, IPC should be discontinued until a noninvasive study, such as an IPG study, can be performed to rule out the formation of a clot during the interruption.
• Encourage the patient to walk with the cuffs in place. The hoses can be disconnected and the cuffs can remain around the calves while the patient is walking.
• Remove the cuffs daily to inspect the skin and provide skin care.
• Document the date and time the IPC cuffs were applied, the pressure settings, the patient's tolerance, and any time the cuffs had to be disconnected.

Home care instructions
• Encourage home use, when applicable. IPC therapy is easy to use and ideal for home care. Codes have been approved to allow for third-party reimbursement of home IPC care.
• Home therapy can be used for recovering surgical patients who won't be fully ambulatory at discharge and are at high risk for thrombophlebitis. It can also be used for cancer patients with chronic lymphedema.
• Teach the patient the reason for this therapy, the importance of increasing ambulation, and the importance of not interrupting therapy for more than 1 hour at a time when used for DVT prophylaxis.
• Explain that the patient can leave the cuffs wrapped around the legs while walking; the hoses connecting the cuffs to the pump can simply be disconnected.

PROGESTINS

The progestins, the natural hormone *progesterone* and its synthetic derivatives, transform a proliferative endometrium into a secretory one. They inhibit the release of pituitary gonadotropins, preventing follicular maturation and ovulation. The progestins also inhibit spontaneous uterine contraction and may demonstrate some estrogenic, anabolic, or androgenic activity.

Because progesterone is relatively inactive in its oral form, the synthetic progestins are more commonly prescribed. In varying degrees, their effects are similar to those of progesterone.

Purpose
• To balance the effects of estrogen in the menstrual cycle by inhibiting the release of luteinizing hormone from the anterior pituitary, inducing secretory changes in the endometrium, relaxing uterine smooth muscle, and thickening cervical mucus
• To reduce the probability of follicular maturation and ovulation by suppressing secretion of pituitary gonadotropins.

Indications

Progestins effectively treat gynecologic conditions that respond to changes in the body's steroid hormone balance. In menstrual disorders caused by hormonal imbalance, *hydroxyprogesterone* or progesterone (both given I.M.) or *norethindrone* (given orally) can induce a normal menstrual cycle. These drugs can also be given to stop dysfunctional uterine bleeding arising from a hyperplastic, nonsecreting endometrium. In addition, norethindrone helps treat endometriosis, and progesterone suppositories help treat premenstrual syndrome. *Norgestrel,* which is used as a contraceptive, is less commonly prescribed than estrogen-progesterone combinations because of its higher incidence of breakthrough bleeding and pregnancy. However, it may be used in patients in whom estrogens are contraindicated.

Progestins are contraindicated in patients with thrombophlebitis, thromboembolic disorders, cerebral hemorrhage, or impaired liver function. They're also contraindicated in known or suspected breast cancer, cancer of the genitalia, undiagnosed vaginal bleeding, or missed abortion. In addition, the synthetic progestins shouldn't be used during the first 4 months of pregnancy.

Progestins should be used cautiously in patients with diabetes mellitus, seizure disorders, migraine headache, cardiac or renal disease, asthma, or mental illness.

Adverse reactions

Adverse reactions to the progestins include breakthrough bleeding, spotting, changes in menstrual flow, amenorrhea, changes in cervical secretions, cervical erosion, breast changes (including tenderness), virilization of the female fetus, edema, weight change, allergic rash with or without pruritus, and acne. A small percentage of patients develop local reactions at the injection site.

Progestins can also cause cholestatic jaundice, chloasma, depression, alopecia, and hirsutism. Thrombophlebitis and pulmonary embolism can also occur.

Care considerations

• Before administering a progestin, check the patient's history for hypersensitivity to these drugs or for disorders that may contraindicate their use.
• Give I.M. injections of progestins deep into the gluteal muscle, and watch for sterile abscess formation.
• Because progestins can cause emboli, be alert for calf tenderness, dyspnea, pleuritic pain, visual disturbances, or paresthesia.
• Observe and palpate the patient's breasts for any changes.

Home care instructions

• Instruct the patient to immediately report severe or sudden headache, loss of coordination, slurred speech, visual changes, and severe depression or irritability. She should also report pain in her chest, groin, or legs, and any shortness of breath, especially if it's unrelated to exertion.
• Tell the patient to report menorrhagia, metrorrhagia, or absence of menstrual bleeding for 45 or more days.
• Advise the patient to take the drug after meals to reduce GI upset.
• If the patient smokes, warn her that smoking increases the risk of thromboembolic disorders; encourage her to stop.
• Teach the patient how to perform breast self-examination. Suggest that she do this monthly and that she report any abnormalities.
• Ensure that the patient knows the signs of pregnancy, and tell her to return to her doctor if she suspects pregnancy; progestins can harm the fetus.
• If the patient is taking minipill progestins as a contraceptive, instruct her

to take the pill every day at about the same time to maintain an effective blood level of the drug.

• If the patient misses a dose, she should take it as soon as she remembers and should take the next pill according to her regular schedule. Advise her to use an alternative method of contraception (such as contraceptive foam, with her partner wearing a condom) whenever she misses a dose. If she misses two doses, she should take only one of the missed doses; then she should resume her regular schedule and use an alternative method of contraception until her next menstrual period.

• Instruct the patient to inform other health care providers that she's taking progestins. Tell her to make an appointment every 6 to 12 months for a pelvic and breast examination and a Papanicolaou test.

• In diabetic patients, glucose tolerance may be decreased. Tell the patient to monitor urine sugar closely and to report any abnormalities.

PROSTATECTOMY

Prostatectomy is the partial or total surgical excision of the prostate gland. Depending on the patient's disease, one of four approaches is used. Transurethral resection of the prostate (TURP), the most common approach, involves insertion of a resectoscope into the urethra. This approach is useful in the treatment of benign prostatic hyperplasia (BPH) with a moderately enlarged prostate and as a palliative measure in prostate cancer. It involves a short hospital stay and doesn't require a surgical incision.

Open surgical methods include suprapubic, retropubic, and radical perineal prostatectomy. These methods are used to treat BPH and prostate cancer if the prostate is too large for transurethral resection and when total removal of the gland is necessary. Su-

prapubic prostatectomy is also used for bladder resections, but it requires a bladder incision and is followed by prolonged and uncomfortable recovery. Retropubic prostatectomy, which does not involve a bladder incision, cannot be used to treat associated bladder disorders. Radical perineal prostatectomy is used if the patient is no longer sexually active because it is associated with a high risk of impotence.

Purpose

• To remove diseased or obstructive prostate tissue

• To restore urine flow through the urethra.

Indications

Prostatectomy is indicated when chronic prostatitis, BPH, or prostate cancer fails to respond to drug therapy or other treatments.

Procedure

The patient receives a general or spinal anesthetic and then, depending on the disease, the surgeon chooses one of four approaches (see *Comparing types of prostatectomy*, pages 524 and 525). If the surgeon chooses the transurethral approach, he passes a resectoscope up the urethra so that he can view the prostate. A heated wire loop or a cutting edge is passed through the resectoscope to cut away as much of the prostate as possible. Pieces of the prostate are washed out through the resectoscope, and the resectoscope is then withdrawn and replaced with an indwelling urinary catheter.

In retropubic or suprapubic approaches, the surgeon makes an abdominal incision to expose the bladder and prostate, and removes the prostate tissue. In radical perineal prostatectomy, the surgeon uses a perineal incision to expose the prostatic tissue. All types of prostatectomy require an indwelling urinary catheter; the su-

(Text continues on page 526.)

Comparing types of prostatectomy

Depending on the patient's disease, the surgeon may perform radical perineal, retropubic, suprapubic, or transurethral resection of the prostate.

Radical perineal prostatectomy

Advantages
- Allows direct visualization of gland
- Permits drainage by gravity
- Has low mortality and decreased incidence of shock

Disadvantages
- High incidence of impotence and incontinence
- Risk of damage to rectum and external sphincter
- Restricted operative field

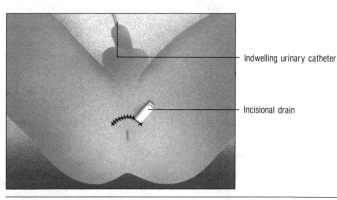

Indwelling urinary catheter

Incisional drain

Retropubic prostatectomy

Advantages
- Allows direct visualization of gland
- Avoids bladder incision
- Requires short convalescence period
- Carries small risk of impotence

Disadvantages
- Can't be used to treat associated bladder disorders
- Increased risk of hemorrhage from prostate venous plexus

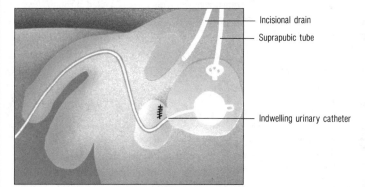

Incisional drain

Suprapubic tube

Indwelling urinary catheter

Suprapubic prostatectomy

Advantages
- Allows exploration of wide area, such as into lymph nodes
- Simple procedure

Disadvantages
- Requires bladder incision
- Hemorrhage control difficult
- Urine leakage common around suprapubic tube
- Prolonged and uncomfortable recovery

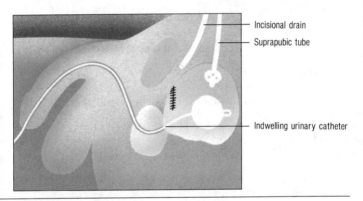

Incisional drain

Suprapubic tube

Indwelling urinary catheter

Transurethral resection of prostate

Advantages
- Safer and less painful and invasive than other prostate procedures
- Doesn't require surgical incision
- Requires short hospital stay
- Carries small risk of impotence

Disadvantages
- Urethral stricture and delayed bleeding may occur
- Not a curative surgery for prostate cancer

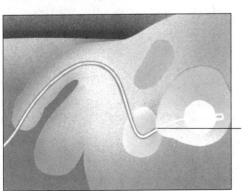

Indwelling urinary catheter

prapubic and retropubic approaches also require an incisional suprapubic drain.

Complications

Severe complications include hemorrhage, infection, urine retention, and epididymitis. Rarely, a patient experiences temporary or permanent impotence after surgery. The radical perineal approach is associated with a high incidence of impotence and incontinence as well as the risk of damage to the rectum and anal sphincter. Transurethral prostatectomy may produce retrograde ejaculation.

Care considerations

Before surgery

• The patient undergoing prostatectomy requires thorough teaching about the surgery and the expected course of recovery. A primary part of this preparation involves emotional and psychological support for the patient to help him overcome his fears and anxieties.

• Review the planned surgery, paying special attention to what the patient knows about the procedure and its aftermath.

• Encourage the patient to ask questions. Provide honest answers and straightforward information to help clear up any misconceptions. Be sure to consider the patient's emotional state as well. Most likely, he'll be worried about the surgery and its effects on his life-style. Encourage him to express his fears; emphasize the positive aspects of the surgery, such as improved urination and prevention of further complications.

• Keep in mind that some types of prostatectomy may cause impotence. Typically, the doctor will discuss this possibility with the patient before surgery. If necessary, arrange for sexual counseling to help the patient cope with this often devastating loss. If the patient is scheduled for TURP, mention that this procedure often causes retrograde

ejaculation but no other impairment of sexual function.

• Administer a cleansing enema, if ordered, and shave the surgical site (unless the patient is scheduled for TURP).

• Explain that the patient will have an indwelling urinary catheter inserted for urine drainage. The catheter may remain in place for 2 to 5 days after TURP and other procedures and will be removed when urine is clear, except after radical prostatectomy; in the latter case, it can be in place for 3 to 4 weeks. Also explain that there may be a tube in his abdomen (suprapubic tube) and possibly an incisional drain.

• Administer antibiotics, as ordered.

After surgery

• Carefully observe the patient for complications. Monitor his vital signs closely, looking for signs of possible hemorrhage and shock.

• Frequently check the incision site for signs of infection, and change dressings as necessary.

• Watch for and report signs of epididymitis: fever, chills, groin pain, and a tender, swollen epididymis.

• Check and record the amount and nature of urine drainage.

• Maintain patency of the indwelling urinary catheter through intermittent or continuous irrigation, as ordered. Watch for catheter blockage from kinking, clot formation, or bladder spasms, and correct, as necessary.

• Maintain the patency of the suprapubic tube, and monitor the amount and character of drainage. Drainage should be amber or slightly blood-tinged; report any abnormalities. Keep the collection container below the level of the patient's bladder to promote drainage, and keep the skin around the tube insertion site clean and dry.

• Expect and report frank bleeding the 1st day after surgery. If bleeding is venous, the doctor may order increasing the traction on the catheter or increasing pressure in the catheter's balloon end. However, if bleeding is arterial (bright red with numerous clots and increased viscosity), it may require surgical intervention.

• Commonly, antispasmodics are prescribed to control painful bladder spasms and analgesics to relieve incisional pain.

• If the patient had a radical perineal prostatectomy, provide emotional support because this procedure usually causes impotence. If possible, arrange for psychological and sexual counseling during recovery.

Home care instructions

• Tell the patient to drink ten 8-oz (240-ml) glasses of water a day, to void at least every 2 hours, and to notify the doctor promptly if he has trouble voiding.

• Warn the patient that he may experience transient urinary frequency and dribbling after catheter removal. Reassure him that he'll gradually regain control over urination.

• Teach the patient catheter care if he will go home with the catheter in place.

• Teach the patient how to perform perineum-tightening (Kegel) exercises to speed the return of sphincter control.

• Suggest that the patient avoid caffeine-containing beverages, which produce mild diuresis.

• Reassure the patient that slightly blood-tinged urine is normal for the first few weeks after surgery. However, instruct him to report bright red urine or persistent hematuria. Tell him that he may see increased bleeding with increased activity.

• Tell the patient to watch for and immediately report any signs of infection, such as fever, chills, and flank pain.

• Warn the patient to avoid sexual intercourse, lifting any object heavier than 10 lb (4.5 kg), performing strenuous exercise (short walks are usually permitted), and taking long car trips until the doctor gives permission. Explain that these activities should usu-

ally be delayed for several weeks (usually 6 weeks) because of the risk of bleeding.

• Advise the patient to keep taking prescribed medications, such as antibiotics, antispasmodics, and stool softeners. Stool softeners are ordered to reduce straining.

PSYCHOTHERAPY

Psychotherapy, a form of counseling, refers to the psychological treatment of mental and emotional disorders. It attempts to uncover the reasons for problem behaviors and promotes effective coping and adaptation skills.

Psychotherapy aims to change a patient's attitudes, feelings, or behavior. To promote such changes, the therapist may use methods such as reinforcement, persuasion, suggestion, reassurance, confrontation, and support. Success of therapy depends largely on the compatibility of patient and therapist, the treatment goals selected, and the patient's commitment. The therapy may be brief or may span several years.

The four approaches to psychotherapy are individual, crisis, group, and family therapy. In individual therapy, the therapist seeks to change the patient's behavior through individual counseling sessions. This involves mutually agreed-upon goals, with the therapist mediating the patient's disturbed patterns of behavior to promote personal health and development. It can be short- or long-term.

In crisis therapy, the patient works on developing adequate coping skills to resolve an immediate, pressing problem. This type of psychotherapy allows the patient to return to the level of function that existed before the crisis. Crisis therapy usually involves just the patient and therapist but may also include the patient's family. Crisis therapy can range from one session to 6 months of treatment.

In group therapy, a group of persons (ideally 4 to 10) with similar emotional problems meet to discuss their concerns as a means of effecting positive behavioral changes and promoting personal growth. Duration of therapy can range from a few weeks to several years.

Family therapy seeks to alter unhealthy relationships within a family to change the problematic behavior of one or more members. Like individual therapy, family therapy can be short- or long-term.

Purpose
• To effect positive changes in a patient's attitudes, emotions, or behavior.

Indications
Psychotherapy is useful for a wide range of mental and emotional problems. Individual therapy may be applied when the patient develops personal distress or dissatisfaction with himself or in his relationships with significant others, coworkers, friends, or family.

Crisis therapy is useful when the patient seems unable to handle an overwhelming current situation. The crisis can be developmental, such as one that follows marriage or the death of a loved one, or situational, such as one that follows a natural disaster or illness.

Group therapy is useful in treating patients with common problems, such as addictions.

Family therapy works to treat adjustment disorders of childhood or adolescence, marital discord, and situations of sexual, physical, emotional, or chemical abuse.

Procedure
Depending on his beliefs and training, the therapist selects an approach to meet the patient's needs. For instance, the therapist may choose reinforcement, which strengthens the appro-

priate behavior by fear of punishment or the anticipation of a reward. Or, if a strong rapport exists between the therapist and patient, the therapist may use suggestion (or persuasion) to implant an idea or belief in the patient's mind as a means of effecting change. The therapist may also direct discussion of the patient's ideas and feelings to achieve abreaction, which is the emotional relief obtained by mentally reliving or bringing into consciousness a long-repressed, painful experience. Abreaction is controversial when it involves the use of sedation. Therapists often combine these and other techniques to achieve treatment goals.

Complications
During therapy, the patient may experience increased distress, depression, anxiety, and restlessness. If the patient feels uncomfortable with the therapy, he may display loss of appetite, irritability, or insomnia. Aggressive or self-destructive impulses may be triggered by the recollection of some memories.

Care considerations
Before therapy
• Review the patient's psychiatric history, treatment history, and current psychiatric status to help assess his needs.
• Explain the therapeutic technique to the patient, and help him establish a treatment goal.
• Maintain the confidentiality of information the patient shares with you, unless he plans to harm himself or someone else. Typically, you'll share only that information that the patient wants shared.
After therapy
• Observe the patient for mood changes, such as increased distress, depression, anxiety, and restlessness. Be alert for loss of appetite, irritability, or insomnia.

• Reassure the patient that talking about his feelings will help relieve distress. Be sure to reinforce any gains the patient has made.
• Assess the patient for suicide potential.

Home care instructions

• Refer the patient to self-help groups, as appropriate.
• Instruct the patient to contact his therapist if distressing symptoms recur.

R

RADIATION THERAPY

Radiation, discovered in the 1890s, offers one of the oldest treatments available for cancer management. Radiation therapy applies high levels of radiation to cancer cells, destroying their ability to grow and multiply. Radiation is thought to either decrease the rate of mitosis or impair the synthesis of deoxyribonucleic acid or ribonucleic acid in these cells.

Preoperatively, radiation can shrink a tumor, thus allowing total excision. Postoperatively, it can eradicate any neoplastic cells that were undetected during surgery. In other curative applications, preliminary surgery may provide access for radiation treatment and chemotherapy. These therapies can also relieve pain and enhance the patient's quality of life in terminal cancer.

Radiation therapy may be delivered externally or internally. External radiation is more widely used and will be discussed here. (For further discussion on internal radiation therapy, see the entry "Radioactive Implants.")

Therapy is given using X-rays or gamma rays that emit a beam of electrons into the target area. Recent advances in external therapy include large-field, large-dose radiation, such as half-body treatments. Large-field, large-dose radiation provides an effective, well-tolerated treatment for patients with metastatic cancer. Total skin electron therapy, another advancement, provides radiation to the entire skin surface and has been successful in managing extensive skin disease. Hyperfractionation, an experimental approach that attempts to achieve better tumor control, delivers more than one radiation treatment per day.

Radiation therapy is contraindicated in pregnant women and should be used cautiously in patients with blood disorders. These patients must have their blood counts monitored closely because radiation therapy can lower hemoglobin, hematocrit, and white blood cell (WBC) and platelet counts.

Purpose

• To destroy or slow the development and growth of abnormal cells.

Indications

Radiation therapy is indicated in the treatment of cancer. Radiation treatments destroy neoplastic cells or curtail their growth. Radiation therapy may be indicated as a curative therapy, as in the management of early-stage Hodgkin's disease. In curative applications, radiation is commonly used preoperatively to shrink a tumor and postoperatively to eradicate residual neoplastic cells. Radiation may also be indicated as palliative therapy that strives to control pain, bleeding, and obstruction.

Procedure

For external radiation, the patient lies immobile on a treatment table or floor (in the case of large-dose radiation) in the X-ray department while a large machine, usually overhead, directs radiation at the target site for the ordered time—usually 1 to 2 minutes.

Complications

Radiation therapy damages normal cells along with cancer cells. Normal cells have a greater ability to recover from radiation than cancer cells; however, numerous complications do occur. The complications or adverse reactions depend on the site receiving the radiation. Such complications include GI disturbances, headaches, reduced sperm count, decreased hormone levels, and reduced WBC and platelet counts. The patient may also suffer feelings of isolation.

Care considerations

Before therapy

• Explain to the patient the type of therapy to be used, including a description of possible adverse reactions.
• Establish baseline WBC and platelet counts.
• Obtain a thorough history, including any previous radiation treatments and adverse reactions to these treatments.
• Radiation therapy can reduce the production of sperm; advise the male patient who desires to have children to deposit his sperm in a sperm bank before initiating therapy.
• In female patients, pelvic radiation can decrease hormone levels, which can lead to infertility and amenorrhea.
• Tell the patient that the radiation therapist may mark the exact areas of treatment on his skin with a pen or dye. Instruct the patient not to remove these markings until after the completion of therapy.
• If positioning will be painful for the patient, provide analgesics, as prescribed.

After therapy

• Monitor the patient's WBC and platelet counts to evaluate myelosuppressive effects.
• Monitor the patient for other effects of radiation treatment, such as erythema and nausea and vomiting.

Home care instructions

• Explain to the patient that the full benefit of radiation treatment may not occur for up to several months.
• Instruct the patient to report adverse reactions to the doctor.
• Stress the importance of keeping follow-up appointments with the doctor.
• Instruct the patient to use mild soap for skin care after radiation treatment and to avoid irritating the radiated area with perfume, powder, or other cosmetics.
• Refer the patient to a community support group, such as the local chapter of the American Cancer Society.

RADICAL NECK DISSECTION

Radical neck dissection is a surgical procedure performed on the head and neck to remove the cervical chain of lymph nodes, the sternocleidomastoid muscle, the fascia, and the internal jugular vein. It may be performed alone or with other head and neck surgery, such as a total laryngectomy.

This procedure causes visible changes in the patient's appearance that may cause profound emotional reactions. It may also cause difficulty eating and, when performed with a laryngectomy, inability to speak. The patient undergoing radical neck dissection will need a strong support system to successfully adapt to his new self-image.

Purpose

• To remove malignant lesions from the tongue, tonsil, lip, nasopharynx, or thyroid
• To prevent or treat metastasis to the cervical lymph nodes.

Indications

Radical neck dissection is indicated in patients with head and neck tumors that may eventually metastasize to the cervical lymph nodes. The procedure is indicated if the cervical lymph nodes are palpable or if metastasis to the nodes is suspected. Radical neck dissection may also be performed if a primary lesion appears in the neck, in an area with a high incidence of neck metastasis, or if metastasis occurs on one or both sides of the neck after laryngectomy.

Procedure

After the patient receives a general anesthetic, the surgeon makes large incisions in the neck, unfolding skin flaps that allow access to the involved area. He then removes muscle and fascia, including the cervical chain of lymph nodes, the internal jugular vein, and the sternocleidomastoid muscle. The spinal accessory nerve is severed, but the carotid artery and the vagus nerve are spared. If necessary, the surgeon may perform a laryngectomy or a tracheotomy at this time. Next, the surgeon may insert drains, protect the carotid artery with a dermal or muscle pedicle graft, and then carefully position skin flaps over the dissected area. The flaps are sutured closed before a dressing is applied to the patient's neck.

Complications

Radical neck dissection can cause several life-threatening complications, including carotid artery rupture and hemorrhage, aspiration and airway obstruction, pharyngeal fistula, infection, necrosis, and pneumothorax. Other complications include facial edema, damage to the larynx resulting in vocal impairment, skin sloughing, shoulder droop due to nerve damage, erosion of the skin and major vessels due to suction tube placement, and Frey's syndrome (excessive sweating of the cheek after eating, which usually occurs when a parotidectomy is also performed).

Radical neck dissection may cause facial disfigurement, leading to changes in the patient's self-perception. As a result, the patient may display intense emotions such as anger, grief, and denial or may exhibit signs of depression, withdrawal, ineffective coping, and negative body image.

Care considerations

Before surgery

• Reinforce the surgeon's explanation of the surgery and the expected postoperative course. Tell the patient what to expect immediately after the surgery, including the presence of tubes and drains, treatment in the intensive care unit, and the inability to talk if laryngectomy or tracheotomy is performed.

• Encourage the patient to express his fears about cancer, the surgery, and his prognosis. Offer emotional support and appropriate reassurance. Involve family members whenever possible. If necessary, refer the patient and family to a mental health professional for additional counseling.

• If the patient is scheduled for a total laryngectomy with a radical neck dissection, discuss the procedure with him and tell him that he'll have a stoma after surgery. Establish a means of communication that the patient will be able to use after surgery (paper and pencil, flashcards, chalk board, or magic slate). Reassure him that he will be able to make his needs and wishes known. Arrange a consultation with a speech therapist.

After surgery

• Postoperatively, elevate the head of the patient's bed 30 to 45 degrees to reduce tension on the suture line, facilitate drainage, and decrease edema.

• Monitor respiratory rate and depth, and check for use of accessory muscles. Regularly auscultate the patient's lungs. Report dyspnea, pulmonary congestion, or increasing edema immediately.

• If the patient has a tracheostomy tube, provide tracheostomy care every 4 hours and as needed. Suction the patient orally or through his tracheostomy tube as needed. Use caution to avoid trauma to the suture line.

• If the patient does not have a tracheostomy tube in place, keep a sterile tracheotomy tray at the bedside in case of airway obstruction. Keep resuscitation equipment nearby.

• Provide frequent oral hygiene to decrease risk of infection and decrease accumulation of old blood and secretions. Use a soft toothbrush and a mild mouthwash to avoid trauma to the oral mucosa.

• Observe skin flap color, and report any hematoma formation at the suture line. Inspect the suture line for redness, swelling, drainage, and separation. Monitor for skin flap necrosis, which may occur if the surgeon was unable to save enough blood vessels to nourish the flap.

• Inspect the patient's neck drains for patency. Usually, they're connected to a closed drainage system. Monitor the amount and character of the drainage.

• Assist the patient to change position by supporting his head and neck; removal of the sternocleidomastoid muscle renders him unable to support his own head.

• Administer analgesics carefully. Remember that opiates depress respiration and inhibit coughing.

• Keep in mind that massive hemorrhage can result if necrosis affects the carotid artery wall. A hemorrhage can also occur 8 to 20 days after a wound infection begins, or sooner as the result of surgical injury or weakening of the artery by preoperative radiation. If hemorrhage occurs, apply pressure, stay with the patient, and call for help.

• If the patient is unable to speak, use alternative means of communication. Reassure the patient that someone is nearby if he needs anything and that you will check on him frequently. Have the patient's call bell and pen and paper within his easy reach.

Home care instructions

• Inform the patient that he may experience shoulder discomfort for months after the surgery. Instruct him to use massage and muscle-strengthening exercises to relieve discomfort. Caution him not to lie on the affected side and not to lift more than 2 lb (about 1 kg) with that arm.

• If the patient has also had a laryngectomy, teach him and a family member stoma and tracheostomy care. Arrange for visits by a speech therapist.

• Emphasize the importance of keeping follow-up doctor's appointments to monitor for possible recurrence of cancer.

• Provide the patient and his family with information about counseling, and encourage membership in a community support group.

RADIOACTIVE IMPLANTS

The implantation of sources of radiation—usually iodine 125 or iridium 192—directly into a tumor site is alternatively known as brachytherapy and implant, intracavity, or interstitial therapy. The advantage of this therapy over conventional external beam radiation therapy is that it delivers a high dose of radiation to the tumor with minimal radiation exposure to the healthy surrounding tissue.

Recently, brachytherapy has been combined with hyperthermia in the treatment of malignant brain tumors in the hope of prolonging the patient's survival. The addition of heat directly before and after radiation implantation is thought to enhance tumor destruction. Preliminary results have not shown significant differences between these patients and those who received brachytherapy alone.

Purpose

• To inhibit growth of a tumor or possibly decrease its size while sparing surrounding healthy tissue.

Indications

Brachytherapy is used for recurrent brain tumors after the patient has received surgery and conventional external beam radiation. Brachytherapy is also used routinely in cervical as well as head and neck cancers, and studies have shown it to be useful in the treatment of breast cancer. Currently, studies are evaluating the effectiveness of brachytherapy in the treatment of lung cancer, esophageal cancer, selected bladder cancers, and early-stage rectal cancer. The use of radioactive implants has shown promising results against selected brain tumors (recurrent malignant gliomas and solitary brain metastasis). Such tumors must be less than 6 cm in diameter, well circumscribed, supratentorial, and unifocal.

Patients who are considered ineligible for brachytherapy are those whose brain tumors are diffuse, multifocal, and larger than 6 cm in diameter, or those whose tumors are located infratentorially (in the brain stem, cerebellum, or thalamus).

Because patients are considered radioactive while the implants are in place, contact with caregivers must be limited. This necessitates that patients be able to perform self-care.

Procedure

To begin intracranial brachytherapy, the neurosurgeon places a stereotactic head frame with the patient under local anesthesia and mild sedation. The patient is then taken from the operating room for a detailed computed tomography (CT) scan of the head. Measurements from the scans are used to determine the three-dimensional coordinates of the tumor; the neurosurgeon makes the determination in consultation with a radiation oncologist and physicist. Catheter placement is also calculated at this time.

After the planning is complete, the patient is returned to the operating room for insertion of catheters into which the radiation sources will later be instilled. (This procedure is called afterloading.) The catheters are inserted and blank sources placed in them. After the patient is stabilized, he is taken for another CT scan to verify the placement of the catheters and blank sources. After confirmation, the blank sources are removed and replaced by the radioactive sources. Insertion of the sources may be performed by either the radiation oncologist or the neurosurgeon, who takes standard radiation precautions.

During radiation therapy, which may last 3 to 7 days, the patient is placed in a private room with limited nursing interventions. Depending on the radioactive source implanted, nursing care may be carried out from behind a lead shield, with the use of lead aprons, or with only a lead helmet worn by the patient. The amount of time persons may spend in the room per day also depends on the type of radioactive isotope used.

After the radiation dose is delivered, the radioactive implants are removed at the bedside. The patient then receives another CT scan to assess the preliminary effects of therapy. The patient is no longer considered radioactive and routine nursing care may be administered. However, the radiation safety department must assess the room with a Geiger counter to verify no radiation spillage.

Complications

Significant complications have been reported during brachytherapy and have occasionally required early removal of the radioactive implants. Complications include worsening of neurologic deficits, increased intracranial pressure, seizures, and infection.

Care considerations
Before therapy
• Explain the procedure to the patient, especially the postoperative phase. Assure him that although he will need to be isolated while the radioactive implants are in place, help will be nearby.
During therapy
• Monitor the patient closely for signs of deteriorating neurologic status and increased intracranial pressure.
• Assess the wound for signs of infection or leakage.
• Keep the patient's head elevated to improve venous drainage and assist in the control of intracranial pressure.
• Administer anticonvulsants, as prescribed, and monitor blood levels. Anticonvulsants are indicated to prevent seizure activity.
• Administer corticosteroids, as prescribed. Corticosteroids reduce cerebral edema, which may be present after the procedure.
• Keep direct nursing care to a minimum, and stand contralateral to the radiation source while caring for the patient. When possible, stand at the foot of the bed or in the doorway to communicate with the patient, thereby increasing distance from the radiation source. If the patient is to wear a helmet, ensure that it is in place before entering the room.
• Be sure to understand and follow the recommended safety standards for the type of radioactive isotope used. If you are unsure, contact the radiation safety department.
• Reassure the patient that isolation is temporary, and remind him that he is not alone. Place his call bell so that it is within his easy reach at all times.
• Monitor and explain to visitors the radiation safety protocols. No children or pregnant women are allowed to visit the patient. Visitors must also follow the radiation protocols for the particular radioactive isotope used.

Home care instructions
• Instruct the patient and family to call the doctor to report such neurologic changes as alterations in level of consciousness, behavior, vision, muscle strength, or sensation as well as seizure activity.
• Tell the patient and family to notify the doctor of continued headache or change in headache, sustained high fever, severe nausea or vomiting, stiff neck (nuchal rigidity), or sensitivity of eyes to light.
• Teach the patient signs and symptoms of wound infection, and tell him to report an infection to his doctor immediately.
• Discuss each of the patient's medications with him, especially corticosteroids and anticonvulsants. Emphasize the importance of taking each as ordered. Warn the patient not to abruptly discontinue any of his medications.
• Inform the patient that he may increase his physical activity as tolerated but should avoid heavy lifting. The patient should discuss with his doctor specific activities of concern.
• Emphasize the importance of follow-up visits and CT scans.

RADIOSURGERY

Radiosurgery is a noninvasive procedure that uses radiation instead of a scalpel or laser to treat a lesion. The radiation is applied to a small intracranial target, such as an arteriovenous malformation or brain tumor, with the intent to destroy or cause a biological effect in the target. Stereotactic location is used; this determines the location of a lesion in the brain using a three-dimensional approach and employs a fixed external reference point (a head frame attached to the patient).

In conventional radiation therapy, the radiation is delivered through one to three portals, limiting the amount of radiation that the patient can receive to protect normal brain tissue from the effects of large radiation dosages. Radiosurgery can deliver high doses of radiation to the lesion and a relatively low dose of radiation to the surrounding normal brain tissue. Because of the delivery method, persons who previously received the maximum conventional brain radiation treatments can receive an additional dose to the lesion using radiosurgery.

Three types of radiosurgery are commonly used: the gamma knife, the linear accelerator (LINAC), and Bragg peak (proton beam or helium ion) therapy. Each uses a slightly different method of delivering radiation to a stereotactically located intracranial lesion.

The *gamma knife* method uses 201 sources of cobalt 60 radiation, arranged in a hemisphere and directed at a single point. Dividing the dosage over 201 points allows each portion of the brain traversed by one beam to receive only 0.05% of the total dosage delivered. This limits the effects on normal brain tissue and increases the amount of radiation delivered to the lesion.

The *linear accelerator* delivers radiation to the target through a series of intersecting arcs. Providing results similar to the gamma knife, LINAC delivers a high dose of radiation to the lesion at the intersection of the arcs, while the surrounding brain receives a relatively low dose of radiation.

Bragg peak therapy, also called proton beam therapy or helium ion therapy, is named for a property of charged particles. As these high-energy particles travel through the brain, their velocity decreases. As their velocity decreases, the amount of energy loss from the particle greatly increases. The energy release is highest at the end of the range of the beam; this energy loss, called the Bragg peak, is what causes the therapeutic effect. When using this technology, the dose is calculated so that the Bragg peak occurs within the targeted lesion.

Purpose

• To inhibit growth of a intracranial tumor or possibly decrease its size
• To cause sclerosing effects in cerebral vessels.

Indications

Radiosurgery is indicated for arteriovenous malformations that are not amenable to surgery because the possibility of neurologic damage, the patient's age, or another medical condition poses a high surgical risk or because the patient refuses surgery. In general, the lesion must be smaller than 3 cm for this procedure to be effective, although some centers have treated larger lesions. Radiosurgery may also be used with embolization procedures to treat arteriovenous malformations.

Radiosurgery is most effective for noninfiltrative tumors that are smaller than 3 cm³, such as acoustic neuromas and meningiomas, although larger lesions have been successfully treated. Radiosurgery may be curative for these tumors when used with or without conventional surgery. Limited use has also been reported in recurrent pituitary tumors and craniopharyngiomas. Recently, radiosurgery has been used to treat malignant gliomas and metastatic brain tumors. In the treatment of gliomas, radiosurgery is an adjunctive treatment after surgery and conventional radiation. The treatment aims to slow progression of the tumor and preserve neurologic function.

Procedure

The patient is usually awake during the entire radiosurgery procedure. The procedure for all three types of delivery systems consists of placing a stereotactic head frame on the patient, followed by radiographic studies such as magnetic resonance imaging (MRI), a computed tomography (CT) scan, or an angiogram. The three-dimensional coordinates of the lesion are determined through calculations based on the radiographic studies. The dosage plan is then calculated by a team consisting of the neurosurgeon, radiation oncologist, and radiation physicist. The radiation is then administered and the head frame removed.

The patient may go home following radiation or be monitored overnight in the hospital.

Complications

Complications of radiosurgery are rare but include vomiting or seizure activity related to cerebral edema secondary to the radiation; these can be relieved with corticosteroids. Vomiting is most often correlated with lesions in the posterior fossa and is controlled by administering antiemetics and corticosteroids before radiation. Seizure activity is controlled by ensuring that anticonvulsant levels are within therapeutic range before the procedure.

Complications that can occur 3 to 6 months after treatment are related to edema and radiation necrosis. They are manifested by changes in neurologic status related to the location of the lesion. Such complications occur most often in tumor patients, are usually temporary, and can be controlled with corticosteroids. If there is a large amount of necrotic tissue, however, surgical removal may be necessary.

Complications in patients with arteriovenous malformations are rare and are usually manifested as seizures. Malformations that are not totally obliterated may bleed, causing neurologic deficits. The risk of bleeding after radiosurgery is approximately 2% per year until the malformation is totally obliterated. This is the same percentage rate as with untreated arteriovenous malformations.

Care considerations
Before the procedure
• Instruct the patient about preparatory procedures, and explain the reasons for preoperative tests, fasting after midnight the night before the procedure, and a preoperative shower.
• Discuss the application of the head frame, including sensations the patient will experience during its application.
• Inform the patient of the sequence of events and approximate time periods for each—head frame placement, radiographic tests, dose planning (several hours), and radiation treatment (5 minutes to 1 hour).
After the procedure
• Monitor neurologic status closely, especially for nausea, vomiting, or seizure activity or for changes in level of consciousness or pupil size. The high dose of radiation given during these procedures may cause cerebral edema. Prompt intervention with corticosteroids is usually sufficient to decrease complications.
• Promote patient comfort, and administer analgesics, as needed. The patient may have mild-to-moderate headache after the head frame is removed.

Home care instructions
• Give the patient a written schedule for postprocedure radiographic studies. Generally, patients with arteriovenous malformations will need an angiogram after 1 year. Patients with tumors will receive a follow-up CT scan or MRI 1 to 3 months after the procedure and then every 3 to 6 months afterward.
• Emphasize that the full effect of the treatment may not be known for up to 2 years, which is why close radiographic follow-up is important.
• Instruct the patient to notify his doctor immediately of any changes in neurologic status, such as seizure activity or changes in level of consciousness, behavior, vision, or muscle strength.
• Tell the patient to notify his doctor of continued headache or change in

headache, severe nausea or vomiting, stiff neck, or sensitivity of eyes to light.
• Inform any patient with arteriovenous malformation that the risk of bleeding will persist until the lesion is completely obliterated.
• Instruct the patient to notify the doctor of any signs of infection at pin sites. Pin sites should be kept clean with soap and water.
• Discuss each of the patient's medications, especially if corticosteroids have been prescribed. Stress the need to *slowly* decrease the corticosteroid dosage.
• Inform the patient that he may perform his normal daily activities as tolerated. There are no restrictions on diet or physical activity related to the radiosurgery procedure.
• If the patient has experienced seizures, tell him to check with his doctor before he resumes driving.

REPLANTATION AFTER TRAUMATIC AMPUTATION

Replantation after traumatic amputation is an emergency attempt to reattach a severed digit, limb, or other body part. Advances in microvascular surgery have resulted in a reported 80% to 90% success rate in the replantation of severed body parts. Even when there is severe injury to the skin, muscle, bone, and blood vessels, replantation may be attempted if the nerves are unscathed or minimally damaged. Patients may then regain a significant degree of function in the replanted body part. Unfortunately, only 20% of patients whose accidentally amputated body parts might be reattached reach a microsurgeon in time for successful replantation.

One of the key factors to successful replantation is minimizing ischemia time, the period of time a body part is without blood supply. Because muscle fibers are sensitive to lack of oxygen

and show microscopic damage after 30 minutes of ischemia, successful replantation requires that ischemia time must be at a minimum and that proper care be taken of the body part. (See *Preserving an amputated body part.*)

Purpose
• To reattach a fully or partially severed body part
• To restore function greater than that provided by a prosthesis.

Indications
Replantation surgery should be considered for all traumatic thumb amputations; multiple digit amputations; all amputations in children; clean amputations at the palm, wrist, or forearm; and any complex injury that may benefit from microvascular surgery. Upper extremity replantation is the most commonly performed. However, successful replantation has also been performed on lower extremities, scalps, ears, and penises.

Procedure
The patient arrives in the operating room with the amputated part preserved in lactated Ringer's or 0.9% sodium chloride solution and packed in ice. It is desirable for a team of surgeons, nurses, and technicians well versed in microvascular surgical techniques to perform the replantation. While one microsurgery team examines, identifies, debrides, and tags structures on the amputated part, another prepares the stump. A vein or tendon graft may be harvested to bridge vessel gaps or stabilize the amputated part. Next, the bone is approximated and stabilized (usually by internal fixation), all clots are removed, and the patency of each vessel is assessed by angiography. The surgeon then repairs the main nerve trunks and creates further meticulous anastomoses. Muscles and tendons are repaired, if possible, and all anastomosed sites are covered with muscle to

Preserving an amputated body part

If you're called upon to preserve an amputated body part for replantation, you must act quickly and correctly.

Protecting a partial amputation
• Treat a partial amputation as you would an open fracture, using a rigid splint to immobilize the extremity.
• Observe the damaged extremity for signs of fracture.
• Palpate the patient's pulse, and check his sensory and motor function distal to the injury. Compare findings to those obtained on the uninjured side.
• Place moist sterile dressings over the site. Don't cover the wound with splinting materials.
• Immobilize at least one joint above and below the level of injury, taking care to pad all bony prominences.
• After splinting, again palpate the patient's distal pulse and test sensory and motor function distal to the injury.
• Keep the extremity cool by covering it with a plastic bag and then enclosing

this in an ice-filled plastic bag. To prevent irreversible tissue damage, always protect the extremity from direct contact with ice. Never use dry ice.

Preserving a severed segment
• Put on sterile gloves, and flush the segment with 0.9% sodium chloride or lactated Ringer's solution. Avoid scrubbing or debriding it.
• Using sterile gauze, gently pat the segment dry. Then wrap it in sterile gauze soaked with 0.9% sodium chloride solution, and cover it with a sterile towel.
• Place the wrapped part in a plastic bag, and seal the bag shut. Then place this bag inside an ice-filled plastic bag, and seal it.
• Label the plastic bag with the patient's name, identification of the amputated segment, and the date and time when cooling began.

allow for optimal capillary and lymphatic regeneration.

After loosely suturing the skin, the surgeon may apply partial-thickness grafts. He may also perform a fasciotomy to prevent ischemia of major repaired vessels from muscle swelling. After completing these procedures, he applies a dressing over the site.

Complications

Postoperative complications include hemorrhage, contractures, and infection. When body parts are replanted after prolonged ischemia, the patient is at higher risk for metabolic acidosis, renal failure, hyperkalemia, and clostridial infection.

Patients may also experience an intolerance to cold in the replanted part, but this usually resolves within 2 years.

Care considerations
Before surgery
• Assess the patient for associated skeletal, neurologic, or visceral injuries as well as compartment syndrome and infection.
• Obtain a detailed medical, surgical, and social history, including circumstances surrounding the injury.
• Keep the patient in a supine position, with the affected extremity elevated and in good body alignment. Monitor vital signs, level of consciousness, and intake and output. Insert a large-bore I.V. needle, and administer fluids, as ordered. Make sure that the patient fasts, and administer analgesics, as ordered.
• Coordinate preoperative diagnostic studies. Schedule an X-ray of the body part to evaluate bone damage, a chest X-ray, a complete blood count, coagulation studies, and routine chemistry. Prepare the patient for type and crossmatch for possible blood transfusion,

and obtain a wound culture and sample for urinalysis.

• If the patient's body part has been completely severed, provide stump care. Make sure the wound is covered with a moist sterile pressure dressing. Place a light ice bag over the stump to control bleeding. Apply pressure if bleeding continues, and keep a tourniquet available if severe bleeding occurs. Note the amount, nature, and location of drainage.

• Ensure that the amputated part has been correctly prepared.

• Administer prophylactic antibiotics, as prescribed. Verify that the patient has had a tetanus immunization within the past 10 years. If ordered, administer an aspirin suppository or heparin for anticoagulation to prevent thrombosis in reanastomosed vessels.

• Provide emotional support and reassurance. Reinforce the surgeon's explanation of the procedure, and emphasize the word "attempted" when discussing the replantation surgery.

After surgery

• Assess the replanted part hourly. Observe color, capillary refill, tissue turgor, and temperature. Be alert for signs of arterial occlusion and venous congestion.

• Monitor vital signs and urine output regularly. Administer I.V. fluids, blood, and volume expanders, as prescribed.

• Regularly check the dressing for excessive bleeding or drainage. If hemorrhage occurs, apply direct pressure and notify the doctor immediately.

• Observe for swelling along fascial planes, a possible sign of compartment syndrome.

• Administer antibiotics and analgesics, as ordered.

• Administer oxygen to correct tissue hypoxia, as ordered.

Home care instructions

• Instruct the patient and his family to watch for and report any unusual pain, bleeding, or signs of infection. Stress the importance of keeping the replantation site clean and dry to avoid skin breakdown, irritation, and infection.

• Stress the importance of not smoking and living in a smoke-free environment for at least 6 weeks postoperatively to avoid smoke-induced vasoconstriction.

• Inform the patient and family that a long and perhaps difficult rehabilitation program will be necessary to recover use of the replanted part, to learn to accept an altered body image, and to resume an independent life-style.

• Refer the patient and his family to a support group or a mental health professional to help them develop coping strategies.

REWARMING TREATMENTS

Rewarming includes a range of strategies from external application of a hot-water bottle to chest intubation and instillation of heated solution to treat hypothermia. Hypothermia is defined as a core body temperature below 95° F (35° C). Below this temperature, the body can no longer generate enough heat to sustain essential body functions.

The type of rewarming ordered depends on the degree of hypothermia and the patient's age and general health. In a healthy patient with mild hypothermia (core temperature of 90° to 94° F [32.2° to 34.4° C]), passive external rewarming, such as use of blankets, is indicated to reduce heat loss by evaporation, convection, and radiation and allow spontaneous rewarming through generation of body heat. Passive rewarming also maintains peripheral vasoconstriction, reducing the risk of vascular collapse.

Active external rewarming, such as use of heating pads or a hypothermia blanket, may be ordered for moderate hypothermia or if passive rewarming fails to raise core temperature at least

1.8° F (1° C) per hour. For severe hypothermia, active core rewarming techniques may be used to raise the patient's temperature rapidly. I.V. infusion of warmed fluids, administration of warmed oxygen, or an instillation of warmed dialysate into the peritoneum may be ordered. In extremely severe hypothermia, a chest tube may be inserted to instill heated 0.9% sodium chloride solution or lactated Ringer's solution into the mediastinum. Extracorporeal blood rewarming may also be initiated.

Purpose
• To restore normal core temperature.

Indications
Rewarming treatments are indicated for hypothermia or in patients with a core temperature below 95° F.

Procedure
For extremely severe hypothermia, the doctor may insert a chest tube and instill warmed 0.9% sodium chloride solution or lactated Ringer's solution into the mediastinum. He may also initiate extracorporeal blood rewarming.

If the patient has severe hypothermia, warmed I.V. fluids are infused to decrease peripheral vasoconstriction and blood viscosity and to improve coronary perfusion, reducing the risk of arrhythmias. Heated, humidified oxygen is given by mask, endotracheal tube, or intermittent positive-pressure breathing device. Mechanical ventilation with heated oxygen and positive end-expiratory pressure may be needed. Peritoneal dialysis, using dextrose 1.5% solution warmed to 110° F (43.3° C), may also be instituted.

If the patient shows signs of frostbite (absence of skin blanching with application of pressure, pain, or possibly loss of sensation), the body part should be handled extremely carefully and quickly immersed in warm water (100° to 108° F [37.8° to 42.2° C]) or wrapped with warmed, moist gauze. Avoid prolonged thawing because it increases cellular damage in frostbite. Avoid rubbing the area to prevent further damage.

If the patient has mild hypothermia, rewarming is begun with a simple measure such as blankets. If the patient's core temperature doesn't rise at least 1.8° F after an hour, active external warming is begun by placing a hot-water bottle or an electric heating pad on the blanket and over the patient's thorax or by immersing the patient in a warm-water bath. A hypothermia blanket may also be ordered.

Complications
Complications during rewarming may include ventricular fibrillation and vascular collapse, and core temperature can plummet after treatment is stopped. However, careful application of rewarming techniques and frequent monitoring help avoid such complications.

Care considerations
Before the procedure
• If possible, explain to the patient that rewarming treatments will restore his body temperature to its normal level. Describe the specific treatment ordered by the doctor. Make sure the treatment room is warm and free of drafts. Have the patient put on a hospital gown without metal snaps to avoid heat injury. Cover him with blankets, and wrap a towel around his head.
• Obtain baseline vital signs and, if the patient has severe hypothermia, continuous electrocardiography.
• Insert an I.V. line, if ordered, and an indwelling urinary catheter to monitor urine output.
• If you're using a hot-water bottle, check it for leaks by filling it with hot water. If no leaks appear, discard the water. Fill the bag about halfway with water heated to 115° to 125° F (46.1° to 51.7° C) for adults or 105° to 115° F (40.6° to 46.1° C) for children and elderly patients.

• If you're using an electrical heating device, check for frayed wires. Also check an aquamatic K pad and hypothermia blankets for leaks, and clear the tubing of air, which could interfere with heat conduction. Cover the device with an absorbent cloth to prevent possible tissue damage.

• If the doctor has ordered a hypothermia blanket, use a single piece of linen as insulation between the patient and the hypothermia blanket. Insert the rectal probe, and tape it in place to avoid dislodgment. Place a blanket over the patient to trap heated air. A second hypothermia blanket may be placed over the patient.

During the procedure

• Reposition the patient every 30 minutes, unless contraindicated, to prevent skin breakdown.

• Monitor vital signs and neurologic status every 5 minutes until core temperature reaches the desired level, then every 15 minutes until the temperature stabilizes or as ordered. Active core rewarming is typically discontinued when core temperature approaches 96° F (35.6° C) to avoid hyperthermia.

• Be alert for other possible complications of rewarming.

• The patient's neurologic status usually improves as core temperature rises. If you don't observe any improvement, assess for an underlying problem.

After the procedure

• After discontinuing rewarming, be alert for falling core temperature. If it occurs, notify the doctor; he may reinstitute rewarming.

Home care instructions

• If appropriate, teach the patient how to prevent recurrence of hypothermia.

• If the patient had severe frostbite, recommend physical therapy.

• Evaluate the patient's home care needs. If you suspect the patient doesn't have adequate shelter or clothing, contact a social service agency. If the underlying cause is drug or alcohol abuse, recommend counseling.

RHINOPLASTY AND SEPTOPLASTY

Rhinoplasty is a surgical procedure that changes the nose's external appearance, correcting congenital or traumatic deformity. Septoplasty corrects a deviated septum, preventing nasal obstruction, thick discharge, and secondary pharyngeal, sinus, and ear problems. These procedures may be performed together or independently.

Purpose

• To correct a deformity and enhance the appearance of the nose

• To correct a deviated septum and restore easy breathing.

Indications

Rhinoplasty is indicated to correct congenital or traumatic nasal deformity. Septoplasty is indicated to prevent nasal obstruction caused by a deviated nasal septum.

Procedure

In both procedures, the patient receives topical and local anesthetics. In rhinoplasty, the surgeon fractures the nasal bones, removes excess tissue, and then repositions the bones. He makes an incision in the groove between the upper and lower nasal cartilages and trims the soft tissue to reshape the tip of the nose. He may also insert a cartilage implant to bolster a saddle-bridge or retracted columella.

In septoplasty, the surgeon makes an incision inside the nose past the mucocutaneous junction. He separates the perichondrium from the cartilage and septal bone and cuts the deviated cartilage into pieces or incises and repositions it midline. Alternatively, in a procedure known as submucous resection, he removes the cartilage entirely except for a small wedge that supports the nose.

After either procedure, the doctor inserts nasal packing.

Complications

Although both procedures are generally well tolerated, they can cause swelling, nasal hemorrhage, and septal hematoma. Other complications include nasal skin necrosis, infection, and septal perforation.

Care considerations

Before surgery

• Reinforce the surgeon's explanation of the procedure. In rhinoplasty, the surgeon will explain the extent of the procedure and how the nose should look postoperatively.

• For both rhinoplasty and septoplasty, tell the patient to expect nasal packing after surgery and that this, along with swelling, may give him an uncomfortable sensation of facial fullness. Warn him against trying to relieve this by manipulating the packing.

• Ensure that the patient has signed a consent form.

After surgery

• Watch closely to make sure the packing doesn't slip and obstruct the airway. Assess airway patency every hour and frequently check the position of nasal pack. If the patient becomes restless or starts to choke, notify the doctor — the nasal pack may have slipped.

• Provide analgesics, as prescribed and needed, to relieve headache.

• Tell the patient that the doctor will remove the packing 24 to 48 hours after surgery.

• Monitor vital signs, and observe for hemorrhage, which may be immediate or delayed. Keep the patient on his side to prevent aspiration of blood, and periodically examine the back of his throat for fresh blood. Also check any sputum or emesis for blood. The patient will probably have a mustache dressing (a folded gauze pad placed under the nose and above the lip and taped to the cheeks). This will need to be changed periodically.

• Help the patient rinse his mouth every 2 to 4 hours, and give him ice chips, as needed. Offer oral fluids 4 hours after surgery, and expect the patient to resume a normal diet the next day.

Home care instructions

• Instruct the patient not to blow his nose for at least 10 days after the nasal packing is removed because this may precipitate bleeding. If he needs to clear his nose, tell him to sniff gently.

• If the patient has a bandage or an external splint in place, tell him not to manipulate it because he may cause misalignment or bleeding.

• If the doctor orders inhalation treatments to reduce swelling and prevent crusting, instruct the patient to place a bowl of hot water before him and to drape a towel over his head, creating a tent. Then he should breathe in the warmed air.

• If the doctor prescribes nose drops, tell the patient how to administer them: He should lie flat on his back, instill the drops, and remain supine for 5 minutes to facilitate absorption by swollen tissues.

• Instruct the patient to take antibiotics and analgesics, as prescribed.

• Tell the patient to avoid bending or heavy lifting for 1 to 2 weeks, as recommended by the doctor.

• Advise the patient to notify the doctor if he develops severe pain, bleeding, or fever to rule out a nasal septal hematoma.

S

SCLERAL BUCKLING

Used to repair retinal detachment, scleral buckling involves application of external pressure to the separated retinal layers, bringing the choroid (a membrane that partially covers the eye between the retina and the sclera) into contact with the retina. Indenting (or buckling) brings the layers together so that an adhesion can form. It also prevents vitreous fluid from seeping between the detached layers of the retina and causing further detachment and possible blindness. When the break or tear is small enough, laser therapy, diathermy, or cryotherapy may be used to seal the retina.

Scleral buckling is successful in about 95% of patients. Its effectiveness depends on the cause, location, and duration of detachment. If the retinal macula is detached, visual acuity may still be poor after surgery.

Purpose
• To seal retinal breaks and reattach the retina.

Indications

Three types of retinal detachments may require scleral buckling: rhegmatogenous detachments, which are associated with holes or tears; tractional detachments, which occur when the fibrous tissue in the vitreous pulls the retina away from the retinal pigment epithelium; and exudative detachments, which are caused by such processes as intraocular inflammation with an accumulation of fluid beneath the retina.

Procedure
The patient's pupil is dilated with medication before surgery; this allows the surgeon access to the internal eye. After the patient receives a local anesthetic, the surgeon makes an incision in the conjunctiva, exposes the sclera, and then tags the rectus muscles with sutures to aid positioning of the eye.

Using a drawing that shows the location of ocular landmarks and the retinal tear, the surgeon locates the retinal tear and marks its position on the sclera by diathermy or cryotherapy. This forms an adhesive, exudative choroiditis at the site of the retinal hole. (As this heals, the scar should keep the retina in place.)

For an explant procedure, the surgeon sutures a scleral silicone sponge over the retinal hole. For an implant procedure, he dissects the scleral bed. Then he drains the subretinal fluid to allow the retina to contact the choroid. He does this by perforating the choroid and, if necessary, indenting the globe to drain the fluid. The surgeon places a silicone sponge in the prepared site and sutures the scleral flaps over the sponge. A band may also be sutured in place around the entire globe.

After scleral buckling, the surgeon may inject gas or air into the posterior cavity to create a bubble that pushes the retina into place against the choroid. Next he inserts antibiotic ointment or drops into the eye, and a patch is applied.

Complications

The two most common complications of scleral buckling are glaucoma and infection. In about 20% of patients, the retina fails to reattach, possibly requiring repeat surgery.

Care considerations

Before surgery

• Stress the importance of bed rest and remaining still to prevent further detachment of the retina.
• Explain the procedure to the patient.
• Instruct the patient to wash his face with an antiseptic solution to prevent infection.
• Administer mydriatic and cycloplegic drugs, as ordered, to dilate the pupils and relax the focusing muscles of the eye. Also administer any ordered sedative.
• Have the patient sign a consent form, and place it in the patient's chart.

After surgery

• After scleral buckling, place the patient in the ordered position. Notify the doctor immediately if you observe any eye discharge or if the patient experiences fever or sudden, sharp, or severe eye pain.
• Because the patient will probably have binocular patches in place for several days, institute safety precautions. Raise the side rails of his bed, and help him when he walks.
• Provide a safe environment. Assist the patient with all meals.
• Keep the patient's room free of obstacles.
• Ensure that the call bell is within easy reach of the patient.
• Advise the patient to avoid activities that increase intraocular pressure, such as hard coughing or sneezing, bending, or straining during defecation.
• Administer antiemetics, as prescribed, if the patient is nauseated because vomiting increases intraocular pressure.
• Emphasize to the patient that he must not rub or squeeze his eyes or squint.

This can rupture the suture line or cause retinal detachment.
• As prescribed, administer mydriatic and cycloplegic eyedrops to keep the pupil dilated and antibiotics and corticosteroids to reduce inflammation and infection. If the patient's eyelid or conjunctiva swells, apply ice packs.

Home care instructions

• Instruct the patient to notify the doctor of any signs of recurring detachment: floating spots, flashing lights, and progressive shadow. He should also report any fever, eye pain, or drainage.
• Stress the importance of avoiding strenuous activity or situations (such as crowds) in which jostling or eye injury could occur. Warn against heavy lifting, straining, or any strenuous activity that increases intraocular pressure.
• Tell the patient to avoid rapid eye movement, as in reading, until the doctor gives permission.
• Encourage the use of sunglasses during the day and an eye shield at night.
• Show the patient how to use prescribed dilating, antibiotic, or corticosteroid eyedrops. Stress the importance of meticulous cleanliness to avoid infection.
• Explain the importance of keeping follow-up medical appointments to check for further retinal detachment, glaucoma, and other complications.

SCLEROTHERAPY, ENDOSCOPIC FOR ESOPHAGEAL VARICES

Endoscopic sclerotherapy is used to treat esophageal varices by injecting the swollen veins with a sclerosant (a strongly irritating solution). The injection causes thrombosis of the mucosal and submucosal veins. Injection into the tissue beside the distended vein produces a fibrotic area and local edema that compresses the vessel. Eradicating the varix stops the variceal bleeding and prevents rebleeding.

Endoscopic sclerotherapy of esophageal varices was first reported in the late 1930s. From 1940 to 1970, this procedure intermittently gained and lost favor as surgical procedures (for example, portacaval shunting) overshadowed endoscopic treatment.

Recent improvements in endoscopic equipment and technique, combined with recognition of the shortcomings of some surgical procedures, have once again made endoscopic sclerotherapy the initial treatment of choice in most institutions.

After the initial treatment to control an acute bleeding episode, the patient is usually scheduled for elective additional endoscopic sclerotherapy treatments. They are usually scheduled at intervals of a few weeks, depending on the risk level and healing rate of the patient. Prophylactic endoscopic sclerotherapy is aimed at preventing rebleeding of the varices.

A similar procedure has been used successfully in treating leg varicosities and hemorrhoids by injecting a sclerosing agent into the distended veins.

Purpose
• To thrombose and obliterate distended esophageal veins
• To decrease the frequency and severity of variceal bleeding.

Indications
Endoscopic sclerotherapy is the current treatment of choice to control hemorrhage from esophageal varices, a condition associated with high morbidity and mortality. The treatment is also used prophylactically to prevent recurrence of variceal bleeding.

Endoscopic sclerotherapy cannot be performed on an uncooperative patient because any unscheduled movement could result in tearing of the varix or perforation of the esophagus with resulting hemorrhage.

Procedure
Before endoscopic sclerotherapy, the patient receives anesthesia in the form of conscious sedation (patient is sedated but awake). The procedure is performed by a doctor under direct visualization through a gastroscope. Following oral passage of the gastroscope, the doctor locates and identifies the variceal channels at or just above the gastroesophageal junction. If a bleeding varix is identified, a sclerosant is injected through a needle injector into the varix or the surrounding tissue. The needle is then withdrawn from the varix into the sheath, and this injection procedure is repeated at various locations to sclerose all variceal columns. The doctor will determine the number of injections and the volume of sclerosant used during each treatment. If no active bleeding is found, prophylactic treatment is initiated at the most distal portion of the esophagus to prevent blood from the injection site from obscuring subsequent target areas.

The sclerosants generally used in the United States are sodium morrhuate (5%), sodium tetradecyl sulphate (1.5% to 3%), absolute alcohol, and ethanolamine oleate.

Complications
Endoscopic sclerotherapy is associated with a 20% to 40% incidence of complications and a mortality rate of 1% to 2%. Transient chest pain, dysphagia, and fever are common, occurring within the first 24 hours after endoscopic sclerotherapy. Allergic reactions to the sclerosants are also possible.

Ulceration at the injection site is common with endoscopic sclerotherapy and may occur in as many as 94% of patients. However, ulceration is not consistently regarded as a complication but as a stage of variceal eradication.

Pulmonary complications include aspiration pneumonia, pleural effusion, pulmonary infiltrates, and adult respiratory distress syndrome. Traumatic esophageal perforation and hemorrhage can also occur and are usually attributable to the endoscopic procedure.

Esophageal stricture formation develops in 2% to 10% of patients and usually responds to conservative dilatation treatment.

Bacteremia occurs in 5% to 50% of patients, but antibiotic prophylaxis is not considered necessary except for patients with prosthetic heart valves.

Care considerations
Before the procedure
• Prepare the patient for perioral endoscopy.
• Record baseline vital signs and other pertinent data.
• Establish and maintain vascular access for I.V. fluids or blood replacement.
• Emphasize to the patient the importance of lying still to prevent injury.
After the procedure
• Observe the patient for signs of blood loss, pulmonary complications, fever, perforation, or other complications.
• Monitor the patient's vital signs.
• Maintain the I.V. line, as ordered.
• Administer additional pain medication, as prescribed.

Home care instructions
• Give the patient written and oral instructions about signs and symptoms of complications.
• Instruct the patient to report any fever, bleeding, respiratory problems, chest pain, or difficulty swallowing to the doctor immediately.
• Tell the patient to use mild analgesics, if prescribed by the doctor, for transient, mild chest pain.

• Instruct the patient about diet restrictions, as ordered by the doctor.

SEMANS' TECHNIQUE

Semans' technique is a procedure that helps treat premature ejaculation. In this technique, the partner manually stimulates the patient's penis, halting just before ejaculation so that the patient becomes more aware of his sexual response. Also called the "start-stop" technique, it was developed by Dr. Semans in 1956. Typically, Semans' technique is combined with sensate focus therapy—nongenital and genital touching exercises between the patient and his partner—to increase communication and reduce sexual anxiety.

Purpose
• To help the patient gradually regain control over ejaculation through serial "stop-start" penile stimulation.

Indications
Semans' technique is indicated for treatment of premature ejaculation.

Procedure
Semans' technique is taught by a sex therapist, doctor, or psychologist but may be reinforced by the nurse. The patient's partner begins by stimulating the patient's penis with her hands until he feels the urge to ejaculate. She then stops the stimulation and waits until the patient's urge to ejaculate passes before she begins stimulating his penis again. This penile stimulation is repeated four times, each time stopping short of ejaculation. Next, the partner stimulates the patient's penis one more time, allowing him to ejaculate. The couple is advised to avoid progressing to intercourse until this controlled manual stimulation has been mastered.

Complications

There are no reported complications associated with this procedure; however, sexual dysfunction can cause feelings of anger, guilt, rejection, avoidance, and insecurity. Therapy to help enhance communication is important.

Care considerations

Before therapy

• Reinforce the instructions given to the patient and his partner by the doctor, psychologist, or sex therapist.
• Emphasize that the patient and his partner may need to practice this technique for as long as several months before the patient can avoid ejaculating prematurely.

After therapy

• Review the instructions for performing Semans' technique, as necessary, to ensure that the couple will practice it correctly at home.

Home care instructions

• Stress the importance of setting aside time to satisfy the partner's sexual needs.
• Encourage the patient and his partner to attend follow-up counseling sessions to discuss their progress in using Semans' technique.
• Encourage honest communication between the patient and his partner.

SENSATE FOCUS THERAPY

Sensate focus therapy involves non-genital and genital touching exercises between the patient and his partner to increase communication and reduce sexual anxiety. Helpful in treating various sexual disorders, sensate focus therapy encourages a couple to relax and express intimacy. This therapy can be one of a variety of methods employed by the therapist to help couples experiencing sexual dysfunction. Initially, vaginal penetration is prohibited during these exercises to encourage each partner to focus on sensual feelings without being burdened by preset goals or performance anxiety. As a result, many couples discover or renew a deep sense of intimacy.

Purpose

• To decrease sexual anxiety by increasing a couple's awareness of touch and sexual intimacy.

Indications

Sensate focus therapy is indicated for patients who suffer from various sexual dysfunctions, especially when personal and emotional difficulties interfere with sexual expression.

Procedure

Sensate focus therapy is taught by a sex therapist, doctor, or psychologist. The nurse may be asked to explain or reinforce the instructions given. The couple removes all their clothes. One partner touches and explores the other's body, except for the genitals and breasts. The two then reverse roles so that each person gives and receives pleasurable sensations. Once they're comfortable performing this exercise, their touching progresses to include the genitals and breasts. They are advised to avoid intercourse until they feel fully at ease.

Complications

Feelings of anger, guilt, frustration, avoidance, rejection, and insecurity can result from or lead to sexual dysfunction. Interpersonal problems may surface during therapy.

Care considerations

Before therapy

• Tell the couple that they may feel uncomfortable or embarrassed when they first practice sensate focus exercises; however, with time, they'll overcome these inhibitions. Stress the importance of letting each other know what feels good and what doesn't.

• Stress the importance of a relaxed, undemanding atmosphere. The focus is on giving pleasure to the partner. There should be no distractions.
• When the couple feels sufficiently at ease to progress to intercourse, mention that intromission without thrusting is the next step. However, they should check with their therapist before taking this step and the next: intromission with thrusting.
• Suggest using moisturizing creams and lotions to enhance the sensation. Also suggest touching with the hands to start, then blowing, sucking, and stroking with objects such as a feather.
• Encourage the partner to concentrate on the pleasurable sensations of being touched.

After therapy
• Clear up any questions the couple may have about sensate focus exercises. Then remind them to set aside an uninterrupted time during the day or evening when they feel relaxed to practice these exercises.

Home care instructions
• Explain how to perform sensate focus exercises so the couple can practice them at home.
• Instruct the couple not to rush sensate focus exercises. Encourage them to repeat each exercise until they feel completely at ease before moving on to the next one. Stress that each couple must progress at its own pace.
• Stress the importance of communication throughout the exercise. Encourage the couple to be assertive and take responsibility for their sexual pleasure by frankly discussing what they find enjoyable and what they find unpleasant.
• Because many couples attempt intercourse too early during therapy, emphasize the importance of concentrating on touch and intimacy in a relaxed, nondemanding atmosphere.
• Encourage the couple to identify feelings of guilt, anxiety, fear, and frustra-tion. These feelings need to be dealt with through therapy in addition to sensate focus exercises.

SHUNT, PORTAL-SYSTEMIC

A portal-systemic shunt is a treatment used to reduce portal pressures and prevent or control bleeding from esophageal varices in patients with intractable portal hypertension. Typically, this surgery is performed only after more conservative measures (diet and drug therapy, endoscopic sclerotherapy) prove ineffective. If possible, it's performed after esophageal bleeding is controlled and the patient's condition is stabilized. However, emergency surgery may be necessary if esophagogastric tamponade or vasopressor drugs can't control hemorrhage from ruptured varices.

Three types of portal-systemic shunting are performed. To create a portacaval shunt (the most common), the surgeon diverts blood from the portal vein to the inferior vena cava, thereby reducing portal pressure. Splenorenal shunting, used in portal vein obstruction and when hypersplenism accompanies portal hypertension, diverts blood from the splenic vein to the left renal vein. Mesocaval shunting, indicated in portal vein thrombosis, previous splenectomy, or uncontrollable ascites, routes blood from the superior mesenteric vein to the inferior vena cava. A fourth type of shunt uses a device, a transjugular intrahepatic portosystemic shunt, and is indicated for patients with variceal hemorrhage secondary to portal hypertension. It uses an expandable balloon stent to shunt blood from the portal vein to the hepatic vein.

Due to complications, portal-systemic shunting has a mortality rate of approximately 25% to 50%. Research suggests that this surgery does little to prolong survival, with patients succumbing to

Hazards of portal-systemic shunting

Careful postoperative assessment can help you detect complications from portal-systemic shunting and perhaps even prevent death. For 48 to 72 hours after surgery, closely monitor the patient's fluid balance. Check his vital signs and record intake and output hourly. Monitor cardiac output and other hemodynamic measurements. Auscultate the patient's lungs at least every 4 hours to detect signs of pulmonary edema, such as crackles.

Watch closely for neurologic changes, such as lethargy, disorientation, apraxia, or hyperreflexia, which may indicate hepatic encephalopathy and developing hepatic coma. As ordered, obtain a serum sample for determination of ammonia levels. (Blood decomposition in the intestinal tract raises serum ammonia levels; a damaged liver may be unable to metabolize the ammonia, resulting in neurotoxic effects.) Also as ordered, obtain blood specimens for liver function and electrolyte studies.

To prevent pulmonary complications, encourage the patient to cough, deep-breathe, and change position at least once hourly. Provide an incentive spirometer, and show him how to use it.

hepatic complications more commonly than to uncontrolled esophageal bleeding.

Purpose

• To reduce portal pressure and control bleeding esophageal varices by shunting blood away from the portal venous system.

Indications

Portal-systemic shunts are indicated for patients with portal hypertension resulting from liver disease.

Procedure

After the patient receives a general anesthetic, the surgeon makes an abdominal incision. In portacaval shunting, he joins the portal vein and the inferior vena cava. An end-to-side anastomosis reduces portal pressure most effectively, but a side-to-side anastomosis allows some portal blood flow through the liver.

In splenorenal shunting, the surgeon joins the splenic vein and the left renal vein. An end-to-side anastomosis involves splenectomy; side-to-side anastomosis may be used in the absence of hypersplenism.

In mesocaval shunting, the surgeon joins the superior mesenteric vein to the inferior vena cava. However, neither the side-to-side anastomosis nor the synthetic graft performs as well as the other shunts, and both carry the risk of thrombosis.

Complications

A delicate and complicated surgery, portal-systemic shunting poses grave risks. (See *Hazards of portal-systemic shunting.*) For example, diversion of large amounts of blood into the inferior vena cava may cause pulmonary edema and ventricular overload. And shunting of blood away from the liver inhibits the conversion of ammonia to urea, possibly causing hepatic encephalopathy, which can progress rapidly to hepatic coma and death. Other possible complications include hemorrhage from a leaking anastomosis, which can cause peritonitis, and respiratory complications.

Care considerations
Before surgery
• Provide the patient with an explanation of the procedure if time permits.
• Stabilize the patient for emergency surgery; assist with measures to control bleeding.

• Inform the patient that he'll return from surgery with a nasogastric tube and chest tube in place. Tell him that he will also be connected to a cardiac monitor and will have pulmonary artery, arterial, and central venous pressure catheters in place to monitor hemodynamic status.

After surgery

• Monitor the patient's fluid balance closely for 48 to 72 hours after surgery.
• Check vital signs and record intake and output hourly.
• Auscultate the patient's lungs at least every 4 hours to detect signs of pulmonary edema.
• Watch closely for neurologic changes, such as lethargy, disorientation, apraxia, or hyperreflexia, which may point to hepatic encephalopathy and developing hepatic coma. As ordered, obtain a serum sample for determination of ammonia levels. (Blood decomposition in the intestinal tract raises serum ammonia levels; the damaged liver may be unable to metabolize the ammonia, resulting in neurotoxic effects.)
• As ordered, obtain blood for liver function and electrolyte studies.
• Encourage the patient to cough, deep-breathe, and change position at least once every hour. Provide an incentive spirometer, and show him how to use it.
• Administer analgesics, as prescribed.

Home care instructions

• Explain to the patient that although surgery has stopped the bleeding and will reduce the risk of future bleeding, it has not corrected the underlying liver disease. Emphasize the importance of complying with ordered diet and drug regimens, including strict abstention from alcohol. Also stress the need for adequate rest to reduce the risk of bleeding and infection.
• Tell the patient and his family to watch for and immediately report disorientation, lethargy, amnesia, slurred speech, tremors, or inability to perform purposeful movements. Explain that these signs and symptoms may herald hepatic encephalopathy, a potentially fatal complication.
• Stress the importance of regular follow-up examinations to evaluate shunt patency and liver function.

SHUNT, VENTRICULAR

Used for adults and children, this surgical treatment for hydrocephalus involves insertion of a catheter into the ventricular system to drain cerebrospinal fluid (CSF) into another body space, where it can be absorbed. The shunt extends from the cerebral ventricle to the scalp, where it's tunneled under the skin to the appropriate cavity. Typically, ventricular shunts consist of a radiopaque ventricular catheter and a one-way valve to prevent backflow of blood or other secretions.

The ventriculoperitoneal shunt, the most common type, drains CSF into the peritoneal sac. Other types, less commonly used, can drain CSF into the ureters, the right atrium, or the pleural space.

A small percentage of patients with congenital hydrocephalus outgrow the need for the shunt. Most hydrocephalic patients, however, are dependent on the shunt for the rest of their lives.

Purpose

• To relieve increased intracranial pressure (ICP) by draining CSF from the ventricles of the brain.

Indications

Ventricular shunts treat both communicating hydrocephalus (excessive accumulation of CSF in the subarachnoid space) and noncommunicating hydrocephalus (blockage of normal CSF flow from the lateral ventricles to the subarachnoid space).

Procedure

Insertion of a ventricular shunt requires specialized surgical skills. It is usually performed in an operating room with the patient under general anesthesia. The procedure varies according to the type of shunt being inserted.

To implant the ventriculoperitoneal shunt, the surgeon places a catheter into the anterior portion of the lateral ventricle through a burr hole in the skull. The catheter is connected to a one-way valve device, whose purpose is to prevent backflow of blood or other secretions. In order to place the proximal portion of the catheter into the peritoneum, an abdominal incision is made. The peritoneal catheter is then sutured to the ventricular catheter and valve unit, allowing CSF to be drained into the abdominal cavity.

To place a ventriculoatrial shunt, the surgeon runs the catheter from the ventricle through the jugular vein to the right atrium of the heart.

Another type of ventricular shunt can be placed in an operation known as a third ventriculostomy. In this procedure, the surgeon elevates the frontal lobe to expose the third ventricle for catheter insertion. Then the surgeon passes the other end of the catheter into the cistern of chiasma of the subarachnoid space.

The ventriculocisternal shunt differs from other types because it is usually temporary. It is used only occasionally and does not require a craniotomy. Instead, the surgeon makes a small burr hole in the occipital region, inserts a catheter into a lateral ventricle, and passes it under the dura and into the arachnoid canal (cisterna venae magnae cerebri).

Complications

Complications include infections such as ventriculitis and peritoneal infection. Shunt malfunction can result if the shunt becomes blocked or kinked;

this occurs most often in growing children and can result in elevated ICP. Ventricular collapse from improper catheter placement or faulty pumping techniques can also occur. Complications of a ventriculoatrial shunt involve the cardiovascular system and can include cardiac arrhythmia, valvular damage with cardiac perforation due to catheter migration, and thrombus or embolus formation.

Care considerations
Before surgery

• Tell the patient or family that this procedure lowers ICP and helps prevent brain damage. Prepare the patient as you would for a craniotomy. (See the entry "Craniotomy.") Explain that he'll have dressings on his head and, depending on the site of drainage, on his abdomen or chest.

• While the patient awaits surgery, carefully monitor vital signs and neurologic status and watch for signs of increased ICP: headache, vomiting, irritability, visual disturbances, and decreased level of consciousness.

• If the patient is an infant, measure his head circumference daily to detect any increase. Also observe his fontanels for bulging and tenderness.

• Make sure the infant's earlobe is lying flat, and place a sheepskin or rubber foam pad under his head to minimize the development of pressure areas on the scalp.

• To turn the infant, move the head, neck, and shoulders with the body; this reduces strain on the infant's neck.

After surgery

• Keep the patient flat for 3 to 5 days after shunt insertion. This will help him adjust to lowered ICP. Gradually raise his head in stages, about 20 degrees at a time.

• Carefully check vital signs and neurologic status every 2 hours. Immediately report any signs of elevated ICP, which may indicate a blocked or malfunctioning shunt.

• When picking up the child, be sure to support his buttocks. This prevents dislodgment of the drainage tube.

• Continue the child's normal diet. To help prevent constipation, which can cause shunt malfunction, encourage him to eat soft foods and drink plenty of liquids.

• Check for and report any signs of infection, such as fever, headache, nuchal rigidity, and local pain and inflammation. If infection occurs, the doctor will probably prescribe I.V. antibiotics. If the infection doesn't subside within 1 to 2 weeks, the shunt will be removed and replaced.

• To avoid pressure on the shunt suture lines, position the patient on the nonoperative side. This protects against suture abrasion and prevents local dependent edema.

• If ordered, pump the shunt. Use proper technique to avoid excessive CSF drainage from the ventricular system, which can abruptly reduce ICP and lead to ventricular collapse or blood vessel rupture. While pumping, watch for signs of rapidly rising ICP, which may indicate ventricular collapse.

Home care instructions

• Instruct the family to bathe the shunt suture line as they would normally bathe the child's skin.

• Inform the family that reddened skin may be caused by the child lying on the shunt and that they should keep the child from lying on that side for prolonged periods.

• Tell the family to report signs of infection or increased ICP immediately.

• If ordered, teach the family how to pump the shunt. The doctor may ask the patient or family to pump the shunt once or twice a day. Teach them to locate the pump by feeling for the soft center of the device under the skin behind the ear. Tell them to depress the center of the pump with the forefinger and then slowly release it. Advise them to pump only as many times as the doc-

tor has ordered (usually between 25 and 50 times, once or twice a day). Warn that excessive pumping can lead to serious complications.

• After shunt insertion, the doctor may order a 6- to 12-month course of anticonvulsant drug therapy. If so, emphasize the importance of complying with the medication schedule to prevent seizures. Also discuss possible drug reactions—especially those affecting the central nervous system and cardiovascular system—and the need to inform the doctor of any such reactions.

• If the patient is a child, remind the parents that he'll need periodic surgery as he grows to increase the shunt's length and modify its placement.

• Alert the family to signs of infection, such as rectal temperature above 101° F (38.3° C) for more than 6 hours; increased sleepiness; or warm, reddened skin at the incision site. Instruct them to notify the doctor of any of these signs.

• Alert the family to watch for signs of shunt malfunction. Instruct them to call the doctor immediately if they see bulging, tightness, and shining of the soft spots on the child's head, or if the child seems unusually fussy or sleepy, refuses to eat, vomits forcefully, or has difficulty grasping objects.

SINUS SURGERY, ENDOSCOPIC

Endoscopic sinus surgery is a surgical technique that uses fiber-optic endoscopes or telescopes to eradicate chronic and acute sinus disease. The use of fiber-optic endoscopes enhances visualization, because these tubes contain a light source, magnifying devices, and attachments for performing biopsies and brushings.

Purpose

• To establish an adequate sinus drainage system.

Indications

Endoscopic sinus surgery is indicated when medical therapies such as nasal irrigations with 0.9% sodium chloride solution or use of decongestants, antihistamines, or antibiotics fail to eradicate sinusitis. It is also indicated when a persistent obstruction to drainage is present. Conditions that may be improved by endoscopic sinus surgery include chronic and acute sinusitis, nasal polyposis, deviated septum, fungal sinusitis, or an enlarged middle turbinate that obstructs the sinus ostea. It may also be used for foreign body removal, excision of a tumor, or drainage of a periorbital abscess.

Procedure

Endoscopic sinus surgery is performed by a specially trained otolaryngologist. The patient is placed under general or local anesthesia. Then the surgeon injects a local anesthetic into the nasal mucosa to achieve maximum vasoconstriction. This is important because any amount of bleeding decreases the surgeon's ability to see during endoscopic sinus procedures. Using an endoscope, the surgeon opens the natural sinus ostea, which may have closed due to chronic sinus disease or may have become obstructed by polyps or cysts. If the nasal septum is deviated, this is straightened at the time of surgery. Packing will be placed in the nose for approximately 48 hours if a turbinectomy or trimming of the turbinate tissue was performed. The turbinates have a tendency to be bloody; therefore, packing is placed in the nasal cavity to act as a hemostatic dressing. Patients do not experience any visible bruising or discoloration of the nose or surrounding skin. And, because all of the incisions are made inside the nose, there are no external scars.

Complications

Complications resulting from endoscopic sinus surgery include bleeding (1 in 100 patients), infection, leakage of cerebrospinal fluid, loss of smell, scarring of the nasal tissue, and visual disturbances (including blindness). Bleeding and infection are the most common complications.

Care considerations

Before surgery

• Explain the procedure and its potential complications. The patient and family should be informed that endoscopic sinus surgery carries a potential risk to the eye, including the possibility of blindness, diplopia, or partial vision loss.
• Prepare the patient for the postoperative course, including expectations for pain and duration of the recovery period.
• Instruct the patient to fast from all food and fluids after midnight the night before surgery.
• Ensure that the patient has signed a consent form.

After surgery

• Monitor vital signs. Observe for airway problems, epistaxis, or hematemesis.
• Monitor the patient for pain, and administer analgesics, as needed.
• Provide written home care instructions.

Home care instructions

• Arrange for a perioperative nurse to call the patient's home the day after surgery to evaluate his postoperative course.
• Tell the patient to spend the first 24 hours at home resting. He should avoid heavy lifting, straining, and bending over, which increases the pressure within the nose and can cause bleeding.
• Advise the patient to avoid all medications containing aspirin or ibupro-

fen until instructed otherwise by the doctor.

• Tell the patient who has nasal packing in place to begin using a 0.9% sodium chloride nasal spray the day after the packing is removed. He should use the spray five to six times daily to provide moisture and prevent the accumulation of nasal crusts.

• Tell the patient that the nasal packing may be removed at the doctor's office. A young child may need to be under general anesthesia during this procedure.

• Tell the patient that copious amounts of mucus will cause him to feel like he has a cold.

• Reinforce the importance of postoperative follow-up for nasal suctioning.

• Instruct the patient to notify the doctor of fever over 101° F (38.3° C) or increased nasal drainage.

• Instruct the patient to contact the doctor and, if necessary, report to the nearest emergency department if uncontrolled bleeding occurs.

• Ensure that the patient understands dosages and administration of antibiotics and analgesics.

SITZ BATH

A sitz bath, also known as a hip bath, is the immersion of the pelvic area in tepid or hot water.

The tub or device used is usually shaped to allow the legs to remain out of the water. Most health care facilities have sitz bath basins that fit into toilet seats. Disposable sitz bath kits are also available for single-patient use. When special sitz bath devices are not available, a regular bathtub may be used.

Purpose

• To relieve perianal pain, edema, or discomfort

• To enhance healing by cleaning the perineum and anus, increasing circulation, and reducing inflammation

• To promote relaxation of the perianal muscles.

Indications

Sitz baths are commonly used after perianal surgery or childbirth.

Procedure

The patient is assisted to sit in a tub of warm (94° to 98° F [34.4° to 36.6°]) or hot (110° to 115° F [43.3° to 46.1°C]) water.

Usually the patient soaks for 15 to 20 minutes. The water temperature should be checked periodically to ensure that it has not cooled.

A disposable sitz bath kit includes a basin that is filled to the specified line with water and is placed under the toilet seat. An irrigation bag and tubing allow a stream of water to flow continuously over the wound while the patient is positioned in the bath.

Complications

Complications are rare, but occasionally patients develop an irregular or rapid heart rate or experience dizziness when standing up from the bath. These effects are due to vasodilation caused by immersion in hot water.

Care considerations

Before the procedure

• Make sure that the tub is clean and disinfected before each use. Check the water temperature with a bath thermometer before the patient gets in the tub.

• Explain the procedure to the patient.

• Ask the patient to void; then remove and dispose of any soiled dressings.

• Instruct the patient to use the safety rail for balance when getting into the tub.

During the procedure

• Frequently check the water temperature.

Sitz bath: Guide to self-care

Use the following directions when giving yourself a sitz bath.

You will need a sitz bath kit (plastic pan and a plastic bag with a tube attached) or a clean bathtub, medication (if prescribed), access to warm water, and towels.

After assembling all the necessary equipment, raise the toilet seat and fit the plastic pan onto the toilet bowl. The pan should be positioned so that the drainage holes are along the back of the bowl. If the pan is placed correctly, a single hole will be visible in the front.

Then, close the clamp on the bag's tubing and fill the bag with warm water and medication (if prescribed).

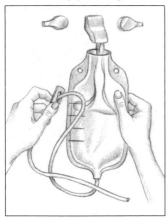

Snap the free end of the tubing into the slot at the front of the pan, and then hang the bag on the door knob or towel bar. Make sure that the bag is higher than the toilet.

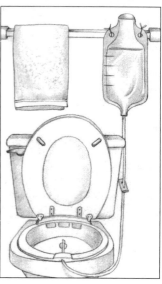

• Assess the patient's color and general condition frequently. If the patient complains of feeling weak, faint, or nauseated or shows signs of cardiovascular distress, discontinue the bath and monitor pulse and blood pressure.

• Cover the patient with a towel or bath blanket to maintain privacy and prevent vasoconstriction due to exposure.

• Place a call bell within easy reach when the patient is unattended.

After the procedure

• Have the patient rise slowly from the bath, using the safety rails for balance.

• Apply clean dressings to the perianal area if necessary.

• Clean and disinfect the tub after each use.

• Assess the patient for dizziness due to vasodilation, and help him to his room.

Carefully lower yourself onto the pan, and open the clamp on the tubing, allowing the warm water to flow from the bag into the pan to fill it. Don't worry if it overflows because excess water will flow out through the drainage holes into the toilet. Remain seated in the pan until the water begins to cool.

After the sitz bath, rise slowly and carefully to a standing position because you may experience fatigue and light-headedness. Then, dry off completely and apply an ointment or dressing, if ordered.

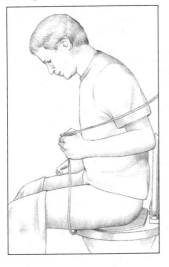

Home care instructions

• Instruct the patient in the use of a regular bathtub as a sitz bath or in the use of a disposable sitz bath kit. (See *Sitz bath: Guide to self-care*.)
• Stress the importance of safety precautions in the home, including a bath thermometer, nonskid bath mat, and safety rails, if available.

SKELETAL MUSCLE RELAXANTS

The skeletal muscle relaxants include *carisoprodol, chlorzoxazone, cyclobenzaprine, diazepam, methocarbamol, baclofen,* and *dantrolene.*

Purpose

• To reduce transmission of nerve impulses from the spinal cord to skeletal muscle (carisoprodol, chlorzoxazone, cyclobenzaprine, and methocarbamol)
• To interfere with intracellular calcium movement by acting directly on skeletal muscle (dantrolene)
• To depress the central nervous system (CNS) at the limbic and subcortical levels (diazepam).

Indications

Carisoprodol, chlorzoxazone, cyclobenzaprine, and methocarbamol are used as adjunctive treatment for painful muscle spasms resulting from acute, self-limiting disorders, such as sprains, strains, or fractures. Baclofen and dantrolene are used to treat severe spasticity associated with chronic disease, such as multiple sclerosis, or spasticity related to spinal cord transection.

Prolonged therapy with skeletal muscle relaxants carries a risk of severe CNS depression. For this reason, these agents are contraindicated in patients with existing CNS depression and in those taking sedatives. Because these drugs are metabolized in the liver and excreted by the kidneys, they should be used cautiously in patients with impaired renal or hepatic function.

Besides these broad guidelines, specific contraindications and precautions apply to individual drugs. For example, carisoprodol is contraindicated in patients with intermittent porphyria or hypersensitivity to related compounds (including meprobamate and diazepam) and in patients with acute angle-closure or chronic open-angle glaucoma, psychosis, or myasthenia gravis.

Baclofen and dantrolene are usually contraindicated in patients who require some degree of muscle spasticity to maintain motor function. Baclofen should also be used cautiously in patients with seizures because of the risk of increased seizure activity.

Adverse reactions

The skeletal muscle relaxants most frequently cause drowsiness, dizziness, and anticholinergic effects such as dry mouth. CNS reactions include vertigo, ataxia, tremor, headache, nervousness, confusion, depressed mood, and hallucinations. Cardiovascular reactions include tachycardia and hypotension. Baclofen may cause seizures or may exacerbate preexisting psychiatric disturbances. Dantrolene may cause abnormal liver function tests and, in some cases, moderate to severe hepatitis.

Care considerations

• Review the patient's drug regimen for possible interactions. Concurrent use with CNS depressants, such as monoamine oxidase inhibitors, narcotic analgesics, tricyclic antidepressants, or parenteral magnesium sulfate, can worsen CNS reactions.
• Some of these drugs have substantial anticholinergic activity, which may result in dry mouth. Have the patient chew sugarless hard candy or gum or use ice chips or artificial saliva. Patients should consult a dentist if therapy will be prolonged because persistent dry mouth is associated with an increase in the incidence of dental caries.
• If severe reactions occur, take precautions to prevent injury, such as raising the side rails of the bed and assisting with ambulation.
• Remember that skeletal muscle relaxants must be discontinued gradually. Abrupt withdrawal may produce

rebound spasticity or milder symptoms such as insomnia, headache, nausea, and abdominal cramps.

Home care instructions

• Instruct the patient never to take a skeletal muscle relaxant with alcohol or any over-the-counter CNS depressants, such as antihistamines or sleeping pills.
• Warn the patient to avoid driving or other hazardous tasks that require alertness, good psychomotor coordination, and visual acuity until the CNS effects of the drug have been established.
• Advise the patient to take baclofen, dantrolene, chlorzoxazone, or methocarbamol with meals or a glass of milk to minimize GI distress. Explain that he can crush chlorzoxazone or methocarbamol tablets and mix them with food or milk to ease swallowing. Tell the patient to take diazepam with food or a full glass of water.
• Instruct the patient to make up a missed dose only if he remembers within an hour or so of the scheduled administration time. If more than an hour has elapsed, he should skip the missed dose and resume taking the drug at the next scheduled administration time. Warn him to never double-dose.
• Emphasize the importance of regular follow-up examinations during long-term therapy.
• As appropriate, explain that chlorzoxazone may turn urine orange or purple; methocarbamol may turn urine green, black, or brown. Reassure the patient that this effect is normal.

SKIN GRAFTS

A skin graft consists of healthy skin taken either from the patient (autograft) or a donor (allograft) and applied to resurface an area damaged by burns, traumatic injury, or surgery.

The graft may be one of several types: split-thickness, full-thickness, or pedicle-flap. A split-thickness graft is the type most commonly used for covering open burns. It includes the epidermis and part of the dermis, and it may be applied as a sheet (usually on the face or neck to preserve the cosmetic result) or as a mesh. A mesh graft has tiny slits that allow the graft to expand up to nine times its original size. Mesh grafts prevent fluids from collecting under the graft and are typically used over extensive full-thickness burns.

A full-thickness graft includes the epidermis and the entire dermis. Consequently, it contains hair follicles, sweat glands, and sebaceous glands, which typically aren't included in a split-thickness graft. Full-thickness grafts are commonly used for small burns that cause deep wounds.

A pedicle-flap graft is a full-thickness graft that includes skin and subcutaneous tissue with subcutaneous blood vessels to ensure a continued blood supply to the graft. Pedicle-flap grafts may be used during reconstructive surgery to cover previous defects.

Purpose
• To restore skin integrity to areas that cannot heal by epithelialization.

Indications
Grafts are indicated when primary closure isn't possible or cosmetically acceptable, when primary closure would interfere with function, or when the defect is on a weight-bearing surface.

Grafts are contraindicated if the defect lacks a sufficient blood supply; for this reason, they can't be applied directly over bare tendon, bone, cartilage, nerves, large fat deposits, or tissue damaged by X-rays. Relative contraindications include arteriosclerosis, venous stasis, previous surgery, and cosmetic considerations; however, in these patients, skin grafts may be the only treatment available to close a large defect.

Procedure
Grafting may be performed under general or local anesthesia, either in the operating room or under sterile conditions at the bedside. Occasionally, grafting may be performed on an outpatient basis for extremely small facial or neck defects.

The thickness of the graft depends largely on the defect to be covered, with thicker grafts used for larger defects. If the blood supply is poor at the recipient site, a thinner graft is used because it requires less time for revascularization.

Autografts are taken from another area of the patient's body with a dermatome. This instrument cuts uniform, split-thickness portions — typically about $0.005''$ to $0.02''$ thick. The graft is then placed on the damaged site, which must be a clean granulating site for revascularization. The graft survives initially by direct contact with the underlying tissue, receiving oxygen and nutrients from the recipient bed through existing lymph, but it eventually will die unless capillary ingrowth develops. In split-thickness grafts, revascularization usually takes 3 to 5 days; in full-thickness grafts, it may take up to 2 weeks. A bulky pressure dressing may be used over the recipient site to enhance vascularization; this dressing will remain in place for 24 to 48 hours.

Complications
Complications include graft failure caused by inadequate blood supply, hematoma formation, poor contact between the graft and wound bed, or infection. Systemic sepsis may develop from infected graft or donor sites, especially in elderly and immunosuppressed patients or in those with poor blood supply.

Care considerations

Before the procedure

• To preserve potential donor sites, provide meticulous skin care. Turn or reposition the patient every 2 hours, provide range-of-motion exercises and massage, maintain good preoperative nutrition, dry donor areas completely after bathing, and watch for reddened areas or other signs of irritation.

• Assess the recipient site. The graft's survival depends on close contact with the underlying tissue; ideally, the recipient site should have healthy granulation tissue that's free of eschar, debris, or infection.

• Provide emotional support, but promote realistic expectations; many patients expect to look better immediately after the surgery. Warn the patient that he won't see the final results for at least a year. Immediately after surgery, normal contours may be distorted by tissue reaction, suture lines may be red, and the color of the newly transplanted skin may differ somewhat from that of surrounding skin. Also tell members of the patient's family what to expect, and enlist their help in providing psychological support for the patient.

• Explain postoperative routines. Tell the patient that you'll be inspecting the graft frequently after surgery to ensure that it's adhering to the underlying tissue, and warn that he'll be immobilized after the grafting procedure to keep the graft in place. Also tell him that the original, rather bulky dressing will remain in place for 1 or 2 days.

• Follow the surgeon's recommendations or the hospital's policy to prepare the donor and recipient sites for surgery. In many hospitals, the donor site is washed twice with soap and water, with the final shave and scrub done in the operating room; the recipient site may receive three or more dressing changes before grafting, with the last one including application of a topical antibiotic.

• If the grafting is being done at bedside, gather the required equipment, including a local anesthetic, dermatome, surgical tray, and dressing materials. Drape the donor site and, if provided, administer the local anesthetic; be careful not to raise wheals.

After the procedure

• The donor site may be covered with fine-mesh gauze or an ointment-impregnated dressing and left open to the air. In some cases, it will be covered with a synthetic adhesive dressing to promote moist wound healing.

• Meticulous postoperative care is vital for graft survival. Position the patient so that he's not lying on the graft, and keep the graft area elevated and immobilized. Modify nursing care to protect the graft; never use a blood pressure cuff over a graft site, for example. For burn patients, omit hydrotherapy while the graft heals.

• The donor site will be more painful than the recipient site. Administer analgesics, as necessary, and help the patient use nonpharmacologic pain-reduction techniques.

• The doctor removes the outer pressure dressing on the graft, usually 24 to 48 hours postoperatively, and may change the graft dressings on the 3rd to 5th postoperative day to assess the graft.

• Use sterile technique when changing a dressing, and work gently to avoid dislodging the graft. Clean the graft site with warm 0.9% sodium chloride solution and cotton-tipped applicators, leaving the fine-mesh gauze intact to prevent dislodging the graft.

• If hematomas, exudate, or purulent drainage are observed, notify the doctor and carefully remove the fine-mesh gauze with sterile forceps. Soak the gauze with warm 0.9% sodium chloride solution to facilitate removal. Then gently clean the area.

• The donor site dressing should be changed, using aseptic technique, every 6 to 8 hours until oozing stops.

Then, if dry exposure is used, an over-bed cradle should be used to tent the sheets.

• If a heat lamp has been ordered for the donor site, keep the lamp at least 2′ (0.6 m) away from the wound. Apply heat lamp therapy for 20 minutes three or four times a day.

• Apply the prescribed cream daily to the healed donor site to keep it pliable.

• Special beds may be required for patients whose graft or donor sites are on the posterior surfaces. Low-air loss or air-fluidized beds that preserve capillary filling pressures facilitate healing and promote comfort.

Home care instructions

• If grafting is done as an outpatient procedure, emphasize to the patient that the graft site must be immobilized to promote healing.

• Tell the patient not to disturb the dressings on the graft or donor site for any reason. If the dressings must be changed, the patient should call the doctor.

• After dressings have been removed, teach the patient to apply cream to the healed graft several times a day to keep the skin pliable and aid scar maturation.

• Because sun exposure can affect pigmentation of the graft, tell the patient to limit exposure to direct sunlight and to use a sunscreen on all grafted areas.

• If applicable, explain that after scar maturation is complete, additional plastic surgery may be needed to improve the graft's appearance.

SQUEEZE TECHNIQUE

Developed by sex therapists Masters and Johnson, the squeeze technique is the treatment of choice for premature ejaculation. In this technique, the patient's partner briefly squeezes the penis just below and above the coronal ridge when the patient feels the urge to ejaculate. This delays ejaculation and helps the patient gradually gain control over it.

Purpose

• To prevent premature ejaculation.

Indications

The squeeze technique is the treatment of choice for premature ejaculation.

Procedure

This technique is taught by a psychologist, doctor, or sex therapist and may be reinforced by a nurse. The partner manually stimulates the patient's penis. The patient lets the partner know when he feels the urge to ejaculate. The partner then positions her fingers around the penis and squeezes firmly for 3 to 4 seconds. This will cause slight flaccidity and forestall ejaculation.

Complications

The squeeze technique may cause temporary impotence, but this is uncommon.

Care considerations
Before therapy

• Begin by reviewing the anatomy of the penis and the physiology of erection and ejaculation.

• Reinforce appropriate instructions, and reassure the patient and his partner that this technique is painless and is usually successful. However, they may require several months of therapy to achieve success.

• Mention that the couple will require follow-up counseling, perhaps for as long as 2 years, because relapse is common.

• Tell the couple to wait 15 to 30 seconds before resuming penile stimulation. Each time the patient nears ejaculation, have the partner apply the squeeze technique until the patient can control ejaculation on his own.

• Once the patient achieves control, tell him to progress to inserting his penis into his partner's vagina but to avoid thrusting. As he develops control, he can attempt thrusting, gradually increasing speed. Have his partner use the squeeze technique as necessary to delay ejaculation to the optimal time.
• Encourage the patient and his partner to express their feelings throughout the activity.

After therapy
• Encourage and reinforce correct performance of the technique.
• Emphasize that timing and hand placement are the keys to success.
• Provide encouragement and support because the couple may have to practice the technique for months before achieving success.

Home care instructions
• Stress the importance of setting aside time to satisfy the partner's sexual needs.
• Encourage the patient and his partner to attend follow-up counseling sessions to discuss their progress in using this technique.

STAPEDECTOMY

Stapedectomy is the surgical removal of all or part of the stapes, the innermost of the three sound-conducting bones of the middle ear. It is usually performed to restore hearing loss due to otosclerosis, in which overgrowth of spongy bone causes the stapes to become immobile. Laser stapedotomy is a more recently developed procedure with fewer complications than stapedectomy and can be performed on an outpatient basis, which decreases hospitalization from 1 to 2 days to 2 to 4 hours. Because otosclerosis is usually bilateral, stapedectomy is usually performed twice—first in the ear with the greatest hearing loss and then, a year or so later, in the other ear.

Purpose
• To remove all or part of the stapes and restore hearing.

Indications
Stapedectomy is indicated in the treatment of otosclerosis. However, patients with a congenital fixation of the stapes, osteogenesis imperfecta, or traumatic dislocation of the stapes may also benefit from stapedectomy.

Stapedectomy is contraindicated in external otitis media and inner ear disease. It should be performed cautiously, if at all, in patients with complete hearing loss in the other ear because of the risk of complications.

Procedure
The patient receives general or local anesthesia. The surgeon may perform a total or a partial stapedectomy, depending on the extent of otosclerotic growth. (See *Understanding types of stapedectomy*, page 563.) In a total stapedectomy, the surgeon removes both the superstructure and the footplate of the stapes and then inserts a graft and prosthesis to bridge the gap between the incus and the inner ear. In a partial stapedectomy, he may sever and remove the anterior crus (arch) and the anterior portion of the footplate or remove the entire superstructure and leave the footplate in place, drilling it and fitting it with a piston.

In laser stapedotomy, the surgeon vaporizes the two crura (arches) of the stapes and the stapedius tendon using a laser. He then creates a small opening in the footplate of the stapes with the laser and places a prosthesis in the opening.

Complications
Complications include sudden sensorineural hearing loss, which can occur if the prosthesis slips into the vestibule

Understanding types of stapedectomy

Stapedectomy may be total or partial, depending on the extent of otosclerotic growth. It may also be performed using various techniques. Two types of stapedectomy are shown below.

Normal middle ear

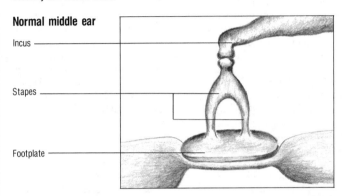

Incus

Stapes

Footplate

Partial stapedectomy
Wire-Teflon prosthesis

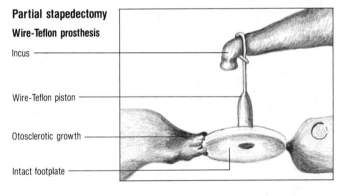

Incus

Wire-Teflon piston

Otosclerotic growth

Intact footplate

Total stapedectomy
Vein graft and strut prosthesis

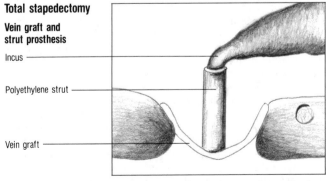

Incus

Polyethylene strut

Vein graft

or if fibrosis develops at the site. Other possible complications include transient vertigo, nausea, and vomiting. Facial nerve paralysis can result from the surgery or the local anesthetic. Rejection of the graft or prosthesis or complete closure of the oval window may allow perilymph fluid to leak. The patient may also develop a perilymph fistula, resulting in tinnitus, vertigo, and fluctuating hearing loss.

Care considerations

Before surgery

• Explain the procedure. Tell the patient whether he'll be receiving local or general anesthesia, and that prostheses are inserted with both procedures.
• Mention that hearing may not be improved for several weeks after surgery because ear packing and edema may mask any initial improvement. Packing is usually removed after 1 week; if absorbable gelatin foam is used, it will dissolve and does not require removal.
• Tell the patient that vertigo, nausea, and vomiting may occur after surgery but that he'll receive medication for these symptoms and for pain. Explain that he can minimize these symptoms by changing position slowly.
• Mention that activity may be restricted after surgery and that the patient may have to lie in one position to keep the prosthesis from dislodging.
• Prepare the patient for surgery, as appropriate, which may include washing his hair or shaving around the auricle. Give eardrops, ointments, irrigations, and hot or cold compresses, as ordered, to decrease any inflammation or relieve discomfort.
• Insert ear wicks loosely into the external ear to remove any drainage by capillary action.

After surgery

• The patient may lie on his operated ear to facilitate drainage, on his opposite ear to avoid graft displacement, or in the most comfortable position. Advise the patient to move slowly and without bending when changing position; this will help to prevent vertigo and nausea.
• Administer antiemetic drugs, as prescribed, if the patient develops vertigo, and keep the bed's side rails up at all times. If the patient experiences vertigo, assist with ambulation. Consider that vertigo may also indicate labyrinthitis or an inner ear reaction.
• Provide pain medication, as needed.
• Monitor for other signs of complications, such as fever, headache, ear pain, or persistent facial nerve paralysis. If facial paralysis results from the surgery, facial nerve decompression or corticosteroid therapy may be necessary.
• Use aseptic technique when changing the patient's dressings. Replace soiled or bloody pledgets in the ear canal as needed, and be sure to keep the ear dry.
• Tell the patient to refrain from coughing, sneezing, or blowing his nose because these actions could dislodge the prosthesis and graft.

Home care instructions

• Instruct the patient to inform the doctor immediately if he experiences fever; pain; purulent drainage; prolonged vertigo; a constant, loud buzzing or ringing; significant decrease in hearing; or sudden hearing loss. These signs may indicate infection or displacement of the prosthesis.
• Inform the patient that ear drainage may be reddish brown in color but usually becomes clear and disappears within 1 to 2 weeks.
• Tell the patient to protect his ear from cold drafts for 1 week and to avoid contact with people who have colds, influenza, or other contagious illnesses. Encourage compliance with prescribed antibiotics. Tell him to report any signs of respiratory infection immediately.
• Advise the patient to postpone washing his hair for 1 to 2 weeks and then,

for the next 4 weeks, to avoid getting water in his ears. Recommend placing a cotton ball in the ear canal and applying petroleum jelly over the cotton to form a seal when washing his hair.
• Tell the patient not to swim for 6 weeks and to wear a sweatband to prevent perspiration from getting into the ear during hot weather or exercise.
• To avoid displacement of the prosthesis, warn the patient to avoid blowing his nose for at least 1 week after surgery, to keep his mouth open when he sneezes, to avoid blowing up balloons and playing wind instruments for 1 month, and to avoid air travel for 6 months.
• Explain that the patient's taste sensation will be slightly altered for several weeks or months because the nerve for taste passes through the ear.
• Inform the patient that hearing may improve or fade at times during the first 3 weeks after surgery and that it's normal to hear cracking, popping, and sounds as if his head is "in a barrel."

SULFONAMIDES

Developed in the mid-1930s, sulfonamides were the first systemic antibacterials used in humans. Short-acting systemic sulfonamides, such as *sulfisoxazole*, are quickly absorbed and rapidly eliminated; intermediate-acting drugs, such as *sulfamethoxazole*, are absorbed and excreted more slowly.

Systemic sulfonamides are usually given orally, because they can precipitate out of I.V. solutions and irritate tissues.

Purpose
• To curb bacterial cell multiplication by inhibiting folic acid production.

Indications
Sulfonamides are effective against both gram-positive and gram-negative organisms, and although increased microbial resistance has limited their usefulness, they're still the drugs of choice for treating urinary tract infections. They're secondary drugs for other conditions, such as trachoma and toxoplasmosis. Topical sulfonamides are also used to prevent burn infections and treat ocular, vaginal, and other soft-tissue infections.

Sulfonamides should be avoided during late pregnancy and lactation and in premature infants and newborns. They easily cross the placenta and are excreted in breast milk, and they can cause kernicterus by displacing bilirubin from binding sites on albumin. These drugs should be used cautiously and in reduced dosage in patients with impaired renal or hepatic function, porphyria, intestinal or urinary obstruction, blood dyscrasias, allergies, or asthma.

Adverse reactions
Hypersensitivity reactions are among the most severe reactions to sulfonamides and include Stevens-Johnson syndrome. GI reactions include nausea, vomiting, diarrhea, impaired folic acid absorption, and hepatitis. Headache, vertigo, tinnitus, peripheral neuropathy, seizures, ataxia, and hallucinations have also been reported. Hematologic reactions include agranulocytosis, anemia, leukopenia, and thrombocytopenia as well as hemolytic anemia in patients with glucose-6-phosphate dehydrogenase deficiency. Sulfonamides can also cause hematuria, crystalluria, proteinuria, nephrotic syndrome, oliguria, and anuria in patients with normal renal function.

Care considerations
• Tell the patient to take the drug on an empty stomach and to drink plenty of fluids throughout therapy to prevent crystalluria.

• Monitor the patient's complete blood count, urinalysis, and intake and output.
• Watch for signs of erythema multiforme; if they occur, the drug should be discontinued.
• Review the patient's drug regimen for possible interactions. For example, methenamine compounds, urine acidifiers, and paraldehyde may cause precipitation of sulfonamides, leading to renal damage.
• Watch for hypoglycemia (caused by pancreatic stimulation) and suppressed thyroid function.

Home care instructions

• Stress the need to complete the full course of prescribed therapy, even after symptoms disappear.
• Instruct the patient to watch for signs of blood dyscrasias, such as sore throat, fever, mucosal ulcers, or jaundice. If these signs occur, the patient should stop the drug and contact the doctor immediately.
• If not contraindicated, encourage the patient to drink at least eight full glasses (8-oz [240-ml]) of water daily to prevent formation of urine crystals. If necessary, have him record his intake and output to monitor hydration.
• Tell the patient who's using a topical sulfonamide to stop using it if he notices local irritation or other allergic signs.
• Warn the patient to avoid prolonged exposure to sunlight because photosensitivity reactions may occur. Recommend wearing protective clothing and applying a sunscreen to exposed areas when outdoors.

SULFONYLUREAS

Developed in the 1950s, sulfonylureas are classified as first- or second-generation drugs. First-generation sulfonylureas include *tolbutamide, chlorpropa-* *mide, acetohexamide,* and *tolazamide;* second-generation drugs include *glyburide* and *glipizide.* (A third-generation group, the biguanides, is used in Europe. *Phenformin,* a biguanide that was once available in the United States, was removed from distribution because of concerns about lactic acidosis.) Both first- and second-generation sulfonylureas work equally well; some clinicians prefer the second-generation drugs because of their lower incidence of adverse effects, especially hyponatremia.

Purpose

• To normalize blood glucose levels by stimulating pancreatic beta cells to produce more insulin; by reducing hepatic glucose output; and by increasing the number of insulin receptors, which improves the insulin sensitivity of extrapancreatic tissues.

Indications

Sulfonylureas are the pharmacologic treatment of choice for Type II (noninsulin-dependent) diabetes mellitus. These oral hypoglycemic drugs work most effectively for patients whose diabetes is mild, nonketotic, uncontrollable by diet alone, and usually associated with obesity. However, they may also prove effective for patients whose diabetes requires dietary modifications and insulin dosages of 40 units/day or less.

Sulfonylureas are contraindicated in patients with Type I (insulin-dependent) diabetes because these patients lack functional beta cells. They're also contraindicated during pregnancy and lactation and for diabetic patients undergoing severe stress (such as from surgery or acute infection). They're usually not recommended in patients with hepatic or renal disease.

Adverse reactions

The primary adverse reactions to the sulfonylureas include hypoglycemia and hypersensitivity reactions such as pruritus, rash, and facial flushing. Increased gastric acid secretion may also cause GI symptoms such as heartburn, nausea, vomiting, abdominal pain, or diarrhea. Long-term therapy may increase the risk of death from cardiovascular disease.

Care considerations

• Review the patient's medication regimen because many drugs interact with sulfonylureas. Cimetidine, nonsteroidal anti-inflammatory drugs, and monoamine oxidase inhibitors may increase the hypoglycemic effects of the sulfonylureas; oral contraceptives, calcium channel blockers, thiazide diuretics, and alcohol may decrease the hypoglycemic effects of the sulfonylureas.

• Give sulfonylureas 30 minutes before meals to reduce postprandial blood glucose levels. Dividing the daily dose improves GI tolerance.

• If the patient is transferring from insulin therapy to an oral sulfonylurea, check urine glucose and ketone levels at least three times daily, before meals. Collect a double-voided specimen.

• If the patient is taking chlorpropamide, monitor his serum sodium level for hyponatremia and be alert for dysuria, anuria, hematuria, or other signs of renal insufficiency. Because this drug has a long duration of action (36 hours), monitor the patient for 3 to 5 days to detect hypoglycemia. If it occurs, I.V. dextrose may be required.

• If the patient is elderly, debilitated, or malnourished, be alert for an increased response to sulfonylureas, which may require reduced dosage.

Home care instructions

• Explain to the patient that sulfonylurea therapy represents only part of his diabetes care plan. Emphasize that the drug may be effective only temporarily or even ineffective if he fails to follow his prescribed diet and exercise program.

• Warn the patient not to take other medications without medical approval.

• If the patient is taking chlorpropamide or tolbutamide, warn him to avoid alcohol. Even small amounts of alcohol can induce chlorpropamide-alcohol flush, a disulfiram-like reaction that's characterized by extreme discomfort with facial flushing, light-headedness, pounding headache, nausea, vomiting, tachycardia, shortness of breath, and photosensitivity. Explain that these symptoms can last for up to an hour.

• Tell the patient that he'll need continued follow-up care and that he shouldn't discontinue this medication without medical approval. Instruct him to take his medication at the same time each day, as prescribed, to help stabilize his blood glucose levels. Tell him to take a missed dose as soon as he remembers, unless it's almost time for his next dose; he should not double-dose.

• Teach the patient how to test his blood or urine glucose levels. Explain that if blood glucose remains uncontrolled after several months of therapy or if it becomes uncontrolled after initial successful control by sulfonylureas, he may require insulin therapy. The patient may need insulin during an acute infection or traumatic injury or if surgery is required.

• Tell the patient to wear a medical identification bracelet containing information about his condition and the prescribed drug.

• Teach the patient how to recognize the signs and symptoms of hypoglycemia. If they occur, he should immediately notify his doctor and ingest a quick-acting sugar, such as hard candy, orange juice, or table sugar.

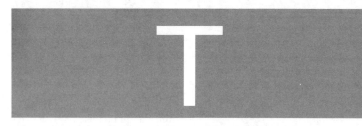

TARSORRHAPHY

Tarsorrhaphy is the intermarginal closure of the eyelids with sutures. It may be a temporary or a permanent procedure. Tarsorrhaphy is now rarely performed because of the availability of eyedrops and contact lenses to lubricate and protect the eye.

Purpose

• To reduce the width of the palpebral fissure (the space between the upper and lower eyelids) and therefore protect the eye from exposure
• To correct deformity of the eyelid.

Indications

Tarsorrhaphy may be indicated to protect the cornea from exposure caused by exophthalmos, neuroparalytic eyelids, exposure keratitis, superficial ulcerative keratitis, wounds, burns with scarring, or entropion. It's also performed to protect a disfigured or blind eye that doesn't require enucleation.

Procedure

Tarsorrhaphy is typically performed as an outpatient procedure. After administering a local anesthetic, the surgeon sutures the eyelids closed, leaving small portions of the palpebral fissure open for drainage of secretions (typically, the medial corner of the eyelids). An antibiotic ointment is then applied, and the eye is patched.

Complications

Complications of tarsorrhaphy are few and minor. They include superficial infection and eyelid edema.

Care considerations
Before surgery

• Reinforce the surgeon's explanation of the procedure. Encourage the patient to verbalize his feelings about the surgery; offer emotional support and reassurance.
• Emphasize to the patient that it is important he remains still during the procedure.
• Explain that after the entire eyelid is closed with sutures the patient will have monocular vision, reduced depth perception, and partial loss of peripheral vision on the affected side. He will need to move about cautiously until he adjusts to these visual limitations.
• Ensure that the patient has signed a consent form.

After surgery

• To ensure safety, help the patient get up and walk around until he adjusts to his altered vision.

Home care instructions

• Instruct the patient to take an analgesic, such as acetaminophen, to relieve mild discomfort. Tell the patient to contact the doctor if pain is severe or persistent.
• After a temporary tarsorrhaphy, inform the patient that the doctor will remove the sutures in 2 weeks. If eyedrops or ointments will be used after discharge, teach the patient or caregiver how to instill them properly. (See *How to instill eyedrops after tarsorrhaphy*.)
• Warn the patient to avoid rubbing the affected eye and to avoid wearing eye makeup until approved by the doctor. If tearing occurs, tell the patient to dab, rather than wipe, the tears.

How to instill eyedrops after tarsorrhaphy

Before giving eyedrops, verify the contents of the bottle and the strength of the medication. Also check the expiration date. Then follow these directions.

- Wash your hands.
- Have the patient lie down and turn his head sideways to allow gravity to pull the drops down and into the eye. (If you're putting drops in the right eye, turn his head to the right; if you're putting them in the left eye, turn it to the left.)
- Identify the small opening at the medial corner of the eyelid; then squeeze the

prescribed number of drops into the opening, taking care not to touch the eyelid with the dropper.
- Have the patient remain in position for 60 seconds after instillation so that the drops will flow inside the opening.
- Finally, using a tissue, gently remove excess medication. Wash your hands again.

• Tell the patient to notify the doctor if the affected eye becomes irritated or if a foreign particle becomes lodged in it. The patient should not try to treat these conditions himself.

• Give the patient and family members instructions for accommodating the patient's visual limitations in daily activities. Suggest placing dishes and beverages on the unaffected side because loss of peripheral vision may interfere with eating. To avoid spills when pouring liquids, advise the patient to touch the pouring container to the receiving container; when setting objects down, to release them only when they've contacted the surface.

• Caution family members to keep pathways clear of obstacles and to inform the patient before rearranging furniture.

• Instruct the patient to exercise caution in assessing the height of curbs or stairs. Reduced depth perception may impair his judgment.

• Instruct the patient to turn his head fully when crossing the street because peripheral vision is decreased.

• Advise the patient to avoid driving or other hazardous tasks that require normal vision until the doctor has given permission. Advise the patient who must drive to compensate for vision changes

by turning his head farther or relying more closely on the car's mirrors.

TETRACYCLINES

The tetracycline antibiotics include the drugs *demeclocycline, doxycycline, minocycline, oxytetracycline,* and *tetracycline hydrochloride.* Tetracyclines are available for systemic, ophthalmic, and topical use. They are rarely given by the I.M. route because they are very irritating to tissues.

Purpose

• To treat infections caused by susceptible organisms
• To treat the syndrome of inappropriate antidiuretic hormone secretion (demeclocycline).

Indications

Tetracyclines are used to treat infections caused by sensitive gram-positive and gram-negative organisms, including those of the genera *Rickettsia* (Rocky Mountain spotted fever, Q fever), *Mycoplasma,* and *Chlamydia* (lymphogranuloma venereum, psittacosis, trachoma). However, because of widespread microbial resistance (for ex-

Preventing tetracycline malabsorption

A patient who experiences GI upset during tetracycline therapy might be inclined to drink a glass of milk or take some stomach-soothing product, such as an antacid. Unfortunately, taking milk or an antacid with tetracyclines significantly reduces blood levels — and therefore the effectiveness — of these drugs. The calcium, magnesium, or aluminum in these substances interacts with tetracycline to form insoluble complexes.

To prevent GI upset while promoting proper drug absorption, tell the patient to take each dose with a full glass of water on an empty stomach. Also, review the patient's history for the following foods or drugs that interfere with tetracycline absorption:

• milk
• calcium supplements
• antacids that contain calcium, magnesium, or aluminum
• iron preparations, such as vitamins containing iron
• other products that contain magnesium, including sodium bicarbonate and milk of magnesia
• colestipol.

Advise the patient to take any of these at least 1 hour before or 2 hours after taking tetracycline.

ample, by *Proteus* and *Pseudomonas* organisms), tetracyclines are rarely the drugs of first choice.

Demeclocycline treats gonorrhea and infections caused by sensitive gram-negative and gram-positive organisms, including those of the genera *Rickettsia* and *Chlamydia*. Doxycycline, which can be used safely in renal impairment, treats infections caused by sensitive gram-positive and gram-negative organisms, including those of the genera *Rickettsia*, *Mycoplasma*, and *Chlamydia*. Minocycline proves effective for asymptomatic carriers of *Neisseria meningitidis* (but is not

recommended for meningococcal infections), gonorrhea, syphilis, or chlamydial infections. A naturally derived tetracycline, oxytetracycline treats urinary tract infections. As a substitute for penicillin, it may be used in brucellosis, syphilis, and gonorrhea. Tetracycline hydrochloride, the most widely used and least expensive tetracycline, is commonly used for acne, gonorrhea, syphilis, and chlamydial infections.

Tetracyclines should be avoided in patients with renal impairment because they increase tissue breakdown and therefore increase levels of waste products in the blood. They're also contraindicated during pregnancy because they may permanently discolor the teeth of the fetus. In children under age 8, they may cause permanent tooth discoloration and enamel defects and impede bone growth.

Adverse reactions

Hepatotoxicity may result from high doses of tetracyclines or from use in patients with renal impairment. Photosensitivity reactions have been reported with all tetracyclines but appear to be less frequent with demeclocycline and minocycline. Transient light-headedness and vertigo can occur in patients taking minocycline. Other adverse reactions include nausea, vomiting, loose stools, hairy tongue, *Candida* overgrowth, and skin pigmentation. Rarely, Stevens-Johnson syndrome (with minocycline) and pseudotumor cerebri may occur; infants may display bulging fontanels. Demeclocycline may cause a diabetes insipidus-like syndrome.

Care considerations

• Avoid giving oral tetracyclines with dairy products, antacids, iron preparations, multivitamins with iron, or laxatives. (See *Preventing tetracycline malabsorption*.) If both oral tetracycline and an iron preparation are prescribed, doses must be scheduled as far apart as possible because iron (as well

as other metallic ions, such as magnesium and zinc) combines with tetracyclines to inhibit absorption.
• Watch for overgrowth of nonsusceptible organisms, evidenced by mycotic infections of the mouth, throat, and vagina. The patient may experience a sore mouth, black hairy tongue, oral thrush, and rectal and perineal itching. To help relieve these symptoms, provide meticulous skin care in the affected areas two to three times daily.
• If the patient has diarrhea, carefully evaluate it to rule out gastroenteritis resulting from superinfection; this can be life-threatening and usually requires discontinuation of the drug.
• If the patient is receiving I.V. tetracycline, infuse the drug slowly in a well-diluted solution.
• During long-term use, monitor complete blood count and blood urea nitrogen level for evidence of blood dyscrasias.
• Watch for signs of diabetes insipidus, such as polyuria and polydipsia, in patients taking demeclocycline.
• Oral tetracyclines irritate the GI mucosa, causing nausea, vomiting, and flatulence. Giving the drug with water minimizes such GI irritation. If discomfort persists, give the drug with a light snack, such as crackers, although this may slightly reduce absorption.

Home care instructions

• Instruct the patient to take tetracycline at least 1 hour before or 2 hours after ingesting dairy products, antacids, or laxatives. To prevent GI upset, advise taking the drug with a glass of water.
• Warn the patient to avoid intense or prolonged exposure to sunlight. If exposure is unavoidable, advise him to wear protective clothing and use a sunscreen to prevent photosensitivity.
• Warn the patient that his stools may be loose during tetracycline therapy. Emphasize that he should report diarrhea and abdominal cramps to his doctor immediately.

THORACENTESIS

Thoracentesis is the aspiration of fluid or air from the pleural space by means of a needle or catheter inserted through the chest wall. The underlying cause of such fluid accumulation must be identified and corrected, or the pleural effusion is likely to recur.

Purpose

• To aid the identification of diseases of the pleura
• To relieve pulmonary compression and respiratory distress
• To instill medication into the pleural space.

Indications

Thoracentesis may be indicated in patients with pleural effusions caused by emphysema, tuberculosis, cancer, or chylothorax.

Thoracentesis must be performed with extreme caution in patients with a bleeding disorder because of the risk of hemorrhage.

Procedure

Thoracentesis is typically performed by a doctor at the bedside with a nurse's assistance. The nurse commonly assists with fluid drainage, specimen collection, and administration of drugs during the procedure.

After the patient is properly positioned (see *Positions for thoracentesis,* page 572) and the skin is prepared, the doctor administers a local anesthetic at the puncture site. Next, using sterile technique, he inserts the thoracentesis needle through the chest wall and into the pleural space. A 50-ml syringe is attached to the stopcock of the needle (a hemostat may be used to hold the needle in place and to prevent a pleural tear or lung puncture). The doctor may introduce a Teflon catheter into the needle, remove the needle, and attach

Positions for thoracentesis

Below are possible positions in which patients may be placed when thoracentesis is performed.

Leaning on a table

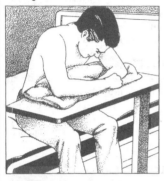

Straddling a chair

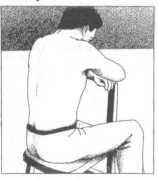

Semi-Fowler's position in bed

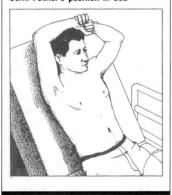

a stopcock and syringe or drainage tubing to the catheter. The doctor then slowly and carefully aspirates the pleural fluid and, after the needle or catheter is removed, applies pressure to the puncture site before applying a sterile dressing.

Complications

Complications of thoracentesis include pneumothorax, tension pneumothorax, fluid reaccumulation, mediastinal shift, and hypovolemic shock. Air embolism, a rare complication, may occur if air enters a superficial pulmonary vessel from injury to the visceral pleura. Infection may result if contamination occurs during the procedure.

Care considerations
Before the procedure
• Reinforce the doctor's explanation of the procedure. Encourage the patient to verbalize his feelings about the procedure, and offer emotional support and reassurance. Administer sedation, as prescribed.
• Advise the patient that he may feel a stinging sensation during injection of the local anesthetic and some pressure during needle insertion and fluid withdrawal. Stress the importance of remaining still during the procedure to reduce the risk of lung injury.
• Arrange for a chest X-ray or ultrasonography to identify the exact location of the fluid. Obtain copies of the results.
• Assess the patient's respiratory function and vital signs as a baseline. Review the patient's blood coagulation studies.
• Keep a chest tube setup, oxygen, and resuscitation equipment nearby.
• Prepare laboratory request slips to be sent with the specimens for analysis.
• If necessary, shave the needle insertion site and clean the area with an antiseptic solution.

During the procedure
• Position the patient as appropriate.
• Remind the patient not to move suddenly, cough, or breathe deeply.
• Continue to provide emotional support during the procedure.
• As appropriate, collect specimens, drain fluid, and administer drugs.
• Monitor the patient's vital signs, respiratory status, and color. Be alert for signs of mediastinal shift, which may cause labored breathing, arrhythmias, and sudden hypotension.

After the procedure
• Assist the patient to a comfortable position.
• Monitor the patient's vital signs and respiratory status every 15 minutes for 1 hour, every 30 minutes for the next 2 hours, every hour for the next 4 hours, and then as ordered. Be alert for signs of pneumothorax or rapid fluid reaccumulation (hemoptysis, respiratory distress, and a persistent, irritable cough), which may occur after the needle has been removed from the pleural cavity.
• Check the puncture site for excessive leakage. Be alert for signs of hypovolemic shock if a large amount of fluid was withdrawn. Change the dressing as needed.
• Arrange for a postprocedure chest X-ray and for any collected specimens to be sent to the laboratory for analysis.

Home care instructions
• Instruct the patient and family to notify the doctor if fever, dyspnea, or tachycardia develop.

THROMBOLYTICS

The thrombolytic enzymes *streptokinase* and *urokinase* and the newer agents *anistreplase and alteplase* (also known as tissue plasminogen activator) provide rapid correction of acute and extensive thrombotic disorders. For example, alteplase, streptokinase, or urokinase infusion can serve as an alternative to surgery in massive pulmonary emboli.

Each patient must be carefully evaluated before thrombolytic therapy, and the anticipated benefits must be weighed against the potential risks. Factors to consider when evaluating a patient include recent (within 10 days) major surgery or obstetrical delivery, organ biopsy, serious GI bleeding, puncture of noncompressible vessels, cerebrovascular disease, acute pericarditis, hemostatic defects (including those secondary to hepatic or renal disease), and advanced age (over age 75).

Purpose
• To degrade fibrin clots, fibrinogen, and other plasma proteins by activating plasminogen and converting it to plasmin.

Indications
Streptokinase, which has replaced urokinase as the drug of choice for most thrombotic disorders, also helps dissolve acute deep vein and arterial thrombi.

Anistreplase, alteplase, and streptokinase are used for lysis of thrombi obstructing coronary arteries in patients with acute myocardial infarction (MI). Such treatment should begin as soon as possible after the onset of acute MI. The goal of therapy is to reduce the infarct size and ultimately reduce the mortality associated with this condition.

Streptokinase is contraindicated in patients with ulcerative wounds, recent internal injuries, visceral or intracranial cancer, ulcerative colitis or diverticulitis, severe hypertension, hepatic or renal insufficiency, uncontrolled hypocoagulation, chronic pulmonary disease with cavitation, subacute bacterial endocarditis or rheumatic disease, or recent cerebral embolism, thrombosis, or hemorrhage. It's also contraindicated for at least 10 days after any surgery or intra-arterial diagnostic procedure. It should be used carefully when treating arterial emboli originating in the left side of the heart because of the risk of cerebral infarction.

Adverse reactions

Thrombolytics may cause severe, sudden external or internal bleeding or oozing from puncture sites. The risk of bleeding may be further increased by the concomitant use of heparin therapy.

Thrombolytics may also cause mild allergic reactions; serious anaphylactic reactions are more common with streptokinase. Febrile reactions have been reported; they should not be treated with aspirin or antiplatelet drugs. Rapid lysis of coronary artery thrombi may be associated with a reperfusion-related cardiac arrhythmia, which is usually transient but occasionally requires treatment.

Thrombolytics may cause hypotension unrelated to bleeding or anaphylaxis. This hypotension is usually transient but may require reduction of the drug dosage.

Care considerations

• Before beginning thrombolytic therapy, draw serum samples for blood typing and crossmatching and for determination of prothrombin time and partial thromboplastin time.
• Obtain a baseline electrocardiogram (ECG) as well as electrolyte, arterial blood gas, blood urea nitrogen, creatinine, and cardiac enzyme levels. Check subsequent findings against these baselines throughout therapy.
• At the start of streptokinase or anistreplase therapy, watch for signs of hypersensitivity: hypotension, shortness of breath, wheezing, a feeling of tightness and pressure in the chest, and angioedema. Keep emergency resuscitation equipment readily available.
• Throughout therapy, continuously monitor the patient's ECG and compare

it with baseline readings to detect arrhythmias. Be prepared to administer antiarrhythmics as ordered.
• Monitor the patient for signs of bleeding; check every 15 minutes for the 1st hour, every 30 minutes for the next 7 hours, and every 8 hours thereafter. If you detect bleeding, the drug should be discontinued during clinical evaluation. Ensure that packed red blood cells, whole blood, and aminocaproic acid are readily available to treat possible hemorrhage.
• Check the patient's vital signs frequently, and monitor pulses, color, and sensory function in the extremities every hour. If the patient develops fever (a common effect of streptokinase), administer acetaminophen, not aspirin.
• Because the patient is prone to bruising during thrombolytic therapy, handle him gently and as little as possible. Keep invasive procedures and venipunctures to a minimum, and pad the side rails of his bed to prevent injury.
• Expect to administer anticoagulants to prevent recurrence of thrombosis.

Home care instructions

• Encourage the patient to keep follow-up appointments with his doctor.
• Remind the patient who is receiving anticoagulants to keep laboratory appointments for bleeding time assessments.

THYROIDECTOMY

Thyroidectomy is the surgical removal of part (subtotal) or all (total) of the thyroid gland. Total thyroidectomy eliminates the possibility of recurrent thyrotoxicosis but requires lifetime thyroid hormone replacement therapy. Subtotal thyroidectomy removes up to 80% of the gland; the remaining 20% supplies enough thyroid hormone for normal function.

Purpose
- To remove hyperfunctioning tissue and thereby decrease circulating thyroid hormone levels
- To remove enlarged thyroid tissue and relieve respiratory obstruction
- To remove thyroid cancer.

Indications
Thyroidectomy is the treatment of choice for thyroid cancer, goiter, and hyperthyroidism unresponsive to antithyroid medication, and when radiation therapy is contraindicated.

Procedure
Thyroidectomy is performed while the patient is under general anesthesia. The patient is placed in the dorsal position, with sandbags or an air pillow under his shoulders, and his neck hyperextended. The surgeon makes an incision ⅜″ to ¾″ (1 to 2 cm) above the clavicles, creating skin flaps to the area. The thyroid gland is then exposed and excised. Drains are inserted, and the wound is closed with clips or staples before a dressing is applied.

Complications
Complications are rare after thyroidectomy if the patient has been prepared with thyroid hormone antagonists before surgery. Potential complications include thyroid storm; hemorrhage; parathyroid damage, resulting in postoperative hypocalcemia or tetany; and laryngeal nerve damage, causing hoarseness or permanent voice change. (See *Guarding against hazards of thyroidectomy*, page 576.)

Care considerations
Before surgery
- Reinforce the surgeon's explanation of the surgery. Offer emotional support and reassurance. Encourage the patient to verbalize his feelings about the surgery.
- Ensure that the patient has followed the prescribed preoperative regimen of antithyroid drugs (to accomplish a euthyroid state) and iodine preparations (to decrease excessive vascularity of the thyroid gland).
- Encourage the patient to maintain an adequate caloric intake; about 4,000 to 5,000 calories daily may be necessary to regain and maintain weight lost due to the effects of excess thyroid hormone.
- Because hyperthyroidism causes increased nervousness and anxiety, promote a calm and restful environment. Remind the patient to avoid caffeine and other stimulants. Administer tranquilizers as appropriate.
- Inform the patient what to expect in the immediate postoperative period. Tell him that he will have dressings and drains in place, and that he may experience some hoarseness, sore throat, or temporary difficulty speaking.

After surgery
- Monitor vital signs frequently. Assess respiratory status; be alert for signs of upper airway obstruction, such as stridor, dyspnea, cyanosis, or "crowing." Keep a tracheotomy tray and emergency equipment nearby. Suction the patient's mouth and trachea as needed. Steam inhalation may be used to promote expectoration of secretions.
- Keep the patient in semi-Fowler's position to promote venous return from the head and neck, facilitate drainage, and decrease edema. Support the patient's head and neck with sandbags or pillows. Apply an ice collar to the patient's neck to promote comfort and decrease edema.
- Check for laryngeal nerve damage, and assess speech and swallowing periodically.
- Check the dressing frequently, especially the posterior portion, where drainage may pool dependently. Note the amount, location, and characteristics of drainage. Check the patency of incisional drains; expect only scant drainage after 24 hours.
- Monitor the patient's incision. Note any redness, swelling, hematoma, or

Guarding against hazards of thyroidectomy

Thyroidectomy has many benefits and relatively few complications. However, some complications can be life-threatening if not promptly recognized and corrected.

Thyroid storm

This rare but severe form of thyrotoxicosis can occur in a patient who has received inadequate preoperative treatment with thyroid hormone antagonists. Its symptoms include high fever; hot, flushed skin; tachycardia and tachyarrhythmias; agitation and restlessness; confusion; and frank psychosis. Without treatment, hypotension, coma, and vascular collapse may follow.

If you detect thyroid storm, infuse fluids, apply a hypothermia blanket, and give acetaminophen. Also give saturated solution of potassium iodide (SSKI), propranolol, and hydrocortisone I.V. Instill propylthiouracil through a nasogastric tube to block thyroid hormone synthesis and release. If the patient develops respiratory distress, administer oxygen and ensure a patent airway. Treat extreme restlessness with sedatives, as prescribed, and monitor vital signs, cardiac rhythm, and serum thyroid hormone levels.

Hypocalcemia

Inadvertent damage to the parathyroid glands during surgery may cause transient hypoparathyroidism with resulting hypocalcemia. To detect it, check for early signs of hypocalcemia (such as paresthesia in the extremities) every 2 to 4 hours postoperatively. Test for positive Chvostek's and Trousseau's signs. Be alert for later signs of hypocalcemia: muscle cramps, tetany, sei-

zures, stridor, dyspnea, diplopia, and abdominal pain, and urinary frequency. If the patient develops acute hypocalcemic tetany, administer I.V. calcium gluconate. Expect emergency tracheotomy if stridor and vocal cord paralysis lead to respiratory obstruction.

Hemorrhage

In the initial hours after surgery, hemorrhage may appear in the confined space of the deep cervical fascia, causing acute airway obstruction with increasing respiratory distress and restlessness. Maintain airway patency and, if necessary, assist with emergency tracheotomy. The patient may require surgery to reopen the wound, relieve the pressure, and correct the hemorrhage.

Nerve injury

Inadvertent damage to the recurrent laryngeal nerves can cause temporary or permanent voice change or permanent paralysis. Assess the patient's voice as he awakens from anesthesia and for 2 days after surgery. Unilateral nerve damage causes initial hoarseness and a nonexplosive cough, improving until the patient has a normal voice that tires easily. Bilateral injury causes early postoperative stridor and ineffective respirations. The patient may need reintubation for 7 to 10 days and eventually, if no improvement occurs, a tracheotomy. Be prepared to relieve respiratory distress.

separation. Administer analgesics as appropriate.
• Monitor serum calcium levels. Test for Chvostek's and Trousseau's signs, indicators of neuromuscular irritability from hypocalcemia. Keep calcium gluconate available for emergency I.V. administration.
• Be alert for signs of thyroid storm.

• Teach the patient to prevent strain on the neck muscles when rising to a sitting position; tell him to support his head with a pillow and put his hands together behind his neck as he rises.

Home care instructions

• Stress the importance of regularly taking prescribed thyroid hormone replacement. Teach the patient to recognize and report signs of hypothyroidism, hyperthyroidism, and infection.

• If parathyroid damage occurred during surgery, explain the need for calcium supplements. Teach the patient the warning signs of hypocalcemia.

• Teach the patient how to keep the incision site clean and dry.

• Recommend appropriate coping strategies for the patient to deal with his altered appearance. Suggest loosely buttoned collars, high-necked blouses, or scarves, which can hide the incision until it has healed. Recommend using a mild body lotion to soften the healing scar and improve its appearance.

• Encourage adequate rest and nutrition to promote healing and regain or maintain weight.

• Stress the importance of keeping follow-up appointments to monitor serum thyroid hormone levels.

THYROID HORMONE ANTAGONISTS

Two classes of thyroid hormone antagonists—the stable iodines and the thioamides—are currently used. A third class, represented by the drug *ipodate*, has been found to reduce serum triiodothyronine levels rapidly. The stable iodines, such as *potassium iodide*, were once the only therapy available for hyperthyroidism. These drugs suppress thyroid hormone secretion and reduce the gland's vascularity and size. Although they effectively combat thyrotoxic crisis in adults, they're now used less commonly than the thioamides because they're not as long acting. Chronic use of iodides may cause reversible iodism, a toxic condition characterized by skin eruptions, swelling and inflammation of the mucous membranes, conjunctivitis, fever, edema, and irritability.

The thioamides, the mainstay of antithyroid drug therapy, inhibit formation of thyroid hormone.

The thyroid hormone antagonists don't permanently affect the thyroid gland, but they inhibit hormone production until spontaneous remission of hyperthyroidism occurs. Because they decrease thyroid vascularity, they're also used before thyroidectomy to prevent hemorrhage and thyroid storm.

Purpose

• To provide temporary euthyroidism in the hyperthyroid patient

• To reduce thyroid vascularity and hormone levels before surgery.

Indications

Thyroid hormone antagonists are the primary treatment for patients with transient hyperthyroidism (from Graves' disease, multinodular goiter, or thyroiditis), for those who refuse iodine 131 treatment, and for those in whom thyroidectomy is contraindicated.

Propylthiouracil (PTU) is the preferred thioamide when rapid action is desired, as in severe hyperthyroidism or thyroid storm. Longer acting *methimazole* can be given once daily and is preferred for treating mild-to-moderate hyperthyroidism. (A similar drug, *carbimazole*, is used widely in Europe but has not yet been approved for use in the United States.)

Thyroid hormone antagonists should be given cautiously during pregnancy. When they're needed, PTU is usually prescribed because methimazole has been linked with aplasia cutis congenita.

Adverse reactions

Therapeutic doses of thyroid hormone antagonists can cause fever, chills, sore throat, weakness, backache, swelling of the ankles or feet, and joint pain. Toxic doses can cause constipation; cold intolerance; dry, puffy skin; headache;

sleepiness; muscle aches; and unusual weight gain.

Methimazole and PTU may cause agranulocytosis, aplastic anemia, hepatitis, or exfoliative dermatitis.

Care considerations

• If administering potassium iodide, first check the patient's history for iodine allergies. If none exist, dilute the solution in juice or milk to counteract its metallic taste and have the patient sip it through a straw to avoid discoloring his teeth. Give this solution after meals to prevent gastric irritation.

• If the patient is receiving potassium iodide for a prolonged period, check for signs of iodism—a brassy taste or burning sensation in the mouth, skin eruptions, conjunctivitis, fever, edema, and irritability. A rare but serious hypersensitivity reaction, marked by angioedema, hemorrhagic skin lesions, and serum sickness, may occur when iodine is given I.V. To deal with this reaction, make sure that resuscitation equipment is available at the patient's bedside.

• If the patient is receiving a thioamide, monitor for signs of hypersensitivity, which may require a decreased dosage. Monitor the patient's complete blood count (CBC) periodically to detect leukopenia and granulocytopenia, which may occur 4 to 8 weeks after therapy begins. The drug may be continued if leukopenia is mild, but it must be withdrawn if the patient develops granulocytopenia. Continue to monitor CBC until leukocyte production returns to normal, usually within 1 to 2 weeks after discontinuing the drug.

• Monitor serum thyroid hormone levels to determine response to therapy. If the patient is taking PTU, expect hormone levels to return to normal in 14 to 60 days.

Home care instructions

• If the patient is receiving thyroid hormone antagonists in preparation for surgery, explain the intended effects and the importance of maintaining the medication schedule.

• If the patient is receiving thyroid hormone antagonists for hyperthyroidism, stress the importance of maintaining the medication schedule to prevent recurrence. Warn that he may not notice improvement for several weeks, until he exhausts his stores of thyroid hormones. Mention that symptoms related to increased sympathetic activity, such as tachycardia, diaphoresis, and tremors, may disappear rapidly. (If not, the beta blocker propranolol may be prescribed.) However, improvement of symptoms related to catabolic activity, such as weight loss, hypercalcemia, and myopathy, will take longer.

• If the patient is taking a thioamide, tell him to watch for hypersensitivity reactions and to report skin eruptions immediately. Emphasize the importance of promptly reporting a sore throat, fever, or mouth sores, especially during the 4th to 8th week of therapy.

• Warn the patient not to stop taking the prescribed drug without medical approval; abrupt withdrawal may precipitate thyroid storm.

• Tell the patient to take his medication at the same time each day.

• Explain diet restrictions, such as limitation of iodine-rich foods during therapy.

• Instruct the patient to take a missed dose as soon as possible; however, if it's almost time for his next dose, he should take both together. If he misses two doses, he should call his doctor for specific instructions.

• Tell the patient to store the medication in its original light-resistant container. Warn him not to take any over-the-counter drugs (especially decongestants and cough medications, which may contain iodine) without medical approval.

• Advise the patient to inform all doctors or dentists of his medication regimen before any invasive procedures to minimize the risk of thyrotoxicosis.

THYROID HORMONES

Thyroid hormone replacements were first used to treat hypothyroidism in the 1890s. These extracts of animal thyroid hormone, such as desiccated thyroid and thyroglobulin, are still in use despite concerns about variations in their ratio of triiodothyronine (T_3) to thyroxine (T_4) from batch to batch. However, purified synthetic preparations, such as *liothyronine, levothyroxine,* and *liotrix,* are now more commonly used.

Purpose

• To restore hormonal and metabolic balance in a patient with deficient endogenous thyroid hormone levels.

Indications

Liothyronine, a rapidly acting T_3, is used for treating myxedema or myxedema coma, mild hypothyroidism, and simple (nontoxic) goiter. However, dosage regulation is difficult, and the hormone's rapid action may cause cardiotoxic effects or abrupt metabolic changes. Levothyroxine (synthetic T_4), the drug of choice for long-term therapy, possesses a longer half-life than liothyronine. As a result, it can be administered once daily, improving compliance. Liotrix, a combination of T_3 and T_4, isn't prescribed frequently because T_4 is converted to T_3 in peripheral tissues, and patients receiving adequate doses of T_4 alone have normal T_3 levels; administering this drug may result in excessively high T_3 levels.

Thyroid hormones should be used with extreme caution in patients with atherosclerosis and other heart diseases because they can precipitate angina pectoris or myocardial infarction. They should also be given cautiously to patients with adrenal insufficiency because they can increase tissue demand for adrenal hormones, causing adrenal crisis. Thyroid hormones can be given safely during pregnancy but must be used cautiously during lactation because small amounts are excreted in breast milk.

Adverse reactions

Adverse reactions are usually dose related and resolve when the dosage is reduced or the drug is discontinued. The most common adverse reaction is hyperthyroidism, which is most likely due to therapeutic overdose. Common symptoms include nervousness, insomnia, tremor, tachycardia, nausea, and headache. Other reactions include weight loss, menstrual irregularities, sweating, heat intolerance, and fever.

Care considerations

• Before giving thyroid hormones, ask the patient about hypersensitivity to aspirin. An aspirin-sensitive patient may be allergic to tartrazine dye, which is present in some preparations of liotrix and levothyroxine. Also check for lactose intolerance, which may forewarn of sensitivity to levothyroxine.

• Review the patient's medication regimen for possible interactions. Concurrent use of cholestyramine or colestipol, for example, can impair absorption of thyroid hormones, requiring separation of doses by 4 to 5 hours. Use of digitalis glycosides requires careful monitoring because of the increased risk of digitalis toxicity.

• When the patient begins therapy, monitor serum total or free T_4 levels. Expect an improvement in 1 to 3 days if the patient is taking liothyronine; in 1 to 3 weeks if he's taking levothyroxine.

• Be alert for symptoms of hyperthyroidism, especially in elderly patients or those with cardiac disease.
• Watch for GI reactions, such as diarrhea, abdominal cramps, weight loss, and increased appetite.
• Check for cardiovascular effects, such as palpitations, chest pain, sweating, tachycardia, increased pulse and blood pressure, angina, and arrhythmias. Also note such other effects as headache, nervousness, heat intolerance, tremors, and insomnia. Any of these symptoms may require dosage reduction.

Home care instructions
• Inform the patient that thyroid hormone replacement doesn't cure his disease – it only relieves his symptoms – and therefore must be taken continuously, although he'll feel better in a few weeks.
• Emphasize to the patient that adherence to the medication schedule is extremely important. He should take the drug at the same time each day to maintain constant hormone levels. Instruct him to take a missed dose as soon as possible unless it's almost time for his next dose; he shouldn't double-dose. Tell him to call his doctor if he misses two or more doses.
• Warn the patient to report symptoms of hypothyroidism or hyperthyroidism immediately because such symptoms indicate a need for dosage adjustment.
• Instruct the patient to keep his medication in its original container and to protect it from light and moisture. Tell him to store it in a cool place (below 40°F [4.4°C]).
• Advise the patient to use the same brand of medication because the bioavailability of different brands may not be the same.

TOCOLYTICS

The beta agonists *ritodrine* and *terbutaline* relax uterine muscles to suppress premature labor. Currently, only ritodrine has the Food and Drug Administration's approval for inhibiting preterm labor. However, clinicians used terbutaline for this purpose before the introduction of ritodrine and some continue to prefer it.

The tocolytics usually are administered by I.V. infusion until uterine contractions stop. After discharge, the patient may continue with oral doses until the delivery of a mature infant is assured. Alternatively, some doctors prescribe a 5-day treatment course, which avoids prolonged maternal and fetal exposure to the drug. Infusion may be repeated if premature labor recurs.

Purpose
• To decrease the frequency, intensity, and duration of uterine contractions.

Indications
Tocolytics are indicated when conservative treatments (such as hydration or bed rest) fail to halt uterine contractions, diagnosis of premature labor is certain, gestation is less than 34 weeks, the cervix is dilated less than 4 cm, and no contraindications exist for their use.

The adverse cardiovascular and metabolic effects of these drugs are most severe with I.V. administration. They occur in both the mother and the fetus but can usually be controlled by reducing the drug dosage.

Tocolytics shouldn't be used when continuation of the pregnancy presents a greater hazard than premature delivery. Such conditions include pregnancy-induced hypertension, hemorrhage, intrauterine fetal death, maternal cardiac disease, and hypothyroidism. They should be used cautiously in patients with cardiovascular disease, diabetes mellitus, and hyperthyroidism and with concurrent administration of corticosteroids.

Adverse reactions

Tocolytics may cause nervousness, anxiety, headache, tremor, dose-related alterations in blood pressure, palpitations, tachycardia, electrocardiogram (ECG) changes, pulmonary edema, nausea, vomiting, hyperglycemia, hypokalemia, rash, and erythema.

Care considerations

• Carefully monitor the patient during therapy. If a tocolytic will be given I.V., perform a baseline ECG and connect the patient to a fetal monitor. Also collect serum samples for a complete blood count and electrolyte and glucose studies, as ordered. During therapy, monitor these laboratory studies, usually at 6-hour intervals, to detect hypokalemia, hypoglycemia, or decreased hematocrit. Report abnormal findings to the doctor.

• Monitor the patient's cardiac status continuously for any arrhythmias. Check blood pressure and pulse every 10 to 15 minutes initially, then every 30 minutes or as ordered. If her pulse rate exceeds 140 beats/minute or her blood pressure falls 15 mm Hg or more, drug intolerance may necessitate a dosage adjustment. Be sure the patient remains in the left lateral position to provide increased blood flow to the uterus.

• If the patient complains of palpitations, chest pain, or tightness in the chest, decrease the drug dosage and notify the doctor immediately. Keep emergency resuscitation equipment nearby.

• Assess pulmonary status every hour during I.V. therapy, and monitor intake and output. Fluid overload may lead to pulmonary edema, especially if the patient is receiving concurrent

corticosteroids. Auscultate her lungs, and report any crackles or increased respirations; also report urine output that drops below 50 ml/hour. If signs of pulmonary edema develop, place the patient in high Fowler's position and administer oxygen, as ordered.

• Check the patient's temperature every 4 hours during I.V. infusion. Report any fever to the doctor.

• Note the frequency and duration of uterine contractions. Check the fetal heart rate on the monitor every 10 to 15 minutes initially and then every 30 minutes or as appropriate. Immediately notify the doctor if the fetal heart rate exceeds 180 beats/minute or falls below 120 beats/minute.

• For 1 to 2 hours after I.V. therapy, monitor fetal heart sounds as well as the patient's vital signs and intake and output. Perform serial ECGs as ordered, and assess for uterine contractions. Immediately report tachycardia, hypotension, decreased urine output, or diminished or absent fetal heart sounds.

Home care instructions

• Reassure the patient that the drug should have minimal effects on the infant—for example, mild hypoglycemia for the first 24 hours after birth.

• Tell the patient to notify her doctor immediately if she experiences sweating, chest pain, or increased pulse rate. Teach her to check her pulse before taking the drug. If her pulse exceeds 130 beats/minute, she should skip the dose and notify the doctor promptly.

• Emphasize to the patient the importance of immediately reporting any contractions, low back pain, cramping, or increased vaginal discharge.

• Tell the patient to notify the doctor about headache, nervousness, tremors, restlessness, nausea, or vomiting; such reactions will probably necessitate reduction of drug dosage. She should also notify the doctor if her urine output decreases or if she gains more than 5 lb (2.3 kg) in a week.

• Tell the patient to take her temperature every day and to report any fever. This may be a sign of infection.

• Advise the patient to take oral doses of the drug with food (to avoid GI upset) and to take the last dose several hours before bedtime (to avoid insomnia).

• Instruct the patient to maintain bed rest as much as possible. Also tell her not to prepare her breasts for breast-feeding until about 2 weeks before her due date because this can stimulate the release of oxytocin and initiate contractions.

• Emphasize to the patient the importance of keeping follow-up appointments so that the doctor can monitor her progress with laboratory tests and fetal monitoring.

TONSILLECTOMY AND ADENOIDECTOMY

Tonsillectomy is the surgical removal of the palatine tonsils; adenoidectomy is the surgical removal of the pharyngeal tonsils. Both procedures were once performed routinely on school-age children but are now less commonly used. Instead, systemic antibiotics are prescribed to treat tonsils and adenoids enlarged by bacterial infection.

Tonsillectomy is most commonly performed on children over age 3. In rare circumstances an adult may require this procedure. Adenoidectomy is performed almost exclusively in children because adenoid tissue usually atrophies by adolescence.

Purpose

• To remove the palatine and pharyngeal tonsils.

Indications

Either or both of these procedures may be indicated when enlarged tonsillar tissue obstructs the upper airway, causing hypoxia or sleep apnea. Tonsillectomy is the preferred treatment for peritonsillar abscess and chronic tonsillitis that causes more than seven acute attacks within 2 years. Adenoidectomy may be performed to prevent recurrent otitis media, although some experts dispute its effectiveness.

Tonsillectomy and adenoidectomy are contraindicated in patients with acute tonsillar infection, active tuberculosis, hemophilia, or leukemia. They are also contraindicated in cleft palate because removal of this tissue allows air to escape through the nose and may create severe speech problems in these patients.

Procedure

Both surgeries may be performed as inpatient or outpatient procedures. For tonsillectomy, a child typically receives a general anesthetic; an adult patient may receive a local anesthetic. The surgeon removes tonsillar tissue by dissection and snare. In an adenoidectomy or adenotonsillectomy, the child receives a general anesthetic. Adenoidectomy is usually performed before tonsillectomy. The child is placed in Rose's position (head hyperextended), and the surgeon removes adenoidal tissue with a gentle, sweeping motion, using an adenoid curette or adenotome. If necessary, he then removes the palatine tonsillar tissue.

Complications

The most serious complication of these surgeries is hemorrhage, which may occur within 24 hours after surgery or up to 10 days later, when the healing tissue formed at the operative site begins to slough off. Other complications include pain that interferes with adequate hydration and problems with airway patency from edema or accumulated secretions.

Care considerations
Before surgery
• Reinforce the surgeon's explanation of the surgery. Encourage the child and his parents to verbalize their feelings, and offer emotional support and reassurance.
• Arrange for the child and family to tour the operating and postanesthesia rooms. Explain hospital routines, and answer questions simply and honestly.
• If the child is scheduled for an adenoidectomy, evaluate his speech and articulation. If necessary, arrange for an evaluation by a speech therapist.
• Assess the child for the presence of loose teeth, which can become dislodged during surgery.

After surgery
• Position the child recovering from anesthesia on his side or abdomen to facilitate drainage of secretions. Suction cautiously. Position the adult (under local anesthesia) with his head up at a 45-degree angle.
• Monitor vital signs, level of consciousness, and respiratory status.
• With a flashlight, assess the throat and check for bleeding. Frequent swallowing may indicate blood seeping down the back of the throat. Vomiting of dark brown emesis, caused by blood swallowed during surgery, is common. Watch for bright red blood, which indicates new bleeding at the operative site.
• As the patient becomes more alert, offer fluids to soothe the throat and prevent dehydration. Start with ice chips, and progress to ice pops and clear cold fluids. Ensure adequate fluid intake (1 to 2 liters/day for a child; 2 to 3 liters/day for an adult).
• Warn the patient not to attempt to cough or clear the throat to avoid dislodging clots. Avoid using straws or other utensils placed in the mouth.
• Medicate with acetaminophen as appropriate (avoid analgesics that contain aspirin, which may cause bleeding).
• Provide an ice collar or cool compresses to relieve sore throat.

Home care instructions
• Instruct the patient or the parents to report any bleeding or fever immediately. Advise them to watch for frequent swallowing, especially during sleep. Note that the risk of bleeding continues until 7 to 10 days after surgery, when the white membrane formed at the operative site begins to slough off.
• Instruct the patient or parents to limit diet to liquids and soft foods for 1 to 2 weeks to avoid dislodging clots or precipitating bleeding. Stress the importance of maintaining an adequate fluid intake to avoid dehydration and to soothe the throat.
• Inform the patient or parents that minor discomfort, such as ear pain (especially on swallowing), a sore throat, and voice changes, may persist for 1 to 2 weeks after surgery. Instruct them to avoid medications that contain aspirin and to use acetaminophen as needed.
• Encourage the patient to brush his teeth gently, to use a mild mouthwash, and to avoid vigorous brushing, gargling, and irritating liquids for several weeks.
• Advise the patient to avoid vigorous activity for 5 to 7 days after discharge. A child typically returns to school after 10 to 14 days. The patient should avoid exposure to persons with colds or other contagious illnesses for at least 2 weeks.

TRABECULECTOMY

A surgical filtering procedure, trabeculectomy removes part of the trabecular meshwork of the eye to allow aqueous humor to bypass blocked outflow channels and flow safely away from the eye. An iridectomy is performed at the same time to prevent the iris from prolapsing into the new opening and obstructing the flow of aqueous humor.

Purpose
• To create a new path for aqueous humor outflow
• To prevent the buildup of intraocular pressure.

Indications
Trabeculectomy is the procedure of choice in primary and secondary open-angle glaucoma.

Procedure
After the patient has received a local anesthetic, the surgeon dissects a flap of sclera and removes a portion of the trabecular meshwork. He then performs a peripheral iridectomy to create a filtering bleb, or opening for aqueous humor outflow, under the conjunctiva. An antibiotic ointment is then applied before the eye is patched.

Complications
Complications of trabeculectomy include a temporary rise in intraocular pressure, collapse of the filtering bleb, severe inflammatory reaction, infection, early cataract formation, and hyphema.

Care considerations
Before surgery
• Reinforce the surgeon's explanation of the surgery. Encourage the patient to verbalize his feelings about the surgery, and offer emotional support.
• Emphasize to the patient that this procedure will probably prevent further visual impairment but that it can't restore vision that's already lost. Explain that it will temporarily affect depth perception and peripheral vision on the operative side.
• Administer prescribed antiglaucoma drugs until the patient leaves for the operating room.

• Warn the patient to avoid any activities that could increase intraocular pressure, such as bending, vigorous coughing or sneezing, or straining during defecation.
• Tell the patient what to expect in the immediate postoperative period. Tell the patient that an eye patch or shield will be in place, tell him that periodic tonometry measurements will be taken, and warn him that he will experience blurred vision.

After surgery
• Observe the eye for excessive bleeding from the affected area.
• Monitor the patient for nausea and administer antiemetics because vomiting can raise intraocular pressure.
• Administer prescribed eyedrops: miotics, such as pilocarpine, will be given immediately after surgery; mydriatics, such as atropine, after 3 to 4 days. Also give corticosteroids to reduce iritis, analgesics to relieve pain, and antiglaucoma drugs to reduce pressure in the unaffected eye.
• Remind the patient to avoid activities that increase intraocular pressure, to not sleep on the affected side until approved by the doctor, and to use an eye shield at night.
• Because the patient's depth perception may be affected after surgery, remind him to ask for help when rising from bed or walking.

Home care instructions
• Instruct the patient to immediately report sudden onset of severe eye pain, photophobia, excessive lacrimation, inflammation, or vision loss.
• Explain that glaucoma isn't curable but can be controlled by taking prescribed drugs regularly.
• Warn the patient to avoid wearing constrictive clothing around his neck or torso because it can increase intraocular pressure.
• Emphasize to the patient that changes in his vision can present safety hazards. Show him how to use up-and-down

head movements to compensate for loss of depth perception. To help him overcome the loss of peripheral vision, teach him to turn his head fully to view objects on his side.
• Instruct the patient to avoid excessive fluid intake, heavy lifting, and undue straining, all of which raise intraocular pressure.
• Warn the patient to avoid driving or other hazardous tasks that require normal vision until the doctor gives permission.
• Stress the importance of regular medical follow-up for periodic monitoring of peripheral vision and intraocular pressure. Urge family members to have regular eye examinations, because glaucoma is usually familial.

TRACHEOTOMY

A tracheotomy is the surgical creation of an opening into the trachea through the neck. An incision is made between the tracheal rings, and a tube is inserted through the opening to allow the passage of air and removal of secretions. A tracheotomy may be temporary or permanent, depending on the patient's condition.

Purpose
• To provide access to the lower airway, permitting ventilation and removal of secretions.

Indications
A tracheotomy is most commonly performed to provide an airway for the intubated patient who needs prolonged mechanical ventilation. It may also be performed to bypass upper airway obstruction caused by trauma, burns, epiglottitis, or a tumor or to help remove lower tracheobronchial secretions in a patient who can't clear them. Although endotracheal intubation is the treatment of choice in an emer-

gency, a tracheotomy may be performed if intubation is impossible. After laryngectomy, the patient has a permanent tracheostomy, in which the skin and the trachea are sutured together to create the necessary stoma.

Procedure
In an emergency, a tracheotomy may be performed at the bedside. Elective, permanent tracheotomy is performed in the operating room with the patient under general anesthesia. The patient is placed in the dorsal position, with the neck hyperextended. The surgeon makes a vertical incision in the midline of the neck from the lower border of the thyroid cartilage to slightly above the suprasternal notch. The trachea is exposed, and a second vertical incision is made between the third and fourth tracheal rings. Next, a tracheostomy tube is inserted to permit access to the airway. Selection of a specific tube depends on the patient's condition and the doctor's preference. (See *Comparing tracheostomy tubes*, page 586.) After controlling bleeding and suctioning excess secretions, the surgeon applies a dressing around the tube and insertion site before loosely fastening tracheostomy ties around the patient's neck.

Complications
A tracheotomy can cause serious complications. Within 48 hours after surgery, the patient may develop hemorrhage at the site, bleeding or edema within the tracheal tissue, aspiration of secretions, pneumothorax, pneumomediastinum, cardiac tamponade, or subcutaneous emphysema. After 48 hours, subsequent complications may include stomal or pulmonary infection, ischemia and hemorrhage, airway obstruction, hypoxia, and arrhythmias. (See *Managing complications of tracheotomy*, pages 588 and 589, for details on preventing or recognizing such complications.)

Comparing tracheostomy tubes

Tracheostomy tubes are made of plastic or metal and may be cuffed, uncuffed, or fenestrated. Tube selection depends on the patient's condition and the doctor's preference. These commonly used tracheostomy tubes have the following advantages and disadvantages.

TUBE TYPE	ADVANTAGES	DISADVANTAGES
Uncuffed (plastic or metal) 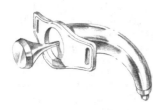	• Permits free flow of air around tube and through larynx • Reduces risk of tracheal damage • Recommended for children because it doesn't require a cuff	• In adults, absence of the cuff increases the risk of aspiration • Adapter may be necessary for ventilation
Cuffed (low pressure and high volume) 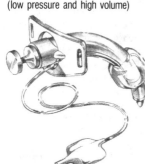	• Disposable • Cuff is bonded to tube; won't detach accidentally inside the trachea • Cuff pressure is low and evenly distributed against tracheal wall; no need to deflate periodically to lower pressure • Reduces risk of tracheal damage	• May be costlier than other tubes
Fenestrated 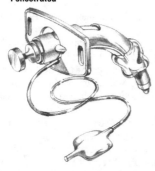	• Permits speech through upper airway when external opening is capped and cuff is deflated • Allows breathing by mechanical ventilation with inner cannula in place and cuff inflated • Inner cannula can be easily removed for cleaning	• Fenestration may become occluded • Inner cannula can become dislodged

Care considerations

Before surgery

• For an emergency tracheotomy, briefly explain the procedure to the patient, if possible, and quickly obtain supplies or a tracheotomy tray.

• For a scheduled tracheotomy, reinforce the surgeon's explanation of the procedure. Encourage the patient to verbalize his concerns. Offer emotional support and reassurance.

• Establish a communication system with the patient, such as a letter board, magic slate, or flash cards, and have him practice using it so he can communicate comfortably while his speech is limited.

• Tell the patient what to expect in the immediate postoperative period. Tell the patient that he will have dressings in place, will require frequent suctioning, and will lose the ability to speak and the sense of smell.

• Arrange for the patient to meet someone who has undergone a similar procedure and has adjusted well to tube and stoma care.

• Arrange for diagnostic studies as appropriate.

After surgery

• Monitor the patient's vital signs, color, and level of consciousness closely. Check the operative site for bleeding.

• Auscultate the patient's breath sounds every 2 hours after a tracheotomy is performed, noting crackles, rhonchi, or diminished sounds. Turn the patient every 2 hours to prevent pooling of tracheal secretions. Note the amount, consistency, color, and odor of secretions.

• Provide chest physiotherapy to help mobilize secretions.

• Provide humidification to reduce the drying effects of oxygen on mucous membranes and to thin secretions. Expect to deliver oxygen through a T-piece connected to a nebulizer or heated cascade humidifier. If the patient is an infant or a young child, be sure to warm the oxygen.

• Monitor arterial blood gas results, and compare them with baseline values to help determine if oxygenation and carbon dioxide removal are adequate. As appropriate, also monitor the patient's arterial oxygen saturation using pulse oximetry.

• Using sterile equipment and technique, suction the tracheostomy as needed to remove excess secretions. Use a suction catheter no larger than half the diameter of the tracheostomy tube, and minimize oxygen deprivation and tracheal trauma by keeping the bypass port open while inserting the catheter. Use a gentle, twisting motion on withdrawal to help minimize tracheal and bronchial mucosal irritation.

• Apply suction for no longer than 10 seconds at a time, and discontinue suctioning if the patient develops respiratory distress. (Before suctioning, ventilate the patient with 100% oxygen.) Also monitor for arrhythmias, which can occur if suctioning decreases partial pressure of oxygen in arterial blood (PaO_2) below 50 mm Hg. Evaluate the effectiveness of suctioning by auscultating breath sounds.

• A cuffed tube, usually inflated until the patient no longer needs controlled ventilation or is no longer at risk for aspiration, can cause tracheal stenosis from excessive pressure or incorrect placement. Prevent trauma to the interior tracheal wall by using pressures lower than 18 mm Hg and minimal leak technique when inflating the cuff. Reduce the risk of trauma to the stomal site and internal tracheal wall by using lightweight corrugated tubing for the ventilator or nebulizer and providing a swivel adapter for the ventilator circuit.

• Make sure the tracheostomy ties are secure but not overly tight. Refrain from changing the ties unnecessarily until the stomal track is stable, thereby helping to prevent accidental tube dislodgment or expulsion. Observe carefully for any tube pulsation, which may

Managing complications of tracheotomy

COMPLICATION	PREVENTION
Aspiration	• Evaluate patient's ability to swallow. • Elevate patient's head, and inflate the cuff during feeding and for 30 minutes afterward.
Bleeding	• Don't pull on the tracheostomy tube; don't allow ventilator tubing to do so. • If dressing adheres to the wound, wet it with hydrogen peroxide and remove gently.
Infection	• Always use strict aseptic technique. • Thoroughly clean all tubing. • Change nebulizer and humidifier jar and all tubing daily. • Collect sputum and wound drainage specimens for culture.
Pneumothorax	• Assess for subcutaneous emphysema, which may indicate pneumothorax. Notify the doctor if this occurs.
Subcutaneous emphysema	• Make sure that cuffed tube is patent and properly inflated. • Avoid displacement by securing tracheostomy ties and using lightweight ventilator tubing and swivel valves.
Tracheomalacia	• Avoid excessive cuff pressures. • Avoid suctioning beyond the end of the tube.

indicate proximity to the innominate artery, predisposing the patient to hemorrhage.
• Using aseptic technique, change the tracheostomy dressing when soiled or once per shift. Observe the amount and characteristics of any drainage. Assess the stoma and the surrounding skin, noting any swelling, erythema, bleeding, or skin breakdown.
• Keep a sterile tracheostomy tube (with obturator) at the patient's bedside, and be prepared to assist the doctor should he need to replace an expelled or contaminated tube. Also have available a sterile tracheostomy tube (with obtu-

DETECTION	TREATMENT
• Assess for dyspnea, tachycardia, rhonchi, crackles, excessive secretions, and fever.	• Obtain chest X-ray, if ordered. • Suction excessive secretions. • Give antibiotics if necessary.
• Check dressing regularly; slight bleeding is normal, especially if the patient has a bleeding disorder.	• Keep cuff inflated to prevent edema and aspiration of blood. • Administer humidified oxygen. • Document rate and amount of bleeding; check for prolonged clotting time. • As ordered, assist with application of an absorbable gelatin sponge or ligation of small bleeding vessels.
• Check for purulent, foul-smelling drainage from stoma. • Be alert for other signs of infection: fever, malaise, increased white blood cell count, and local pain.	• Obtain culture specimens and administer antibiotics. • Inflate tracheostomy cuff to prevent aspiration. • Suction frequently, maintaining sterile technique; avoid cross-contamination. • Change dressing whenever soiled.
• Auscultate for decreased or absent breath sounds. • Check for tachypnea, pain, and subcutaneous emphysema.	• Prepare for chest tube insertion as appropriate. • Obtain chest X-ray to evaluate pneumothorax or to check placement of the chest tube.
• Expect to find in mechanically ventilated patients. • Palpate neck for crepitus, listen for escape of air around tube cuff, and check for excessive swelling at the wound site.	• Inflate cuff correctly or use a larger tube. • Suction patient and clean tube to remove blockage. • Document extent of crepitus.
• Be alert for dry, hacking cough and blood-streaked sputum when the tube is being manipulated.	• Minimize trauma from tube movement. • Keep cuff pressure below 18 mm Hg.

rator) that's one size smaller than the tube currently being used because the trachea begins to close after tube expulsion, making insertion of the same size tube difficult.

• Explain all procedures carefully, and assure the patient that he will be closely monitored. Place the call bell as well as pen and paper within easy reach of the patient.

• Monitor the patient's hydration and nutritional status. Evaluate his ability to swallow. Arrange for a consultation with a dietitian to modify his diet as needed.

• To allow oral communication, deflate the cuff and instruct the patient to temporarily occlude the tracheostomy opening with his finger or a plug. Arrange for a consultation with a speech therapist so the patient can learn esophageal or other alternative methods of speech.

Home care instructions

• Tell the patient to promptly report any breathing problems, chest or stoma pain, or any change in the amount or color of his secretions.
• Teach the patient and family how to care for his stoma and tracheostomy tube. Include instructions about suctioning, wound care, humidification, changing tracheostomy ties, where to purchase supplies, and scheduling of follow-up visits.
• Emphasize to the patient the importance of not getting water in his stoma. Advise him to avoid swimming and to wear a stoma shield or direct the water below his stoma when showering.
• Tell the patient to place a foam filter over his stoma in winter, thereby warming inspired air, and to wear a bib over the filter.
• Teach the patient to bend at his waist during coughing to help expel secretions. Tell him to keep a tissue handy to catch expelled secretions.
• Assist the patient to develop coping strategies to deal with his altered body image. Suggest wearing loosely buttoned collars or scarves to disguise the stoma.
• Refer the patient and his family to a community support group.

TRACTION

Mechanical traction exerts a pulling force on a part of the body – usually the spine, pelvis, or long bones of the arms and legs. Either skin or skeletal traction may be used. Skin traction is applied directly to the skin and thus indirectly to the bone. In skeletal traction, an orthopedic surgeon inserts a pin or wire through the bone and attaches the traction equipment to the pin or wire to exert a direct, constant, longitudinal pulling force.

Purpose

• To exert a pulling force on an injured or deformed part of the musculoskeletal system and thereby restore anatomic alignment.

Indications

Traction devices are used to reduce fractures, treat dislocations, correct or prevent deformities, improve or correct contractures, or decrease muscle spasms. The type of traction is determined by the doctor according to the patient's condition, age, and weight as well as the condition of the skin, the duration of traction, and the purpose of traction.

Skin traction is contraindicated in severe injury with open wounds, and in patients with an allergy to tape or other skin traction equipment, circulatory disturbances, dermatitis, or varicose veins. Infections such as osteomyelitis contraindicate skeletal traction.

Procedure

The surgeon may use skin traction or skeletal traction, depending on the injury or condition. (See *Comparing traction types.*) Skin traction may be applied at the bedside. It is usually used when a light, temporary, or noncontinuous pulling force is required. The amount of weight most often used is 5 to 10 lb (2.2 to 4.5 kg). Types of skin traction include Buck's traction, pelvic traction with pelvic belt, and cervical traction with cervical halter.

Skeletal traction involves placement of wires, pins, or tongs into or through the bones; these may be inserted under local, general, or spinal anesthesia in aseptic conditions. Skeletal traction is

Comparing traction types

Traction therapy restricts movement of a patient's affected limb or body part and may confine the patient to prolonged bed rest. The limb is immobilized by pulling with equal force on each end of the injured area—an equal mix of traction and countertraction. Weights provide the pulling force. Countertraction is produced by using other weights or by positioning the patient's body weight against the traction pull.

Skin traction

This procedure immobilizes a body part intermittently over an extended period through direct application of a pulling force to the patient's skin. The force may be applied using adhesive or nonadhesive traction tape or other skin traction devices such as a boot, belt, or halter. Adhesive attachment allows more continuous traction; nonadhesive attachment allows easier removal for care.

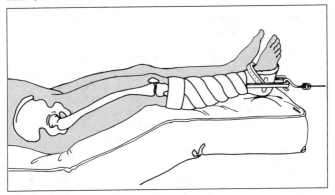

Skeletal traction

This technique immobilizes a body part for prolonged periods by attaching weighted equipment directly to the patient's bones. This may be accomplished with pins, screws, wires, or tongs. Skeletal traction allows more prolonged traction with heavier weight than skin traction.

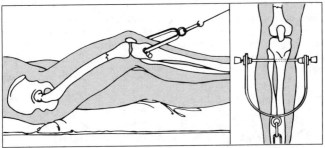

most often used for fractures of the femur, humerus, tibia, or cervical spine. The usual amount of weight is 25 to 40 lb (11.3 to 18 kg). Types of skeletal traction include balanced skeletal traction, overhead arm traction, and cervical traction with tongs. Skeletal traction may be kept in place 3 to 4 months. Pads, slings, or pushers may be combined with the traction to reduce the fracture.

Complications

Immobility during traction may result in pressure ulcers, muscle atrophy, weakness, contractures, and osteoporosis; it can also cause GI disturbances, such as constipation; urinary problems, including urinary stasis and renal calculi; respiratory problems, such as stasis of secretions and hypostatic pneumonia; and circulatory disturbances, including circulatory stasis and thrombophlebitis. Prolonged immobility, especially after traumatic injury, may promote depression or other emotional disturbances. Skeletal traction may cause osteomyelitis originating at the pin or wire sites. Non-union or delayed union, as well as pin breakage, may occur.

Care considerations
Before therapy
• Clarify the purpose of traction to the patient and family. Emphasize the importance of maintaining proper body alignment.
• Teach the patient how to use an overhead trapeze to assist with position changes.
• Have all appropriate traction equipment transported to the patient's room on a traction cart.
• Set up the traction frame according to the policy of the health care facility.
During therapy
• Assist with the skin traction procedure as needed. When using skin traction, apply ordered weights slowly and

carefully to avoid jerking the affected extremity.
• Support the patient.
• Show the patient how much movement he's allowed, and instruct him not to readjust the equipment. Tell him to report any pain or pressure from the traction equipment.
• Assess for signs and symptoms of immobility complications.
• In patients with skeletal traction, monitor for signs of infection, such as elevated temperature, increase in redness, drainage, or swelling at pin sites.
• Provide meticulous pin care.
• Unwrap skin traction every shift to assess for signs of skin breakdown, such as redness, warmth, and blisters.
• Add traction weights as ordered.
• About every 2 hours, check the patient for proper body alignment and reposition him as necessary.
• Provide skin care and change of position frequently; examine bony prominences for signs of irritation and pressure. Encourage coughing and deep-breathing exercises, and assist with range-of-motion exercises for unaffected extremities. Apply elastic support stockings as appropriate.
• Monitor the patient's elimination pattern, and provide dietary fiber and sufficient fluids to prevent constipation; administer stool softeners, laxatives, or enemas as needed.
• Regularly monitor vital signs and neurovascular status.
• Administer analgesics and antibiotics as prescribed.
• Inspect traction equipment regularly: assess for wrinkles in the elastic bandages or foam pads and for kinks or knots in the ropes. Make sure weights hang freely and do not touch the floor.
• Tell the patient that traction must be continuous to be effective.
• Encourage the patient to perform as much self-care as possible to reestablish a positive self-concept.

Home care instructions

• Instruct the patient on traction basics if traction will be used at home.
• Notify a home health care agency, as necessary, for follow-up care.

TRANSCUTANEOUS ELECTRICAL NERVE STIMULATION

A useful method for relieving both acute and chronic localized pain, transcutaneous electrical nerve stimulation (TENS) uses a mild electric current to stimulate nerve fibers and block the transmission of pain impulses to the brain. This method is based on the gate theory of pain, which proposes that painful impulses pass through a "gate" in the spinal cord.

The TENS unit, available by prescription, is a portable, battery-powered generator that transmits painless electric current through electrodes placed on the skin at points determined to be related to the pain. Treatments may be given three or four times daily for 30 to 45 minutes, for periods of 6 to 8 hours, or intermittently at the patient's discretion. The TENS unit is easy for the patient to use and permits normal activity.

A second-generation TENS unit, a "pain suppressor," utilizes electrodes with water as the conducting substance. The electric current, not felt by the patient, causes an elevation of serotonin levels in the systemic circulation, which enhances the response to endogenous endorphins. With this unit, treatments are administered only for short intervals several times a day.

Purpose

• To reduce pain by sending electrical impulses to the skin and underlying tissues.

Indications

TENS is used to treat chronic back pain and pain after knee, hip, or lower back surgery. Other indications include dental pain, pain from peripheral neuropathy or nerve injury, postherpetic neuralgia, reflex sympathetic dystrophy, musculoskeletal trauma, arthritis, and phantom limb pain.

TENS is contraindicated in patients with pacemakers. The electric current may also interfere with electrocardiography or cardiac monitoring. TENS shouldn't be used for pain of unknown etiology because it may mask a new pathology. The electrodes should never be placed over the carotid sinus nerves, over laryngeal or pharyngeal muscles, or on the eyes. They should never be placed on a pregnant patient's abdomen because safety during pregnancy has not been determined.

Procedure

The physical therapist or specially prepared nurse performs treatments with TENS. The skin at the electrode sites is cleaned with an alcohol sponge and dried well. The area may be shaved, if necessary. A small amount of electrode gel is applied to the bottom of each electrode (unless the electrodes are pregelled) to improve conductivity. The electrodes are placed on the skin at least 2″ (5 cm) apart and are usually secured with tape (some are self-adhering). (See *Positioning TENS electrodes*, pages 594 and 595.) The unit is turned on and the intensity adjusted until the patient feels a tingling sensation. Most patients select stimulation frequencies between 60 and 100 Hz.

Complications

The few adverse effects of TENS therapy relate to skin irritation and pruritus caused by the electrodes, the conductive gel, or the adhesive used to secure the electrodes. Electrical burns can result from improper placement of electrodes.

Care considerations
Before therapy
• Show the patient the TENS unit. Inform him that he will have electrodes attached to his skin and will feel a tingling sensation when the controls are turned on. Explain that the controls will be adjusted to specified settings or to those most comfortable and effective. Advise him to use the unit for at least a week before deciding if it helps reduce his pain.

• Assess the patient's level of pain to use as a baseline. Then assemble the TENS unit, lead wires, and electrodes, making sure that alcohol sponges, electrode gel, and tape are available. Determine the locations for electrode placement, and be sure to rotate sites. Proper positioning is crucial and can mean the difference between pain relief or increased pain.

• Make sure the TENS unit is off before beginning treatment.

During therapy
• Assess the patient for signs of excessive or inadequate stimulation. Muscle twitching may indicate overstimulation, whereas absence of any tingling sensation may mean that the electric current is too low.

Positioning TENS electrodes

In transcutaneous electrical nerve stimulation (TENS), electrodes placed around peripheral nerves (or an incision site) transmit electrical impulses to the brain. The electric current is thought to block pain impulses. The patient can influence the level and frequency of his pain relief by adjusting the controls on the device.

Typically, electrode placement varies even among patients who may have similar complaints. Electrodes can be applied by covering the painful area or surrounding it, as for muscle tenderness or painful joints, or by "capturing" the painful area between the electrodes, as for incisional pain.

In nerve injury, electrodes should be placed proximal to the injury (between the brain and the injury site) to avoid increasing pain. Placing electrodes in a hypersensitive area also increases pain. In an area lacking sensation, electrodes should be placed on adjacent dermatomes.

The illustrations show combinations of electrode placement (black squares) and areas of nerve stimulation (shaded) for low back and leg pain.

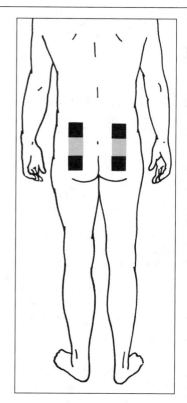

• If the patient complains of pain or intolerable paresthesia, check the settings, connections, and electrode placements; adjust them if necessary. If you must relocate the electrodes during treatment, first turn off the TENS unit.

After therapy

• Evaluate the patient's response to each TENS trial, and compare the results. Also use your baseline assessment to evaluate the effectiveness of the procedure.

Home care instructions

• If the patient will be using the TENS unit at home, have him demonstrate the procedure, including electrode placement, the setting of the unit's controls, electrode removal, and proper care of the equipment. Advise him to rotate sites of electrode placement.

• Advise the patient to adhere strictly to the ordered settings and electrode placements. Warn against using high voltage, which may increase pain, and against using the unit for pain of unknown cause. Also tell the patient to notify the doctor if pain worsens or develops at another site.

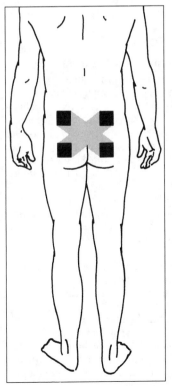
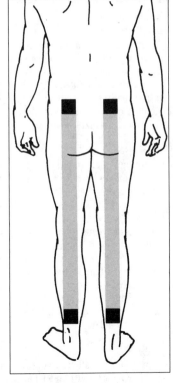

• If skin irritation occurs, instruct the patient to keep the area clean and apply soothing lotion. However, if his skin breaks down, he should notify the doctor. Explain that irritation may be decreased by leaving the electrodes in place during the day between treatments. Inform him that nonallergenic electrodes, such as those made with karaya gum, are available if skin irritation worsens.

• Make sure the patient understands that he should remove the unit before coming in contact with water to avoid possible electrocution (unless he is using a battery-powered unit).

TRANSHEPATIC BILIARY CATHETERIZATION

Transhepatic biliary catheterization is the insertion of a catheter through the abdominal wall and liver into the bile duct to relieve obstruction of bile flow. The flow of bile may be reestablished into the duodenum, or it may be diverted externally to a drainage bag. Although not curative, this procedure permits a more normal life-style.

Purpose

• To relieve signs and symptoms of biliary obstruction and reduce the associated risk of sepsis.

Indications

The most common cause of biliary obstruction requiring drainage is nonresectable cancer of the liver, pancreas, or bile duct. This procedure may also be indicated to treat stones in the common bile duct, surgical injuries to the bile duct, or strictures of the duct resulting from cholangitis.

Procedure

Transhepatic biliary catheterization is performed by a radiologist under fluoroscopic guidance. The radiologist inserts a sheathed needle percutaneously through the liver and into the bile duct. Utilizing a guide wire, he inserts a catheter into the duct. If possible, the catheter is positioned in the duodenum to eventually reestablish downward bile flow. External drainage may be necessary until edema caused by the catheter subsides. With complete obstruction, the distal end of the catheter may be positioned above the obstruction and the bile drainage permanently diverted into an external collection bag. The catheter may be secured with skin sutures.

Complications

The most common complication of transhepatic biliary catheterization is hemorrhage resulting from puncture of the highly vascular liver. Sepsis may also occur as a result of manipulation of the bile duct. The catheter may become blocked with debris or may be dislodged.

Care considerations
Before the procedure

• Monitor the results of blood coagulation studies, and notify the radiologist of abnormalities indicating bleeding disorders because of the risk of bleeding from penetration of the liver.

• Clarify the procedure with the patient and family. Explain what to expect before, during, and after the procedure. Be sure to inform the patient that the procedure may take several hours and may cause pain. Tell the patient that pain medication will be available.

• Withhold food and fluids the day of the procedure.

• Ensure that the patient has signed a consent form.

After the procedure

• Monitor vital signs frequently for indications of hemorrhage or sepsis.

• Keep the patient on complete bed rest for at least 6 hours to reduce the risk of bleeding.

• Check the consistency and odor of the fluid in the external drainage bag. Also check the amount; drainage that exceeds 1,500 ml in 24 hours may mean retrograde flow of duodenal contents secondary to intestinal obstruction.

• Monitor for excessive blood in the drainage bag, which may indicate displacement of the catheter into a hepatic blood vessel.

• After edema has subsided and if ordered, cap the catheter to allow bile to drain into the duodenum.

• Assess for cramping, pain, or leakage of fluid around the catheter; this may indicate blockage of the catheter or displacement from the bile duct.

• Irrigate the catheter through the external port every 8 hours or as otherwise ordered to maintain patency; use aseptic technique to introduce 5 to 10 ml of sterile 0.9% sodium chloride solution with gentle pressure.

• Do not aspirate during flushing; this may result in the introduction of duodenal contents into the catheter or bile duct. Do not force irrigant through the catheter.

• Change the dressing over the catheter daily, and observe the skin at the catheter insertion site for local signs of infection or irritation.

• Apply a protective dressing to the skin surface, if needed, to prevent excoriation from bile leakage.

Home care instructions

• Teach the family caregiver the correct method of irrigating the tube and changing the dressing. (The position of the catheter usually makes self-care difficult.) Provide written instructions and an opportunity for supervised practice before discharge.

• Obtain a referral to a home health care agency to ensure that the proper technique is used in the home.

• Instruct the patient and the family caregiver to report the following signs of problems: fever and shaking chills, severe pain, excessive leakage around the catheter, and redness or tenderness around the catheter insertion site. Also tell them to report inability to flush the catheter or accidental removal of the catheter.

• Inform the patient that follow-up visits to check the placement of the catheter will be scheduled with the radiologist.

TRICYCLIC ANTIDEPRESSANTS

Tricyclic antidepressants (TCAs) are currently the drugs of choice for treating major depression. These drugs include *amitriptyline, amoxapine, clomipramine, desipramine, doxepin, imipramine, maprotiline, protriptyline,* and *trimipramine.* Clomipramine is also used to treat obsessive-compulsive disorder, and imipramine is also used to treat enuresis in children age 6 and older. TCAs, especially amitriptyline, desipramine, doxepin, imipramine, and nortriptyline, are useful in the management of severe chronic pain.

Newer alternatives to TCAs include *bupropion, fluoxetine, isocarboxazid, phenelzine, sertraline, tranylcypromine,* and *trazodone.* These agents are also used to treat depression. Fluoxetine is the drug of choice for short-term management of depression.

Purpose
• To relieve depression.

Indications
TCAs are indicated in the treatment of major depression and dysthymic disorder.

Bupropion should be used cautiously in patients with a history of head trauma or seizure disorder because the incidence of seizures associated with this drug is greater than that of the other antidepressants.

TCAs should be administered cautiously to suicidal patients because an overdose can occur with as little as 10 times the regular daily dose. They should also be given cautiously to patients with acute angle-closure glaucoma, benign prostatic hyperplasia, cardiovascular disorders, or urine retention.

Adverse reactions

Adverse reactions associated with TCAs include dizziness, drowsiness, dry mouth, constipation, hypertension, tachycardia, orthostatic hypotension, electrocardiogram (ECG) changes, urine retention, and sweating.

Care considerations

• Expect some patient improvement in 10 to 14 days after the start of therapy; full effect usually takes 30 days. However, keep in mind that adverse reactions, such as dry mouth, dizziness, and drowsiness, can begin immediately.
• Monitor the depressed patient with a psychotic disorder for worsened hallucinations or delusions. If symptoms worsen, reduce the dose of the TCA as ordered. Also observe the patient for mood swings or suicidal tendencies.
• Check the patient's alertness and psychomotor coordination, and warn against driving or other hazardous activities requiring alertness and fine-motor coordination.
• If the patient is elderly, be alert for increased sensitivity to the sedative and hypotensive effects of TCAs.
• If the TCA causes constipation, increase the patient's fluid intake and administer a stool softener, as prescribed.
• Check the patient's vital signs, watching for orthostatic hypotension, tachycardia, and hypertension. Instruct the patient to rise slowly from a sitting or lying position and to sit momentarily before rising.
• Monitor the patient's ECG for any changes during therapy.

• Review the patient's medications for possible interactions. Concurrent use of barbiturates, for example, can diminish the TCA's antidepressant effect. Monoamine oxidase inhibitors may cause severe excitation, seizures, and hyperpyrexia, especially in high doses. Corticosteroids, oral contraceptives, and methylphenidate all potentiate the effect of TCAs. Observe the patient receiving these drugs, and adjust dosages as ordered.

Home care instructions

• Inform the patient that adverse reactions usually subside within 2 to 3 weeks after therapy begins. Encourage him to continue taking the drug as long as the reactions don't worsen. Warn against stopping the drug abruptly.
• Suggest hard candy or sugarless gum to relieve dry mouth.
• If drowsiness is a problem, the entire daily dose may be taken at bedtime.
• Tell the patient to take a missed dose if he remembers within 2 hours of the scheduled time; otherwise, he should skip the missed dose.
• Warn the patient to avoid alcohol while he is taking a TCA because the combination can cause severe central nervous system depression.
• Advise the patient to consult with his doctor before taking any over-the-counter drug.
• Weight gain can present a problem in the patient on TCA therapy because TCAs increase appetite while decreasing metabolism. Tell the patient to weigh himself weekly; if he gains weight too rapidly, suggest that he reduce his caloric intake.
• Inform the patient that depression may take 2 to 4 weeks to subside.

U

ULTRASOUND THERAPY

For the past 60 years, ultrasonography – high-frequency sound waves – has been used to produce heat in soft tissue. Ultrasonic waves penetrate deeply and significantly elevate tissue temperature to depths of 2″ (5 cm). The greatest increase in temperature occurs in tissues with a high protein content, such as muscle, bone, and joint capsules. Thus, ultrasound therapy is an effective way to selectively deliver heat to injured soft tissue.

Purpose
• To increase blood flow to injured soft tissue
• To reduce pain and muscle spasm
• To aid in the stretching of joint contractures and scar tissue.

Indications

Ultrasound therapy is useful for the management of tendonitis, bursitis, muscle spasm, soft-tissue contractures, joint contractures, scar tissue, and soft-tissue or joint pain. Ultrasound therapy is usually used by the physical therapist as an adjunct to strengthening, mobilization, or range-of-motion exercises in the treatment of these conditions.

Ultrasound therapy is contraindicated over areas of vascular insufficiency, acute inflammation, or thrombophlebitis. It should be used cautiously over areas of decreased pain or temperature sensation. An ultrasound transducer should not be applied over the heart because it can cause ST-segment elevation. It should not be applied directly over the eye because this can cause retinal damage; over malignant tissue, because it increases the possibility of metastasis and can accelerate tumor growth; over the pregnant uterus, because it could injure the fetus; or over the testes, because it can cause temporary sterility. Furthermore, epiphyseal areas in children should receive only minimal exposure to ultrasonic waves.

Procedure
Ultrasound therapy is usually administered by physical therapists, physical therapy assistants, or athletic trainers. Ultrasound treatments are performed in hospital physical therapy departments, outpatient physical therapy clinics, and athletic training facilities. Ultrasonic waves are delivered to the patient through a transducer. Piezoelectric crystals within the transducer generate the ultrasonic waves. Air between the transducer and the surface to be treated is eliminated by means of a conduction gel so that sound waves can be transmitted to the surface. The conduction gel usually consists of mineral oil and water-soluble gels. Treatments involve slow, sweeping motions of the transducer over the area to be treated and typically take 5 to 10 minutes.

Complications
Correctly used, ultrasound therapy is safe and has few complications. It is important that soft tissue not be overheated because ultrasonic waves can cause thermal injury. The therapist depends on patient feedback about any

changes in pain and temperature during treatment. For this reason, ultrasound therapy must be used cautiously over areas of insensitive skin.

Care considerations

• Assess the sensitivity of the patient's skin before treatment.
• Determine the status of the patient's circulation to minimize the possibility of thermal injury.
• The patient's skin should be clean, dry, and free from oils and creams.
• Instruct the patient to inform the therapist of pain or any changes in tissue temperature.
• Apply the conduction gel between the transducer and the patient's skin.
• Use ultrasound therapy as an adjunct to other therapeutic procedures to achieve rehabilitative goals.

Home care instructions

• Instruct the patient to supplement the beneficial effects of ultrasound therapy with an exercise program.

ULTRAVIOLET LIGHT TREATMENTS

Ultraviolet (UV) light, administered through sources that may include projectors, xenon arc lamps, fluorescent bulbs, or lasers, is used to treat various skin disorders. UV light depresses deoxyribonucleic acid synthesis and therefore decreases the rate of cell division in the epidermis. New and experimental UV light treatments (photopheresis and photodynamic therapy) are being used for palliation and as a potential cure in the treatment of some cancers.

Ultraviolet light is categorized as UVA, UVB, and UVC light, depending on its wavelength. UVC (long waves) light is used in germicidal lamps but is not used therapeutically because it carries the risk of serious burns and cancer. UVB (middle-length waves) light, the component of sunlight that causes sunburn, has been successfully used in the treatment of psoriasis for over 50 years. UVA (short waves) light alone has little effect on normal skin, but oral methoxsalen tablets (psoralens) or topical tripsoralen or methoxsalen creates an artificial sensitivity to UVA light. The combination of psoralens and UVA is known as photochemotherapy or PUVA therapy.

Purpose

• To decrease cell proliferation
• To induce mild desquamation and clearing of the skin
• To stimulate melanocytic activity in depigmented areas of the skin.

Indications

Ultraviolet light treatment is indicated in patients with psoriasis, mycosis fungoides, atopic dermatitis, vitiligo, and uremic pruritus. Photodynamic laser therapy may be indicated in cancers of the esophagus, endobronchus, oropharynx, bladder, retina and choroid, cervix and vagina, and head and neck, and in subcutaneous and cutaneous lesions.

Contraindications to PUVA and UVB therapy include photosensitivity disease, use of photosensitivity-inducing drugs, a history of skin cancer, previous skin irradiation, cataracts, or loss of a lens due to cataract surgery.

Procedure

Ultraviolet light therapy may be performed in the hospital, in a doctor's office, or at home. Typically, the light source is a bank of high-intensity fluorescent bulbs set into a reflective cabinet. The therapy may be delivered in full body cabinets, smaller cabinets (to treat localized lesions), or by natural sunlight. Appropriate dosage is determined according to the patient's skin type and pigmentation.

The patient disrobes and puts on a gown that bares only the area to be treated; vulnerable areas of the skin are protected by towels and sunscreen. The patient wears protective goggles. After the prescribed dosage of UV light has been administered, the patient may continue daily activities with appropriate precautions to minimize further exposure to UV light.

Complications

Overexposure of the skin to UV light can result from prolonged treatment, inadequate distance between the patient and light source, use of photosensitizing drugs, or sensitive skin. Cataracts and corneal and retinal damage may result if the eyes are not protected during the treatment and for 24 hours after treatment with psoralens. Long-term effects of treatment are essentially the same as those of excessive sun exposure: atrophy and aging of the skin and an increased risk for skin cancer.

Care considerations

Before therapy

• Reinforce the doctor's explanation of the treatment. Explain that UV light treatments produce a mild sunburn that will help clear up skin lesions. With UVB therapy, the erythema appears within 4 to 6 hours; with PUVA therapy, it may not become evident for 48 to 72 hours. In either case, it should disappear within another 24 hours. Inform the patient that mild dryness and desquamation will follow within 1 to 2 days.
• Thoroughly assess the patient's skin and medical history. Check for a history of photosensitivity diseases, skin cancer, or radiation treatments. Ask about current use of photosensitizing drugs, such as anticonvulsants, certain antihypertensives, phenothiazines, salicylates, sulfonamides, tetracyclines, tretinoin, and various cancer chemotherapeutic drugs.

• Instruct the patient undergoing PUVA therapy to take psoralens with food 2 hours before treatment.

During therapy

• Assist the patient to disrobe and to put on a hospital gown. Once inside the phototherapy unit, have the patient remove the gown or expose the area to be treated. Make sure the patient is wearing protective goggles and that vulnerable areas of his skin are protected by a sunscreen, towels, or the gown.
• If the patient is standing, instruct him to report any dizziness.
• If the patient is undergoing local UVB treatment, make sure he's positioned at the correct distance from the sunlamp or hot quartz lamp. For facial exposure with a sunlamp, position the patient's face 12″ (30 cm) from the lamp. For exposure of body areas, and if using a quartz lamp, position the patient about 30″ (76 cm) away from the lamp.

After therapy

• After delivering the prescribed UVB dose, help the patient out of the phototherapy unit.
• Observe the treated area for marked erythema, blisters, peeling, or other signs of overexposure 4 to 6 hours after UVB therapy and 24 to 48 hours after PUVA therapy. If overexposure occurs, treatment is usually withheld for a few days and then reinstituted at a lower level of exposure.
• If the doctor has prescribed tar preparations with UVB therapy, watch for signs of sensitivity, such as erythema, pruritus, or eczematous reactions.

Home care instructions

• Advise the patient to use emollients and a mild soap to combat dry skin. Warn him to avoid hot baths or showers, which also promote dry skin.
• If the patient is having PUVA treatments, review the schedule for taking psoralens. Explain that any deviation from the schedule could result in burns or ineffective treatment. Emphasize the

importance of wearing UV-opaque sunglasses outdoors for at least 12 hours after taking psoralens.
• Emphasize the need for an annual eye examination to detect possible formation of cataracts.
• Instruct the patient to seek medical approval before taking any drug, including aspirin, to prevent heightened photosensitivity.
• Instruct the patient who is using a sunlamp at home to first allow the lamp to warm up for 5 minutes and then to limit exposure to the time ordered. Instruct him to protect his eyes with goggles and to use a dependable timer or have someone else monitor exposure time.
• Emphasize the importance of never using a sunlamp when tired; falling asleep under the warmth of the lamp can cause severe burns.
• Advise the patient to relieve a localized burn by applying cool water soaks for 20 minutes or until skin temperature is cool; have him notify the doctor of larger burns.
• Instruct the patient to limit exposure to natural light, to use a sunscreen with a skin protection factor (SPF) rating of 15 or greater, and to wear a hat, long sleeves, and sunglasses when outdoors.
• Instruct the patient to inform the doctor immediately of any suspicious lesions.

URETERAL STENTS

A ureteral stent is a hollow tubular device designed for placement within the ureter. The stent has side holes that allow urine to drain unimpeded from the renal pelvis to the bladder. Typically made of soft, flexible silicone, the stent may be temporary or permanent. It is inserted intraoperatively, transcystoscopically, or percutaneously through a nephrostomy site.

Ideally, a ureteral stent provides free, unobstructed flow of urine; remains in position; and causes few, if any, symptoms. Many different types are available, and the urologist carefully chooses the stent design, diameter, and length needed for each patient. For example, double-J stents have a J-shaped curve at each end to prevent migration of the tube upward or downward; double pigtail stents have a coil at each end that allows the upper coil to be positioned in the renal pelvis and the lower coil at the ureteral orifice. The Smith Universal stent is used for external drainage after certain procedures until it is clamped off to allow urinary drainage down the ureter to the bladder.

Purpose
• To maintain ureteral flow in patients with ureteral obstruction
• To promote healing
• To maintain the caliber and patency of the ureter after surgery.

Indications
Ureteral stents may be used to maintain ureteral flow in patients with obstruction caused by renal calculi, edema, stricture, or tumor. Ureteral stents can also be used if significant mucosal trauma, submucosal tunneling, or ureteral perforation occurs during endourologic procedures. Ureteral and uretero-vaginal fistulas can be treated by placement of an indwelling stent to maintain patency while the ureter heals. After surgery, such as manipulation of a renal calculi, stents may be used to maintain the caliber and patency of the ureter. Stents may be inserted intraoperatively to identify the ureter and prevent ligation and are often used after extracorporeal shock-wave lithotripsy to ensure urine drainage and facilitate passage of calculi fragments. Stents may also be used after ureteral trauma.

Procedure

The type of anesthesia used is at the discretion of the urologist and anesthesiologist. For transcystoscopic or retrograde placement of a ureteral stent, the patient is placed in a modified lithotomy position. Cystoscopy is performed, and a guide wire is passed through the cystoscope up the ureter. The stent is placed over the guide wire and advanced up the ureter under fluoroscopic guidance. When the correct position is confirmed by X-ray or fluoroscopy, the guide wire is removed; the stent will resume its original configuration and secure itself.

A stent may also be placed through a percutaneous nephrostomy. The patient is placed in a prone oblique or supine position for this procedure. A guide wire is passed through the nephrostomy down the ureter, and the stent is passed over this wire under fluoroscopic guidance. The stent's position is checked before the guide wire is removed. Intraoperative placement during open surgery on a ureter may not require an X-ray to confirm position.

Complications

Complications include inflammation or infection from a foreign body. Rarely, stents may become obstructed from clot formation or encrustation. Other complications include migration or dislodgment of the tube; reportedly, perforation or erosion of a stent through the ureter has caused fistula formation.

Care considerations

Before surgery

• Explain the procedure. If possible, show the patient what the stent will look like.
• Tell the patient what to expect postoperatively, and describe necessary care.
• Involve the family, and arrange for visits from a home health care nurse if the patient will have a stent with external communication.
• Ensure that the patient has signed a consent form.

After surgery

• Administer I.V. fluids and I.V. antibiotics, as ordered.
• Monitor the patient's vital signs, and observe for bleeding. Expect pink-tinged urine, but report dark- or bright-red urine to the doctor.
• Monitor the patient's intake and output. Keep in mind that decreased urine output and colicky pain with chills, nausea, and vomiting may indicate stent dislodgment or obstruction.
• Assess the patient for fever or, as appropriate, for purulent drainage at the insertion site or in the drainage bag.
• Observe the surgical wound for leakage of urine; this may indicate stent dislodgment or obstruction.

Home care instructions

• Instruct the patient discharged with a ureteral stent in place how to observe for signs and symptoms of complications, and tell him what action to take if any should occur.
• Instruct the patient who has a stent with external communication about the procedures for care of the stent entry site and for dressing changes.
• Advise the patient to take showers rather than baths.
• Encourage intake of at least eight 8-oz. (240-ml) glasses of fluid daily.
• Discuss resumption of sexual activity.
• Encourage the patient to keep follow-up appointments with the doctor. Stent replacements will be necessary.

URINARY DIVERSION SURGERY

A urinary diversion provides an alternative route for excretion of urine when pathology impedes the normal flow of urine through the bladder. A permanent urinary diversion is indicated in any condition that requires a total cystectomy. In conditions requiring temporary urine drainage or diversion, a suprapubic or ureteral catheter is usually inserted to divert the flow of urine temporarily. The catheter remains in place until the incision heals.

Several types of permanent urinary diversion surgery can be performed. Most require the patient to wear a urine-collecting appliance and to care for the stoma created during surgery.

The two most common types of urinary diversion surgery are cutaneous ureterostomy and ileal conduit. Cutaneous ureterostomy offers several advantages. It is a shorter and easier-to-perform surgery than ileal conduit diversion and can be performed successfully on chronically dilated, thick-walled ureters. Unlike an ileal conduit, it doesn't involve intestinal anastomoses and thus carries little risk of peritoneal and intestinal complications caused by intestinal absorption of urine contents.

Ileal conduit diversion involves intestinal (ileum) anastomoses. Because the ileum allows for creation of a much larger stoma than can be created from a ureter, an ileal conduit is usually easier to care for than a ureterostomy.

Continent urinary diversion procedures provide alternative methods of drainage that eliminate the need for external devices. The Koch pouch is a small-bowel reservoir for urine. In this diversion, the surgeon creates nipple valves to prevent reflux. Intermittent catheterization is usually required to empty urine from the pouch. Alternative types of urinary diversion include the Indiana, Mainz, or UCLA pouches. For these procedures, the more muscular walls of the large bowel create the urine reservoir, and the ileocecal valve forms the continence mechanism.

Purpose

• To provide an alternative route for excretion of urine when bladder dysfunction or removal doesn't allow normal drainage.

Indications

Most commonly performed in patients who have had total or partial cystectomy, urinary diversion may also be performed in patients with congenital urinary tract defects; severe, unmanageable urinary tract infections that threaten renal function; injury to the ureters, bladder, or urethra; obstructive cancer; or neurogenic bladder.

Procedure

The patient receives general anesthesia, and the surgeon chooses the most appropriate type of urinary diversion.

In the simplest type, cutaneous ureterostomy, the surgeon dissects one or both ureters from the bladder and brings them out through the skin surface on the flank or the anterior abdominal wall to form one or two stomas. The surgeon can choose among five approaches to this procedure: unilateral, bilateral, flank loop, and double-barrel ureterostomy as well as transureteroureterostomy.

In an ileal conduit procedure, the surgeon anastomoses the ureters to a small portion of the ileum excised especially for the procedure. He then creates a stoma from one end of the ileal segment.

In continent urinary diversion, the surgeon uses a portion of the small bowel to create both a reservoir for urine and reflux-preventing nipple valves. (See *Types of permanent urinary diversion,* pages 606 and 607.)

Complications

Because the intestinal mucosa is delicate, an ill-fitting appliance can cause bleeding, especially with an ileal conduit.

The peristomal skin may become reddened or excoriated from too-frequent changing or improper placement of the appliance, poor skin care, or an allergic reaction to the appliance or adhesive. Constant leakage around the appliance can result from its improper placement or poor skin turgor.

Care considerations

Before surgery

• Teach the patient proper collection and stoma management techniques.

• To improve patient compliance, provide emotional support as the patient adjusts to the changes in his self-image brought about by the stoma and the collection device.

• Review the planned surgery with the patient, reinforcing the surgeon's explanations as necessary. Use an anatomic diagram to enhance your discussion, and provide printed information from the United Ostomy Association or other sources if possible. Tell the patient that he'll receive a general anesthetic and will have a nasogastric (NG) tube in place after surgery.

• Prepare the patient for the appearance and location of the stoma: for an ileal conduit, the stoma will be located somewhere on the lower abdomen, probably below the waistline; for a cutaneous ureterostomy, the stoma site typically is chosen during surgery, depending on the length of patent ureter available.

• Review the enterostomal therapist's explanation of the urine collection device the patient will use after surgery. Encourage the patient to handle the device to ease acceptance of it. Reassure him that he'll receive complete training on how to use it after surgery.

• If possible, arrange for a visit by a well-adjusted ostomy patient, who can provide a firsthand account of the operation and offer some insight into the realities of stoma and collection device care.

• As appropriate, include the patient's family in all aspects of preoperative teaching—especially if they'll be providing much of the routine care after discharge.

• Ensure that the patient or a responsible family member has signed a consent form.

• Before surgery, prepare the bowel to reduce the risk of postoperative infection from intestinal flora. As appropriate, maintain a low-residue or clear-liquid diet, ensure that the patient has fasted 8 hours before surgery, and administer a cleansing enema and an antimicrobial drug such as erythromycin or neomycin. Other preparatory measures may include total patenteral nutrition (TPN) or fluid replacement therapy for debilitated patients and prophylactic I.V. antibiotics.

After surgery

• Monitor vital signs. Carefully check and record intake and output; report any decrease in output, which could indicate obstruction from postoperative edema or ureteral stenosis. Observe urine drainage for pus and blood; keep in mind that urine is usually blood-tinged initially but should clear rapidly. Urine is also tinged with mucus because the bowel normally produces mucus.

• Record the amount, color, and consistency of drainage from the incisional drain and NG tube. Notify the doctor of any urine leakage from the drain or suture line; leakage may signal developing complications such as hydronephrosis. Watch for signs of peritonitis (fever, abdominal distention, and pain), which can develop from intraperitoneal urine leakage.

• Check the patient's dressings frequently, and change them as appropriate. (The surgeon will probably perform the first dressing change.) When changing dressings, check the incision for redness, swelling, and drainage.

• Maintain fluid and electrolyte balance, and continue I.V. replacement therapy as appropriate. Provide TPN if necessary to ensure adequate nutrition.

Types of permanent urinary diversion

The types of permanent urinary diversion with stomas include ureterostomy, ileal conduit, and continent urinary diversion.

Ureterostomy

A stoma or stomas are formed when ureters are diverted to the abdominal wall or flank. There are five different types of ureterostomy.

Flank loop ureterostomy

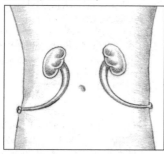

Ureters loop as they are brought to the skin surface.

Double-barrel ureterostomy

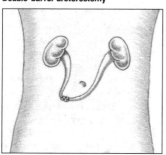

Both ureters are brought to the skin surface, forming a stoma.

Transureteroureterostomy

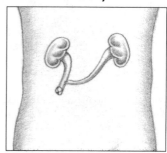

One ureter is anastomosed to the other, which is then brought to the skin surface to form a stoma.

Bilateral ureterostomy

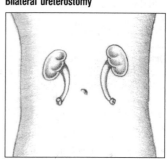

Both ureters are brought to the skin surface to form stomas.

• If continent urinary diversion surgery has been performed and a neo-bladder is present, irrigate with 0.9% sodium chloride solution as appropriate (usually 30 ml every 4 hours) to prevent excessive mucus formation.
• Perform routine pouch maintenance as applicable. Make sure the device fits tightly around the stoma; allow no more than a ⅛" margin of skin between the stoma and the device's faceplate. Regularly check the appearance of the stoma and peristomal skin. The stoma should appear bright red; if it becomes deep red or bluish, suspect impaired blood flow and notify the doctor. The stoma

Unilateral ureterostomy

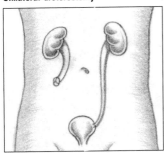

One ureter is brought to the skin surface to form a stoma.

Ileal conduit

A segment of the ileum is excised, and the two ends of the ileum that result from excision of the segment are sutured closed. Then the ureters are dissected from the bladder and anastomosed to the ileal segment. One end of the ileal segment is closed with sutures; the opposite end is brought through the abdominal wall, thereby forming a stoma.

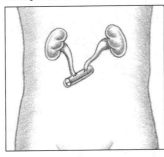

Continent urinary diversion

After total cystectomy, an 8″ (22-cm) segment of the ileum is used to create the urine reservoir (Kock's pouch). Additional segments of ileum form the afferent and efferent limbs, which act as reflux-preventing nipple valves.

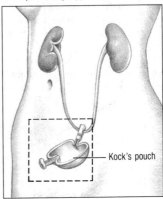

Kock's pouch

Kock's pouch

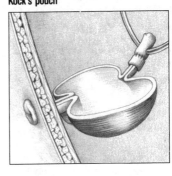

should also be smooth; report any dimpling or retraction, which may point to stenosis. Check the peristomal skin for irritation or breakdown. Remember that the main cause of irritation is urine leakage around the edges of the collection device's faceplate. If you detect leakage, change the device, taking care to apply the skin sealer to ensure a tight fit.

• If skin breakdown occurs, clean the area with warm water and pat it dry; then apply a light dusting of karaya powder and a thin layer of protective dressing. If you detect severe excoriation, notify the doctor.

• Provide emotional support throughout recovery.
• Help the patient adjust to his altered body image and, if applicable, to the stoma and collection device.

Home care instructions

• If applicable, make sure the patient and family know how to perform stoma care and how to change the pouch.
• If the patient will be discharged with an indwelling urinary catheter, ensure that the patient and family know how to care for it.
• Instruct the patient and family to watch for and report signs of complications, such as fever, chills, flank or abdominal pain, and pus or blood in the urine.
• Stress the importance of keeping scheduled follow-up appointments with the doctor and the enterostomal therapist to evaluate stoma care and make any necessary changes in equipment. For instance, stoma shrinkage, which usually occurs within 8 weeks after surgery, may require a change in pouch size to ensure a tight fit.
• Tell the patient that he should be able to return to work soon after discharge unless his work requires heavy lifting; in that case, he should have medical approval before resuming work. Explain that he can safely participate in most sports, even such strenuous ones as skiing, skydiving, and scuba diving. However, suggest that he avoid contact sports, such as football and wrestling.
• Refer for sexual counseling any patient who expresses doubts or insecurities about his sexuality related to the stoma and pouch.
• Assure the female patient that pregnancy should cause her no special problems, but urge her to consult with her doctor before pregnancy.
• If applicable, refer the patient to a support group such as the United Ostomy Association.

V

VALSALVA'S MANEUVER

Valsalva's maneuver is a procedure in which the patient forces an expiration against a closed glottis. This maneuver can correct supraventricular tachycardias and atrial arrhythmias and has been known to relieve angina by triggering vagal stimulation of the heart.

The physiologic response from Valsalva's maneuver involves an initial rise in intrathoracic pressure from its normal level of 3 to 4 mm Hg to levels of 60 mm Hg or higher. This increase in pressure is transmitted directly to the great vessels and the heart, causing decreased venous return, stroke volume, and systolic pressure. Within seconds, the baroreceptors stimulate the medulla by increasing the heart rate and causing peripheral vasoconstriction. When the patient exhales at the end of the maneuver, blood pressure begins to rise. But peripheral vasoconstriction is still present, and the combination of rising blood pressure and vasoconstriction causes vagal stimulation, which in turn slows the heart rate. The slowed heart rate is believed to be responsible for relieving angina pectoris. In some situations, cough cardiopulmonary resuscitation (CPR) may help convert potentially lethal arrhythmias. (See *Cough CPR and ventricular arrhythmias*, page 610.)

Purpose
• To help correct supraventricular tachycardia and atrial arrhythmias

• To assist with diagnosis of cardiac abnormalities during echocardiography.

Indications

Valsalva's maneuver should be initiated only by a doctor. Valsalva's maneuver is indicated as therapy for patients with rapid atrial arrhythmias and supraventricular tachycardias. It can also be used for patients with mild coronary disease suffering from angina pectoris, but this is rare.

Valsalva's maneuver is contraindicated for patients with severe coronary artery disease, acute myocardial infarction, or moderate-to-severe hypovolemia.

Procedure

Because Valsalva's maneuver can be complicated by severe bradycardia, when it is first performed the patient should be placed on a cardiac monitor with emergency equipment nearby; an I.V. line is usually in place. To perform Valsalva's maneuver in the traditional manner, have the patient lie supine and ask him to inhale deeply and bear down, as in defecation. If no syncope, dizziness, or arrhythmias occur, he should continue to hold his breath and bear down for 10 seconds. Then he should exhale and breathe quietly. If the maneuver is successful, the patient's heart rate will begin to slow before he exhales.

Complications

Valsalva's maneuver can cause mobilization of venous thrombi, bleeding, ventricular arrhythmias, and asystole.

Care considerations
Before the procedure
• Explain to the patient what Valsalva's maneuver is and, in simple terms, what it's intended to accomplish. If the patient has angina, tell him that the maneuver will diminish his heart's work load and will thereby relieve the pain. For the patient with an atrial arrhythmia, explain that the maneuver temporarily raises the blood pressure and that the heart responds by beating more slowly. Explain how the maneuver is done (you can describe it as trying to exhale while holding one's breath), and briefly demonstrate it yourself.
• Warn the patient that he may feel faint or dizzy during the procedure.

During the procedure
• Ensure patency of the I.V. line, and take vital signs. Attach a 12-lead electrocardiogram (ECG), and gather resuscitation equipment and medications.
• Monitor the patient's ECG and continue to record it throughout the procedure.
• If the patient develops dizziness or syncope, check to be sure he is in a supine position.

After the procedure
• Assess the ECG and vital signs when the procedure is completed. Monitor the patient's ECG continuously for at least 12 hours to ensure that arrhythmias don't return. If an atrial arrhythmia doesn't resolve, drug therapy will probably be prescribed.

Home care instructions
• The patient may be instructed to perform Valsalva's maneuver at home. When teaching Valsalva's maneuver, instruct the patient to lie down to prevent fainting or dizziness and to perform the maneuver for 10 seconds.
• Tell the patient to call his doctor immediately if the maneuver doesn't relieve symptoms.

Cough CPR and ventricular arrhythmias

Like Valsalva's maneuver, a simple cough may help convert potentially lethal arrhythmias to normal sinus rhythm. Whereas Valsalva's maneuver is used for *atrial* arrhythmias, cough cardiopulmonary resuscitation (CPR) can disrupt *ventricular* arrhythmias. By closing the epiglottis and strongly contracting the respiratory muscles, coughing greatly increases intrathoracic pressure. The compressive force of this pressure increase promotes coronary perfusion.

Researchers believe that coronary perfusion also improves as a result of increased aortic pressure and reflex coronary vasodilation secondary to baroreceptor activation. So far, cough CPR has been used mainly in cardiac catheterization laboratories, where researchers have found that continuous, forced coughing spurts, 1 to 3 seconds apart and beginning just before or at the onset of ventricular tachycardia or fibrillation, can help patients maintain consciousness for up to 30 seconds. Cough CPR buys time for defibrillation by maintaining cerebral perfusion. In addition, it's a technique that heart patients can potentially use on their own, even after they've left the hospital.

VASCULAR SURGICAL REPAIR

Vascular surgical repair includes procedures that bypass obstructions or replace, remove, or reinforce portions of a diseased vessel. They are performed to improve circulation. Types of surgical vascular repair include aneurysm resection, carotid endarterectomy, bypass grafting, embolectomy, interruption of vena cava blood flow, and vein stripping. Surgical vascular repair can be an emergency procedure, for example for life-threatening dissecting or ruptured aortic aneurysms or limb-threatening acute arterial occlusion.

Patients who do not qualify as candidates for vascular surgery include those whose underlying disease puts them at too great of a surgical risk and those whose vascular disease is too mild to warrant surgery. The latter group may benefit from percutaneous trans-arterial angioplasty, laser surgery, or atherectomy.

Purpose
• To restore vessel patency.

Indications
Vascular surgery may be used to treat vessels damaged by atherosclerotic or thromboembolic disorders such as aortic aneurysm or arterial occlusive disease. Other indications include vascular trauma, infections, or congenital defects. Vascular surgery may also be used for patients with obstructions that severely compromise circulation or for patients whose vascular disease does not respond to drugs or such non-surgical treatments as balloon catheterization.

Procedure
The specific surgical procedure used depends on the type, location, and extent of vascular occlusion or damage. Types of vascular surgery include aneurysm resection, carotid endarterectomy, bypass grafting, embolectomy, replacement with vascular prostheses, vena cava clipping or ligation, and vein stripping. (See *Understanding types of vascular surgery*, pages 612 and 613.)

These procedures are performed under general anesthesia; some may necessitate use of cardiopulmonary bypass.

Complications
All vascular repair procedures have the potential for serious complications, such as vessel trauma, emboli, hemorrhage, and infection. Pulmonary complications such as pneumonia may result from immobility or intubation. Grafting carries added risks: The graft may occlude, narrow, dilate, or rupture.

Care considerations
Before surgery
• If the patient requires emergency surgery, briefly explain the procedure if possible. If time allows, make sure that the patient and family understand the doctor's explanation of the surgery and its possible complications.
• Explain that an I.V. line will be in place to provide access for fluid and drugs, electrocardiograph (ECG) electrodes will allow for continuous cardiac monitoring, and an arterial line or a pulmonary artery catheter will provide continuous blood pressure monitoring.
• Know that an indwelling urinary catheter may be inserted for accurate measurement of fluid output.
• If appropriate, explain to the patient that he will be intubated and placed on mechanical ventilation and that his vital signs and incision site will be checked regularly.
• Perform a complete vascular assessment the day before surgery. Take vital signs to provide a baseline. Record the temperature of the extremities, their sensitivity to motor and sensory stimuli, and any pallor, cyanosis, or redness.
• Instruct the patient to restrict food and fluids for at least 12 hours before surgery. Tell him that he probably will receive a sedative to help him relax and sleep the night before surgery.
• Ensure that the patient has signed a consent form.
• If the patient is awaiting surgery for repair of an aortic aneurysm, be alert for symptoms of acute dissection or rupture. Especially note sudden, severe pain in the chest, abdomen, or lower back; severe weakness; diapho-

(Text continues on page 614.)

Understanding types of vascular surgery

Aortic aneurysm repair

Purpose
To reinforce the wall of the aorta or to remove an aneurysmal segment of the aorta

Procedure
The surgeon first makes an incision to expose the aneurysm site. If necessary, the patient is placed on a cardiopulmonary bypass machine; then, the surgeon clamps the aorta above the aneurysm. Depending on the severity of the aneurysm and on whether it is ruptured, he wraps the weakened arterial wall with synthetic material to reinforce it or replaces the damaged portion with a prosthetic graft. The illustration at right shows a wrapped arterial wall.

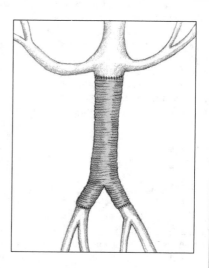

Bypass grafting

Purpose
To bypass an arterial obstruction resulting from atherosclerosis

Procedure
After exposing an affected artery, the surgeon anastomoses a synthetic or autogenous graft to divert blood flow around the occluded arterial segment. The graft may be synthetic or may be a vein harvested from elsewhere in the patient's body.

The illustration at right shows a femoropopliteal bypass.

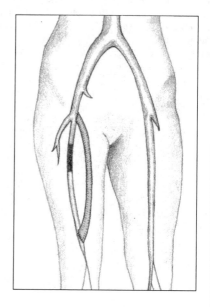

Understanding types of vascular surgery *(continued)*

Embolectomy

Purpose
To remove an embolus from an artery

Procedure
The surgeon inserts a balloon-tipped Fogarty catheter into the artery and passes it through the thrombus (top). He then inflates the balloon and withdraws the catheter to remove the thrombus (bottom).

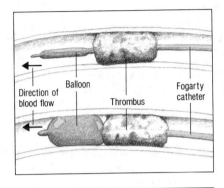

Direction of blood flow • Balloon • Thrombus • Fogarty catheter

Surgical interruption of the vena cava

Purpose
To block circulation through the vena cava

Procedure
The surgeon makes a flank incision. He then uses a catheter to insert a filter or an umbrella device (shown at right) into the vein. Alternatively, the vein may be ligated or clipped externally.

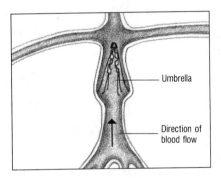

Umbrella

Direction of blood flow

Vein stripping

Purpose
To treat varicosities by removing the saphenous vein and its branches

Procedure
The surgeon ligates the saphenous vein. He then threads the stripper into the vein, secures it, and pulls it back out, bringing the vein with it.

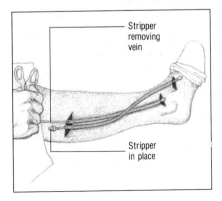

Stripper removing vein

Stripper in place

resis; tachycardia; or a precipitous drop in blood pressure. If any such symptoms occur, emergency surgery may be required to save the patient's life.

After surgery

• Check and record the patient's vital signs every 15 minutes until his condition stabilizes and every 30 minutes to 1 hour thereafter.

• Monitor the patient's ECG for abnormalities of heart rate or rhythm. Also monitor other pressure readings, and carefully record intake and output.

• Check the patient's dressing regularly for excessive bleeding.

• Position the patient as appropriate, and instruct him on recommended levels of activity during early stages of recovery. Provide analgesics, as prescribed, for incisional pain.

• Frequently assess peripheral pulses, using Doppler ultrasonography if palpation proves difficult. Check all extremities for muscle strength and movement, color, temperature, and capillary refill time.

• Throughout the recovery period, assess frequently for signs of complications. Fever, cough, congestion, or dyspnea may indicate pulmonary infection. Low urine output and elevated blood urea nitrogen and serum creatinine levels may point to renal dysfunction. Severe pain and cyanosis in a limb may indicate occlusion. Hypotension, tachycardia, restlessness and confusion, shallow respirations, abdominal pain, and increased abdominal girth may signal hemorrhage. Notify the patient's doctor immediately of any of these signs.

• Frequently check the incision site for drainage and signs of infection.

• As the patient's condition improves, help wean him from the ventilator, if appropriate. To promote good pulmonary hygiene, encourage frequent coughing, turning, and deep-breathing exercises.

• Assist the patient with range-of-motion exercises for his legs to help prevent thrombus formation.

Home care instructions

• If appropriate, instruct the patient to check his pulse in the affected extremity before rising from bed each morning. If the patient can't check his own pulse, teach a family member to do it. Tell the patient to notify the doctor if he can't palpate his pulse or if he develops coldness, pallor, or pain in the extremity.

• Explain the importance of strict compliance with any prescribed medication. Make sure the patient understands the schedule and the expected adverse effects of all prescribed medications.

• Emphasize to the patient the importance of regular medical follow-up to monitor his condition.

VASOCONSTRICTORS, OPHTHALMIC

Ophthalmic vasoconstrictors are commonly available as over-the-counter eyedrops. The most commonly used ophthalmic vasoconstrictors include *naphazoline, phenylephrine, ephedrine,* and *tetrahydrozoline*. These agents are available in varying strengths and combinations.

Purpose

• To temporarily relieve eye itching and redness
• To produce vasoconstriction.

Indications

Vasoconstrictors are indicated to relieve the itching and redness associated with eye irritation and inflammation caused by pollen-related allergies, colds, dust, smog, swimming, and contact lenses. They also provide relief from eye strain caused by reading or driving.

These agents are contraindicated in acute angle-closure glaucoma and should be used cautiously in hyperthyroidism, heart disease, hypertension, or diabetes mellitus because toxic reactions are possible. Vasoconstrictors should be used with extreme caution, if at all, in infants and children because they may produce severe central nervous system depression. Also, their variable systemic absorption may cause a severe drop in body temperature.

Adverse reactions

Vasoconstrictors may cause mild, transient eye stinging. They may also cause headache, dizziness, irregular heartbeat, and excessive drowsiness. Systemic effects are less likely but may follow excessive use.

Care considerations

• Review the patient's drug regimen for possible interactions. Concurrent use of ophthalmic vasoconstrictors and monoamine oxidase inhibitors, for instance, may trigger a hypertensive crisis. Use of tricyclic antidepressants can cause toxic effects.
• During therapy, monitor the patient's vital signs and mental status. Report symptoms of toxicity, such as tachycardia, headache, and excessive drowsiness.

Home care instructions

• Instruct the patient to report symptoms of toxicity: headache, dizziness, irregular heartbeat, or excessive drowsiness.
• Teach the patient how to correctly administer his own eyedrops. Emphasize that he shouldn't touch the tip of the dropper to the eye or surrounding tissue. Tell him to apply gentle pressure to the inside corner of the eye during administration and for 1 minute afterward to prevent drug absorption through the tear duct.

• Emphasize that the drug usually shouldn't be used for more than 4 days. Longer use may actually worsen eye irritation as well as increase the risk of adverse reactions.
• Warn the patient against exceeding the recommended dose, which can cause rebound irritation and inflammation.
• Tell the patient not to use the solution if it changes color, becomes cloudy, or develops a precipitate.

VASOPRESSORS

By stimulating the sympathetic nervous system, vasopressors rapidly raise blood pressure and increase cardiac output, thereby improving perfusion to vital organs. In patients with traumatic multisystem injuries, vasopressors provide prompt stabilization and deter development or worsening of shock. As a result, they can sustain life until emergency treatments can correct the underlying problem. However, vasopressors should typically be given after hypovolemia has been corrected to prevent peripheral vascular damage.

The four vasopressors used routinely are *dopamine, epinephrine, norepinephrine,* and *phenylephrine.* Other agents used in this category are *dobutamine, isoproterenol,* and *metaraminol* (see *Comparing vasopressors,* pages 616 and 617).

Because of their vasoconstrictive effects, vasopressors must be diluted and their doses titrated precisely to prevent peripheral vascular damage and subsequent loss of digits. They should be given cautiously because extravasation into the surrounding tissue can cause necrosis. During injection or infusion, they require careful monitoring to detect blood pressure or pulse rate changes and other adverse reactions.

Comparing vasopressors

DRUG, ROUTE, AND INDICATIONS	CONTRA-INDICATIONS	ADMINISTRATION TIPS
Dopamine I.V.: to treat shock and correct hemodynamic imbalances	Ventricular fibrillation, uncorrected tachyarrhythmias, pheochromocytoma	• Mix just before use with 0.9% sodium chloride solution, dextrose 5% in water (D_5W), or a combination of these. Discard after 24 hours or if discoloration occurs. Don't mix with alkaline solutions, and don't give alkaline drugs through I.V. line containing dopamine. • Use a microdrip or infusion pump to control rate. Use large vein to reduce risk of extravasation. If it occurs, stop infusion and call doctor. • If diastolic pressure rises disproportionately, decrease infusion rate.
Epinephrine I.V., into endotracheal tube, or intracardiac: to restore cardiac rhythm in cardiac arrest S.C., I.M., or I.V.: to treat bronchospasm, hypersensitivity, and anaphylaxis	Acute angle-closure glaucoma, shock (except for anaphylactic shock), coronary insufficiency, organic brain damage	• Mix just before use with 0.9% sodium chloride solution, D_5W, or a combination of these. Store in light-resistant container. Discard after 24 hours or if discoloration or precipitation occurs. • Avoid I.M. injection of oil solution into buttocks because gas gangrene may occur. • Massage site after injection to counteract possible local vasoconstriction. • If blood pressure rises too rapidly, give a fast-acting vasodilator.
Norepinephrine I.V.: to restore blood pressure in acute hypotension	Mesenteric or peripheral vascular thrombosis, pregnancy, profound hypoxia, hypercapnia, hypotension caused by blood volume deficits, or during cyclopropane or halothane anesthesia	• Mix just before use with 0.9% sodium chloride solution and D_5W; don't mix solely with 0.9% sodium chloride solution. Discard solution after 24 hours. • Use a microdrip or infusion pump to control rate. Use large vein to minimize risk of extravasation. If it occurs, stop the infusion and call the doctor. Check for blanching along the course of the infused vein. • Keep atropine available to correct bradycardia and propranolol to correct arrhythmias. • During infusion, check blood pressure every 2 minutes until stable, then every 5 minutes.

Comparing vasopressors *(continued)*		
DRUG, ROUTE, AND INDICATIONS	**CONTRA- INDICATIONS**	**ADMINISTRATION TIPS**
Phenylephrine I.V.: to treat severe hypotension and shock	Acute angle-closure glaucoma, ventricular tachycardia, severe cardiovascular disease	• Mix with 0.9% sodium chloride solution, D₅W, or a combination of these. • Monitor blood pressure frequently. Adjust infusion rate to maintain blood pressure slightly below patient's normal level, if known.

Purpose
• To raise blood pressure
• To increase cardiac output.

Indications

Except for epinephrine, vasopressors have similar indications: They correct acute hypotension caused by shock. Epinephrine, the drug of choice for treating anaphylactic shock, can also restore cardiac rhythm after cardiac arrest.

Adverse reactions

Adverse reactions include decreased urine output, widened pulse pressure, hypertension, extravasation, headache, nausea, vomiting, nervousness, restlessness, insomnia, arrhythmias, bradycardia, and palpitations.

Care considerations

• Be sure to dilute the prescribed vasopressor in the correct solution.
• If possible, review the patient's medications for possible interactions. For example, use of monoamine oxidase inhibitors in a patient receiving dopamine or phenylephrine may trigger hypertensive crisis. Similarly, used of tricyclic antidepressants with epinephrine or norepinephrine may worsen cardiac adverse effects. Concomitant use of epinephrine with drugs that have alpha-adrenergic blocking properties (such as phenothiazines)

may result in "epinephrine reversal"— a drop in blood pressure. Concurrent use of phenytoin with dopamine may cause sudden hypotension and bradycardia.
• During therapy with vasopressors, monitor the patient's blood pressure, heart rate, and electrocardiogram continuously. Be alert for decreased urine output, altered cardiac output, tachycardia, widened pulse pressure, and hypertension. If any of these occur, notify the doctor immediately. Such reactions may require dosage adjustment or discontinuation of the drug.
• When administering norepinephrine or dopamine, be especially alert for signs of extravasation, such as pain, swelling, blanching, or discoloration at the infusion site. If extravasation occurs, stop the infusion immediately and estimate the amount of extravasated solution. Using a tuberculin syringe, the doctor will slowly and gently aspirate as much as possible of the infiltrated solution from the subcutaneous tissue and then will order instillation of phentolamine. This drug combats the vasoconstrictive effects of norepinephrine and dopamine by dilating the peripheral vessels; it must be administered as soon as possible after extravasation to act as an antidote. Dilute 5 to 10 mg of phentolamine in 10 ml of 0.9% sodium chloride solution; then instill the solution into the area of ex-

travasation. Apply warm compresses to the area for 24 hours or as appropriate. This will promote vasodilation and reduce pain. Because tissue damage may be severe, obtain a plastic surgery consultation as appropriate.

• After treating extravasation, continue to monitor for signs of tissue necrosis and sloughing: discoloration, pain or loss of sensation, swelling, or coldness at the site. Tell the patient to report any of these signs.

• Check the patient's extremities frequently for changes in skin color and temperature and for the presence of distal pulses. Be especially alert if the patient has a history of occlusive vascular disease that puts him at risk for distal necrosis and tissue sloughing.

• When discontinuing I.V. administration of vasopressors, decrease the infusion rate gradually and monitor the patient for sudden onset of hypotension. Continue to monitor vital signs for several hours after the drug is discontinued.

Home care instructions

• Teach the patient how to monitor his blood pressure and heart rate if he is receiving a vasopressor at home.

• Advise the patient and family to be alert for signs of extravasation and to notify a home health care nurse or doctor if it occurs.

VENTRICULAR ASSIST DEVICE

A temporary life-sustaining treatment for heart failure, the ventricular assist device (VAD) is used to decrease myocardial work load while maintaining systemic pressure and cardiac output. Ventricular assistance allows the heart to rest and recover adequate ventricular function and is considered a bridge to heart transplantation or implantation of a mechanical or artificial heart.

Used most commonly to assist the left ventricle, this device may also be used to assist the right ventricle or both ventricles. It works by diverting systemic blood flow from the diseased chamber into a pump and then returning it to the aorta (in the case of a left VAD) or to the pulmonary artery (in the case of a right VAD). Currently available VADs include Hemopump, Heart Mate, the left ventricular assist device by Thermo Cardiosystems, Inc. (TCIVAD), Symbion Acute VAD, and Thorate VAD System.

VADs have much in common with the artificial heart. The main differences are that VADs assist the heart rather than replace it and are used temporarily rather than permanently. Because of these differences, the VAD doesn't have to be as compact as the artificial heart. Nevertheless, recent developments in VADs have reduced their size. For example, the Heart Mate is fully implanted except for a wire that connects to a battery pack.

Purpose

• To temporarily reduce ventricular work, promote myocardial rest, and improve contractility.

Indications

Candidates for a VAD include patients with cardiogenic shock after a massive myocardial infarction; patients who cannot be weaned from cardiopulmonary bypass despite fluids, pharmacologic support, or use of an intraaortic balloon pump; and patients with acute myocarditis who are in cardiogenic shock refractory to conventional treatment. VADs are sometimes used for patients awaiting heart transplantation who have also been unresponsive to other treatment options, including fluids and drugs. VADs may also be indicated for a patient who rejects a heart transplant. They are also used for patients undergoing high-risk percutaneous transluminal coronary angioplasty, such as patients with multiple-vessel coronary artery disease and severe left ventricular dysfunction who are not candidates for bypass grafting.

Patients who are poor candidates for a VAD include those with concurrent severe renal failure; severe cerebrovascular, pulmonary, or hepatic disease; cancer with metastasis; or significant blood dyscrasias. Another option for these patients may be dynamic cardiomyoplasty. (For more information about this treatment, see *Dynamic cardiomyoplasty: Treatment for CHF*, pages 620 and 621.) Other contraindications include a body surface area of less than 1 m² or difficult catheter placement.

Procedure

VAD insertion is usually performed in the operating room. With the patient under general anesthesia, the surgeon makes an incision in the chest. If the patient will be receiving a left VAD, the surgeon places the catheters in the left atrium and aorta; for a right VAD, in the right atrium and pulmonary artery. After suturing the catheters in place, the surgeon connects them to tubing that is attached to the pump head of the VAD. Usually, the pump itself remains outside the body, and the synthetic tubing enters the chest through the incision. Finally, the surgeon turns on and adjusts the pump, checks that it is functioning properly and that the sutures aren't leaking, and applies an occlusive dressing.

Most VADs require an open-chest surgical procedure for implantation; however, the Hemopump can be inserted via the femoral artery or via a transthoracic or retroperitoneal approach. To insert the Hemopump, the pump-assembly catheter is advanced up the aorta until it passes the aortic valve and rests in the left ventricle. The part of the catheter that contains the pump rests inside the descending aorta.

Complications

The VAD carries a high risk of complications. Hemorrhage is a frequent surgical complication; coagulation disorders result from prolonged cardiopulmonary bypass. Other complications include hemidiaphragm paralysis, acute respiratory failure, renal failure, multisystem organ failure, and VAD failure. The device can damage blood cells, thereby causing thrombus formation and subsequent pulmonary embolism or cerebrovascular accident. If the VAD hasn't improved ventricular function in 96 hours, heart transplantation may be considered.

Care considerations
Before surgery
• Explain the procedure, and answer any questions the patient or his family may have. Be sure that informed consent has been obtained and that the patient understands the risks of the treatment.
• Explain that food and fluids will be restricted before surgery and that cardiac function will be monitored continuously using an electrocardiograph, a pulmonary artery catheter, and an arterial catheter.
• If time allows, the patient's chest may be shaved and scrubbed with an antiseptic solution.
• Place an air mattress or sheepskin on the patient's bed. This will help the patient's postoperative positioning and help prevent skin breakdown.
After surgery
• The patient returns to an intensive care unit (ICU) with the VAD in place.
• Expect the patient to show the residual effects of the general anesthetic when he arrives on the ICU; usually the anesthetic isn't reversed as a sedative measure. As the anesthetic wears off, administer analgesics, as prescribed.
• Keep the patient immobilized while the VAD is in place to prevent accidental extubation, contamination, or

Dynamic cardiomyoplasty: Treatment for CHF

Some patients with congestive heart failure (CHF) may benefit from dynamic cardiomyoplasty, an investigational surgical procedure. In this procedure, part of the patient's own skeletal muscle and its associated neurovascular supply is used to repair the cardiac defect. After the skeletal muscle and heart are grafted together, a pacemaker stimulates the muscle to contract in synchrony with the heart to augment its compromised pumping action. Although skeletal muscle has long been recognized as a potential myocardial substitute, attempts to use it have usually failed because skeletal muscle tires rapidly. However, electrical conditioning techniques now in use allow the muscle to contract repeatedly like the heart. With such conditioning, researchers have successfully used a patient's latissimus dorsi as an overlay to assist cardiac function after resection of diseased myocardium or in diffuse cardiomyopathy and CHF.

Because dynamic cardiomyoplasty uses the patient's own muscle, it avoids the risk of tissue rejection and donor organ shortages. And because the muscle acts as a

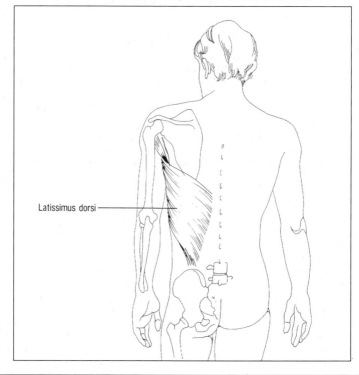

Latissimus dorsi

disconnection of the device. Use soft restraints on the patient's hands.
• Monitor for signs of bleeding by noting increased chest tube drainage or bloody drainage from incisions or catheter insertion sites.

• Monitor hemodynamic parameters. If you're authorized to adjust the device's pump, maintain cardiac output at 5 to 8 liters/minute, pulmonary capillary wedge pressure at 10 to 20 mm Hg, central venous pressure at 8 to 16 covering flap, the ventricle's original size remains unchanged. Besides avoiding many of the risks of human or artificial heart transplantation, this procedure is also less costly.

To perform the procedure, the surgeon first isolates the patient's latissimus dorsi, preserving its neurovascular supply. Then, he prepares the muscle for its new function by implanting a proximal pacing electrode where the neurovascular bundle divides and a distal electrode near the free edge of the muscle flap. To check function, he stimulates the muscle with a pacemaker.

Next, the surgeon brings the muscle with its attached leads under the patient's arm into his chest cavity through an incision in the third or second rib and then attaches it to the left ventricle. This done, he implants a sensing epicardial electrode on the right ventricle. After a suitable recovery period and electrical conditioning, the muscle is stimulated to contract synchronously with the heart.

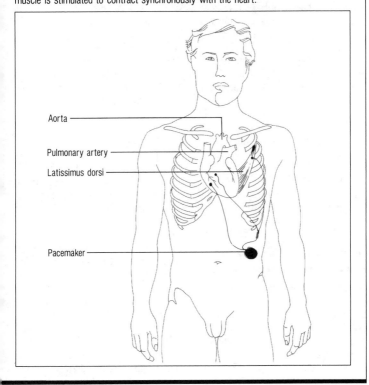

mm Hg, and left atrial pressure at 4 to 12 mm Hg. Monitor for signs of poor perfusion and ineffective pumping: arrhythmias, hypotension, cool skin, slow capillary refill, oliguria or anuria, confusion, restlessness, and anxiety.

• Administer heparin, as prescribed, to prevent clotting in the pump head and thrombus formation. Check for bleeding, especially at the operative sites. Every 4 hours, monitor prothrombin time, partial thromboplastin time, and hemoglobin and hematocrit levels. Notify the doctor of abnormal findings.

• Because of the patient's debilitated status, watch for infection. Assess incisions and the catheter insertion site for signs of infection, and culture any suspicious exudate. Monitor the patient's white blood cell count and differential.

• Monitor oxygenation, renal function, and neurologic status.

• If the patient receives the VAD as a bridge to transplantation, he will go to surgery when a donor heart becomes available.

• Patients who are not awaiting heart transplants will be weaned from ventricular assistance when they have been stabilized with the VAD.

• Weaning from the VAD can begin by turning the device off for a few minutes once a day to evaluate ventricular function.

• After the patient is weaned from the VAD, he usually receives support with an intra-aortic balloon pump or drug therapy.

Home care instructions

• Encourage the patient to keep follow-up appointments with his doctor.

VENTRICULOSTOMY

A ventriculostomy is insertion of a catheter into the ventricle of the brain to help lower intracranial pressure (ICP) while monitoring that pressure. A device known as a subarachnoid screw also provides ICP monitoring, but is less effective for lowering ICP.

The decision whether to use a ventricular catheter or subarachnoid screw is based on several factors. The ventricular catheter provides more accurate ICP measurement and allows for continuous cerebrospinal fluid (CSF) drainage. The subarachnoid screw is used when a ventriculostomy is not possible. It can be-

come occluded more readily but is easier to insert, especially in patients with midline shifting or collapsed ventricles. Because the device requires a firm skull for anchoring, it isn't typically used in young children or in patients whose skull integrity may be compromised.

Purpose

• To lower ICP
• To provide access for monitoring ICP.

Indications

This procedure is indicated in conditions that involve increased ICP, such as hematomas, abscesses, tumors, aneurysms, and cerebral edema. It is also indicated for conditions that increase intracranial blood volume: hyperemia, hypercapnia, and obstructions to venous outflow. Conditions that benefit from ICP drainage include communicating hydrocephalus and subarachnoid hemorrhage.

Procedure

The patient receives a general anesthetic. The surgeon makes a burr hole in the patient's skull, inserts an intraventricular catheter into the burr hole, and sutures the catheter in place. He then connects the catheter to tubing filled with 0.9% sodium chloride solution and connects it to a transducer that converts ICP into electrical impulses that are relayed to the monitor. If CSF will be drained, stopcocks and a collection bag can be attached to the tubing.

Complications

Excessive CSF drainage is a potential complication of ventriculostomy and may result in collapsed ventricles, tonsillar herniation, and medullary compression. Cessation of drainage may indicate clot formation. If drainage is blocked, the patient may develop signs of increased ICP. Another possible complication is infection, which can cause meningitis.

Care considerations
Before the procedure
• If the patient is alert and communicative, explain that the device will be inserted to check ICP and to drain excessive CSF.
• Explain the insertion procedure and how the device works. Tell the patient that his head will be shaved over the insertion site and that a sterile dressing will be placed over the site after the device is secured to guard against infection. If a ventricular catheter is to be inserted, explain that the catheter will be sutured in place onto the scalp.
• Administer a sedative, if ordered.

After the procedure
• Check ICP, neurologic reflexes, and vital signs frequently. Be alert for early signs of increased ICP: headache, pupillary changes, vision disturbances, focal neurologic deficits, and changes in respiratory patterns.
• Observe CSF drainage, and note the amount, color, clarity, and presence of any blood or sediment. If appropriate, send daily drainage specimens to the laboratory for culture and sensitivity studies; white blood cell count; and protein, glucose, or chloride levels.
• Monitor for signs of excessive CSF drainage, which may include headache, tachycardia, diaphoresis, and nausea. If drainage accumulates too rapidly, clamp the system and notify the doctor immediately. This is a neurosurgical emergency.
• Decreased CSF drainage may indicate clot formation. If you can't quickly identify the cause of the obstruction, notify the doctor immediately.
• Take precautions to prevent further increases in ICP. For example, keep the patient's room softly lit and quiet. Enforce bed rest, and raise the patient's head 30 to 45 degrees to promote drainage. Instruct him to exhale while moving or turning in bed. Provide help if the patient needs to sit up, and tell him not to flex his neck or hips or push against the footboard. Give ox-

ygen before suctioning and proceed carefully. Give stool softeners, as prescribed, to prevent straining.
• Watch for signs of infection, and use strict aseptic technique when caring for the insertion site. Administer prophylactic antibiotics, if prescribed, and check the patient's temperature.
• Check that the external drain is at the correct height to maintain sufficient pressure for drainage. Check the drain whenever the patient changes his position; also check the tubing for kinks or obstructions. Avoid putting pressure on the tubing to ensure adequate drainage and to prevent accidental dislodgment.
• When the patient's neurologic status has stabilized, ICP monitoring and CSF drainage will be discontinued and the device removed. Usually, the device remains in place for 5 to 7 days; if the patient needs it longer, it will be replaced by a new one. When the new device is in place, continue periodic neurologic assessments and maintain accurate intake and output records. Continue to monitor for signs of meningitis.

Home care instructions
• Teach aseptic technique to the patient and his family. Emphasize the need for proper care of the suture and insertion sites until healing is complete.

VITAMIN SUPPLEMENTS

Vitamin supplements are organic compounds that are commonly prescribed when dietary sources fail to provide adequate vitamins.

Vitamin supplements are widely promoted for various conditions, ranging from the common cold to cancer. However, controlled clinical studies haven't substantiated these claims. In fact, vitamin supplements are not necessary for well-nourished, healthy in-

(Text continues on page 627.)

Understanding vitamin supplements

Most people know that vitamins are essential for growth and development. But how they're stored and given can greatly influence their intended effects. And how they act can depend on the patient's condition, use of prescription or over-the-counter drugs, and other factors. When administering a vitamin supplement, review the information below.

Vitamin A
- Don't give by oral route to patients with malabsorption syndrome. However, if malabsorption results from inadequate bile secretion, oral route may be used with concurrent administration of bile salts. Vitamin A is also contraindicated in hypervitaminosis A.
- Don't give vitamin A by I.V. route, except for special water-miscible forms intended for infusion with large parenteral volumes. Never give any form of vitamin A by I.V. push because death can occur.
- Don't give vitamin A or carotene (its precursor) with mineral oil, cholestyramine resin, or colestipol. These drugs can impair vitamin absorption.
- Because of the potential for additive toxicity, vitamin A should be used cautiously with isotretinoin.
- In severe hepatic dysfunction, diabetes, or hypothyroidism, use vitamin A rather than carotene. However, if carotene is prescribed, dosage should be doubled.
- To ensure adequate vitamin A absorption, make sure that patient has suitable protein intake and adequate secretion of bile; also administer concurrent doses of the recommended daily allowance of vitamin E and zinc.
- Know that absorption is fastest and most complete with water-miscible preparations, intermediate with emulsions, and slowest with oil suspensions.
- Watch for symptoms of hypervitaminosis, such as bone pain and irritability.
- Closely monitor for skin disorders because high doses may induce chronic toxicity.
- Carefully evaluate vitamin A intake from fortified foods, dietary supplements, and drugs to help avoid toxicity. Discourage self-administration of megadoses.
- In pregnant women, avoid doses exceeding the recommended daily allowance.
- Liquid preparations are available if nasogastric administration is necessary. This vitamin may be mixed with cereal or fruit juice.
- Document the patient's eating and bowel habits. Report abnormalities to the doctor.
- Protect vitamin A from light and heat.

Vitamin B₁ (thiamine)
- Perform sensitivity tests before giving large I.V. doses. During administration, keep epinephrine readily available to treat anaphylaxis.
- In a patient with Wernicke's syndrome, give thiamine before I.V. glucose to prevent worsening of symptoms.
- Don't add thiamine to alkaline I.V. solutions; it will decompose.
- Rotate I.M. injection sites to reduce discomfort.

Vitamin B₂ (riboflavin)
- Before riboflavin is absorbed, it must be combined with phosphorus. Administer with dairy products.
- Because riboflavin supplements are sensitive to light, store them in an opaque container.
- Don't give riboflavin with alkaline substances.

Understanding vitamin supplements *(continued)*

Vitamin B₃ (niacin)

- Don't give niacin to patients with active peptic ulcer, hepatic dysfunction, severe hypotension, hemorrhage, or arterial bleeding. Use cautiously in patients with gallbladder disease, diabetes mellitus, or gout.
- Give I.V. only for severe niacin deficiency. Use slow injection.
- Begin therapy with small doses to minimize adverse effects; increase dosage gradually. Initial therapeutic response usually occurs within 48 hours.
- Administer niacin supplements with meals to reduce GI upset. Tell the patient to avoid taking niacin with hot beverages because of increased vasodilation.
- Inform the patient that tingling, itching, headache, or a sensation of warmth — especially around the head, neck, and ears — can occur shortly after administration but that such effects usually subside with continued therapy. Niacinamide or timed-release niacin may be given to minimize these effects.
- Monitor hepatic function and blood glucose levels frequently.
- Warn the patient against prolonged exposure to bright sunlight. Also warn against engaging in hazardous activities because he may experience dizziness or weakness, particularly early in the course of therapy.

Vitamin B₆ (pyridoxine)

- Consider that pyridoxine requirements may be increased in patients taking isoniazid, cycloserine, oral contraceptives, hydralazine, or penicillin.

Vitamin B₉ (folic acid)

- Don't give folic acid to patients with normocytic or aplastic anemias; to treat methotrexate, pyrimethamine, or trimethoprim overdose; or to treat refractory anemia. Folic acid should never be used to treat undiagnosed anemia because it can correct the hematologic manifestations of vitamin B₁₂ deficiency (pernicious anemia) without altering the progression of the neurologic damage.
- Note that prolonged folic acid therapy may decrease serum levels of vitamin B₁₂.
- If the patient has a sore mouth and tongue, provide soft, bland foods or liquids.
- Don't mix folic acid with other medications for I.M. administration.
- Protect folic acid from light and heat.

Vitamin B₁₂ (cyanocobalamin)

- To prevent impaired vitamin absorption, don't give neomycin, colchicine, para-aminosalicylic acid, or chloramphenicol with cyanocobalamin. Don't administer parenterally to a patient with a hypersensitivity to cobalt. Don't mix with other parenteral medications.
- Because I.V. administration may cause an anaphylactic reaction, give by this route only when other routes are ruled out.
- Protect cyanocobalamin from light and heat.
- Closely monitor serum potassium levels for first 48 hours. Give potassium if necessary.

Vitamin C (ascorbic acid)

- Don't give to infants by I.M. injection because tissue necrosis can occur.
- Give I.V. doses of vitamin C slowly; rapid injection can cause dizziness and syncope. Administer cautiously to patients with renal insufficiency because excess amounts are excreted in urine.
- Protect parenteral solution from light.
- Avoid giving sodium-containing preparations of vitamin C to patients on sodium-restricted diets. Similarly, avoid giving preparations containing calcium to patients receiving digitalis glycosides because cardiac disturbances may result.

(continued)

Understanding vitamin supplements *(continued)*

Vitamin D
- Don't give to patients with hypercalcemia, hypervitaminosis A, or renal osteo-dystrophy with hyperphosphatemia because of the risk of metastatic calcification. Use cautiously in renal impairment.
- If I.V. route is necessary, use only water-miscible solutions intended for dilution in large parenteral volumes. Use cautiously in cardiac patients, especially if they're receiving digitalis glycosides.
- Monitor eating and bowel habits; dry mouth, nausea, vomiting, metallic taste, and constipation can herald toxicity.
- If the patient has hyperphosphatemia, enforce dietary phosphate restrictions and give binding agents to avoid metastatic calcification and renal calculi.
- When high doses are used, monitor serum and urine calcium, potassium, and urea levels. Doses of 60,000 units/day can cause hypercalcemia.
- Malabsorption due to inadequate bile salts or to hepatic dysfunction may require addition of exogenous bile salts to oral vitamin D. Space doses. Use together cautiously.
- Use I.M. injection of vitamin D dispersed in oil in patients unable to absorb the oral form.
- Because this vitamin is fat-soluble, warn the patient against increasing dosage without medical approval.
- Tell the patient to restrict intake of magnesium-containing antacids.

Vitamin E
- Use cautiously with aluminum-containing antacids because large amounts of aluminum hydroxide may precipitate bile acids in the upper small intestine, thereby decreasing absorption of fat-soluble vitamins. Also use cautiously with antihyperlipemics, iron supplements, and vitamin A.
- Know that water-miscible forms are more completely absorbed in GI tract than other forms and adequate bile is essential for absorption.
- Be aware that vitamin E requirements increase with rise in dietary polyunsaturated acids.
- Because it is an antioxidant, vitamin E may be combined with other vitamins.

Vitamin K
- Use cautiously, if at all, during last weeks of pregnancy to avoid toxic reactions in neonates, and in patients with glucose-6-phosphate dehydrogenase deficiency to avoid hemolysis. Use large doses cautiously in severe hepatic disease because doing so may impair hepatic function.
- Use cautiously with other drugs. Concurrent use of antihyperlipemics, for instance, may decrease vitamin K absorption.
- Administer I.V. over 2 to 3 hours. Mix in 0.9% sodium chloride solution, dextrose 5% in water, or dextrose 5% in 0.9% sodium chloride solution. Observe patient closely for flushing, weakness, tachycardia, and hypotension.
- Note that failure to respond to vitamin K may indicate coagulation defects.
- In severe bleeding, don't delay other measures, such as transfusion.
- Protect parenteral products from light. Wrap infusion container with aluminum foil.
- I.V. injections have more rapid onset of effects but shorter duration than S.C. or I.M. injections.
- Monitor prothrombin time to determine dosage effectiveness.
- Phytonadione (vitamin K_1) therapy in infants causes fewer adverse reactions than therapy with other vitamin K analogues.

dividuals; excessive or inappropriate use may cause such adverse effects as anorexia, headache, nausea, and vomiting.

Purpose
• To help correct vitamin deficiency
• To supplement dietary intake in patients with high vitamin requirements.

Indications
Vitamin supplements are most commonly needed by pregnant and lactating women, infants, strict vegetarians, elderly persons, and those who are on a calorie-restricted diet. Vitamin supplements are also indicated for postoperative patients and those undergoing treatment for cancer, alcoholism, GI disturbances, anorexia, or hyperthyroidism.

Care considerations
• Vitamins vary greatly in their routes of administration, their adverse effects, and their interactions. (See *Understanding vitamin supplements*, pages 624 to 626.)

Home care instructions
• Warn the patient about the dangers of taking megadoses of vitamins. Encourage him to eat a well-balanced diet instead.
• To preserve water-soluble vitamins, instruct the patient to steam vegetables and not overcook them.
• Explain that synthetic vitamins are no less effective than natural vitamins despite their lower cost.

VITRECTOMY

This microsurgical procedure removes part or all of the vitreous humor—the transparent gelatinous substance that fills the cavity behind the lens of the eye. The surgical instruments used have advanced to fiber-optic and laser delivery systems. This procedure is usually done in combination with other eye surgeries.

Purpose
• To remove vitreous opacities
• To allow access to the retina
• To allow removal of foreign bodies.

Indications
A vitrectomy helps treat vitreous hemorrhage and other opacities, traction retinal detachment, retinal detachment with vitreous contraction (as may occur in severe diabetic proliferative retinopathy), and chronic posterior uveitis. It's also used to remove foreign bodies.

Procedure
An eye surgeon who specializes in vitreous humor or retinal disorders typically performs this procedure. (See *Understanding vitrectomy*, page 628.) It may be done under local or general anesthesia and usually takes 2 to 3 hours; it is typically performed on one eye at a time. The surgeon makes two incisions into the sclera—one for the insertion of vitrectomy instruments and the other to provide an opening for the fiber-optic light. He then cuts and aspirates the membranes and vitreous humor and infuses 0.9% sodium chloride solution into the vitreous cavity to maintain intraocular pressure. Air or sulfur hexafluoride gas may be injected to hold the retina in place until a firm adhesion develops. Finally, antibiotics are administered and both eyes are patched. The patient is typically discharged within 3 to 5 days.

Complications
Complications of vitrectomy include endophthalmitis (requiring intravitreous and systemic antibiotics and possibly a second vitrectomy), iatrogenic cataracts (requiring later removal), vitreous hemorrhage (which may clear spontaneously or may require laser

Understanding vitrectomy

The illustration below demonstrates the placement of vitrectomy instruments during this surgical procedure.

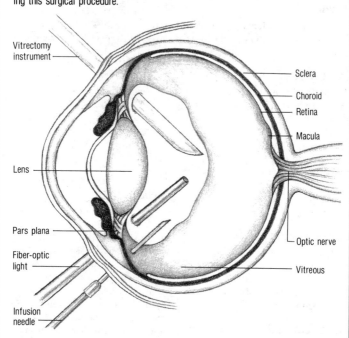

Vitrectomy instrument

Lens

Pars plana

Fiber-optic light

Infusion needle

Sclera

Choroid

Retina

Macula

Optic nerve

Vitreous

photocoagulation), and retinal detachment (which may require scleral buckling). Additionally, the patient may experience temporary decreased vision until the eye is healed. After laser treatment, peripheral vision may be permanently impaired. Because the patient is using only one eye, depth perception will a problem.

Care considerations

Before surgery

• Orient the visually handicapped patient to his surroundings, and ease his anxiety. Tell him that before the procedure he'll receive mydriatic and cycloplegic drugs to dilate the pupil and perhaps antibiotics to prevent infection.

• Ensure that the patient has signed a consent form.

• If general anesthesia is indicated, ensure that the patient does not eat or drink anything within 6 to 8 hours before surgery.

• Administer preoperative medication as appropriate. Routine preoperative preparation may include facial washing (with antiseptic soap) and eyedrops the morning of surgery.

After surgery

• Closely monitor the patient's blood pressure because prolonged hypotension can affect retinal artery circulation. Administer antiemetics, as prescribed, to prevent vomiting. Tell the patient to avoid coughing and straining during defecation, which elevate intraocular pressure and thereby compromise the sclerotomy incision.

• The patient who received injections of air or gas during surgery must maintain a certain position, usually face down, to keep the gas bubble in place over the retina. If air was infused, this may take several days; if gas was infused, 7 to 10 days. Postoperative positioning depends on the retinal work done by the surgeon. The surgeon will have the patient positioned so that the air bubble places pressure on a particular retinal area. Inform the patient that he must maintain this position for several days but will be allowed to sit upright for meals and to stand to use the bathroom. Suggest diversions such as listening to a radio or having a family member read to him to help pass the time.

• If the patient has continued bleeding or hemorrhage, notify the doctor. If the patient has had gas injected to hold the retina in place during surgery, place him in semi-Fowler's position to allow the blood to pool inferiorly and to keep the visual axis clear.

• As appropriate, administer I.M. or oral analgesics, instill mydriatic and cycloplegic eyedrops to maintain pupil dilation, and give antibiotic and corticosteroid eyedrops to prevent infection and control edema. Apply cold compresses as appropriate to manage eyelid and conjunctival edema.

• Expect moderate drainage for 48 hours, but report any unusual color or large amounts of discharge.

Home care instructions

• Tell the patient who's had a gas bubble injected into his eye to avoid air travel until the bubble is completely absorbed.

• Instruct the patient not to stoop, lift heavy objects, exercise strenuously, or dive into water. He may read, watch TV, go up and down stairs, and take walks.

• Suggest wearing dark glasses if photosensitivity develops.

• Emphasize the importance of instilling eyedrops for up to 6 weeks, as ordered, to prevent infection and inflammation.

• Remind the patient to schedule a follow-up appointment after discharge.

• Instruct the patient to sleep with his head elevated on several pillows, as indicated by the surgeon, to prevent further hemorrhage.

W-Z

WOUND IRRIGATION

Wound irrigation is the application of fluid under pressure to a wound site in order to clean tissues; remove contaminants; loosen devitalized tissue; and flush particulate matter, cellular debris, and possible infective bacterial inoculum. Irrigation with an antiseptic solution helps the wound heal properly from the inside tissue layers outward to the skin surface. It also helps prevent premature surface healing over an abscess pocket or infected tract.

Performed correctly, wound irrigation uses strict sterile technique. Universal precautions must be followed because of the risk of infection from splashing and aerosolization of debris. After irrigation, open wounds usually are packed to absorb additional drainage.

Wound irrigations are usually performed in the hospital setting but may be required during home care of chronic, slow-healing wounds. The home environment has fewer pathogenic organisms than a hospital or nursing home, so the risk of infection is somewhat lessened during home care.

Choice of irrigant is important. An appropriate wound irrigating solution has the following characteristics:

• strong enough to remove bacteria and debris

• nontoxic and isotonic, to avoid tissue damage

• sterile, to minimize risk of infection

• nonirritating and painless to the patient because nerve endings may be exposed in the wound.

Purpose

• To enhance wound healing
• To reduce the risk of infection
• To treat an established infection.

Indications

Wound irrigation is used primarily in three situations: trauma, surgery, and postoperative care. Traumatic wounds are considered contaminated. Irrigation is undertaken to reduce the risk of subsequent wound infection in patients with crush injuries, bites, avulsions, and lacerations, for example. During surgery, the wound may be irrigated with an antibacterial solution just before closure. In postoperative and nonsurgical patients, open wounds are often irrigated to treat or prevent infection—for example, in patients with pressure ulcers, abscess pockets, or infected tracts.

Procedure

In the emergency department, wound irrigation is usually carried out as part of wound closure, with irrigation occurring after local anesthesia has been achieved. In the surgical patient, irrigation is carried out by the surgeon as part of the operative procedure. Other wound irrigations are usually performed by a nurse. At home, the patient or family member may be responsible for wound irrigation.

Three typical methods of wound irrigation include use of bulb syringe, use of a piston irrigating syringe, and a new technology that uses 0.9% sodium chloride solution under pressure.

The use of the bulb syringe has been popular but is no longer recommended because it does not deliver the irrigant under sufficient pressure. It's also associated with a risk of aspirating debris into the syringe, causing contamination.

When using a piston irrigating syringe and tip, the irrigating pressure is determined by the size of the syringe and the size of the catheter tip. A pressure of 8 pounds per square inch (psi) is recommended for optimal cleaning with minimal wound damage, and that can be accomplished with a 35-ml syringe and a 19 G catheter. To perform wound irrigation, the syringe is filled with irrigant and then the catheter is connected to the syringe. A slow, steady stream of irrigant is instilled into the wound until the syringe empties. The catheter is pinched closed before the syringe is withdrawn. The syringe is refilled, reconnected to the catheter, and the irrigation is repeated. It's important to reach all areas of the wound. The procedure is continued until the prescribed amount of solution is delivered or until the solution returns clear.

The new Irrijet is a spring-loaded, self-refilling system that allows quick, efficient wound irrigation. A splash shield helps protect the health care worker performing the irrigation. Another new system is the Dey-Wash skin wound cleaner. It consists of an aluminum pouch filled with 0.9% sodium chloride solution suspended in a cylindrical aluminum can. The solution is dispensed by depressing a valve on top of the can. The solution can be dispensed with the can in any position, including upside down. This system is designed to provide a continuous stream approximating the use of a 19 G catheter at a pressure of 8 psi.

Complications

Complications are rare. Careful choice of irrigant will minimize wound or skin irritation and cell damage.

Care considerations

Before the procedure

• Assemble all equipment in the patient's room. Check for allergies, especially to povidone-iodine or other topical medications or solutions.
• Explain the procedure, provide privacy, and position the patient correctly for the irrigation procedure, so that irrigant will flow away from the wound.
• Place a linen-saver pad under the patient, and place a basin below the wound, so that irrigant flows from the wound into the basin; do not let contaminated fluid collect on the patient's linens.

During the procedure

• Maintain a sterile field for irrigating equipment.
• Follow universal precautions, including use of mask, gloves, and goggles, due to the risk of splashing and aerosolization of contaminated irrigant.
• Irrigate until the fluid returns clear or until the appropriate amount of irrigant has been used.

After the procedure

• Keep the patient positioned to allow further wound drainage into the basin.
• Clean the area around the wound to promote local circulation and help prevent skin breakdown and infection.
• Pack the wound if appropriate, and apply a sterile dressing.
• Properly dispose of contaminated materials, wound dressings, and fluids.
• Carefully monitor the size and appearance of the wound.

Home care instructions

• Teach the patient or family member how to perform the procedure. Ask for a return demonstration of the technique, and provide written instructions.
• Arrange for home health supplies and nursing visits, as appropriate.
• Urge the patient to inform the doctor promptly of any signs of infection.

Selected references and index

Selected references

Alt, T. "Dermabrasion," in *Cosmetic Surgery of the Skin: Principles and Techniques.* Edited by Coleman, W., et al. St. Louis: Mosby-Year Book, Inc., 1991.

American Heart Association, Emergency Cardiac Care Committee and Subcommittees. "Guidelines for Cardiopulmonary Resuscitation and Emergency Cardiac Care," *JAMA* 268(16):2172-83, October 28, 1992.

Andrus, C. "Intracranial Pressure: Dynamics and Nursing Management," *Journal of Neuroscience Nursing* 23(2):85-92, April 1991.

Arriaga, M.A., and Myers, E.N. "The Surgical Management of Chronic Parotitis," *The Laryngoscope* 100(12):1270-75, December 1990.

Ashby, D. "Total Laryngectomy and Radical Neck Dissection," *Journal of Post Anesthesia Nursing* 5(3):190-91, June 1990.

Baird, S.B., et al. *Cancer Nursing: A Comprehensive Textbook.* Philadelphia: W.B. Saunders Co., 1991.

Ball, K.A. "The Basics of Laser Technology," *Nursing Clinics of North America* 25(3):619-34, September 1990.

Bardakjian, V.B., et al. "Pulse Oximetry for Vascular Monitoring in Burned Upper Extremities," *Journal of Burn Care and Rehabilitation* 9(1):63-65, January-February 1988.

Bayley, E. "Wound Healing in the Patient with Burns," *Nursing Clinics of North America* 25(1):205-22, March 1990.

Beckermann, S., and Galloway, S. "Elective Resection of the Liver: Nursing Care," *Critical Care Nurse* 9(10):40-47, November-December 1991.

Beersma, D.G. "Do Winter Depressives Experience Summer Nights in Winter?" *Archives of General Psychiatry* 47(9):879-80, September 1990.

Beery, J. "Phacoemulsification," *AORN Journal* 50(6):1230-34, December 1989.

Bernstein, M., et al. "Interstitial Brachytherapy for Malignant Brain Tumors: Preliminary Results," *Neurosurgery* 26(3):371-80, March 1990.

Blehar, M., and Rosenthal, N. "Seasonal Affective Disorders and Phototherapy," *Archives of General Psychiatry* 46(5):469-74, May 1989.

Bobak, I., et al. *Maternity and Gynecologic Care: The Nurse and the Family,* 4th ed. St. Louis: C.V. Mosby Co., 1989.

Bucci, M.N., et al. "Mechanical Prophylaxis of Venous Thrombosis in Patients Undergoing Craniotomy: A Randomized Trial," *Surgical Neurology* 32(4):285-88, October 1989.

Campbell, A. "Pneumatic Compression Stockings: Preventing Deep Vein Thrombus and Pulmonary Embolus," *Today's OR Nurse* 12(7):4-9, July 1990.

Caprini, J.A., et al. "Role of Compression Modalities in a Prophylactic Program for Deep Vein Thrombosis," *Seminars in Thrombosis and Hemostasis* 14(suppl.):77-87, 1988.

Carabott, J., et al. "Teaching Families Tracheotomy Care," *Canadian Nurse* 87(3):21-22, March 1991.

Carney, M. "Hypothermic Conditions," *Emergency* 23(3):46-49, March 1991.

Chernecky, C. *Cancer, Diagnostics and Chemotherapy: A Reference Manual.* Philadelphia: W.B. Saunders Co., 1991.

Chopin, D. "Cotrel-Dubousset Instrumentation (CDI) for Adolescent and Pediatric Scoliosis," in *The Textbook of Spinal Surgery.* Edited by Bradwell, K., and DeWald, R. Philadelphia: J.B. Lippincott Co., 1991.

Clark, R.F., and Shufflebarger, C. "Electrical Interventions," *Topics in Emergency Medicine* 11(2):42-51, July 1989.

Cohen, S., et al. *Maternal, Neonatal, and Women's Health.* Springhouse, Pa.: Springhouse Corp., 1991.

Coleman, W. "Liposuction," in *Cosmetic Surgery of the Skin: Principles and Techniques.* Edited by Coleman, W., et al. St. Louis: Mosby-Year Book, Inc., 1991.

Cook, N. "Pearls for Practice: Quick and Easy Ear Cleaning," *Journal of the American Academy of Nurse Practitioners* 1(3):98, July-September 1989.

Crosby, W. "A History of Phlebotomy Therapy for Hemochromatosis," *American Journal of the Medical Sciences* 301(1):28-31, January 1991.

Davis, J.C., and Hunt, T.K. *Problem Wounds: The Role of Oxygen.* New York: Elsevier Science Publishers, Inc., 1989.

Degroot, K.D., and Damato, M.B. *Critical Care Skills.* East Norwalk, Conn.: Appleton & Lange, 1987.

DeLisa, J.A., ed. *Rehabilitation Medicine: Principles and Practice.* Philadelphia: J.B. Lippincott Co., 1988.

Denson, C. "Ureteral Stents," *AORN Journal* 51(5):1293-1306, May 1990.

Derkay, C.S., et al. "Pediatric Endoscopic Sinus Surgery," *AORN Journal* 54(5):989-1001, November 1991.

Dire, D.J., and Welsh, A.P. "A Comparison of Wound Irrigation Solutions Used in the Emergency Department," *Annals of Emergency Medicine* 19(6):704-08, June 1990.

Drummond, B. "Preventing Increased Intracranial Pressure: Nursing Care Can Make the Difference," *Focus on Critical Care* 17(2):117-22, April 1990.

Dugan, L. "What You Need to Know About Permanent Pacemakers," *Nursing91* 21(6):46-52, June 1991.

Eckhout, G.V., and Willbanks, O.L. "Silastic Ring Vertical Banded Gastroplasty," in *Surgery for the Morbidly Obese Patient.* Edited by Deitle, M. Philadelphia: Lea & Febiger, 1989.

Edwards, J. "Lasers in Gynecology," *Nursing Clinics of North America* 25(3):673-84, September 1990.

Eisenstadt, R. "Therapeutic Phlebotomy," in *Principles of Transfusion Medicine.* Edited by Rossi, E., et al. Baltimore: Williams & Wilkins Co., 1990.

Emergency Procedures. Clinical Skillbuilders Series. Springhouse, Pa.: Springhouse Corp., 1991.

"Endocrine Problems," in *NurseReview,* vol. 2, 3rd ed. Springhouse, Pa.: Springhouse Corp., 1991.

Evarts, C.M. *Surgery of Musculoskeletal System,* 2nd ed. New York: Churchill Livingston, 1990.

Ferrante, F.M., et al. *Patient-Controlled Analgesias.* Boston: Blackwell Scientific Publications, 1990.

Fogel, C., and Lauver, D. *Sexual Health Promotion.* Philadelphia: W.B. Saunders Co., 1990.

Folkes, M.E. "Transfusion Therapy in Critical Care Nursing," *Critical Care Nursing Quarterly* 13(2):15-28, September 1990.

Friedman, W. "LINAC Radiosurgery," *Neurosurgery Clinics of North America* 1(4):991-1008, October 1990.

Gadacz, T., and Talamini, M. "Traditional Versus Laparoscopic Cholecystectomy," *American Journal of Surgery* 161(3):336-38, March 1991.

Gallagher, N.M. "Peritoneal Dialysis: Monitoring and Evaluating Therapy: Review of Clinical Indicators and Use of Data Collection Tools," *American Nephrology Nurses' Association Journal* 18(3):284-87, June 1991.

Goldenberg, R., et al. "Laser Stapedotomy," *AORN Journal* 55(3):759-72, March 1992.

Goucke, C.R. "Prophylaxis Against Venous Thromboembolism," *Anesthesia and Intensive Care* 17(4):458-65, November 1989.

Gray, M. *Genitourinary Disorders.* St. Louis: Mosby-Year Book, Inc., 1992.

Groenwald, S.L., et al. *Cancer Nursing: Principles and Practice,* 2nd ed. Boston: Jones & Bartlett Pubs., 1990.

Habib, K. "A Promising New Use for UV Light," *RN* 53(11):72-74, November 1990.

Hayek, N., and Tyler, L. "Caring for a Patient with a Ventriculostomy," *Nursing91* 21(3):32C-32H, March 1991.

Hensley, M., and Rogers, S. "Shedding Light on 'SAD'ness," *Archives of Psychiatric Nursing* 1(4):230-35, August 1987.

Hoffman, R., et al., eds. *Hematology: Basic Principles and Practice.* New York: Churchill Livingston, 1991.

Hudak, C.M., et al. *Critical Care Nursing: A Holistic Approach,* 5th ed. Philadelphia: J.B. Lippincott Co., 1990.

Ignatavicius, D., and Bayne, M. *Medical-Surgical Nursing: A Nursing Process Approach.* Philadelphia: W.B. Saunders Co., 1991.

Illustrated Manual of Nursing Practice. Springhouse, Pa.: Springhouse Corp., 1991.

I.V. Therapy. Clinical Skillbuilders Series. Springhouse, Pa.: Springhouse Corp., 1991.

Jackson, P. "Primary Care Needs of Children with Hydrocephalus," *Journal of Pediatric Health Care* 4(2):59-71, March-April 1990.

Johns Hopkins Medical Letter. "Incontinence: A Problem You Can Cure," *Health After Fifty* 3(3):4-6, May 1991.

Johnson, S., and Anderson, B. "Carotid Endarterectomy: A Review," *Critical Care Nursing Clinics of North America* 3(3):499-506, September 1991.

Kaplan, H.I., and Sadock, B.J. *Comprehensive Textbook of Psychiatry.* Baltimore: Williams & Wilkins Co., 1989.

Kasper, S., et al. "Phototherapy in Individuals with and without Subsyndromal Seasonal Affective Disorder," *Archives of General Psychiatry* 46(9):837-44, September 1989.

Kern, H.E., and Lewy, A. "Corrections and Additions to the History of Light Therapy and Seasonal Affective Disorder," *Archives of General Psychiatry* 47(1):90-91, January 1990.

Kerr, I., et al. "Continuous Narcotic Infusion with Patient-controlled Analgesia for Chronic Cancer Pain in Outpatients," *Annals of Internal Medicine* 108(4):554-57, April 1988.

Kirby, D.F. "Management of Esophageal Varices: A Review of Treatment Options and the Role of the Gastroenterology Nurse and Associate," *Gastroenterology Nursing* 12(1):10-14, Summer 1989.

Kitt, S., and Kaiser, J. *Emergency Nursing: A Physiologic and Clinical Perspective.* Philadelphia: W.B. Saunders Co., 1990.

Kozier, B., et al. *Fundamentals of Nursing: Concepts, Process, and Practice,* 4th ed. Reading, Mass.: Addison-Wesley Publishing Co., 1991.

Krause, E.A., et al. "Radiosurgery: A Nursing Perspective," *Journal of Neuroscience Nursing* 23(1):24-28, February 1991.

Langer, B., et al."Selective or Total Shunts for Variceal Bleeding," *The American Journal of Surgery* 160(1):75-79, July 1990.

Larson, D., et al. "Stereotaxic Irradiation of Brain Tumors," *Cancer* 65(3 suppl.):792-99, February 1, 1990.

Lazarus, J., et al. "Recombinant Human Erythropoietin and Phlebotomy in the Treatment of Iron Overload in Chronic Hemodialysis Patients," *American Journal of Kidney Disease* 16(2):101-08, August 1990.

Leahy, P.F. "Technique of Laparoscopic Appendicectomy," *British Journal of Surgery* 76(6):616, June 1989.

Lehr, P. "Surgical Lasers: How They Work, Current Applications," *AORN Journal* 50(5):972-77, November 1989.

Lewellyn, C. "Emergency Care of the Replant Patient," *Critical Care Nursing Quarterly* 13(1):13-18, June 1990.

Lewis, J., et al. *Substance Abuse Counseling: An Individual Approach.* Monterey, Calif.: Brooks-Cole Publishing Co., 1988.

Lewis-Cullinan, C., and Janken, J. "Effect of Cerumen Removal on the Hearing Ability of Geriatric Patients," *Journal of Advanced Nursing* 15(5):594-600, May 1990.

Lichtenstein, I., et al. "Hernia Repair with Poly-propylene Mesh: An Improved Method," *AORN Journal* 52(3):559-65, September 1990.

Lingeman, J.E., et al."Kidney Stones: Acute Management," *Patient Care* 24(13):20-38, August 15, 1990.

Lingeman, J.E., et al. "Lithotripsy," *Patient Care* 24(13):51, August 15, 1990.

Long, T.D., and Jerome, M.S. "Outpatient Hernia Repair: The Shouldice Technique," *AORN Journal* 52(4):801-16, October 1990

Ludwig, L. "The Role of Hyperbaric Oxygen in Current Medical Care," *Journal of Emergency Nursing* 15(3):230, May-June 1989.

Lukanich, J.M., and Stiegmann, G.V. "Endoscopic Management of Esophageal Variceal Hemorrhage," *Endoscopy Review* 8(4):34-48, 1991.

Lunsford, L.D., et al. "Stereotactic Gamma Knife Radiosurgery: Initial North American Experience in 207 Patients," *Archives of Neurology* 47(2):169-75, February 1990.

Marlow, D., and Redding, B. *Textbook of Pediatric Nursing*, 6th ed. Philadelphia: W.B. Saunders Co., 1988.

McCaffery, M., and Beebe, A. *Pain: Clinical Manual for Nursing Practice*. St. Louis: C.V. Mosby Co., 1989.

McCaughan, L. "Lasers in Photodynamic Therapy," *Nursing Clinics of North America* 25(3):725-38, September 1990.

McCord, A.S. "Teaching for Tonsillectomies: Details Mean Better Compliance," *Today's OR Nurse* 12(6):11-14, June 1990.

McDermott, M., et al. "Interstitial Brachytherapy," *Neurosurgery Clinics of North America* 1(4):801-24, October 1990.

Meeker, R.M., and Rothrock, J.C. *Alexander's Care of the Patient in Surgery*, 9th ed. St. Louis: Mosby-Year Book, Inc., 1991.

Messer, M.S. "Wound Care," *Critical Care Nursing Quarterly* 11(4):17-27, March 1989.

Meusch, R., and Lillis, P. "Liposuction: The Tumescent Technique," *Dermatology Nursing* 3(4):255-60, August 1991.

Meyers, W., and Jones, R. *Textbook of Liver and Biliary Surgery*. Philadelphia: J.B. Lippincott Co., 1990.

Mooney, N.E. "Pain Management in the Orthopedic Patient," *Nursing Clinics of North America* 26(1):73-87, March 1991.

Mygind, N. "Nasal Polyposis," *The Journal of Allergy and Clinical Immunology* 86(6, part 1):827-29, December 1990.

Nash, J. "Digital Replantation: Using the Ninety-Ninety Intraosseous Wiring Technique," *Today's OR Nurse* 12(3):22-35, March 1990.

Neatherlin, J.S., and Brent, V.A. "The Gamma Knife: Implications for Nursing Practice and Patient Education," *Journal of Neuroscience Nursing* 23(1):71-74, February 1991.

Newman, D.K., et al. "Restoring Urinary Continence," *AJN* 91(1):28-36, January 1991.

Nursing Procedures. Springhouse, Pa.: Springhouse Corp., 1992.

O'Hara, M., and Lineaweaver, W. "Microsurgical Replantation: Development and Current Status," *Critical Care Nursing Quarterly* 13(1):1-11, June 1990.

Oleinik, S. "Care of the Critically Ill Child After Liver Transplantation,"*AACN Issues in Critical Care Nursing* 17(4):300-07, August 1990.

Peters, V.J., and Ferkel, R.D. "Arthroscopic Surgery of the Ankle," *Orthopedic Nursing* 8(5):12-19, September-October 1989.

Phipps, W., et al. *Medical-Surgical Nursing: Concepts and Clinical Practice*, 4th ed. St. Louis: Mosby-Year Book, Inc., 1991.

Preventing Lead Poisoning in Young Children. Atlanta: Centers for Disease Control and Prevention, 1991.

Price, J., and Mattox, D., eds. *Atlas of Head and Neck Surgery*, vol. 1. St. Louis: Mosby-Year Book, Inc., 1990.

Rakel, R., ed. *Conn's Current Therapy*. Philadelphia: W.B. Saunders Co., 1992.

Rapid Assessment. Clinical Skillbuilders Series. Springhouse, Pa.: Springhouse Corp., 1991.

Rauscher, J., et al. "Camey Procedure," *AORN Journal* 54(1):34-44, July 1991.

Respiratory Support. Clinical Skillbuilders Series. Springhouse, Pa.: Springhouse Corp., 1991.

Richardson, J., et al. "Social Environment and Adjustment after Laryngectomy," *Health and Social Work* 14(4):283-92, November 1989.

Rockwood, C., and Green, D. *Fractures in Adults*, 3rd ed. Philadelphia: J.B. Lippincott Co., 1991.

Rodts, M.F. "Nursing Care for the Spinal Surgery Patient," in *The Textbook of Spinal Surgery.* Edited by Bradwell, K., and DeWald, R. Philadelphia: J.B. Lippincott Co., 1991.

Rosenthal, N.E. "Light Therapy," in *Treatment for Psychiatric Disorders*, vol. 3. Washington, D.C.: American Psychiatric Association, 1989.

Sabiston, D.C. *Textbook of Surgery: The Biological Basis of Modern Surgical Practice*, 14th ed. Philadelphia: W.B. Saunders Co., 1991.

Sack, R., et al. "Morning Versus Evening Light Treatment for Winter Depression," *Archives of General Psychiatry* (47)4:343-51, April 1990.

Sauter, S. "Cleft Lips and Palates: Types, Repairs, Nursing Care," *AORN Journal* 50(4) 813-24, October 1989.

Sawyer, D., and Bruya, M. "Care of the Patient Having Radical Neck Surgery or Permanent Laryngostomy: A Nursing Diagnostic Approach," *Focus on Critical Care* 17(2):166-73, April 1990.

Schroeder, S.A., et al. *Current Medical Diagnosis and Treatment*. East Norwalk, Conn.: Appleton & Lange, 1990.

Schwartz, S.I., and Ellis, H., eds. *Maingot's Abdominal Operations*, vol. 1, 9th ed. East Norwalk, Conn.: Appleton & Lange, 1989.

Shapiro, P. "Pelviscopy for Ectopic Pregnancy: A Safer and Quicker Alternative," *Today's OR Nurse* 12(6):6-30, June 1990.

Sheehy, S.B. *Mosby's Manual of Emergency Care*, 3rd ed. St. Louis: Mosby-Year Book, Inc., 1990.

Sheets, L. "Liver Transplantation," *Nursing Clinics of North America* 24(4):881-89, December 1989.

Smith, J.R., et al. "Surgical Management of Epilepsy," *Southern Medical Journal* 82(6):736-41, June 1989.

Smith, M.C., et al. "Neurosurgery of Epilepsy," *Seminars in Neurology* 9(3):231-48, September 1989.

Sneed, P., et al. "Interstitial Irradiation and Hyperthermia for the Treatment of Recurrent Malignant Brain Tumors," *Neurosurgery* 28(2):206-15, February 1991.

Sommers, M. "Rapid Fluid Resuscitation: How to Correct Dangerous Deficits," *Nursing90* 20(1):52-60, January 1990.

Spadoni, D., and Cain, C.L. "Facial Resurfacing: Using the Carbon Dioxide Laser," *AORN Journal* 50(5):1007-13, November 1989.

Spencer, S., et al. "Corpus Callosum Section," in *Surgical Treatment of the Epilepsies*, 2nd ed. Edited by Engel, J. New York: Raven Press, 1993.

Steiner, L. "Stereotactic Radiosurgery with the Cobalt-60 Gamma Unit in the Surgical Treatment of Intracranial Tumors and Arteriovenous Malformations," in *Operative Neurosurgical Techniques*, 2nd ed. Edited by Schnidek, H., and Sweet, W. New York: Grune & Stratton, 1988.

Steur, K. "Hepatic Resection: Indications, Procedures, Patient Care," *AORN Journal* 52(2):230-50, August 1990.

Steves, J. "Step-by-step Implementation of PCA Therapy," *Nursing Management* 20(12):35-40, December 1989.

Strohl, R. "Radiation Therapy: Recent Advances and Nursing Implications," *Nursing Clinics of North America* 25(2):309-29, June 1990.

Suddarth, D.S., ed. *The Lippincott Manual of Nursing Practice*, 5th ed. Philadelphia: J.B. Lippincott Co., 1991.

Torres, G.M., et al. "Extracorporeal Shock-wave Lithotripsy: Initial Experience," *Applied Radiology* 18(12):24-26, December 1989.

Treatments. Nurses' Reference Library. Springhouse, Pa.: Springhouse Corp., 1988.

Tunis, S.R., et al. "The Use of Angioplasty, Bypass Surgery, and Amputation in the Management of Peripheral Vascular Disease," *The New England Journal of Medicine* 325(8):556-62, August 22, 1991.

USPDI, 12th ed. Rockville, Md.: United States Pharmacopeial Convention, Inc., 1992.

Wei, W.I., et al. "The Efficacy of Fiber-optic Endoscopic Examination and Biopsy in the Detection of Early Nasopharyngeal Carcinoma," *Cancer* 67(12):3127-30, June 15, 1991.

Weilitz, M. "New Modes of Mechanical Ventilation," *Critical Care Nursing Clinics of North America* 1(4):689-95, December 1989.

Welsh, D., and Chapman, D. "A Stereotactic Technique for Volumetric Interstitial Implantation in the Brain," *Journal of Neuroscience Nursing* 22(4):245-49, August 1990.

Whiteman, K., et al. "Liver Transplantation," *AJN* 90(6):69-72, June 1990.

Williams, S.R. *Nutrition and Diet Therapy*, 6th ed. St. Louis: Times Mirror-Mosby College Publishing, 1989.

Willis, D., and Harbit, M. "Transcatheter Arterial Embolization of Cerebral Arteriovenous Malformation," *Journal of Neuroscience Nursing* 22(5):280-84, October 1990.

Wilson, J., et al. *Harrison's Principles of Internal Medicine*, 12th ed. New York: McGraw-Hill Book Co., 1991.

Witherell, C.L. "Questions Nurses Ask About Pacemakers — How They Work and What to Do When They Don't," *AJN* 90(12):20-28, December 1990.

Wooden, S.R., and Sextro, P.B. "The Ankle Block: Anatomical Review and Anesthetic Technique," *AANA Journal* 58(2):105-11, April 1990.

Zemel, G., et al. "Percutaneous Transjugular Portosystemic Shunt," *JAMA* 266(3):390-93, July 17, 1991.

Zickefoose, S. "Nasal Surgery: Using Lasers with Endoscopy Surgery," *AORN Journal* 50(5):979-88, November 1989.

Zimmaro, D.M. "Catheter Ablation of Ventricular Tachycardia and Related Nursing Intervention," *Critical Care Nurse* 7(4):20-29, July-August 1987.

Index

i refers to illustration; t refers to table

i refers to illustration; t refers to table

i refers to illustration; t refers to table

i refers to illustration; t refers to table

Implantable cardioverter defibrilla-
tor, 373-375
Implant therapy, 533-535
Incentive spirometry, 375-376
Incision and drainage, 376-377
Individual psychotherapy, 527, 528.
See also Psychotherapy.
Indomethacin. *See* Nonsteroidal anti-
inflammatory drugs.
Indwelling catheter, 152-153. *See
also* Catheterization.
Infection
as bone marrow transplantation
complication, 110
as tracheotomy complication,
588-589t
Infertility management, 377-379
Inotropics, 379, 382
comparison of, 380-383t
Insulin infusion pumps, 386-387i.
See also Insulin injection, sub-
cutaneous.
Insulin injection, subcutaneous,
382-390
patient instructions for, 388-389i
Insulins, 382-383
comparing types of, 384-385t
Interferon alfa, 94, 96t. *See also*
Biotherapy.
Interferon gamma-1b, 94, 96t. *See
also* Biotherapy.
Interleukins, 96t. *See also* Biother-
apy.
Interleukin-2, 96t, 97. *See also*
Biotherapy.
Interleukin-3, 96t. *See also* Biother-
apy.
Intermittent mandatory ventilation,
440t. *See also* Mechanical venti-
lation.
Intermittent pneumatic compression,
520-521
Intermittent pneumatic compression
stockings, 47
Intermittent self-catheterization,
155-156i
Internal fixation methods, 314i. *See
also* Open fracture reduction.

Interpositional reconstruction of
joint, 394. *See also* Joint re-
placement.
Interstitial therapy, 533-535
Intoxication. *See* Detoxification *and*
Drug intoxication, treating.
Intracapsular cataract removal, 150i
Intracavity therapy, 533-535
Intracerebral hematoma, 390. *See
also* Intracranial hematoma, as-
piration of.
Intracranial hematoma, aspiration
of, 390-392
In vitro fertilization, 378. *See also*
Infertility management.
IPC stockings. *See* Intermittent
pneumatic compression stock-
ings.
Ipodate, 577. *See also* Thyroid hor-
mone antagonists.
Iron supplements, 446, 447. *See also*
Mineral supplements.
Isocarboxazid, 449, 597. *See also*
Monoamine oxidase inhibitors.
Isoflurophate. *See* Miotics.
Isokinetic exercises, 294. *See also*
Strengthening exercises.
Isometric exercises, 294. *See also*
Strengthening exercises.
Isopropamide iodide. *See* Choliner-
gic blockers.
Isoproterenol, 10, 380-381t. *See also*
Adrenergics *and* Inotropics.
Isosorbide dinitrate. *See* Nitrates.
Isotonic exercises, 294. *See also*
Strengthening exercises.

J

Jejunoileal bypass, 472. *See also*
Obesity, surgical treatment for.
Jejunostomy, enteral nutrition and,
273. *See also* Enteral nutrition.
Joint movement, types of, 292i
Joint replacement, 393-395
alternatives to, 394
Joint resection, 394. *See also* Joint
replacement.

i refers to illustration; t refers to table

Postural drainage, 179-180, 183. *See also* Chest physiotherapy.
  positioning patients for, 181-182i
Potassium intoxication, multiple transfusions and, 105t
Potassium iodide, 577, 578. *See also* Thyroid hormone antagonists.
Potassium-sparing diuretics, 257-258t. *See also* Diuretics.
Potassium supplements, 446, 447. *See also* Mineral supplements.
PPN. *See* Peripheral parenteral nutrition.
Pramoxine, 22
Pravastatin, 57-58
Prazosin, 31t. *See also* Antiadrenergics.
Prednisolone. *See* Corticosteroids.
Prednisone, 171. *See also* Chemotherapy, cancer, *and* Corticosteroids.
Pressure-controlled inverse ratio ventilation, 441t. *See also* Mechanical ventilation.
Pressure-cycled ventilators, 438. *See also* Mechanical ventilation.
Pressure support ventilation, 440t. *See also* Mechanical ventilation.
Primidone, 41, 43t. *See also* Anticonvulsants.
Probucol, 57-58
Procainamide, 32t. *See also* Class IA antiarrhythmics.
Procaine. *See* Nerve blocks.
Procarbazine, 171. *See also* Chemotherapy, cancer.
Procyclidine. *See* Cholinergic blockers.
Progesterone, 521. *See also* Progestins.
Progestins, 521-523
Promethazine. *See* Antihistamines.
Propafenone hydrochloride, 34-35t. *See also* Class IC antiarrhythmics.
Propantheline bromide. *See* Cholinergic blockers.
Prophylthiouracil, 577, 578. *See also* Thyroid hormone antagonists.

Propoxyphene. *See* Analgesics, opioid.
Propranolol, 35t, 92. *See also* Beta-adrenergic blockers *and* Class II antiarrhythmics.
Prostatectomy, 523-527
  types of, 524-525i
Prosthetic heart valves, 340i. *See also* Heart valve replacement.
Protein-modified diet, 249-251
Prothrombin complex
  administering, 302
  indications for, 301
Proton beam therapy, 536. *See also* Radiosurgery.
Protriptyline. *See* Tricyclic antidepressants.
Pseudoephedrine. *See* Decongestants.
Psychotherapy, 527-529
Psyllium, 411. *See also* Laxatives.
PTCA. *See* Percutaneous transluminal coronary angioplasty.
PTU. *See* Propylthiouracil.
PUVA therapy, 600, 601. *See also* Ultraviolet light treatments.
Pyloroplasty, vagotomy with, 324i. *See also* Gastric resection.
Pyrethrins, 504. *See* Pediculicides.
Pyridostigmine, 60-61
Pyridoxine supplements, 625. *See also* Vitamin supplements.

Q

Quazepam. *See* Benzodiazepines.
Quinestrol. *See* Estrogens.
Quinidine, 33t. *See also* Class IA antiarrhythmics.

R

Radial keratotomy, 396-397
Radiation therapy, 530-531
Radical neck dissection, 531-533
Radioactive implants, 533-535
Radiosurgery, 535-538
  types of, 536
Ramipril. *See* Angiotensin-converting enzyme inhibitors.
Range-of-motion exercises, 290-291
  types of, 290

i refers to illustration; t refers to table

i refers to illustration: t refers to table

WXY

Z

i refers to illustration; t refers to table